Lecture Notes in Computer Science 3337

Commenced Publication in 1973
Founding and Former Series Editors:
Gerhard Goos, Juris Hartmanis, and Jan van Leeuwen

José M. Barreiro
Fernando Martin-Sanchez Víctor Maojo
Ferran Sanz (Eds.)

Biological and Medical Data Analysis

5th International Symposium, ISBMDA 2004
Barcelona, Spain, November 18-19, 2004
Proceedings

Springer

Volume Editors

José M. Barreiro
Polytechnical University of Madrid
School of Computer Science
Artificial Intelligence Department
Campus de Montegancedo s/n, 28660 Boadilla del Monte, Madrid, Spain
E-mail: jmbarreiro@fi.upm.es

Fernando Martin-Sanchez
Institute of Health Carlos III
Department of Medical Bioinformatics
Ctra. Majadahonda a Pozuelo, km. 2, 28220 Majadahonda, Madrid, Spain
E-mail: fmartin@isciii.es

Víctor Maojo
Polytechnical University of Madrid
School of Computer Science
Artificial Intelligence Lab
Boadilla del Monte, 28660 Madrid, Spain
E-mail: vmaojo@infomed.dia.fi.upm.es

Ferran Sanz
University Pompeu Fabra
Municipal Institute of Medical Research (IMIM)
Research Unit on Biomedical Informatics (GRIB)
Passeig Marítim de la Barceloneta 37-49
08003 Barcelona, Spain
E-mail: fsanz@imim.es

Library of Congress Control Number: 2004115460

CR Subject Classification (1998): H.2.8, I.2, H.3, G.3, I.5.1, I.4, J.3, F.1

ISSN 0302-9743
ISBN 3-540-23964-2 Springer Berlin Heidelberg New York

Springer is a part of Springer Science+Business Media

springeronline.com

Printed in Germany

Typesetting: Camera-ready by author, data conversion by Olgun Computergrafik
Printed on acid-free paper SPIN: 11362128 06/3142 5 4 3 2 1 0

Preface

This year, the 5th International Symposium on Medical Data Analysis has experimented an apparently slight modification. The word "biological" has been added to the title of the conferences. The motivation for this shift goes beyond the wish to attract a different kind of professional. It is linked to recent trends to produce a shift within various biomedical areas towards genomics-based research and practice. For instance, medical informatics and bioinformatics are being linked in a synergic area denominated biomedical informatics. Similarly, patient care is being improved, leading to concepts and areas such as molecular medicine, genomic medicine or personalized healthcare.

The results from different genome projects, the advances in systems biology and the integrative approaches to physiology would not be possible without new approaches in data and information processing. Within this scenario, novel methodologies and tools will be needed to link clinical and genomic information, for instance, for genetic clinical trials, integrated data mining of genetic clinical records and clinical databases, or gene expression studies, among others.

Genomic medicine presents a series of challenges that need to be addressed by researchers and practitioners. In this sense, this ISBMDA conference aimed to become a place where researchers involved in biomedical research could meet and discuss. For this conference, the classical contents of former ISMDA conferences were updated to incorporate various issues from the biological fields. Similarly to the incorporation of these new topics of the conference, data analysts will face, in this world of genomic medicine and related areas, significant challenges in research, education and practice.

For this conference, after a peer-review process, we selected the scientific papers that are now published in this issue. The editors would like to thank all the participants for their outstanding contributions and Springer for publishing the proceedings of this conference. Finally, we would like to acknowledge the collaboration of Prof. Rüdiger Brause, who was the first chair of the ISMDA conferences. Without his inspiration and support, this idea would not have been possible.

November 2004

Jose M. Barreiro
Victor Maojo
Fernando Martin-Sanchez
Ferran Sanz

Organization

Executive Committee

Chair	Fernando Martin-Sanchez, Institute of Health Carlos III, Spain
Scientific Committee Coordinators	Victor Maojo, Polytechnical Univ. of Madrid, Spain. Ferran Sanz, IMIM-Univ. Pompeu Fabra, Barcelona, Spain

Steering Committee

J.M. Barreiro (Polytechnical Univ. of Madrid, Spain)
R. Brause (J.W.G.-University, Frankfurt, Germany)
M. García-Rojo (Complejo Hospitalario Ciudad Real, Spain)
C. Kulikowski. (Rutgers University, USA)

Scientific Committee

J. Ares (Univ. of A Coruña, Spain)
H. Billhardt (Univ. Rey Juan Carlos, Spain)
V. Breton (CNRS, France)
J.M. Carazo (CNB, Spain)
A. Colosito (Univ. of Rome "La Sapienza", Italy)
M. Dugas (Univ. of Munich, Germany)
A. Giuliani (Nat. Inst. of Health, Italy)
R. Guthke (Hans-Knoell Inst., Germany)
P. Larranaga (Univ. of the Basque Country, Spain)
N. Lavrac (J. Stefan Institute, Slovenia)
L. Ohno-Machado (Harvard Univ, USA)
E. Medico (IRCC, Italy)
X. Pastor (IDIBAPS, Spain)
A. Pazos (Univ. of A Coruña, Spain)
P. Perner (IBaI Leipzig, Germany)
G. Potamias (Institute of Computer Science, FORTH, Greece)
W. Sauerbrei (Univ. of Freiburg, Germany)
J. Sima (Academy of Sciences of the Czech Republic)
A. Silva (Polytechnical Univ. of Madrid, Spain)
A. Sousa (Univ. Aveiro, Portugal)
B. Zupan (Univ. of Ljubljana, Slovenia)
J. Zvárová (Charles Univ. and Academy of Sciences, Czech Republic)

Local Committee

Members of the Executive Board of SEIS, the Spanish Society of Health Informatics.

Table of Contents

Data Analysis for Image Processing

RF Inhomogeneity Correction Algorithm in Magnetic Resonance Imaging 1
Juan A. Hernández, Martha L. Mora, Emanuele Schiavi, and Pablo Toharia

Fully 3D Wavelets MRI Compression 9
Emanuele Schiavi, C. Hernández, and Juan A. Hernández

A New Approach to Automatic Segmentation of Bone in Medical Magnetic Resonance Imaging 21
Gabriela Pérez, Raquel Montes Diez, Juan A. Hernández, and José San Martín

An Accurate and Parallelizable Geometric Projector/Backprojector for 3D PET Image Reconstruction 27
Roberto de la Prieta

Data Visualization

EEG Data and Data Analysis Visualization 39
Josef Rieger, Karel Kosar, Lenka Lhotska, and Vladimir Krajca

A Web Information System for Medical Image Management 49
César J. Acuña, Esperanza Marcos, Valeria de Castro, and Juan A. Hernández

Reliable Space Leaping Using Distance Template 60
Sukhyun Lim and Byeong-Seok Shin

Decision Support Systems

A Rule-Based Knowledge System for Diagnosis of Mental Retardation 67
R. Sánchez-Morgado, Luis M. Laita, Eugenio Roanes-Lozano, Luis de Ledesma, and L. Laita

Case-Based Diagnosis of Dysmorphic Syndromes 79
Tina Waligora and Rainer Schmidt

Bayesian Prediction of Down Syndrome Based on Maternal Age and Four Serum Markers 85
Raquel Montes Diez, Juan M. Marin, and David Rios Insua

SOC: A Distributed Decision Support Architecture for Clinical Diagnosis 96
Javier Vicente, Juan M. Garcia-Gomez, César Vidal, Luís Marti-Bonmati, Aurora del Arco, and Montserrat Robles

Decision Support Server Architecture for Mobile Medical Applications 105
Marek Kurzynski and Jerzy Sas

Ordered Time-Independent CIG Learning 117
David Riaño

SINCO: Intelligent System in Disease Prevention and Control.
An Architectural Approach 129
Carolina González, Juan C. Burguillo, Juan C. Vidal, and Martin Llamas

Could a Computer Based System for Evaluating Patients
with Suspected Myocardial Infarction Improve Ambulance Allocation? 141
Martin Gellerstedt, Angela Bång, and Johan Herlitz

On the Robustness of Feature Selection with Absent and Non-observed Features . 148
Petra Geenen, Linda C. van der Gaag, Willie Loeffen, and Armin Elbers

Design of a Neural Network Model as a Decision Making Aid
in Renal Transplant 160
Rafael Magdalena, Antonio J. Serrano, Agustin Serrano, Jorge Muñoz, Joan Vila, and E. Soria

Learning the Dose Adjustment for the Oral Anticoagulation Treatment 171
Giacomo Gamberoni, Evelina Lamma, Paola Mello, Piercamillo Pavesi, Sergio Storari, and Giuseppe Trocino

Information Retrieval

Thermal Medical Image Retrieval by Moment Invariants 182
Shao Ying Zhu and Gerald Schaefer

Knowledge Discovery and Data Mining

Employing Maximum Mutual Information for Bayesian Classification 188
Marcel van Gerven and Peter Lucas

Model Selection for Support Vector Classifiers via Genetic Algorithms.
An Application to Medical Decision Support 200
Gilles Cohen, Mélanie Hilario, and Antoine Geissbuhler

Selective Classifiers Can Be Too Restrictive:
A Case-Study in Oesophageal Cancer 212
Rosa Blanco, Linda C. van der Gaag, Iñaki Inza, and Pedro Larrañaga

A Performance Comparative Analysis Between Rule-Induction Algorithms
and Clustering-Based Constructive Rule-Induction Algorithms.
Application to Rheumatoid Arthritis 224
J.A. Sanandrés-Ledesma, Victor Maojo, Jose Crespo, M. García-Remesal, and A. Gómez de la Cámara

Domain-Specific Particularities of Data Mining: Lessons Learned 235
Victor Maojo

Statistical Methods and Tools for Biological and Medical Data Analysis

A Structural Hierarchical Approach to Longitudinal Modeling of Effects of Air Pollution on Health Outcomes 243
Michael Friger and Arkady Bolotin

Replacing Indicator Variables by Fuzzy Membership Functions in Statistical Regression Models: Examples of Epidemiological Studies 251
Arkady Bolotin

PCA Representation of ECG Signal as a Useful Tool for Detection of Premature Ventricular Beats in 3-Channel Holter Recording by Neural Network and Support Vector Machine Classifier 259
Stanisław Jankowski, Jacek J. Dusza, Mariusz Wierzbowski, and Artur Oręziak

Finding Relations in Medical Diagnoses and Procedures 269
David Riaño and Ioannis Aslanidis

An Automatic Filtering Procedure for Processing Biomechanical Kinematic Signals 281
Francisco Javier Alonso, José María Del Castillo, and Publio Pintado

Analysis of Cornea Transplant Tissue Rejection Delay in Mice Subjects 292
Zdenek Valenta, P. Svozilkova, M. Filipec, J. Zvarova, and H. Farghali

Toward a Model of Clinical Trials 299
Laura Collada Ali, Paola Fazi, Daniela Luzi, Fabrizio L. Ricci, Luca Dan Serbanati, and Marco Vignetti

Time Series Analysis

Predicting Missing Parts in Time Series Using Uncertainty Theory 313
Sokratis Konias, Nicos Maglaveras, and Ioannis Vlahavas

Classification of Long-Term EEG Recordings 322
Karel Kosar, Lenka Lhotska, and Vladimir Krajca

Application of Quantitative Methods of Signal Processing to Automatic Classification of Long-Term EEG Records 333
Josef Rieger, Lenka Lhotska, Vladimir Krajca, and Milos Matousek

Semantic Reference Model in Medical Time Series 344
Fernando Alonso, Loïc Martínez, César Montes, Aurora Pérez, Agustín Santamaría, and Juan Pedro Valente

Control of Artificial Hand via Recognition of EMG Signals 356
Andrzej Wolczowski and Marek Kurzynski

Bioinformatics: Data Management and Analysis in Bioinformatics

SEQPACKER: A Biologist-Friendly User Interface
to Manipulate Nucleotide Sequences in Genomic Epidemiology 368
Oscar Coltell, Miguel Arregui, Larry Parnell, Dolores Corella, Ricardo Chalmeta, and Jose M. Ordovas

Performing Ontology-Driven Gene Prediction Queries
in a Multi-agent Environment 378
Vassilis Koutkias, Andigoni Malousi, and Nicos Maglaveras

Protein Folding in 2-Dimensional Lattices
with Estimation of Distribution Algorithms 388
Roberto Santana, Pedro Larrañaga, and José A. Lozano

Bioinformatics: Integration of Biological and Medical Data

Quantitative Evaluation of Established Clustering Methods
for Gene Expression Data 399
Dörte Radke and Ulrich Möller

DiseaseCard: A Web-Based Tool for the Collaborative Integration
of Genetic and Medical Information 409
José Luís Oliveira, Gaspar Dias, Ilídio Oliveira, Patrícia Rocha, Isabel Hermosilla, Javier Vicente, Inmaculada Spiteri, Fernando Martin-Sánchez, and António Sousa Pereira

Biomedical Informatics:
From Past Experiences to the Infobiomed Network of Excellence 418
Victor Maojo, Fernando Martin-Sánchez, José María Barreiro, Carlos Diaz, and Ferran Sanz

Bioinformatics: Metabolic Data and Pathways

Network Analysis of the Kinetics of Amino Acid Metabolism
in a Liver Cell Bioreactor 427
Wolfgang Schmidt-Heck, Katrin Zeilinger, Michael Pfaff, Susanne Toepfer, Dominik Driesch, Gesine Pless, Peter Neuhaus, Joerg Gerlach, and Reinhard Guthke

Model Selection and Adaptation for Biochemical Pathways 439
Rüdiger W. Brause

NeoScreen: A Software Application for MS/MS Newborn Screening Analysis . . . 450
Miguel Pinheiro, José Luís Oliveira, Manuel A.S. Santos, Hugo Rocha, M. Luis Cardoso, and Laura Vilarinho

Bioinformatics: Microarray Data Analysis and Visualization

Technological Platform to Aid the Exchange of Information and Applications Using Web Services 458
Antonio Estruch and José Antonio Heredia

Visualization of Biological Information with Circular Drawings 468
Alkiviadis Symeonidis and Ioannis G. Tollis

Gene Selection Using Genetic Algorithms 479
Bruno Feres de Souza and André C.P.L.F. de Carvalho

Knowledgeable Clustering of Microarray Data 491
George Potamias

Correlation of Expression Between Different IMAGE Clones from the Same UniGene Cluster 498
Giacomo Gamberoni, Evelina Lamma, Sergio Storari, Diego Arcelli, Francesca Francioso, and Stefano Volinia

Author Index 507

RF Inhomogeneity Correction Algorithm in Magnetic Resonance Imaging

Juan A. Hernández, Martha L. Mora,
Emanuele Schiavi, and Pablo Toharia

Universidad Rey Juan Carlos, Móstoles, Madrid, Spain
{j.hernandez,mlmora,e.schiavi,ptoharia}@escet.urjc.es

Abstract. MR images usually present grey level inhomogeneities which are a problem of significant importance. Eliminating these inhomogeneities is not an easy problem and has been studied and discussed in several previous publications. Most of those approaches are based on segmentation processes. The algorithm presented in this paper has the advantage that it does not involve any segmentation step. Instead, a interpolating polynomial model based on a Gabor transform was used to construct a filter that can be used in order to correct these inhomogeneities. The results obtained are really good and show that the grey-level inhomogeneities can be corrected without segmentation.

1 Introduction

Magnetic Resonance Imaging (MRI) is a powerful technique in diagnostic medicine. In the last years the radiological sciences have highly expanded in different modalities, such as X-Ray Mammography, X-Ray Computed Tomography (CT), Single Photon Computed Tomography (SPECT), Positron Emission Tomography (PET) and functional Magnetic Resonance Imaging fMRI)[1]. The appearance of new scanners of Magnetic Resonance Imaging (MRI) with a high field (3 Tesla) and faster and more intense gradients, has given rise to the acquisition of new images of the brain that shows its physiology with a greater degree of detail and amplitude.

Additionally to structural type anatomical images, brain functional activity images are now arising, such as water molecules diffusion tensor imaging, perfusion imaging and blood oxygenation level dependent imaging (BOLD)[2].

Reconstruction techniques, processing and data analysis are development of radiological digital imaging. These techniques require a complex mathematical analysis which can be traced back to the theory of partial differential equations (PDE) and to linear and non linear diffusion processes.

The main difficulty in the analysis the MR[1] images is to locate and correct their inhomogeneities, it is to say, the regions with different levels of grey known as intensity artifacts in MR images. To correct them, it is necessary to employ complex algorithms.

[1] Magnetic Resonance

J.M. Barreiro et al. (Eds.): ISBMDA 2004, LNCS 3337, pp. 1–8, 2004.

Many different approaches to correct low-frequency grey level inhomogeneity in MR images have been published and described. All of them use a segmentation step of MR image. DeCarli [3] compares local correction of MRI[2] spatially dependent image pixel intensity specific tissue classes. Tincher [4] approach used a polynomial model of the RF[3] coil in order to decrease the inhomogeneity in MR images. Cohen [5] described a method for compensating purely intensity-based effects, using simple and rapid correction algorithms. Arnold [6] Qualitative and quantitative evaluation of six algorithms for correcting intensity non-uniformity effects. Gispert [7] Inhomogeneity images by minimization of intensity overlapping. Gispert [8] method for bias field correction of brain TI - Weighted Magnetic Resonance images minimizing segmentation error.

Our approach is simple and effective whereas we have developed a correction method that avoids the problems of intensity artifacts in MR images. This method is based on the theory of PDE and uses a multiscale low-pass filter based on a Gaussian kernel to extract the artifact (or a smoothed version of it) from the initial image which can be considered as a function $u_0 : \Omega \subset I\!R^2 \rightarrow I\!R$, being $u_0(x, y)$ the pixel (nodal) intensity values[4]. This allows us to study the fundamental structure of the artifact and to deduce a model for the grey level distribution. This has been calculated in the filtered, smoothed image, say $u_s(x, y)$, fitting the nodal values by using interpolating polynomial functions. The initial image u_0 can be then corrected with a low pass filter in the image domain using a (linear) diffusion attenuation model.

This paper is organized as follows. In Section 2 the algorithm is presented, explaining the details of the development. Section 3 shows the results obtained with real images. At last, in Section 4 conclusion and future works to improve the algorithm are presented.

2 Materials and Methods

The goal of the work presented in this paper is to determine a grey level attenuation correction algorithm. The MR image of the scanned brain is made up with a set of N slices and each slice is extracted from a three dimensional (3D) gradient echo (SPGR) acquisition (using $\alpha = 30^o$, $TR = 20$, $TE = 5$). Each image is represented, in a computational grid which discretize the image domain $\Omega \subset I\!R^2$, by a $n \times m$ matrix, where n is the number of nodes along the width and m is the number of nodes along the height of the slices. The matrix coefficients represents the grey level intensity at each pixel $(x_i, y_j) \in \Omega \subset I\!R^2, \forall i = 1 \ldots n, j = 1 \ldots m$.

Grey-scale attenuation in our images is caused by a coil smaller than usual head coil in the occipital area in order to obtain a good signal-noise ratio in visual areas of the brain but losing signal from frontal areas. It is usually used in Brain activity studies.

---

[2] Magnetic Resonance Imaging

[3] Ratiofrequency

[4] In this communication we are not interested in the mathematical details of the analysis. Nevertheless it is well known ([9]) that a grey-scale image u can be represented by a real-valued mapping $u \in L^1(I\!R^2)$

In Fig. 1 an example of three different slices from the same brain is shown. As can be noticed the three of them are affected by the inhomogeneity artifact. Below each image its histogram is depicted.

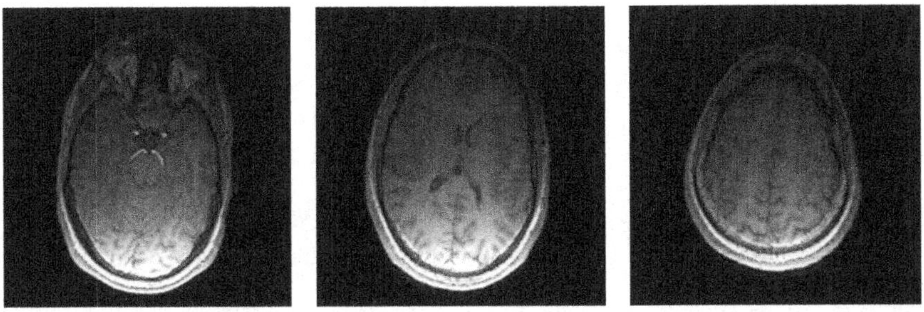

(a) Slice 50 (b) Slice 86 (c) Slice 120

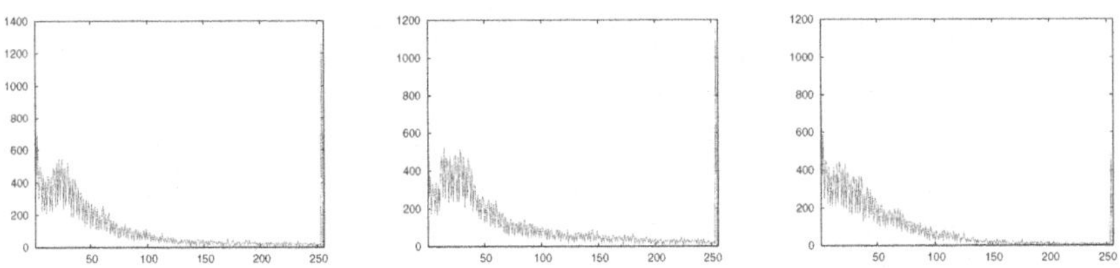

(d) Slice 50 histogram (e) Slice 86 histogram (f) Slice 120 histogram

Fig. 1. Three different slices from the same brain acquisition

The implemented algorithm involve 3 different steps, as can be seen in Fig. 2. In the following, each step is described.

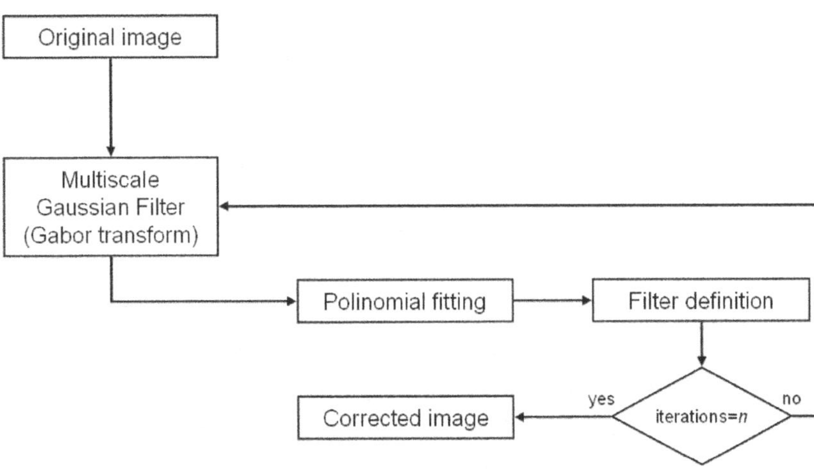

Fig. 2. Blocks diagram describing the algorithm

2.1 Multiscale Gaussian Filter

The first step is done in order to get a new, smoothed image u_s. Indeed, according to Shannon's theory, an image can be correctly represented by a discrete set of values, the samples, only if it has been previously smoothed. This simple remark, that smoothing is a necessary part of image formation, leads us to the theory of PDE [10] and linear diffusion.

The new image represents how is the illumination artifact, i.e., the distribution of the grey level inhomogeneity. This smoothing process is done using a low-pass filter based on a Gaussian kernel of the form:

$$K(x,y) = \frac{1}{2\pi\sigma^2}\exp\left(-\frac{|(x,y)|}{2\sigma^2}\right) \tag{1}$$

where $\sigma > 0$ is the width (standard deviation). This filter attenuates high frequencies in a monotone way. It is well known, [9], that this is equivalent to linear diffusion filtering where smoothing structures of order σ requires to stop the diffusion process at time $T = \sigma^2/2$.

In a similar way we generate a pyramidal decomposition in a multiscale approach named Gabor Transform [11, 12]. The *evolution* of the image under this Gaussian scale–space like–process allows a *deep structure analysis* (see [9]) which provides useful information for extracting semantic information from an image, i.e, finding the most relevant scales (scales-section, focus-of-attention) of the artifact.

This method is justified from the nature of the artifact, because it is a low-frequency effect. The goodness of Gabor transform comes from the fact of having the best resolution in terms of frequency and spatial localization.

2.2 Artifact Polynomial Modelling

Once the artifact distribution is obtained it is necessary to infer a mathematical model of it. Several models can be used (exponential, Rayleigh, etc.) but in order to get the best approximation of the artifact behaviour a polynomial interpolation was used was used to exploit the spatial distribution of u_s and the discrete nature of the data.

For each image column an interpolation is computed, so that the whole artifact model for each slice is composed of n interpolating polynomials. Fig. 3(b) shows the n polynomials as a unique interpolating surface.

2.3 Filter Definition

The mathematical model that we used to solve our restoration problem is based on Gaussian distribution of phases and produces an exponential attenuation of the signal (cutting-off the high frequencies). The result is that additional attenuation can be writen using a diffusion model of the form [13]:

$$A(D) = e^{-bD} \tag{2}$$

(a) Illumination artifact

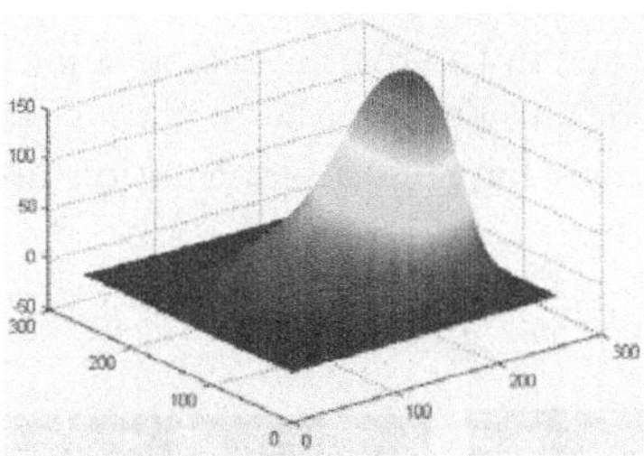

(b) Artifact model

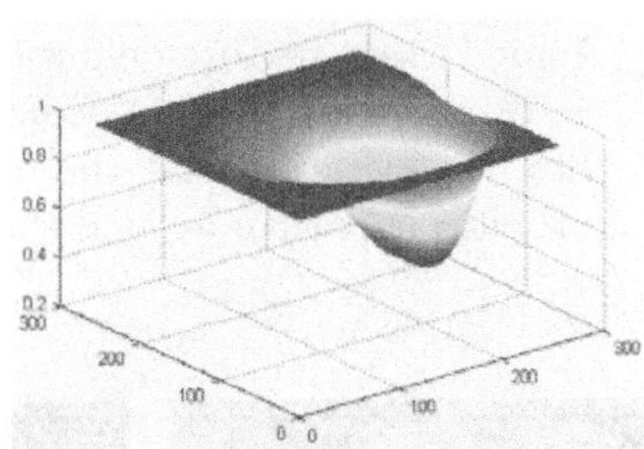

(c) Filter

Fig. 3. (a) Illumination artifact extracted from the Gabor tranform, (b) 3D representation of the artifact and (c) the 3D representation of the built filter

This expression describes the signal attenuation, where D represents the local tissue diffusion coefficient and b-factor depends on the amplitude and timing parameters of the gradient pulses used in the acquisition step of the initial data.

Empiric observations have proven that the diffusion coefficient can be replaced with the polynomial artifact model, while the b-factor has been replaced by a constant we called k. Using this notation Equation 2 can be written as follows:

$$A(P_i) = e^{-kP_i(y)}, \quad i = 1 \ldots n \tag{3}$$

This means that the mathematical model used in molecular diffusion MRI can be also used to correct the grey level inhomogeneity. Based on this idea we defined the image filter (in the image domain) $e^{-kP_i(y_j)}$ to obtain the basic formula:

$$u_f(x_i, y_j) = u_s(x_i, y_j)e^{-kP_i(y_j)} \tag{4}$$

where u_f is the final, corrected image, u_0 is the original image with the inhomogeneity, P_i is the interpolating polynomial the i column and k is the constant previously mentioned.

In Fig. 3(c) a 3D representation of a filter example can be seen.

3 Results and Discussion

As said previously, the problem discussed within this paper is the correction of grey scale inhomogeneities in MR images. The original images affected with this intensity artifact can be seen in Fig. 1 while corresponding corrected images are depicted in Fig. 4. Comparing both figures it can be observed that the intensity artifact has been corrected, giving rise to homogeneous images.

Also, the following observations can be pointed out:

- In the corrected images new structures not clearly evident in the original images appear, such as the fat in the frontal and lateral-front parts.
- A good tissue texture definition can be seen in the rear or occipital part and a worse definition in the frontal of the brain. This can be explained taking into consideration that the original images have more information around occipital part than around the frontal part.

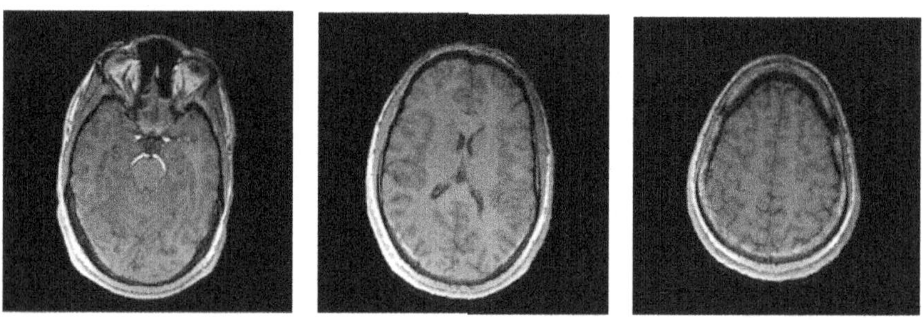

(a) Corrected slice 50 (b) Corrected slice 86 (c) Corrected slice 120

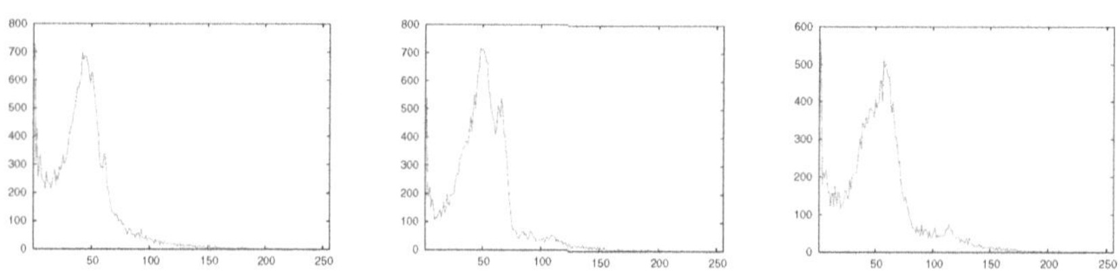

(d) Corrected slice 50 histogram (e) Corrected slice 86 histogram (f) Corrected slice 120 histogram

Fig. 4. Images from Fig. 1 after running the correction algorithm

In the other hand, looking at the original histograms (see Figure 1) it can be pointed out the presence of a great concentration of pixels in highest intensity values. Those pixels represent the intensity artifact. Comparing it with the corrected histograms can be observed that this concentration has dispersed. While the original histograms have two peaks (corresponding to background and artifact) and a distribution of quite dark pixels (representing the rest of the structure) the corrected ones only present two distributions corresponding to the background and the structure.

The correction of the inhomogeneity artifact in MR images has a lot of utilities in different fields. The most important are:

1. **Visualization:** the image quality improvement will enable the physician to study the brain information not only on the RF affected part but the whole brain information.
2. **Segmentation:** the correction algorithm presented in this papers can be used as a previous step to brain segmentation algorithms, not being necessary to include an artifact modelling step in its process.
3. **Brain activity:** as a result of the better visualization of the whole brain and the homogeneous textures, brain activity can be detected in a more accurate way.
4. **3D rendering:** artifact images are not suitable for 3D rendering processes while corrected images can be used as a good input for this kind of techniques. In next figure (Fig. 5) we can observe one axial slice after 3D rendering with the artifact (Fig. 5(a)) and without the artifact (Fig. 5(b)).

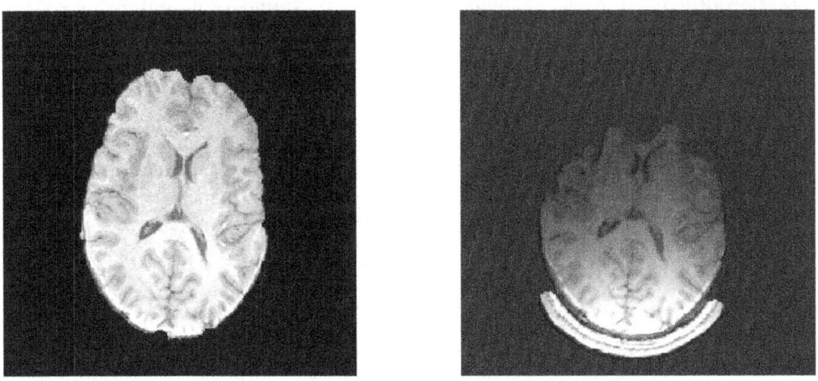

(a) 3D corrected (b) 3D non corrected

Fig. 5. One axial slice after 3D rendering with the artifact (a) and without the artifact (b)

4 Conclusions and Further Work

In this paper a method to correct the inhomogeneity in MRI has been presented. The main advantage of our method is that we don not need any segmentation step for restoration. As a result of this, our algorithm is simpler than the rest and our results are less affected by numerical errors.

A remarkable feature of the presented technique is the analogy with diffusion molecular model, where the diffusion coefficient has been replaced by a polynomial artifact model.

In future work we aim to exploit this analogy. Specifically we are interested in a non linear diffusion model where diffusion coefficient depends on the intensity of the illumination artifact. This can lead to a new approach where the RF artifact inhomogeneity is more realistic modelled.

Acknowledgments

This work was partially granted by the Spanish Commission for Science and Technology with the project number TIC2001-0175-C03-03 titled "Statistic Reconstruction of Positron Emission Tomography Based on High Performance Computation Techniques" and "Research on Molecular and Multimodality Medical Imaging Network" of the Health Institute Carlos III. Also, the authors would like to thank Ruber International Hospital and neuroradiologist Dr. Juan Linera.

References

1. Dhawan, A. P.: Medical Image Analysis. Wiley Intersciense. (2003)
2. Buxton, R. B.: Introduction to functional magnetic resonance imaging. Cambridge University Press. (2002)
3. DeCarli, D., Murphy, D.G.M., Tran, M. and Teichberg, D.: Local histogram correction of MRI spatially dependent image pixel intensity nonuniformity. J. Magn. Reson. Imag. **6** (1996) 519–528
4. Tincher, M., Meyer, C.M., Gupta, R. and Williams, D.M.: Polynomial modelling and reduction of RF body coil spatial inhomogeneity in MRI. IEEE Trans. Med. Imag. **12** (1993) 361–365
5. Cohen, M.S., DuBois R.M. and Zeineh, M.M.: Rapid and effective correction of RF inhomogeneity for high field magnetic resonance imaging. Human Brain Mapping. **10** (2000) 204–211
6. Arnold, J.B., Liow, J.S., Schaper, K.A., Stern, J.J., Sled, J.G., Shattuck, D.W., Worth, A.J., Cohen, M.S., Leahy R.J., Mazziotta, J.C., and Rottenberg, D.A.: Qualitative and quantitative evaluation of six algorithms for correcting intensity nonuniformity effects. NeuroImage. **13** (2001) 931–943
7. Gispert, J.D., Reig, S., Pascau, J., Martinez Lazaro, R., Vaquero, J.J. and Desco, M.: Inhomogeneity images by minimization of intensity overlapping. IEEE **02** (2003) II–847–850 vol. 3
8. Gispert, J.D., Reig, S., Pascau, J., Martinez Lazaro, R., Vaquero, J.J. and Desco, M.: Method for bias field correction of brain TI – Weighted Magnetic Resonance images minimizing segmentation error. Human Brain Mapping. **22** (2004) 133–144
9. Weikert, J.: Anisotropic Diffusion in Image Processing. ECMI Series, B.G. Teubner, Stuttgart. (1998)
10. Guichrad, F., Morel, J.M.: Image Analysis and P.D.E.'s. IPAM GBM Tutorials. (2001). `http://www.ipam.ucla.edu/publications/gbm2001/gbmtut_jmorel.pdf`
11. Gabor, D.: Theory of Communication. Instr. Electr. Engin. **93** (1946) 429–457
12. Nestares, O., Navarro, R., Portilla, J., Tabernero, A.: Efficient spatial–domain implementation of a multiscale image representation based on gabor functions. Electronic Imaging, **7** (1998) 166–173
13. LeBihan, D.: Molecular diffusion nuclear magnetic resonance imaging. Magn. Reson. Quart. **8** (1991) 7–30

Fully 3D Wavelets MRI Compression

Emanuele Schiavi, C. Hernández, and Juan A. Hernández

Universidad Rey Juan Carlos, Móstoles, Madrid, Spain
e.schiavi@escet.urjc.es, c.hernandez.m@terra.es, j.hernandez@escet.urjc.es

Abstract. This paper deals with the implementation of 3D wavelets techniques for compression of medical images, specifically in the MRI modality. We show that at the same compression rate a lower loss of information can be obtained by using fully 3D wavelets as compared to iterated 2D methods. An adaptive thresholding step is performed in each sub-band and a simple Run Length Encoding (RLE) method for compression is finally used. A reconstruction algorithm is then implemented and a comparison study of the reconstructed image is then proposed, showing the high performance of the proposed algorithm.

1 Introduction

The application of new technologies in the field of medicine and, more specifically, in medical images is a far reaching issue in the development of new methods of visualization and storing of digital images. Among others, image compression is one of the major issues in three-dimensional (3D) medical imaging. 3D image modalities such as Magnetic Resonance Imaging (MRI), Computed Tomography (CT) or Positron Emission Tomography (PET) routinely provide large quantities of data. For purpose of storage or archiving, data compression is usually necessary whereas it reduces the storage and/or transmission bandwidth requirements of medical images . In many cases, lossless image compression methods (Lempel-Ziv, Reduced-Difference Pyramid, Shape Adaptive Integer Wavelet transform [1] etc.) are mandatory but the compression ratio obtained by these methods is generally low (typically 3:1). Recently it has been observed that, for some applications such as compression and segmentation of 3D MR images of the head (see [7] for a lossy multiresolution approach to interactive brain sulci delineation and merging into functional PET images), lossy compression can be suited, providing good compression levels without significantly altering final results which may influence diagnosis. In this paper we develop an efficient multiresolution algorithm for lossy compression well suited to 3D MR images. It is based on a sub-band adaptive thresholding followed by a simple but effective Run-Length-Method for sub-band coding and a final, decompression step. Our results show that 3D volume data can be better compressed that 2D slice by slice reconstructions and that high compression rates can be obtained with low Mean square errors (MSE) and high signal to noise ratios (SNR).

This paper is organized as follows: Section 2 introduce to the basic material and definitions. The compression algorithms used in the 2D and 3D cases are

J.M. Barreiro et al. (Eds.): ISBMDA 2004, LNCS 3337, pp. 9–20, 2004.

detailed and the reconstruction (decompression) steps are presented. In Section 3 we show the results we have obtained with different levels of multiresolution by using a Haar family of wavelets. Section 4 is devoted to the discussion and future work.

2 Material and Methods

The use of wavelets and multiresolution analysis is becoming a standard tool in digital images processing and reconstruction and represent a new computational paradigm which in many cases outperforms the Fourier transform methods. In fact, wavelet transforms describes multiresolution decomposition in terms of expansion of an image onto a set of wavelet basis functions which are well localized in both space and time. Its roots are found in a variety of disciplines, Mathematics, Signal processing, Computer Vision, Physics. In the early history of wavelets theory we refer to the pioneering papers of Haar (1910, Haar basis, the first wavelet), Gabor (1946, the Gabor transform-short time Fourier Transform), the Calderon's work on singular integral operators which contains the continuos wavelet transform (1964), and to Rosenfeld and Thurston for multi-resolution techniques invented in machine vision (1971).

The recent history of wavelets can be traced back to Morlet and Grossman, 1984, who proposed wavelets and applied them to the analysis of seismic signals, to Mallat and Meyer who developed the fast wavelets algorithm (1986) and to Daubechies (1988) who created a class of wavelets which can be implemented with digital FIR filters. We refers to these papers and books for all the basic notations and definitions.

In this paper we focus in the field of medical images, specifically in MRI, where the successful design of efficient algorithms represent a fundamental and social goal for diagnostic and early detection of diseases and pathologies.

In this kind of modality and in the three dimensional case, the quantity of memory necessary for storage is very big because, usually, we need to store not only a 3D image but a discrete sequence of images taken along an axis. Due to the basic properties of wavelets which appear to be well suited in image processing (see for example [4, 9, 10, 5, 2, 6, 3]), we choose this technique as a basis for our study of compression of 3D volume data. Our study consist of the development and comparison of two algorithms for compression and reconstruction of 3D images. The first algorithm is based on the pyramidal algorithm of decomposition of the 2D wavelet transform (figure 1). The second one it is based on the the pyramidal algorithm of decomposition of the 3D wavelet transform (figure 2). We also choose to use the Haar wavelet basis which, despite of its simpleness is one of the used families for image processing [4, 9, 5, 2, 6, 8], specially for compression tasks.

Our method is a lossy multiresolution compression method. The loss of information is due to an adaptive thresholding step decorrelating the information before coding the decorrelated signal. This kind of technique is well established in image denoising and provides to be extremely effective in compression. In

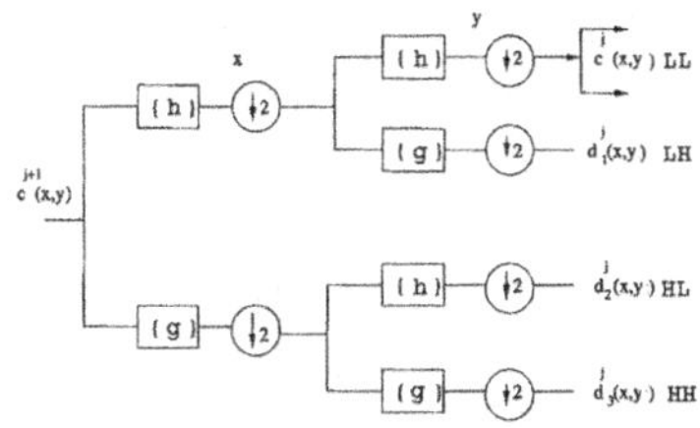

Fig. 1. Pyramidal algorithm for 2D wavelets

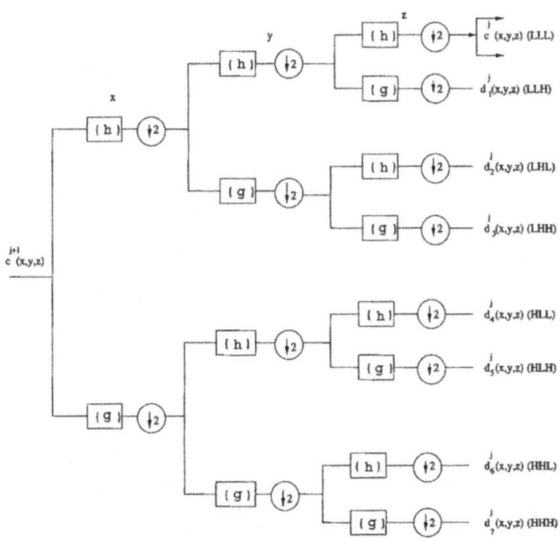

Fig. 2. Pyramidal algorithm for 3D wavelets

particular, the high frequency transform coefficients can be encoded in a coarse manner, since this will produce high-frequency noise.

Our thresholding method is then followed by coding where we choose the Run Length Encoding (RLE) method. Run-length encoding is a data compression algorithm that is supported by most bitmap file formats, such as TIFF, BMP, and PCX. RLE is suited for compressing any type of data regardless of its information content, but the content of the data will affect the compression ratio achieved by RLE. In fact RLE schemes are simple and fast, but their compression efficiency depends on the type of image data being encoded; it is mainly used to compress runs (a repeating string of characters) of the same byte. In our problem this choice is effective because the application of the Haar transform allows to concentrate the energy of the function into the coefficients of scaling while the threshold of the wavelets coefficients generate long runs without modifying excessively the original function energy [8].

The 3D images we used for this study have a resolution of 512x512x128 pixels and a grey scale of 12 bits. Every element of the image is stored as an integer of 16 bits.

2.1 A Compression Algorithm for 2D Wavelets

The compression process we model with this algorithm consists of the individual treatment of the 2D images which make up the volume data, i.e., we compress slice by slice the 3D original image. The basic structure of the algorithm is depicted in figure 3.

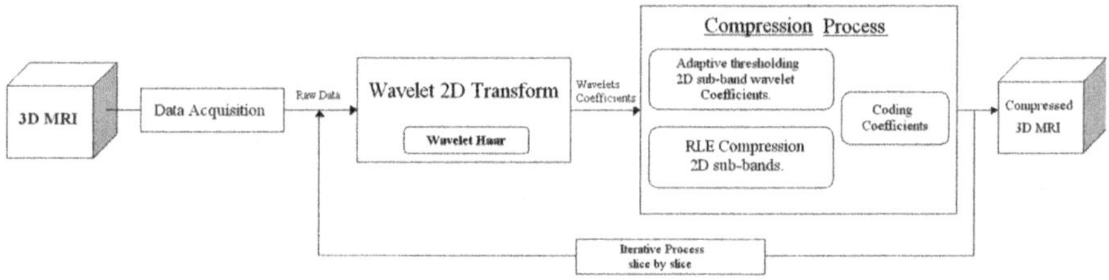

Fig. 3. Compression scheme for 2D Wavelet

The resulting algorithm can be divided into the following stages: 1) 3D data acquisition step, 2) Iterative application of the 2D Haar wavelet transform, 3) Adaptive thresholding of the wavelet coefficients, 4) RLE compression of the 2D sub-bands and 5) Coding the coefficients.

3D data acquisition step. The images were acquired in a SIGNA 3T scanner of GE (General Electric) at Ruber International Hospital (Madrid, Spain). The acquisition sequence was a 3D SPGR (Spoil-Gradient) of GE. The spatial resolution was 512x512x128 for 1mmx1mmx1mm of pixel size.

At the beginning the data volume representing the 3D MR image is read from the hard disk and stored in memory for future manipulation.

Iterative application of the 2D Haar wavelet transform. This stage correspond to the (iterative) application of the 2D Haar wavelet transform on every slice (2D image) of the 3D MR image. In this way every slice is decomposed into a 2D sub-band (for the scaling coefficients) and, say n, 2D sub-bands of wavelets coefficients, depending on the number n of iterations. The results can be seen in figures 4.

Adaptive thresholding of the wavelet coefficients. The elimination of the low energy wavelets coefficients by our adaptive sub-band thresholding is shown in figure 1, and it consists of the following steps: We consider the 2D image decomposed into n sub-bands as provided by the previous stage. We just apply the thresholding to the sub-bands corresponding to the wavelet coefficients.

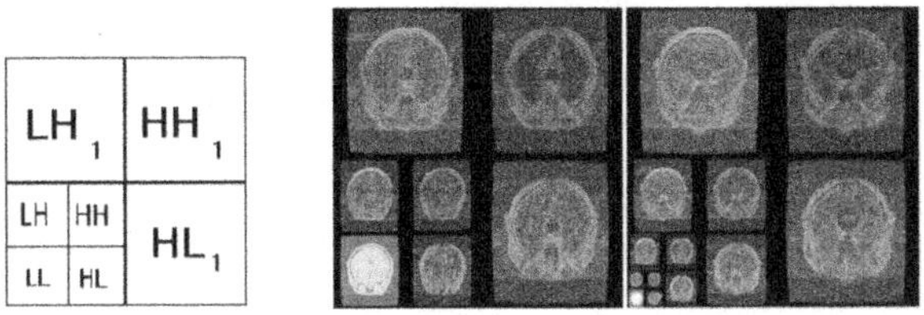

Fig. 4. 2D wavelet decomposition scheme, 2o Level. (on the left). 2o Level in the original image (center). 4o Level in the original image (right)

In every sub-band we have an independent thresholding corresponding to the following steps: 1) To select and extract from the coefficients matrix the corresponding sub-band, 2) To compute the minimum (positive) coefficient (in absolute value) in the selected sub-band. This generate every, independent, sub-band threshold value, 3) To parameterize the previous sub-band threshold value multiplying by a constant value to tune the elimination process. To realize the corresponding adaptive hard thresholding and 4) To actualize the modified coefficients of the selected sub-band in the coefficients matrix.

RLE compression of the 2D sub-bands. The compression stage is adapted on every 2D sub-band of every 2D slice of which it consist of the volume data so that the compression is done image by image.

We next describe the coding coefficients stage (although it is detailed later it is not independent of the previous stage and can be considered as a part of the compression process).

Coding the coefficients. The coding stage is perhaps one of the most critical. The data of which the images consists of are stored with an integer of 16 bits. The wavelet transform generates float type values in the scaling and wavelets coefficients. These values are internally stored by using variables of 32 (float) or 64 (double float) bits, but the storing in the hard disk is done using a format of 16 bits which has been developed to code the float values of the coefficients.

2.2 A Compression Algorithm for 3D Wavelets

In this case we consider the 3D MRI volume data as a whole. The basic structure of the algorithm is as depicted in figure 5.

The algorithm consists of the following different steps: 1) 3D data acquisition step from the initial volume data, 2) Iterative application of the 3D Haar wavelet transform, 3) Adaptive thresholding of the wavelet coefficients, 4) RLE compression of the 3D sub-bands and 5) Coding the coefficients.

3D data acquisition step. This stage is as before and shall not be detailed further.

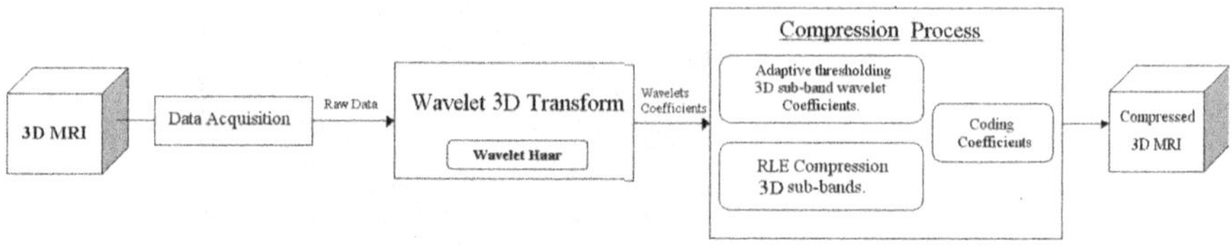

Fig. 5. 3D wavelet compression scheme

Iterative application of the 3D Haar wavelet transform. This stage corresponds to the application of the 3D wavelet transform, using the Haar basis, onto the 3D volume data representing the MRI image. Consequently, the MRI image is decomposed in a sub-band of scaling coefficients and n (the number of iterations) sub-bands of wavelets coefficients. See figures 6, and 7.

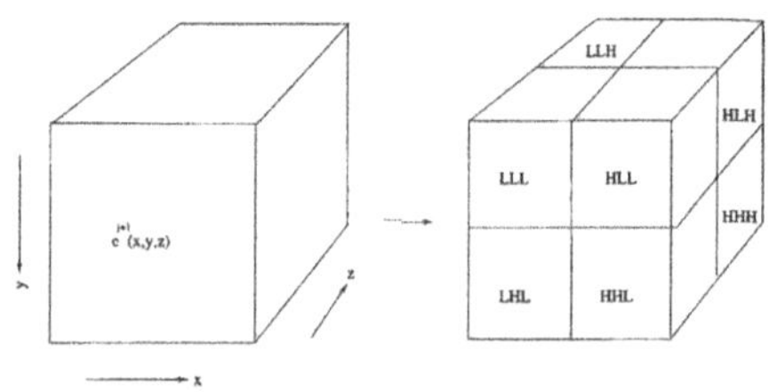

Fig. 6. 3D wavelet decomposition of the data volume

Adaptive thresholding of the wavelet coefficients. The elimination process performed by application of the thresholding of the 3D sub-bands wavelets coefficients is described in figure 2 and it is analogous to the 2D case. It can be done in the following way:

We start with the 3D volume data decomposed into n 3D sub-bands as given by application of the 3D wavelet transform. As in the 2D case, we shall eliminate just the wavelets coefficients leaving unaffected the scaling coefficients.

Each sub-band is considered independently for thresholding in the following manner: 1) To select and extract from the coefficients matrix the corresponding sub-band, 2) To compute the minimum (positive) coefficient (in absolute value) in the selected sub-band. This generate every, independent, sub-band threshold value, 3) To parameterize the previous sub-band threshold value multiplying by a constant value to tune the elimination process. To realize the corresponding adaptive hard thresholding and 4) To actualize the modified coefficients of the selected subband in the coefficients matrix.

RLE compression of the 3D sub-bands. The compression step is performed on every 3D sub-bands. Note that we compress volumes, not slices (as in the 2D case).

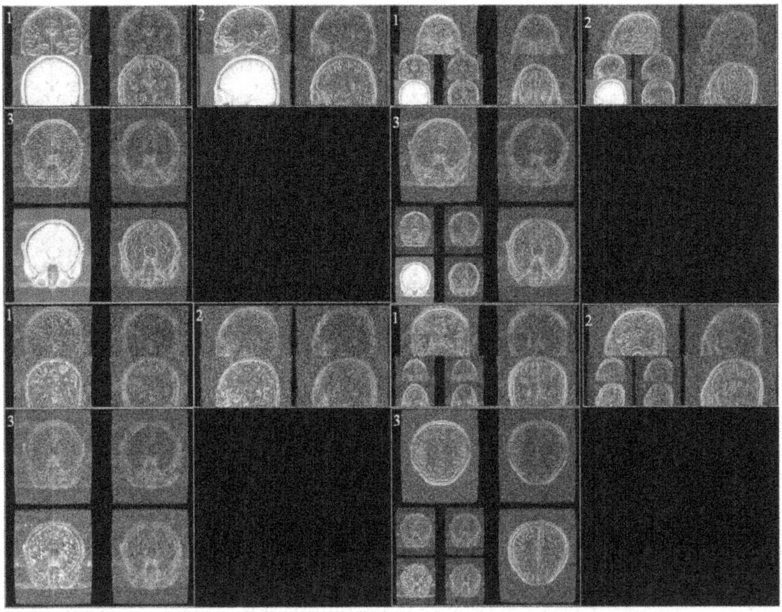

Fig. 7. Coronal (1), Sagital (2) and Transversal (3) sections of the 3D data volume transformed by the first decomposition level(on the left). The second decomposition level (on the right)

Coding the coefficients. It is as in the 2D case (see the corresponding section 2.1).

Once the 3D volumen data has been compressed (using one of previos algorithms) we need to reconstruct the image by means of a decompression algorithm. This is detailed next for both case.

2.3 2D Wavelets Decompression Algorithm

The 3D image reconstruction is done as described in figure 8.

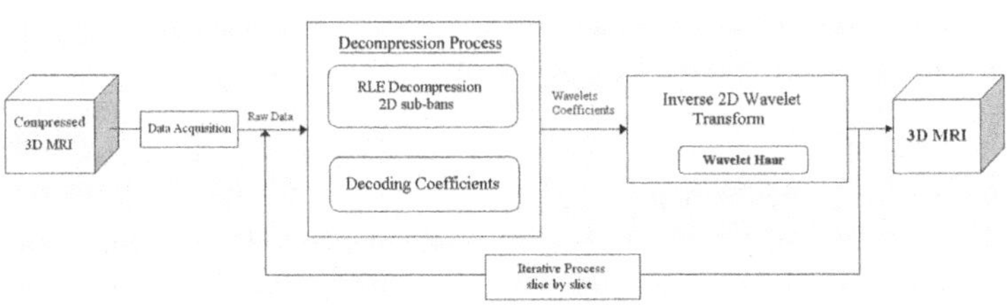

Fig. 8. 2D wavelets decompression scheme

The inverse Haar wavelet transform is applied iteratively depending on the level of decomposition used in the compression process. It is performed slice by slice.

2.4 3D Wavelets Decompression Algorithm

The inverse Haar wavelet transform is applied iteratively depending on the level of decomposition used in the compression process. It is performed using the 3D volume data representing the compressed MR image. The process is described below (figure 9).

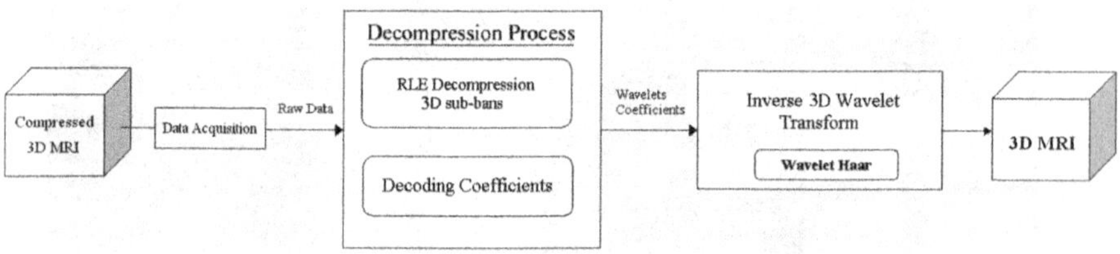

Fig. 9. 3D wavelets decompression scheme

3 Results

Numerical simulations have been done using a 3D MR image of the head and applying the 2D and 3D compression algorithms presented before. In both cases we used different compression rates associated with different resolution levels obtained by application of the corresponding wavelets (2D and 3D). In figures 10, 12, 13, 14, 15 and 16 we show the plots of the results we have obtained. The compression rate is represented on the x axis and the mean square error (MSE) on the y axis. In the caption we indicate the number of iterations (resolution level of the wavelet transform) and the compression algorithm (2D or 3D) we used, i.e.: I3 Wavelet 2D means that we used the 2D wavelet compression algorithm with three iterations. An accurate analysis of these plots (see figure 10) shows that at the same compression rate and for the same number of iterations the 3D algorithm gives better results (when considering the MSE) than the 2D algorithm. Focusing in the 2D case (figure 12) we can appreciate a sustancial improvement in the results when we perform a three level wavelet transform as compared to a one level wavelet transform. This improvement is still evident when we perform a five level wavelet transform if we consider high compression rates. In the 3D case (figure 13) we can still appreciate a sustancial improvement in the results when we perform a three level wavelet transform as compared to a one level wavelet transform. Nevertheless with a five level wavelet transform the improvement is not evident and we need to check directly our data to notice it. We also compared the results in both cases (2D and 3D) when we fix the number of iterations (figures 14, 15 y 16). In all of them we can appreciate that the 3D algorithm is much more efficient.

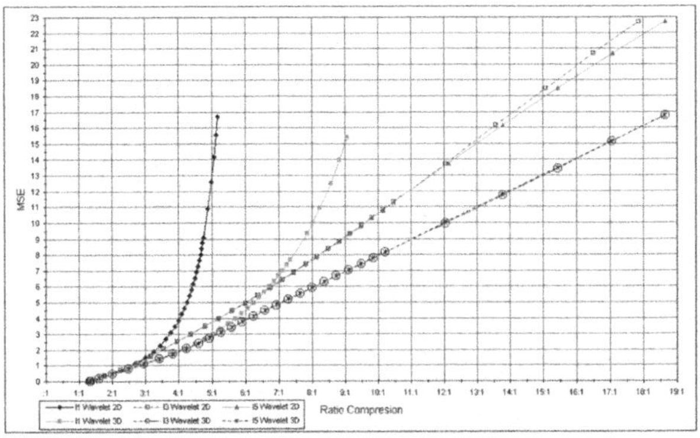

Fig. 10. A global plot representing the results we obtained all together

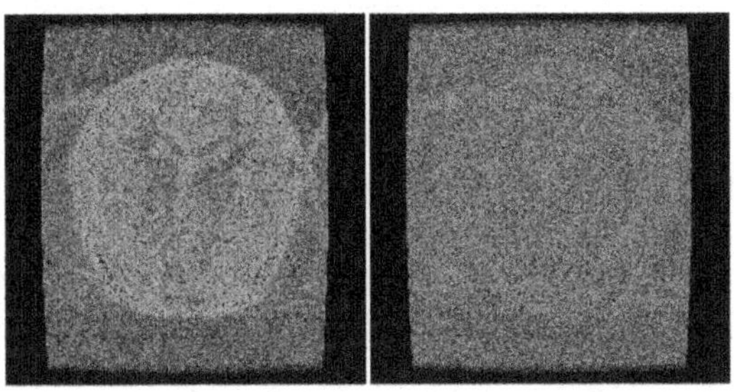

Fig. 11. 2D error image (on the left). 3D error image (on the right)

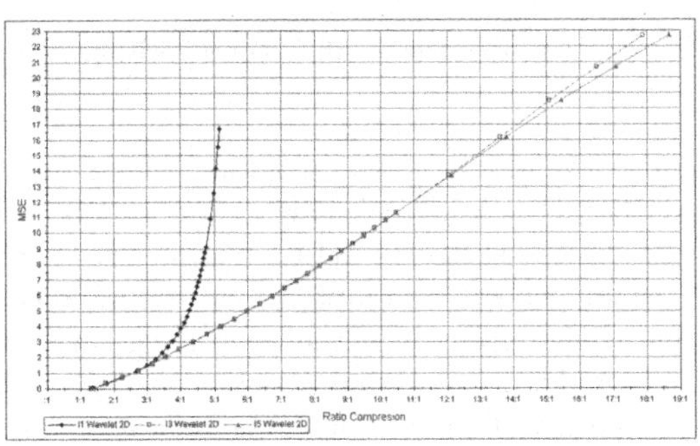

Fig. 12. The results of the 2D algorithm (the image is processed slice by slice)

4 Discussion and Future Work

Our study shows that a fully 3D wavelet lossy compression method can be used efficiently for 3D MR images processing. High compression rates characterized by low MSE and high SNR can be obtained, so outperforming typical lossless

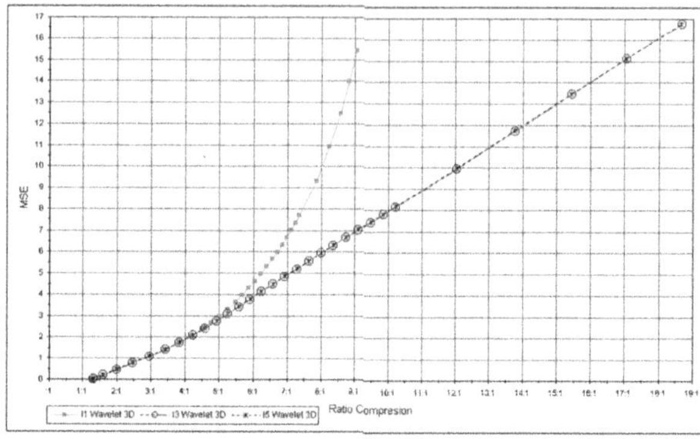

Fig. 13. The results of the 3D algorithm

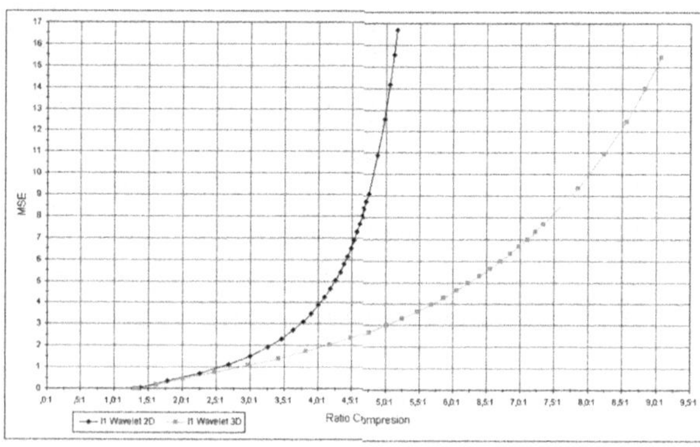

Fig. 14. A comparison between the different algorithms with one iteration

compression schemes. We also demonstrated that the 3D algorithm is far better than the corresponding 2D slice by slice algorithm, an observation by no means obvious. We finally show (see figures 11) that in fact the error image in the 3D case is much more homogeneous and uniformly distributed than the corresponding 2D error image. This implies that the anatomical structures have not been corrupted in the restored image and that a sort of denoising has been achieved by our scheme. Future work will include the implementation, analysis and comparison of others wavelets families with a view to establish the relationship between the image characteristics and the best multiresolution. An improvement in the coding stage as well as other refinements of our algorithm shall also be considered.

Acknowledgements

The work of the first and third authors has been granted by the Spanish Commission for Science and Technology with project number TIC2001-0175-C03-03

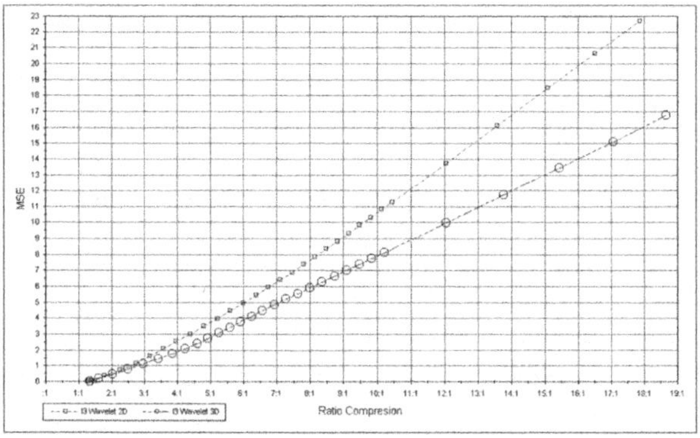

Fig. 15. A comparison between the different algorithms with three iterations

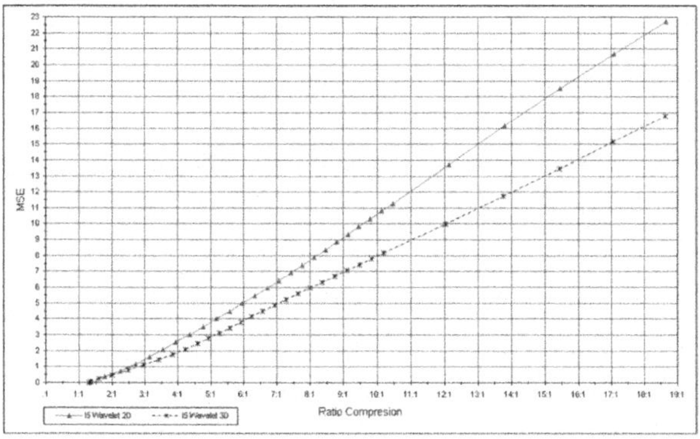

Fig. 16. A comparison between the different algorithms with five iterations

"Statistic Reconstruction of Positron Emission Tomography Base on High Performance Computation Techniques". The second and third authors are granted by "Research on Molecular and Multimodality Medical Imaging Network (IM3)" of the Carlos III Health Institute.

References

1. R. Srinkanth Abhishek Mehrotra and A. G. Ramakrishnan, Shape adaptative integer wavelet transform based coding scheme for 2d/3d mr images, Proceeding of the Data Compresion Conference (DCC'04) (2004 IEEE).
2. Steven Schlicker Edward Aboufadel, Discovering wavelets.
3. J.M. Lina and L. Gagnon, Image enhancement with symmetric daubechies wavelets, (1995).
4. W. Dominguez M. Vidaurrazaga, E. Gonzalez, Mejoramiento de imagenes de resonancia magnética basado en la transformada wavelet, (2001), no. 00260.
5. David Hattery Guinevere Eden Bjorn Jawerth Michael Hilton, Todd Ogden, Wavelet denoising of functional mri data.

6. Rober D. Nowak, Wavelet-based rician noise removal for magnetic resonance imaging, (1998).
7. B. Macq P. Piscaglia, J.P. Thiran and Ch. Michel., Lossy multiresolution compression and segmentation of 3d mr imges of the head., In SPIE Medical Imaging 1996, Newport Beach, California USA (1996).
8. H. Andrea Hijar. Juan Pablo Newman. Mª Angeles Rodríguez. Rafael Peñaliza, Wavelets: Transformada de haar.
9. S. Saha, Image compression - from dct to wavelets: A review, ACM Crossreads Student Magazine (2000).
10. Joaquin Azpiroz Leehan y Sonia Charleston Villalobos, Estudio comparativo de cuatro metodos de compresión para imágenes de resonancia magnética nuclear, (1999).

A New Approach to Automatic Segmentation of Bone in Medical Magnetic Resonance Imaging

Gabriela Pérez, Raquel Montes Diez, Juan A. Hernández, and José San Martín

DIET, URJC, 28933 Móstoles, Spain
{g.perez,r.montes,j.hernandez,jsmartin}@escet.urjc.es
http://www.urjc.es/

Abstract. This paper presents the modelling and segmentation with correction of inhomogeneity in magnetic resonance imaging of shoulder. For that purpose a new heuristic is proposed using a morphological method and a pyramidal Gaussian decomposition (Discrete Gabor Transform). After the application of these filters, an automatic segmentation of a bone is possible despite of other semiautomatic methods present in the literature.

1 Introduction and Background

Magnetic Resonance Imaging (MRI) is a technique used, primarily, as medical diagnosis tool, producing high quality images of organs and structures from human body. MRI provides additional information that cannot be obtained from an X-ray, ultrasound, or CT scan.

In MRI scanning, the area of the human body to study is positioned inside a strong magnetic field. The MRI can detect changes in the normal structure and characteristics of organs and tissues. It also can detect tissue damage or disease, such as a tumor or infection. Information from an MRI scan can be digitally saved and stored in a computer for further study.

The use of computer systems to help physicians has extremely increased in the last years in all medical fields. More important than saving and storing information, orthopaedic specialist will be helped by computers on diagnosis and planning processes that require detailed studies and analysis before exposing a patient to a possible high risk intervention treatment.

We are interested in the 3D MRI clinical modelling in order to shape and to analyze the shoulder. It is necessary to do distinguish the different elements that make up the surgical field of a shoulder as bone, cartilage, ligaments, muscle and skin. Therefore it is necessary to review and to have a thorough knowledge of the different pathologies by means of research, in order to help to prepare and to treat them [1–3].

Our interest focuses on the segmentation of different parts of shoulder and especially on the bone in real MR images. Most muscle-skeletal segmentations are still manually performed by experts, requiring extensive and meticulous analysis, as well as many hours of intense human effort [4]. We investigate on the possibility of automating the segmentation technique and to support and accelerate manual segmentation (semiautomatic) where full automation is not possible.

One obstacle in automatic segmentation performing is the presence of inhomogeneities in the MR images which affect the measured gray level values of pixels in

J.M. Barreiro et al. (Eds.): ISBMDA 2004, LNCS 3337, pp. 21–26, 2004.

different regions of the image, reducing the accuracy of classification algorithms. Gray scale inhomogeneities in MR images may have different causes [5–7] and to characterize the field of inhomogeneity of MR machines is almost impossible since it changes with every sample under different study.

Removing inhomogeneity intensity of MRI is an essential requirement for the image qualitative analysis. It contributes to the strength of the image segmentation. There are many algorithms that allow later illumination correction by means of parametric and nonparametric approach. These methods have been extensively treated in the literature, making evident the importance to approach this problem. Some authors [5] present an exhaustive comparison of six algorithms for this purpose.

Most part of cases comes from of a segmentation of the image with illumination in an implicit or explicit way, though there are methods that not need segmentation [8–13].

In this work we propose a procedure which considers independently both inhomogeneity correction and 2D image segmentation. The illumination artifact correction is based on a homomorphic algorithm with a low step filter. In order to segment the image, we use firstly multiresolution decomposition based on Gaussian Pyramid (Gabor Transform) [14], [15] and the segmentation itself is performed by applying a combination of edge detection algorithm as well as other mathematical morphological algorithms.

2 Materials and Methods

In order to achieve our aim, we are interested on using a scheme of edge detection methods (Canny edge detector) [16] as well as other morphological methods. Our experience show that these methods perform poorly when they are applied on 2D muscle-skeleton MR image automatically, given the complexity of the image. In order to reduce this complexity, we prepare the image in advance, by correcting the illumination inhomogeneity using a homomorphic filter and by decomposing the image into low and high frequencies in the Gabor domain.

The following algorithm is employed:

- Correction of intensity inhomogeneity
- Multiscale Analysis in Gabor domain
- Segmentation
  - o Edge detection
  - o Remove end points of lines without removing small objects completely
  - o Remove isolated pixels (1's surrounded by 0's)
  - o Fill isolated interior pixels (0's surrounded by 1's).

All the different steps in the proposed algorithm were performed by using Matlab software (6.5.1 version).

2.1 Illumination Correction

Firstly, we remove illumination inhomogeneity and other potential problems that may make more difficult the process of automatic segmentation by using a homomorphic filter. The homomorphic filter has been designed to correct intensity inhomogeneities in the frequency domain. This filter compresses illumination conditions brightness and simultaneously, it enhances the contrast between reflection properties of objects. This filter is used when the interference is multiplicative; that is, when the original image is the result of the product of a free noise image by an illumination image. As the illumination component usually dominates the low frequencies and the reflection component dominates high frequencies, the resulting image can be effectively manipulated in the Fourier domain.

Whereas an increment in high frequency component in Fourier image improves the reflection image, the illumination image is attenuated [17–19]. This can be achieved by using the 2D Butterworth filter which approaches the constant magnitude in the step band of an ideal filter.

2.2 Gabor Domain Multiresolution Analysis

Once grayscale inhomogeneity has been removed and in order to break down our image of interest into low and high frequency components, we use the multiscale analysis presented by a previous work [14], where the authors focus on the spatial domain implementation, arguing two important advantages from the Fourier method: it is more plausible one for modelling vision and it permits local processing which is restricted to areas of interest and non rectangular shapes. Their algorithm proposed on [14] improves the original work [15] by (1) incorporating a High-Pass Residual (HPR) covering the high frequencies and (2) improving the quality of the reconstruction by assigning different fixed gains to the Gabor channels before adding them together; and (3) separating one dimensional filter masks with small size (11-tap), resulting in a spatial domain implementation faster than the implementation in the frequency domain via FFT, while maintaining a high fidelity in the filter design. The low frequency image is subjected to the segmentation procedure.

2.3 Segmentation

Segmentation is performed on the basis of edge detection by using canny algorithm [16], [19]. This algorithm concentrates an ideal step edge, represented as a sign function in one dimension, corrupted by an assumed Gaussian noise process. In practice this is not an accurate model but it represents an approximation to the effects of sensor noise, sampling and quantisation. The approach is based on convolution of the image function with Gaussian operators and their derivatives.

In order to improve this edge segmentation, we use a series of morphological operators for multidimensional binary images [19–25], such as removing spurious and isolated pixels and filling regions [26].

3 Results

We present the results obtained by applying the proposed method to a volume magnetic resonance image of shoulder. The image dimensions are 150 X 256 X 92 scans. The image is courtesy of the Ruber International Hospital in Madrid. In order to present results of the different steps proposed we select one of the slides of the image. Figure 1 shows the original image; note the illumination artifact cause by the patient position respect of the acquisition coil.

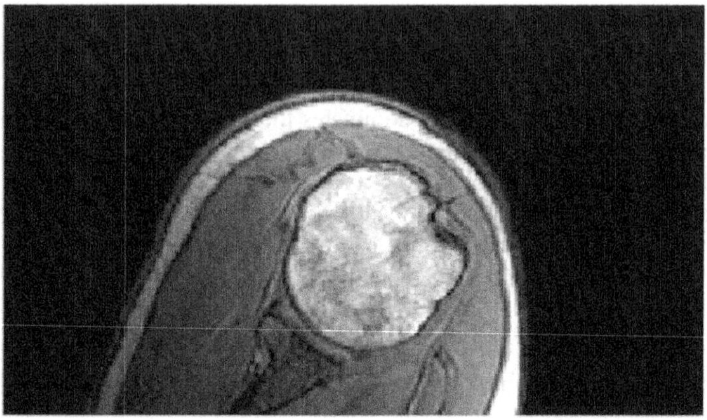

Fig. 1. Original Image

Figure 2a shows the corrected image after applying the homomorphic filter described in 3.1. The image presents now a much more homogeneous appearance of gray levels.

According to the proposed algorithm we next separate our image into low and high frequency images in the Gabor domain. We are interested in obtaining the low frequency image with lower resolution that allows us to segment the object of interest, in this case bone, by applying the Canny method. Figure 2b presents the low frequency component of our image after Gaussian Filter by mean Gabor transform.

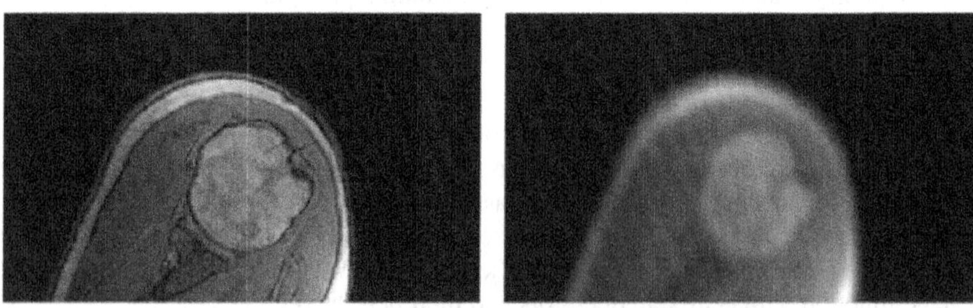

Fig. 2. a) Image corrected y b) Gabor image low frequency

Then, we submit this image to the of edge detection procedure based on the Canny method. Some computational background is necessary in order to determine the threshold to use in this method. For instance, in Figure 3a, a 0.03 threshold has shown to perform satisfactorily.

Once edges haven been detected in the image, we apply morphological algorithms for binary images in order to remove spurious and isolated pixels. Figures 3b and 3c show the resulting image after removing spurious and isolated pixels, respectively. Finally figure 3d shows the slices bone, perfectly segmented after applying a morphological operator to fill in regions of interest.

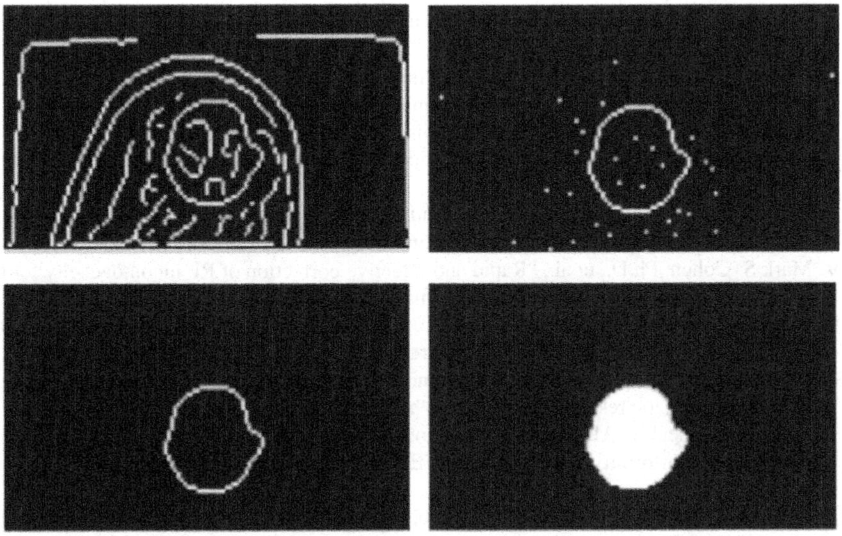

Fig. 3. a) Edges image, b) region of interest with spurious pixels after morphological filter, c) isolated pixels removed d) Segmented bone

4 Discussion and Further Studies

The algorithm proposed allows automating segmentation of the bone in high quality MR images. The algorithm is not capable to deal with other kind of tissues.

We have detected some problems for the automatic segmentation in images with poor signal to noise ratio or in extreme images (far from the acquisition center).

Now, our interest is focus on improving the heuristic to segment soft tissues. Furthermore we are trying to obtain an automatic bone 3D rendering using our automatic segmentation as a previous step.

Acknowledgments

This work was partially granted by the Spanish Commission for Science and Technology with project number TIC2001-0175-C03-03 titled "Statistic Reconstruction of Positron Emission Tomography Based on High Performance Computation Techniques" and "Research on Molecular and Multimodality Medical Imaging Network" of the Carlos III Health Institute.

Finally the authors of the present work would like to thank Ruber International Hospital and neuroradiologist Dr. Juan Linera for their disinterested help.

References

1. Nadia Magnenat, et al., "Problems and solutions for the accurate 3D functional modelling of the hip and shoulder.
2. http://www.bonejointdecade.org/organization/default.html
3. Mirowitz SA, "MR imaging artifacts. Challenges and solutions", Magn Reson Imaging Clin N Am 1999 Nov; 7 (4):717-32.

4. Tina Kapur, et al., "Model based segmentation of clinical Knee MRI. JMRI, 10, 4, 550 – 562, 1999.
5. J.B. Arnold et al., "Qualitative and quantitative evaluation of six algorithms for correcting intensity nonuniformity effects". Neuro-Image, pp. 931 -943, 2001.
6. http://www.hggm.es/umce/imagen/pdfs/Gispert-CASEIB'02.pdf
7. J.D. Gispert, PhD "Segmentación estadística de imagines de Resonancia Magnética", pp. 8-22; 75-96.
8. E. Vokurka, et al.,, 1999 "A fast model independant method for automatic correction of intensy nonuniformity in JMRI, 10, 4, 550-562
9. Mark S. Cohen, Ph.D., et al., "Rapid and effective correction of RF inhomogeneity for high field magentic resonante imaging". In human brain mapping.
10. Brinkmann, B.H., Manduca, A., y Robb, R.A. 1996. Quantitative analysis of statistical methods for grayscale inhomogeneity correction in MR images. In SPIE, pp. 2710.
11. Mark, S. Cohen, Ph.D., et al., "Rapid and effective correction of RF inhomogeneity for high field magnetic resonante imaging, in human brain mapping.
12. Sled J.G. Zijdenbos AP, Evans AC. A nonparametric method for automatic correction of intensity nonuniformity in MRI data. IEEE trans. Med Imaging 1998, 17: 87-97. SPIE vol. 2710.
13. Brinkmann, B.H., Manduca, A., y Robb, R.A. 1998. Optimized homomorphic unsharp masking for MR grayscale inhomogeneity correction. IEEE Transactions on Medical Imaging 17: 161-171.
14. O. Nestares, R. Navarro, J. Portilla and A. Tabernero, Efficient Spatial Domain Implementation of a Multiscale Image Representation Based on Gabor Functions. 1998. Journal of Electronic Imaging, 7(1), pp. 166-173.
15. R. Navarro and A. Tabernero, "Gaussian wavelet transform: two alternative fast implementation for images". Multidimensional system and signal processing, 2421- 436 (1991).
16. J. Canny, "A computational approach to edge detection", IEEE Trans. on Pattern Analysis and Machine Intelligence, 8(6), pp. 679-698 (1986).
17. http://support.erdas.com/documentation/files/spanish_field_guide/5_realces.pdf
18. Gonzalo Pajares y Jesús M de la Cruz. Visión por computador. Imágenes digitales y aplicaciones (2001). Ra - ma.
19. Atam P. Dhawan, "Medical Image Analysis. 2003., IEEE engineering in medicine and biology, Society, Sponsor. Pp. 175-209; 220-241
20. Joseph H. Bosworth and Scott T. Acton. "Morphological image segmentation by local monotonicity". Proceedings of the 1999 Asilomar Conference on Signals, Systems, and Computers, *pp. 53-57.*
21. Chen, C., Luo, J., Parker, K., Image Segmentation via Adaptive K.Mean Clustering and Knowlegde Based Morphological Operations whit Biomedical Applications, 1998, IEEE transactions on Image Processing, Vol, 7 No. 12
22. http://www.tsi.enst.fr/tsi/groups/TII/activite_96/en/
23. http://www.ph.tn.tudelft.nl/Courses/FIP/frames/fip-Morpholo.html
24. Segmentation of ultrasound B-mode images with intensity inhomogeneity correction Guofang Xiao; Brady, M.; Noble, J.A.; Yongyue Zhang; Medical Imaging, 2002. IEEE Transactions on Volume 21, Issue: 1, pp. 48 – 57
25. José Crespo, Ronald W. Schafer, Jean Serra, Cristophe Gratin, Fernand Meyer. "The flat zone approach: A general low-level region merging segmentation method". 1997. Signal Processing volume: 62, Issue 1, pp 37 -60.
26. Karl Heinz Höhne and William A. Hanson. "Interactive 3D Segmentation of MRI and CT Volumes using Morphological Operations". Published in: Journal of Computer Assisted Tomography, 16(2):285-294

An Accurate and Parallelizable Geometric Projector/Backprojector for 3D PET Image Reconstruction*

Roberto de la Prieta

Universidad Rey Juan Carlos
Departamento de Informática, Estadística y Telemática, ESCET, C/Tulipán s/n
28933 Móstoles, Madrid, Spain
rprieta@escet.urjc.es

Abstract. C code for an accurate projector/backprojector for Positron Emission Tomography (PET) image reconstruction has been developed. Iterative PET image reconstruction methods are supported by a projection/backprojection step built inside of any of such algorithms. It is not surprising that a more precise modeling of the forward process of the measurement will yield better results when solving the inverse problem of image reconstruction. Among the factors that can be include in this forward model are γ-ray scatter contributions, attenuation, positron range, photon non-collinearity, crystal characteristics. Currently, we only include the geometric tube of response (TOR) modeling for a generic multi-ring scanner device. The elements in the transition matrix are calculated by a high statistics Monte Carlo simulation, taking advantage of the inherent symmetries and then the nonzero elements stored in a run length encoding incremental fashion. The resulting projector/backprojector is a voxel driven implementation. We show some preliminary results for 3D ML-EM reconstructions on synthetic phantom simulated data.

1 Introduction

Positron Emission Tomography (PET) is an intrinsically three-dimensional (3D) imaging technique. However, it was only 14 years ago that the first fully 3D PET commercial scanner was available. After that, significant effort has been devoted to the development of methodology for the acquisition and reconstruction of PET data in fully 3D mode, the ultimate aim being the maximization of the signal per unit of absorbed radiation dose, i.e. the sensitivity (see [1] for further details and references). There is a price to pay in doing so. First, increased scatter and randoms background. Second, the amount of the data set increases, especially if iterative methods are considered. These kinds of methods, though leading to a much higher computational burden, have shown better performance than analytic or rebinning ones due to their ability of incorporate the discrete nature of

* This work was partially made while the author was visiting UCLA under a grant sponsored by CAM-Fundación URJC

J.M. Barreiro et al. (Eds.): ISBMDA 2004, LNCS 3337, pp. 27–38, 2004.

the measured data, a statistical model of the acquisition process and constraints (positivity, anatomical tissue boundaries information) or a priori/regularization penalization.

In [3] it is argued that the well known iterative algorithm ML-EM is less sensitive than ART to the matrix coefficients computation. However, the properties of any iterative algorithm will always relay to a great extent on that of the projector/backprojector. Several approaches are at hand in order to generate the matrix coefficients. The most simple model is perhaps the "line length of intersection" , leading to fast ray-tracing implementations, such as Siddon algorithm ([2]), and suitable for on-line calculations. Coming from X-ray CT, this model is not totally appropriate for ET and it is known to yield artifacts. Better results for 2D PET reconstructions are to be obtained with a "strip area" system model ([3]) while in 3D, the model of choice seems to be the "angle of view" ([4], [5], [6], [7], [15])

On the other hand, as scanner technology and computer machinery enhance, algorithms improve in both two ways: time performance and in pursuing a better SNR-resolution trade-off characteristic. This calls naturally for including more detailed physical effects in the data acquisition process ([4], [9], [5]). In this situation, it would be advisable to study carefully the effects of geometrical and other forward modeling issues on the reconstruction as in [10].

Following the work in [11] we chose Monte Carlo simulation as the method for calculating the matrix elements. This is easy to implement and has a clear physical meaning. We do not introduce any approximation here in order to get good quality coefficients, provided a sufficiently high number of emissions is used. Another advantage of this approach is that the resulting code is embarrassingly parallel. The main drawback is the speed, especially considering that the acceptance angle of PET scanners is usually relatively small, thus leading to a high number of emissions going undetected. It would be possible to optimize the procedure presented here in several ways.

This paper is organized as follows: Section 2 gives the definitions and notation and describe in some detail the procedure followed to obtain the matrix elements. Section 3 explains how to take advantage of the transition matrix symmetries for this voxel-driven implementation, while section 4 describe the encoding procedure to get rid of the zero elements. Section 5 presents some preliminary results using the projector/backprojector in 2D and 3D ML-EM iterative reconstructions on simulated data. Finally, in Section 6 conclusions are extracted and future work is outlined.

2 Calculation of the Matrix Elements

We consider a generic multi-ring device (see Fig. 1) with a polygonal trans-axial arrangement. This setting allow us to model also the quasi-cylindrical standard geometry, using 1 detector per polygon side. We would like to extend our projector/backprojector to other non standard geometries, especially for dual rotating head experimental small-animal PET scanners of the kind described in [12].

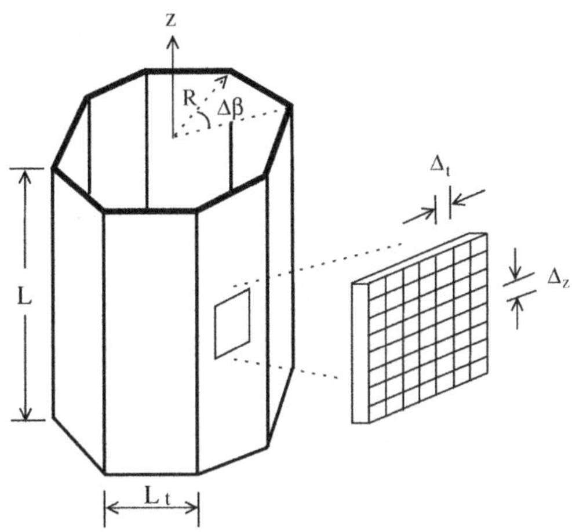

Fig. 1. Schematic of the generic polygonal multi-ring scanner considered here

2.1 Definitions and Notation

The scanner geometry is characterized by the following parameters,
L: length in the z (axial) direction
N_R: number of rings
N_S: number of sides of the trans-axial polygon
N_{DS}: number of (individual) detectors per ring side
N_D: number of (individual) detectors per ring, $N_D = N_{DS}N_S$
L_t: length of the polygon side
Δ_z: detector (crystal) axial length
Δ_t: detector trans-axial length
$\Delta\beta$: polygon angle
β_0: scanner rotation angle (angle of the first vertex)

First, we precalculate and store certain quantities and parameters of frequent use:

The radius of the scanner is given by

$$R = \frac{L_t}{2\sin\left(\frac{\pi}{N_S}\right)}$$

Vertexes of the scanner polygon:

$$\mathbf{V}_j = R\left(\cos(\beta_0 + j\Delta\beta), \quad \sin(\beta_0 + j\Delta\beta)\right) \qquad j = 0, ..., N_S - 1$$

Normal vectors (not necessarily unit) to each axial plane of detectors:

$$\mathbf{N}_j = \mathbf{V}_{j+1} + \mathbf{V}_j$$

Tangential unit vectors to each axial plane of detectors:

$$\mathbf{T}_j = \frac{\mathbf{V}_{j+1} - \mathbf{V}_j}{|\mathbf{V}_{j+1} - \mathbf{V}_j|}$$

The following vectors will be used in next section for the ray generation (see Fig. 2(a)):

$$\mathbf{u}_\varphi = (\cos\varphi, \sin\varphi)$$

$$\mathbf{u}_\theta = (A, B, C)$$

with

$$A = \cos(\theta + \frac{\pi}{2})\cos(\varphi - \frac{\pi}{2}) = -\sin\theta\sin\varphi$$

$$B = \cos(\theta + \frac{\pi}{2})\sin(\varphi - \frac{\pi}{2}) = \sin\theta\cos\varphi$$

$$C = \sin(\theta + \frac{\pi}{2}) = \cos\theta$$

The symbol $\cdot$ will be used to denote the standard Euclidean scalar product, the dimension being clear by the context. For a vector $\mathbf{v} = (v_1, v_2) \in \mathbb{R}^2$, we will also use the notation $\mathbf{v}^\perp = (-v_2, v_1)$

T and I will denote the sets of tubes of response (TOR's) and voxel indexes, respectively.

2.2 Random Sampling and Geometrical Calculations

The physical meaning for the geometric transition matrix generic element $p_{\alpha i}$ is the probability of an emission in the volume of the voxel i being detected in a pair of detectors corresponding to TOR α.

Thus, in order to calculate and store the transition matrix $\mathbf{P} = (p_{\alpha i})_{\alpha \in T, i \in I}$, for each voxel volume $i \in I$, a sequence of uniformly random distributed points,

$$\mathbf{x}^{i,k} = (x^{i,k}, y^{i,k}, z^{i,k}), \quad k = 1, .., N_{emi}$$

is generated inside it. We used the multiplicative linear congruential random generator described in [13].

For each $\mathbf{x}^{i,k}$ we sample angles $\varphi^{i,k}$ from a uniform distribution $U(0, \pi)$ and $\theta^{i,k}$ from $U(-\frac{\pi}{2}, \frac{\pi}{2})$. Then we set $s^{i,k} = x^{i,k}\cos\varphi^{i,k} + y^{i,k}\sin\varphi^{i,k}$. Next, the two sides of interest in the scanner are determined by calculation of the intersection of the straight line and the circle circumscribing the scanner in the trans-axial plane

$$\begin{cases} x\cos\varphi^{i,k} + y\sin\varphi^{i,k} = s^{i,k} \\ x = R\cos\beta, \quad y = R\sin\beta \end{cases}$$

to find

$$\beta_{1,2}(i,k) = \varphi^{i,k} \pm \arccos\left(\frac{s^{i,k}}{R}\right)$$

and the side (or plain of detectors) indexes of current interest

$$j_{1,2}(i,k) = \left\lfloor \frac{\beta_{1,2}(i,k) - \beta_0}{\Delta\beta} \right\rfloor \bmod N_S$$

where $\Delta\beta = \frac{2\pi}{N_S}$ is the scanner trans-axial angle.

Now, for $j = j_1, j_2$ we get the points of intersection of the plain of detectors

$$\mathbf{N}_j \cdot (x,y) = \mathbf{N}_j \cdot \mathbf{V}_j$$

with the ray

$$\begin{cases} \mathbf{u}_{\varphi^{i,k}} \cdot (x,y) = s^{i,k} \\ \mathbf{u}_{\theta^{i,k}} \cdot (x,y,z) = \mathbf{u}_{\theta^{i,k}} \cdot \mathbf{x}^{i,k} \end{cases}$$

The solutions are found to be

$$(\tilde{x}_j^{i,k}, \tilde{y}_j^{i,k}) = \frac{(\mathbf{N}_j \cdot \mathbf{V}_j)\mathbf{u}^{\perp}_{\varphi^{i,k}} + s^{i,k}\mathbf{N}_j^{\perp}}{\mathbf{N}_j \cdot \mathbf{u}^{\perp}_{\varphi^{i,k}}}$$

$$\tilde{z}_j^{i,k} = \frac{1}{\cos\theta^{i,k}} \mathbf{u}_{\theta^{i,k}} \cdot (x^{i,k} - \tilde{x}_j^{i,k}, y^{i,k} - \tilde{y}_j^{i,k}, z^{i,k})$$

and the indexes for the two individual detectors illuminated in the trans-axial plane (see Fig. 2(b)) are

$$d_{1,2} = \left\lfloor \frac{\frac{L_t}{2} + \tilde{\mathbf{x}} \cdot \mathbf{T}_{j_{1,2}}}{\Delta_t} \right\rfloor + j_{1,2} N_{DS}$$

whereas the ring indexes are

$$r_{1,2} = \left\lfloor \frac{\tilde{z}^{i,k}_{j_{1,2}}}{\Delta_z} \right\rfloor$$

If $(r_1 - r_2)\theta^{i,k} < 0$ we permute r_1 and r_2 so for non-negative ring difference we can assume $r_1 \geq r_2$.

2.3 Ray Indexing

The number of view (see Fig. 3) is calculated as

$$n_v = d_1 + d_2 + 1$$

To calculate the trans-axial displacement, first the individual detectors d_1, d_2 are rotated to obtain

$$d'_{1,2} = \left(d_{1,2} - \left\lfloor \frac{n_v}{2} \right\rfloor\right) \bmod N_D$$

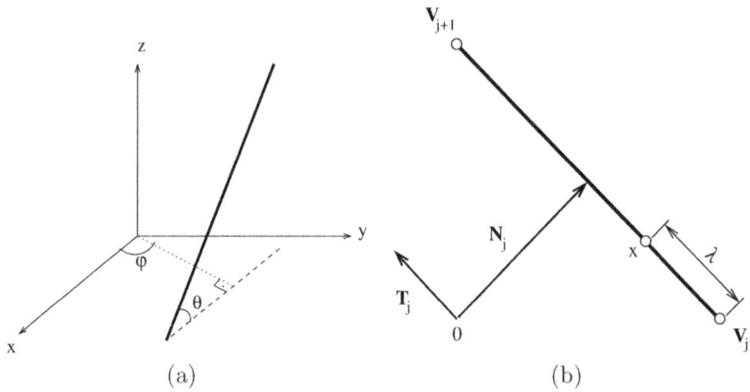

Fig. 2. (a) Ray angles: trans-axial angle $0 \leq \varphi \leq \pi$ and axial angle $-\frac{\pi}{2} \leq \theta \leq \frac{\pi}{2}$ (b) Calculation of the detector position: $\lambda = x \cdot \mathbf{T}_j + \frac{1}{2}\,|\mathbf{V}_{j+1} - \mathbf{V}_j|$

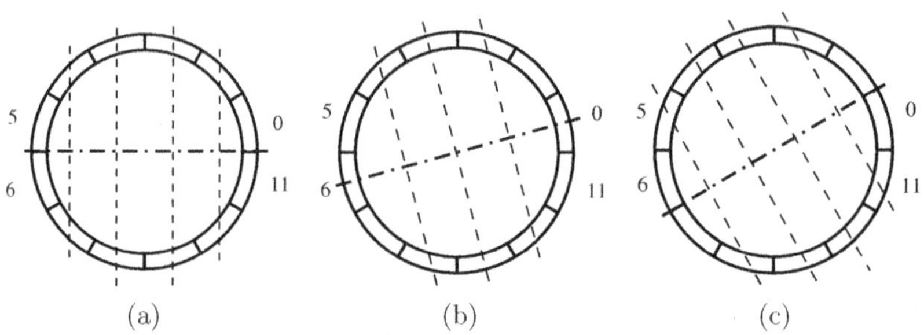

Fig. 3. View and trans-axial displacement indexing for a ring with 12 individual detectors. $\Sigma = d_1 + d_2$, $\Delta = d_1 - d_2$ (properly oriented)3(a) View 0: $\Sigma = 11 \mod 12$, $\Delta = 3, 5, 7, 9$. 3(b) View 1:$\Sigma = 0 \mod 12$, $\Delta = 4, 6, 8$. 3(c) View 2: $\Sigma = 1 \mod 12$, $\Delta = 3, 5, 7, 9$

Thus, we get a new TOR with the same trans-axial displacement but in view 0 or 1, so now we can easily calculate

$$n'_t = \frac{|d'_1 - d'_2| - (n_v \pmod 2 + 1)}{2}$$

and this quantity is shifted to take into account the number of views corresponding to the current field of view (FOV)

$$n_t = n'_t - \frac{\frac{N_D}{2} - N_{Bins}}{2}$$

Only counts in TOR's with $0 \leq n_t < N_{Bins}$ are kept, disregarding the rest. The TOR (r_1, r_2, n_v, n_t) is given an index

$$\alpha = f(r_1, r_2) N_{Views} N_{Bins} + n_v N_{Bins} + n_t$$

and stored in memory. $f(\cdot,\cdot)$ is some ordering function. Currently we use

$$f(r_1, r_2) = r_2 2N_R + r_1$$

Finally, for each voxel i the counts result for each TOR are normalized by N_{emi} to obtain the element $p_{\alpha i}$. It would be also possible to store the count in a short integer (1 or 2 bytes) instead of the float (typical 4 bytes) thus allowing a reduction in the storage requirements. This depends on the counts statistics and have to be checked carefully.

3 Compression and Element Encoding

Once the sinogram for a voxel is generated we save the nonzero elements to hard disk in a sparse vector format, with a header for the voxel index and number of elements and pointers to the element value and index information. This will be one column of the transition matrix **P**. Looking at a typical sinogram set (see Fig. 4) we see that when saving this sequence to disk the most frequent transition will be

$$\Delta r_1 = \Delta r_2 = 0, \quad \Delta n_t = \text{small integer}, \quad \Delta n_v = 0, 1$$

If we do not take into account the truncated sinograms (see Fig. 4(a) 4(b)) these kind of transitions will fail to occur 1 of kN_V times, being k the mean number of active TOR's ($p_{\alpha i} \neq 0$) per sinogram view. With typical data sizes and roughly speaking the failure rate will be less than 1% of the cases. Actually this rate will be slightly greater due to the truncated sinograms.

Bearing this idea in mind an encoding scheme for the indexes is outlined in Fig. 5. A control byte is always included to deal with one of the two cases discussed above. In mode 0, no extra information is needed to decode the index, while in mode 1 some extra information may be included after the control byte. The Δ bits set to 1 indicate a unitary increment in the corresponding variable, while the other bits set indicate that the corresponding variable value is included after the control byte.

4 Matrix Symmetries

To make an efficient algorithm it is important to keep the matrix in memory. However, the matrix size in 3D PET applications is usually huge (see Section 4.4) Fortunately, P is sparse and have lot of symmetries. On the other hand, to carry out the parallelization of this projector/backprojector one must take into account that it is a voxel-driven implementation: the information for a voxel is read and then information for all symmetry-related voxels is calculated. This decoding process will consume an extra time. Thus, to take advantage of all the system memory, each node could store only a part of the matrix and maybe it would be not necessary to use all the symmetries encoding, depending on the problem size and architecture performance. Our versatile code allows for several degrees of freedom in this sense. This and other related issues will be studied in short.

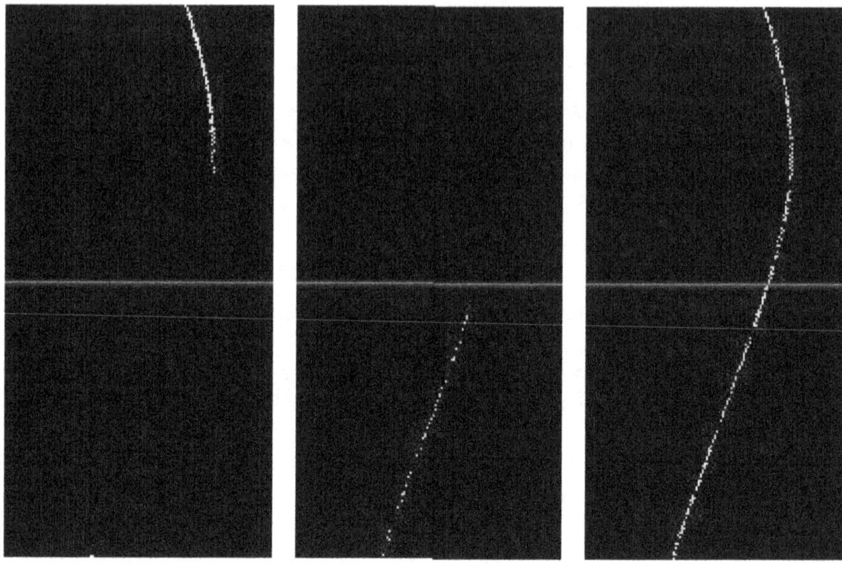

(a) (b) (c)

Fig. 4. Three different sinograms obtained from the same matrix column: (a) and (b) truncated sinograms (c) complete sinogram. The truncation phenomenon appears more strongly in the most oblique sinograms. The accuracy of these three sinograms could be enhaced increasing the parameter N_{emi} in the matrix generation procedure

4.1 Trans-axial Symmetries

The group of movements that leave a regular plain polygon invariant is the symmetry group or dihedral group (see [16])

$$D_n = \{\rho^q \sigma^r : \quad q = 0, \ldots, n-1, \quad r = 0, 1\}$$

where ρ is the rotation of amplitude $\frac{2\pi}{n}$ and σ is a reflection leaving the polygon invariant. Thus the order of the group is $|D_n| = 2n$. If Q_n and R_m are two regular polygons of even n and m number sides, properly arranged, and $n \leq m$ then we can assume that $D_n \subseteq D_m$. Henceforth the factor limiting the exploitation of trans-axial symmetries is, in our case, the rectangular grid of the image discretization. A polar grid, as mentioned in [8], would permit this aim, but it does not seem obvious to set up the patterns and sizes of the resulting voxels. We are currently studying the viability of this approach so we do not pursue this topic here and we confine ourselves to the standard rectangular grid.
In our current implementation of the projector/backprojector we allow free discretization step in the trans-axial image plane. If a square grid is used, trans-axial symmetries allow a reduction in size of the elements to store/compute of $|D_4| = 8$. More concretely, we only have to compute the matrix elements for voxels $i \in O_1$, the first octant.

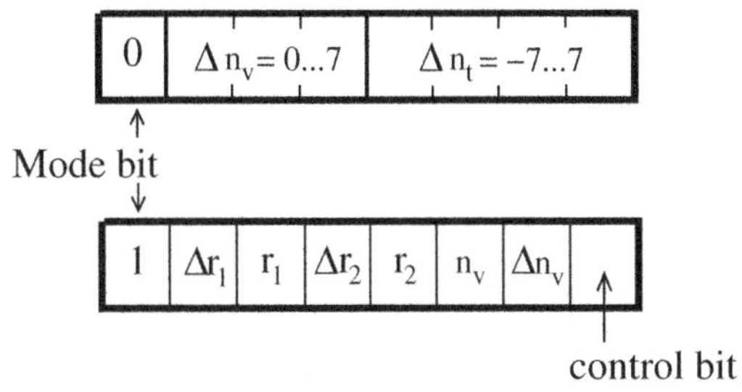

Fig. 5. The two types of control bytes for the index encoding scheme proposed

4.2 Axial Symmetries

In our current implementation we use a fixed axial discretization, namely, $2N_R - 1$ slices. The image planes are shifted such that half of the planes (direct planes) have their z center at the z center of the rings. There are two movements that can be used: First, the translation τ of amplitude $2\Delta_z$ in the z axis of the scanner and second, the symmetry with respect to the axial plane passing through the center of the scanner. This translation has two equivalence classes: even and odd slices, so it is only needed to store/compute two slices, thus achieving a saving factor of

$$\frac{2N_R - 1}{2} \approx N_R$$

The symmetry allows us to compute only nonnegative ring differences thus yielding a saving factor of approximately 2. However, storing ring differences of $2N_R$ is necessary to use τ properly, so the previous factor 2 is then canceled.

4.3 Using the Symmetries in the Projection/Backprojection Step

When reading an element $p_{\alpha i}$ from disk, first the TOR index (r_1, r_2, n_t, n_v) is decoded and the corresponding value is read. With this value we can then compute the contributions related to the set

$$\{p_{\tau^k(\alpha)\tau^k(i)} : \quad k = -\min(r_1, r_2) \ldots N_R - \max(r_1, r_2)\}$$

where $\tau^k = \overbrace{\tau \circ \ldots \circ \tau}^{k}$

Finally, we repeat the above procedure to compute all the contributions

$$\{p_{\xi(\alpha)\xi(i)} : \quad \xi \in D_4\}$$

where we make an abuse of notation to refer the induced applications in the voxel and TOR indexes sets by the movements τ, ξ.

4.4 Projection Matrix Size

For a fully 3D PET acquisition, all ring differences, no span, the total number of elements in the projection matrix $\mathbf{P} = (p_{\alpha i})_{\alpha \in T, i \in I}$ being T and I the set of TOR and voxel indexes is given by

$$|\mathbf{P}| = |T||I| = {N_R}^2 N_{Views} N_{Bins} N_x N_y N_z$$

In commercial human PET scanners, $|\mathbf{P}|$ may range from 10^{12} to 10^{15} (see [1], [14] for further details). Fortunately, the nonzero elements may stay in the range 10^9 to 10^{11} . We get an extra saving factor of $8N_R$ if we use symmetries, in agreement with the ray-driven projector in [14]. Thiese quantities are of course theoretical, for one must also consider the storage format (currently float), encoded indexes and headers information. Nevertheless, we hope to be able to store the matrix in 1 Gb memory in the worse case.

5 Preliminary Results

In order to perform preliminary tests on the projector/backprojector developed, a ML-EM 3D PET code was also developed building inside the decoding projector/backprojector step. Several ML-EM reconstructions (see [3]) have been run on a Pentium 4, 2.8 GHz, 1Gb RAM DDR 400 MHz machine. The code was compiled with gcc 3.2, using optimization for speed, on a Linux Red Hat 8.0 flavor. Two synthetic software phantoms were simulated and reconstructed. First, a Derenzo kind phantom was simulated for a 1 ring device, 512 detectors of 5 mm. axial length, and 128x128 sinogram acquisition. The sinograms were then corrupted with Poisson noise up to a total of $5 \cdot 10^6$ counts. A Matrix with 10^6 emissions per voxel was generated to perform the reconstruction. The result for a ML-EM 128x128 reconstruction is shown in Fig. 6(a).

Next, two cylinders for the 3D case where simulated for a 3 rings device, 256 individual detectors per ring, radius 8.1 cm, 4.6 cm radius of the FOV. The Matrix was generated with 10^5 emissions per voxel. The results for one slice of a 64x64x5 reconstruction is shown in Fig. 6.

The matrix generation consumed several hours heavily depending on the parameter N_{emi}, taking each iteration about 1 min. depending on the data size, but we have to perform more test.

We have observed that, as pointed out by several groups, the speed of convergence in terms of iterations, is remarkably greater in 3D reconstructions (due probably to existence of more redundancies in the data set).

6 Conclusions and Future Work

C code for an accurate projector/backprojector for PET image reconstruction has been developed. A ML-EM reconstruction has been set up using it, and preliminary results show feasibility in performing 3D PET reconstructions, though several aspects have to be improved: code optimization, random sampling

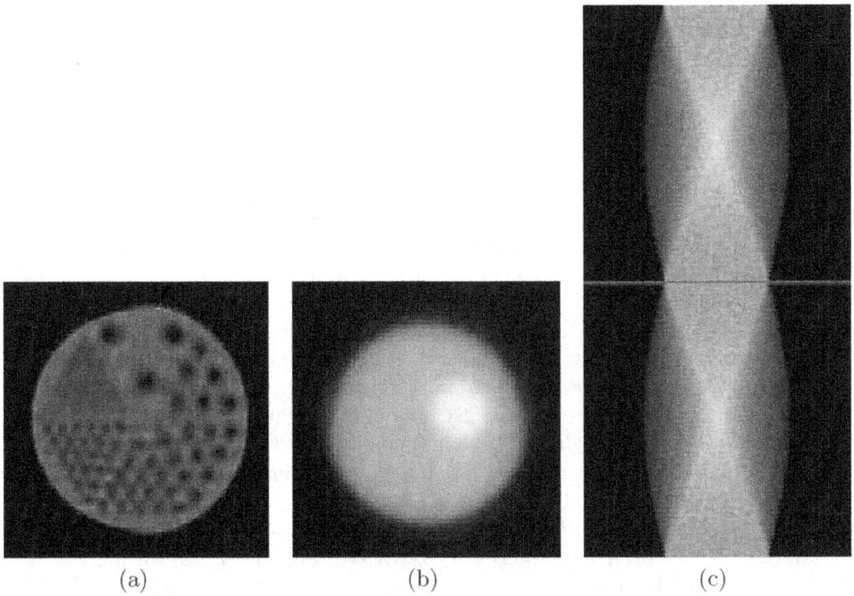

Fig. 6. (a) 2D EM Reconstruction Derenzo phantom, 50 iterations, Poisson noise $5 \cdot 10^6$ counts (b) 3D EM reconstruction of two cylinders (c) Inter-iteration projection step for the 3D reconstruction

scheme, storage (float, short), non-fixed axial resolution, mashing, storage reduction by only computing voxels in the FOV, study of the ordering function in Sect. 2.3, parameters such as maximum ring difference acquired, mashing, different sinogram formats, inter-crystal space, corners, etc. Test on real data sets will be performed soon and also another (iterative) algorithms and probability models different from the ML criterion, that could be relevant in certain cases (precorrected sinograms for randoms and scatter)

Also, multi grid strategies will be eventually considered to speed-up the reconstruction process.We also would like to extend this projector/backprojector to other non standard geometries (small-animal research scanners).

The use of a polar grid to further exploit symmetries have been mentioned previously in Section 4.1.

An active line of research in our group is in penalized/regularized iterative algorithms, namely, by means of non linear diffusion processes which lead us to the study of certain PDE's variational techniques to tackle the problem. This methods can be well combined together with wavelets and in general multi resolution analysis. As this methods will raise the computational cost of the algorithms, we are studying the parallelization of the projector developed. We have to study the convenience of keeping the whole matrix on memory or split it into the nodes, encode symmetries always or take advantage of the versatile backprojector code, whether to implement it on cluster or shared memory multiprocessor architecture. We hope that after that, more accurate and useful 3D PET reconstructions could be performed on real data on clinical acceptable times, and also research scanners could take advantage of our reconstruction tool.

References

1. M. Defrise et al., in Bernard Bendriem, David W. Townsend, Eds. *The Theory and Practice of 3D PET* (Kluwer Academic Publisher, The Netherlands, 1998)
2. R. L. Siddon, "Fast calculation of the exact radiological path for a three-dimensional CT array", Medical Physics, **vol. 12** (1985) March, pp. 252-255
3. L.A.Shepp, Y.Vardi, "Maximum Likelihood Reconstruction for Emission Tomography", IEEE Trans. Med Img., **vol. MI-1, No. 2** (1982), pp.113-122, October
4. A. Terstegge, S. Weber, H. Herzog, H. W. Muller-Gartner, and H.Halling, "High resolution and better quantification by tube of response modeling in 3D PET reconstruction", IEEE Nucl. Sci. Symp., **vol. 3** (1996), pp.1603-1607
5. J.Qi,R.M. Leahy, S.R. Cherry, A. Chatziioannou and T.H. Farquhar, "High resolution 3D Bayesian image reconstruction using the microPET small-animal scanner", Physics in Medicine and Biology, **vol. 22, no. 2** (2003), pp. 258-276
6. C.A. Johnson, Y.Yan, R.E.Carson, R.L Martino, M.E. Daube-Witherspoon,"A system for the 3D reconstruction of retracted-septa PET data using the EM algorithm", IEEE Transactions on Nuclear Science,**Volume: 42, Issue: 4** (1995), pp.1223-1227
7. Chen C.M., Lee S.-Y, "On Parallelizing the EM Algorithm for PET Image Reconstruction" IEEE Transactions on Parallel and Distributed Systems, **Volume 5, no 8** August (1994)
8. Kehren F., Schmitz T., Herzog H., Halling H. "Implementation Aspects of a Fully Iterative, Parallel 3D-Reconstruction-Software for PET Data", International Meeting on Fully Three-Dimensional Image Reconstruction in Radiology and Nuclear Medicine, Egmond aan Zee, Niederlande, June 23-26, (1999)
9. Mumcuoglu E.U., Leahy R.M., Cherry S. R. "Bayesian reconstruction of PET images: Methodology and performance analysis", Physics in Medicine and Biology **Volume 41 (9)** Sept. (1996) pp. 1777-1807
10. J.Qi, R.H. Huesman, "Effect of Errors in the System Matrix on Iterative Image Reconstruction", IEEE Medical Image Conference, Roma 2004, to appear.
11. G.Kontaxakis, L.G. Strauss and G. Tzanakos, "An efficient implementation of the iterative ML-EM image reconstruction algorithm for PET on a Pentium PC platform", Journal of Computing and Information Technology, **7(2)** (1999) pp. 153-163
12. S.Siegel, J.J.Vaquero, L.Aloj, J. Seidel, E. Jagoda, W.R. Gandler, W.C. Eckelman, M.V. Green, "Initial Results from a PET/Planar Small Animal Imaging System", IEEE Nuclear Science Symposium, Conference Record. (1998) **Volume 2**
13. P. L'Ecuyer, "Efficient and Portable Combined Random Number Generators", Communications of the ACM, **Vol 31** (1988) pp. 742-749, 774
14. Kris Thielemans, http://www.hammersmithimanet.com/~kris/PETbasics/projmatrixsizeHTML/, (2001)
15. William A. Worstell, Stephen S. Adler, Haris A. Kudrolli, Hohn D. Nevin, Leonid V. Romanov "Compact Representation of PET 3D System Response Matrices", IEEE International Symposium on Biomedical Imaging (2004) Washington DC
16. S. Xambó, F. Delgado, C. Fuertes, *Introducción al Algebra*, Ed. Complutense, Madrid, (1993) p. 110

EEG Data and Data Analysis Visualization

Josef Rieger[1], Karel Kosar[1], Lenka Lhotska[1], and Vladimir Krajca[2]

[1] Gerstner Laboratory, Czech Technical University in Prague
Technicka 2, 166 27 Prague 6, Czech Republic
lhotska@fel.cvut.cz

[2] University Hospital Bulovka
Budínova 2, 18081 Prague 8, Czech Republic
krajca@fnb.cz
http://cyber.felk.cvut.cz

Abstract. Healthcare technology produces today large sets of data every second. An information overload results from these enormous data volumes not manageable by physicians, e.g. in intensive care. Data visualization tools aim at reducing the information overload by intelligent abstraction and visualization of the features of interest in the current situation. Newly developed software tools for visualization should support fast comprehension of complex, large, and dynamically growing datasets in all fields of medicine. One of such fields is the analysis and evaluation of long-term EEG recordings. One of the problems that are connected with the evaluation of EEG signals is that it necessitates visual checking of such a recording performed by a physician. In case the physician has to check and evaluate long-term EEG recordings computer-aided data analysis and visualization might be of great help. Software tools for visualization of EEG data and data analysis are presented in the paper.

1 Introduction

Visual perception is our most important means of knowing and understanding the world. Our ability to see patterns in things and pull together parts into a meaningful whole is the key to perception and thought. This ability is very closely linked with experience: the more experienced we are the more complex tasks of deriving meaning out of essentially separate and disparate sensory elements we are able to perform. Seeing and understanding together enable humans to discover new knowledge with deeper insight from large amounts of data. The visualization approach integrates the human mind's exploratory abilities with the enormous processing power of computers.

Modern medicine generates huge amounts of data, but at the same time there are often lacking explicit relations among these data and data understanding. Orientation in this amount of data is not always easy and unambiguous. Computation, based on these large data sets, creates content. It frequently utilizes data mining techniques and algorithms. Some of them are difficult to understand and use. Visualization makes data, computation and mining results more accessible to humans, allowing comparison and verification of results.

Visualization techniques are roughly divided into two classes [1], depending on whether physical data is involved. These two classes are scientific visualization and information visualization. Scientific visualization focuses primarily on physical data. Information visualization focuses on abstract, non-physical data such as text, hierarchies, and statistical data.

J.M. Barreiro et al. (Eds.): ISBMDA 2004, LNCS 3337, pp. 39–48, 2004.

In this paper, we focus on scientific visualization in the first place. However, information visualization, namely visualization of intermediate and final results, represents integral part of the developed systems. The software systems being implemented and used in two case studies are described.

2 EEG Data

EEG as one of the available techniques for brain monitoring has several advantages. It provides reasonable spatial resolution and excellent temporal resolution. It is a non-invasive technique. It can be applied in either structural disorders or metabolic/physiological disorders. The introduction of computerized digital recording techniques and data transmission via computer networks has largely eliminated the difficulties associated with bedside use of the EEG in the past, such as excessive paper use and problems in providing real-time review. However, one major problem remains, namely real-time or nearly real-time interpretation of EEG patterns. Speaking in terms of classical "paper" electroencephalography using standard speed of shift of 3 cm/s, 20 minute recording represents length of 36 meters of paper. When studying sleep disorders, length of recording may reach several hundreds meters of paper. During long-term (e.g. 24 hour) monitoring the data load is even much higher. In addition, we do not acquire a single signal but in case of the most frequently used International 10-20 system of electrode placing we acquire 20 parallel signals. Therefore, pure manual visual analysis is impossible. It is necessary to develop such tools for visualization that satisfy several basic requirements: visualization of raw signals, interaction with signal processing techniques (filtration, segmentation, computation of quantitative signal characteristics), visualization of resulting signals and values, possibility to correct the segment borders manually, interaction with data mining techniques, visualization of results in various forms, etc.

3 Case Study I: System for Classification of Comatose (Sleep, Newborn) EEG

The system consists of several basic modules (see Figure 1). Each of the modules enables visualization of data or information it is working with. More detailed description follows.

The main window serves for visualization of the EEG signal and enables access to all functions of the program. Its standard layout is shown in figure 2. It is possible to set up way of visualization and processing of individual electrodes as needed. For example, it is possible to exclude from visualization (and computation) electrodes that are disconnected, having no signal, or inadequate (ECG, EOG), etc. Scale of the signal of individual electrodes as well as joint scale for all electrodes and several other properties for displaying (grid, time stamps, numbering of segments, isoline, etc.) can be set up. The setup can be saved into a file for repetitive use. The window for setup is shown in figure 3.

The program enables relatively detailed setup of segmentation. Most of the control elements serve for adaptive segmentation. The setup can be saved into a file for repetitive use as well. The window for setup of segmentation is shown in figure 4.

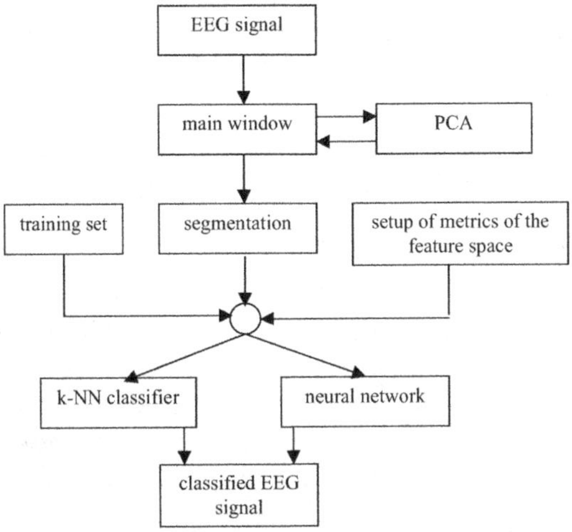

Fig. 1. Structure of the system

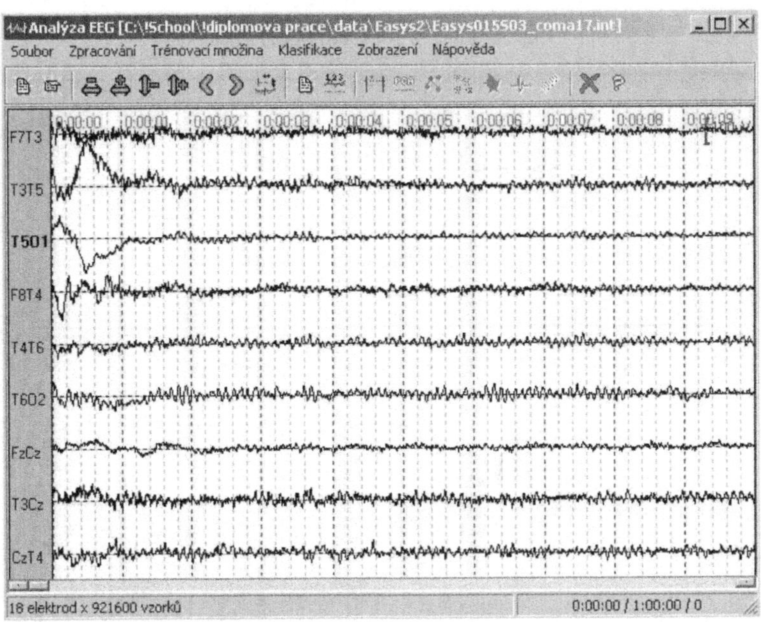

Fig. 2. Main window of the program

The core of the system is the training set used for classification. The user has several options how to create a training set. Therefore the system is flexible and can be used for solving different tasks. The options are the following ones:

- reading the traning set from a file
- generation of the training set by cluster analysis
- generation of the training set manually by moving segments from the main window to corresponding classes of the training set.

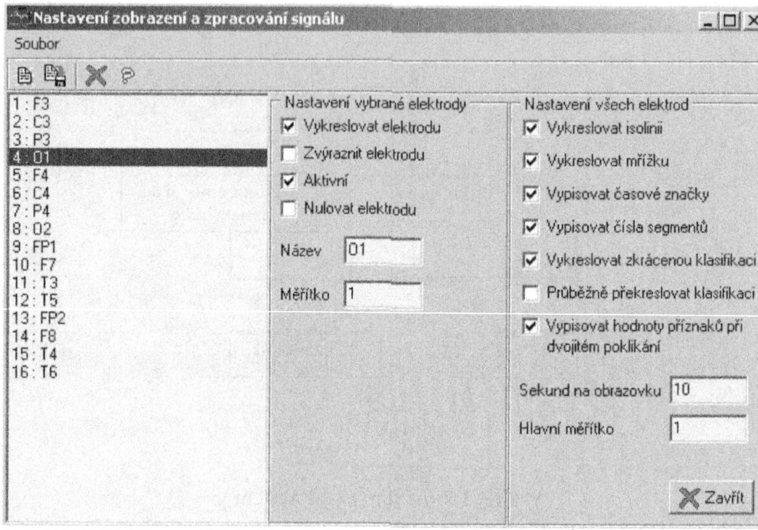

Fig. 3. Window for setup of parameters

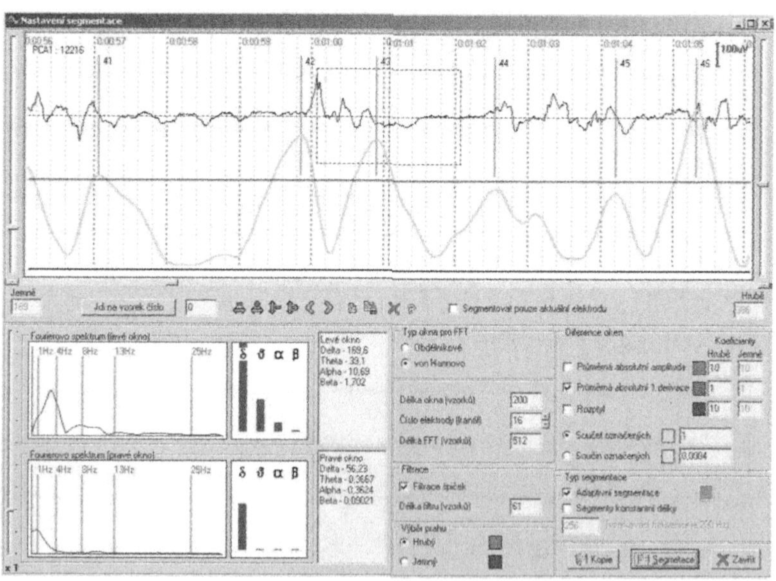

Fig. 4. Window for setup of segmentation

The user can define required number of classes, add and delete classes, set up their colouring, etc. For individual segments of the training set, it is possible to change their scale, sampling frequency, to move them between the classes, delete, or deactivate (segments are not used for classification). The window for setup of the training set is shown in figure 5.

After this setup it is necessary to set up the metric of the feature space: to select feature that will be used and their weights (see Figure 6).

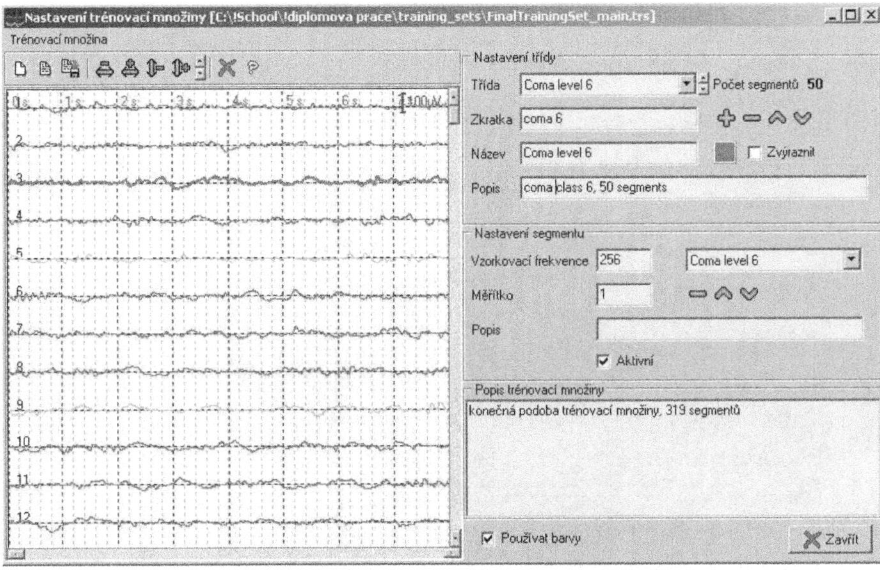

Fig. 5. Window for setup of the training set

As it has been already mentioned, one option for generation of the training set is the application of cluster analysis. In the system, the algorithm of non-hierarchical k-means clustering is implemented. The user can select number of classes, their minimum occupancy (it prevents from creation of empty classes), way of initialization of cluster centre and the source of segments for clustering. Result of the cluster analysis can be copied to the main training set and there successively edited in detail (to move segments between classes, deactivate segments, delete segments, save the resulting training set to a file, etc.). The window for cluster analysis is shown in figure 7.

For classification there are implemented two methods at the moment, namely a k-NN classifier and a multilayer neural network. In both methods, basic parameters can be either set up manually or read from a file.

The classification has been tested using real sleep EEG records. The training set has been generated using cluster analysis and manually modified using expert knowledge. Resulting training set contains 319 pattern segments divided into 10 classes; each segment is 8 second long. For classification the algorithm of nearest neighbour has been used, the result is shown in Figure 8.

Each class of the training set is coloured by a certain basic colour of the spectrum (class 1 - violet, 2 - blue, 3 - green, 4 - yellow, 5 - orange, 6 - red, 7 - violet, 8 - blue, 9 - green, 10 - red). According to classification to the given class, the corresponding segments of the classified EEG signal are coloured and number of the class is attached to the segments. In the lower part of the screen (see Figure 8), there is displayed for fast orientation in EEG signal classification of the whole EEG record (in this case 2 hours). Each classified (active) electrode is represented by one horizontal strip. Classification of 2 hour EEG record has lasted less than two minutes.

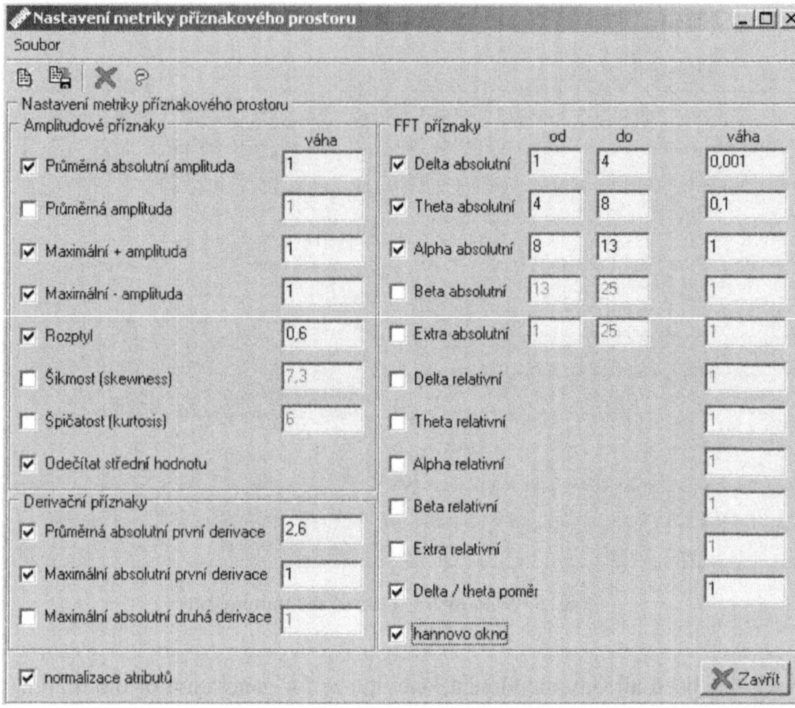

Fig. 6. Window for setup of the metric of the feature space

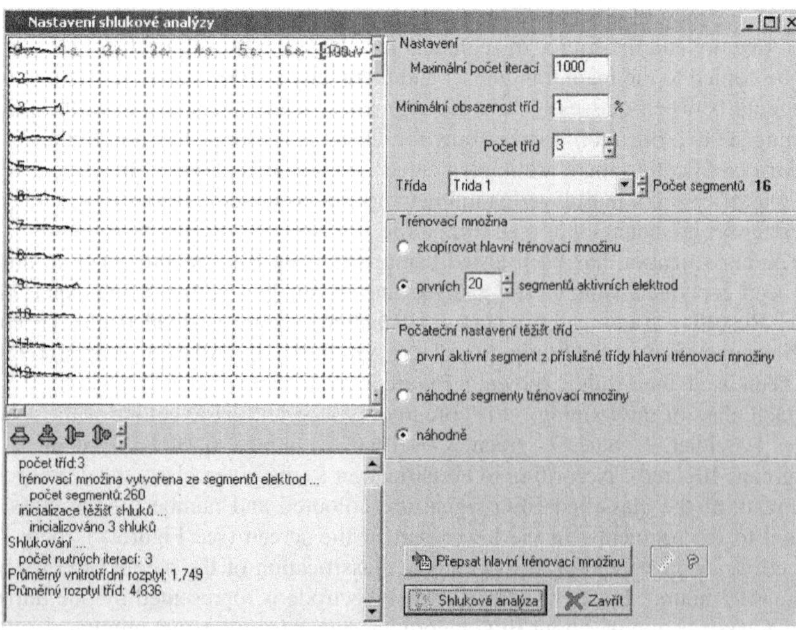

Fig. 7. Window of cluster analysis

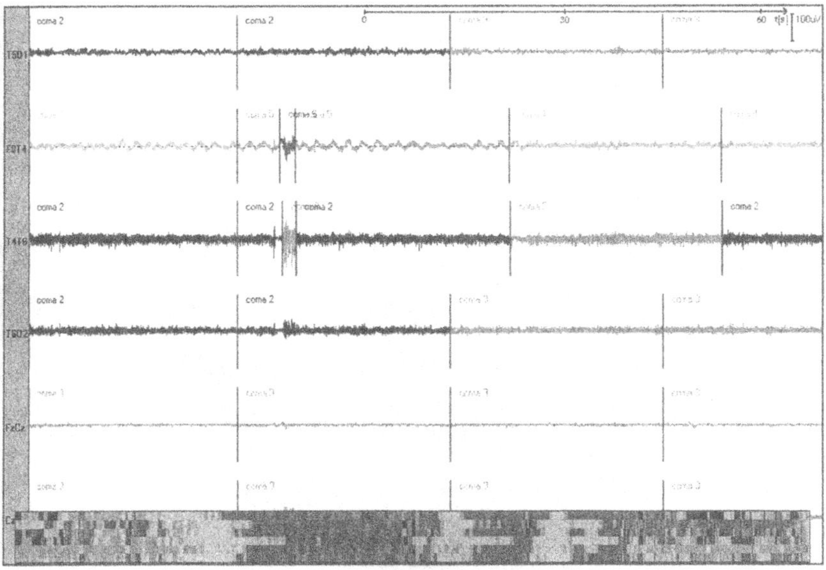

Fig. 8. Classification of real EEG signal

4 Case Study II: Classification of Long-Term EEG (Epileptic) with 3D Imaging

Structure of this implementation is very similar to case study I. However, it is completed with 3D mapping of the brain activity in time based on [2]. The mapping algorithm is based on the existence of 3D model consisting of a set of contour points. The contour points are mutually connected by a system of general n-angles forming an area. The way of interconnection is not important because we are working only with positions of contour points and positions of applied electrodes. Positions of both electrodes and points are normalized in 3D space. The applied algorithm is designed with respect to the real environment where the computation of relatively complex spline curves at each image change could be extremely slow and thus practically unusable. For given placement of electrodes, the values of model coefficients are constant and the computation can be divided into two steps. In the first step (time-consuming), the coefficients of individual electrodes and individual model points are pre-computed. In the next step, the EEG is mapped relatively quickly using the pre-computed coefficients. While the first step is performed only once, the second step is performed for each change of EEG activity. In the application, the most frequent International 10-20 system of electrode placement is considered. The mapping of EEG activity in time domain is shown in Figure 9.

The 3D model of the scull has been developed using reconstruction of MRI images. The algorithm for 3D imaging is able to work in real time on most of present average PCs. The brain activity is converted to different colours. The program contains 4 implicit colour palette directly computed (green-yellow-red, blue-violet-red, green-red, grey scale). However the user can define his/her own colour palettes and save them in files.

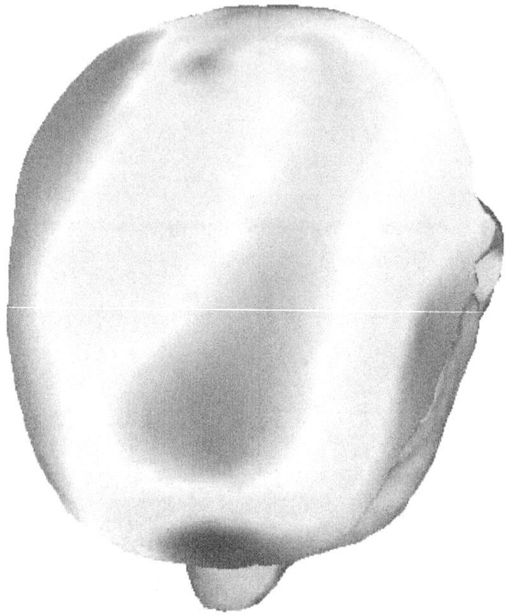

Fig. 9. Mapping of EEG activity in time domain

3D model is displayed in a window after it is activated by an icon in the toolbar, shortcut keys, or menu. The window is shown in Figure 10.

The 3D imaging brings several problems. For example, it is impossible to see the whole head surface in one moment. It is solved by allowing automatic rotation in two axes. The angle changes have been experimentally set up to such values that the model rotates in such a way that it shows maximum of brain part of the head.

The model window has its control elements allowing change model characteristics. The elements are accessible on the toolbar. Each panel serves for different purpose. The numbers in Figure 10 correspond to individual panels. Panel 1 switches between mapping modes. It is possible to map EEG values or sum of spectral activity in specified frequency band. Panel 2 changes size of the model in the window. Panel 3 switches on and off rotation of the model along individual axes. Panel 4 changes different parameters of displaying, namely possibility not to fill planes of the so-called wire model, displaying position of individual electrodes in the model, displaying axis orientation, displaying current colour palette with applied maximum and minimum. Panel 5 enables selection of the colour palette that should be used for the model.

Animation of 3D model. Animation of changes of EEG activity assumes the ability of the program to map the activity in real time. In that case, it is possible to simulate automatic shifting along the time axis of the signal and immediately map corresponding change of EEG. This feature is very suitable especially when the expert processes the signal. It enables the doctor to follow and evaluate changes of EEG characteristics in different time moments even if high speed of shifting is used. That significantly increases efficiency of doctor's work. In animation mode it is possible to control all functions of model imaging as in standard mode. The window Setup (Options/3D Setup) remains open and enables not only control of animation, but also immediate change of parameters of imaging. In addition to functions available in standard mode, there are two functions for animation control. The function Shifting speed allows define number of samples for one shift. Then the program automatically shifts by the given number of samples during animation run. The function Animation control allows shifting along the time axis forward and backward from the current position that is displayed in the title of the model window. The position may be reset to zero or set to required value.

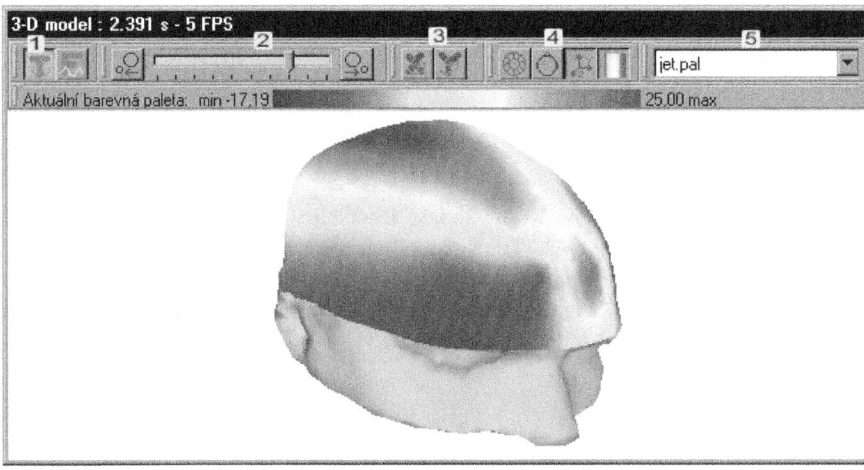

Fig. 10. Window of the 3D mapping

5 Conclusion

Nowadays, intelligent data analysis tools may represent a crucial help to physicians in their decision making process; the interpretation of time-ordered data through the derivation and revision of temporal trends and other types of temporal data abstraction provides a powerful instrument for event detection and prognosis; data visualization is increasingly becoming an essential element in the overall process.

Healthcare technology produces today large sets of data every second. An information overload results from these enormous data volumes not manageable by physicians, e.g. in intensive care. Data visualization tools aim at reducing the information overload by intelligent abstraction and visualization of the features of interest in the current situation. This requires context-aware use of knowledge for proper reduction of the complexity of the data displayed without loosing those parts of information, which are essential and critical in the current situation. Newly developed software tools for visualization should support fast comprehension of complex, large, and dynamically growing datasets in all fields of medicine. These tools should lead to a new generation of software tools, which allow health professionals to cope with the increasing amount of detailed patient data.

In this paper, we have described two case studies illustrating possibilities of visualization of the whole process of data processing and evaluation. The examples used are from a very complex domain of EEG. The implemented systems are simple to use, guiding the user, retrieving all stored data and setups, and executing classification in a minimum number of steps. They present most of the information in graphical form that is most suitable for perception. The main advantage of the systems is that for routine tasks all the setups are defined only once and saved to files. Then the user who may not necessarily know all the subtle details of proper setup starts the corresponding application and evaluates the results. Since it is possible to display classification results of two-hour EEG recording in compressed form on one screen the preliminary visual inspection is very fast. In the next step the user can focus on those segments that indicate serious problems.

It is likely that ongoing refinements and modifications in EEG processing and visualization will enhance its utility and lead to extensive application of EEG monitoring over next years.

Acknowledgement

The research of J. Rieger, K. Kosar and L. Lhotska was supported by the research program No. MSM 210000012 "Transdisciplinary Research in the Area of Biomedical Engineering" of the CTU in Prague, sponsored by the Ministry of Education, Youth and Sports of the Czech Republic. The research of V. Krajca was supported by grants 7511 and 7586 IGA CR.

References

1. Kantardzic M.: Data Mining: Concepts, Models, Methods, and Algorithms. IEEE Press, Piscataway, 2003
2. Perrin F., Pernier J., Bertrand O., Echallier J. F. Spherical splines for scalp potential and current density mapping. Electroencephalography and Clinical Neurophysiology, February 1989, Vol. 72, Issue 2, s. 184-187.

A Web Information System for Medical Image Management

César J. Acuña[1], Esperanza Marcos[1],
Valeria de Castro[1], and Juan A. Hernández[2]

[1] Kybele Research Group
[2] Electronic Technology, Bioengineering and Medical Image Research Group
Rey Juan Carlos University
C/ Tulipán s/n - CP 28933
Móstoles - Madrid - Spain
{cjacunia,emarcos,vcastro,j.hernandez}@escet.urjc.es

Abstract. In the last years, the use of digital images for medical diagnosis and research has increased considerably. For this reason, it is necessary to develop new and better applications for managing in an effective way a large amounts of medical information. DICOM is the standard for the Digital Imaging and COmmunications in Medicine. However, DICOM information is difficult to interchange and integrate out of the scope of medical specialized equipment. This drawback make difficult its use and its integration in a wide context as the Web. XML is the standard for the information exchange and data transportation between multiple applications. As the XML databases are emerging like the best alternative to storage and manage XML documents, in this work we present a Web Information System to store, in an integrated way, DICOM and Analyze 7.5 files in an XML Database. For its development, the XML schemas for both DICOM and Analyze 7.5 formats have been obtained and the architecture for the integration of XML documents in the XML DB has been defined.

1 Introduction

In the last years a considerable increase in the use of digital information has been experienced, mainly of digital images for medical diagnosis and research. The huge quantity of images generated are stored mainly in DICOM format (Digital Imaging and Comunications in Medicine) [2],[21] which is the most widely accepted standard for the interchange of medical images in digital format [18]. In spite of DICOM being the most accepted standard for the exchange of medical image information, it has some drawbacks. On one hand, the DICOM files are generated "individually", difficulting the medical information management. As an example, it is not possible to query all the information related to a same patient, or to select all those images realized with the same acquisition modality (Computed Tomography, Magnetic Resonance, etc.). On the other hand, DICOM represents the information in a specific format, which can only be

J.M. Barreiro et al. (Eds.): ISBMDA 2004, LNCS 3337, pp. 49–59, 2004.

understood by medical imaging equipment conforms to the DICOM standard, without taking into account the medical information interchange and integration in a greater scope. These drawbacks state the necessity of specific software tools development to facilitate the management of this kind of files.

The possible solution to the above problems are based in the following two points:

- To represent DICOM information in XML, improving in this way the interchange and integration of medical information. XML [3] is the standard for the information exchange and data transportation between multiple applications [8]. XML and XML Schema [27] allow to represent all kind of information, also modelling its structure and its semantic constraints.
- To store the DICOM information in a XML database improving the DICOM file management. To solve the problem of the DICOM file management, the obvious solution should be to store DICOM files in a database.

This paper focus in a Web Information System (WIS) development for the management of DICOM files represented in XML and their storage in an XML database. For this purpose, the DICOM information meta-model has been defined in XML Schema from the information model defined in the DICOM Standard. Also, this WIS allows managing and querying, in an integrated way, information from Analyze 7.5 (Analyze, from now on) [15], which is another of the most used formats to store medical images information. Some proposals have appeared addressing the problem of adopting XML technology into medical domain. Specifically [1] tries to overcome the difficulties of medical information integration and compatibility developing using XML DTDs to represent the information of DICOM files. Unfortunately, as it is said in [5], DTDs are not sufficient to represent the semantic constraints defined in DICOM.

The rest of the paper is organized as follows: in section 2 an introduction to the DICOM Standard as well as the Analyze format is presented; in section 3 the proposed WIS is presented, introducing its functionalities, its architecture, the XML database schema and the Web-user interface; finally section 4 sums up the main conclusions and future works.

2 DICOM Standard and Analyze Format

DICOM is the main standard for the medical images interchange in digital format. The standard defines: the data structures for medical images and their related information, the network oriented services (image transmission, query of an image archive, etc.), formats for storage media exchange, and requirements for conforming devices and programs [20].

Internally, a DICOM file is composed by two components:

- The first one is a header which consist of a Data Set. The Data Set has Data Elements. The DICOM header has a plain structure as is depicted in figure 1. A Data Element is uniquely identified by a *Data Element Tag* which is an ordered pair of integers representing a *Group Number* followed by an *Element Number*. *VR* is the *Value Representation* of the *Value Field* and defines its data type. The *Value Length* field define the length of the *Value Field*. Finally the *Value Field* contains the Value(s) of the Data Element. Each data element defines information associated to the medical image. In this way we can find, for example, data elements like: patient name, age, pixel spacing, etc. Due to its organization (in data elements) DICOM information is very similar to XML information, so it is posible to process DICOM files contents in order to store it in a equivalent XML structure.

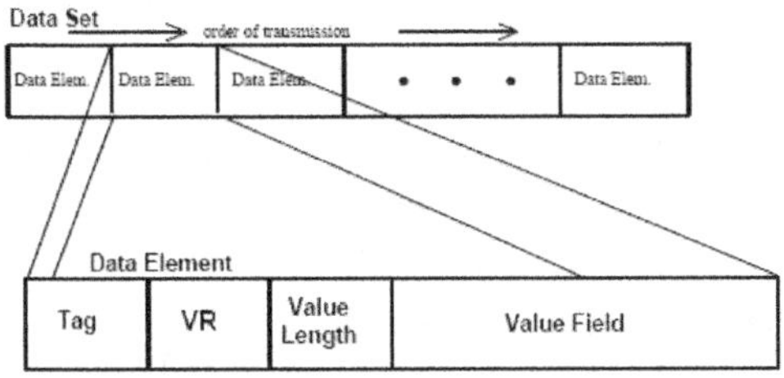

Fig. 1. DICOM header Structure

- The second component contains one or more images, that is to say, the bytes stream that encodes the images themselves. It must not be confuse the Image data (slices, bits allocated, rows, cols, etc.) which are codified in header component.

The information from a DICOM file can only be understood by those software tools and medical imaging equipment conform with the standard. So, it is always necessary to use specialized software tools for storing, managing and querying DICOM files, called PACS (Picture Archiving and Communication System). Each PACS supplier uses his own approach to codify, interchange and store the DICOM files information, making even more difficult the integration and interchange of medical information.

As it's been said before, the proposed WIS in this work, integrates the Analyze file format into the DICOM information Model. That file format is a proprietary format of the image visualization, processing and analysis tool called Analyze. This format is also very used to store medical images information. Unlike DICOM, Analyze splits the medical image information in two files, one of them (with the extension .img) stores the image and the other one (with the extension .hdr) stores the image related information. The .hdr file contains information that is similar to the one contained in the DICOM file header.

3 A Web Information System for Medical Image Management

This section presents the main features of the proposed Web Information System. The objectives of this WIS are:

- To represent DICOM files using XML improving in this way, the interoperability and integration of the medical information in a broader context, as the Web.
- To facilitate the integrated organization, query and retrieval of the DICOM and Analyze files information by means of an XML database.
- To allow a suitable imaging processing and analysis of the Medical Images stored in the database, where the results are also stored together with the original images, in the same database. This images database and its results would use as historical file that could be consulted and used through Internet in future studies and research projects

The main functionalities provided by the WIS, are the following:

- To import DICOM or Analyze files. This process takes the Analyze and DICOM original files, as inputs. Then, these files are transformed into XML documents and inserted in the database.
- To convert formats. The WIS allows to export information from the database to any of the supported formats. For example a DICOM file can be converted in an Analyze File and vice versa. The amount of information of each file format is different so, during the conversion process there will be an inevitable lost of information.
- To make queries and updates over the stored data from the XML database. This web application allows to manage in a efficient way the information, enabling searches by patient, studies, image modalities, among others.
- To process and to statistically analyze the images stored in the database

3.1 Architecture

In figure 2 one can see the Web Information System architecture.

Taking as a reference the architectures for web application development proposed by .NET [16] and J2EE [24], this web application has been structured in three layers:

- **Presentation Layer:** For this layer a Web user interface has been developed. Section 3.4 briefly describe the Web User interface.
- **Behavioural Layer:** In the behavioural layer are placed the main components, this components are described in section 3.2.
- **Persistence Layer:** here is placed the XML database management system, for its implementation, we have chosen the Oracle XML DB extension. This layer is best explained in section 3.3.

3.2 Behavioural Layer

The main components of the WIS are in the behavioural layer. Next, we describe each one of them:

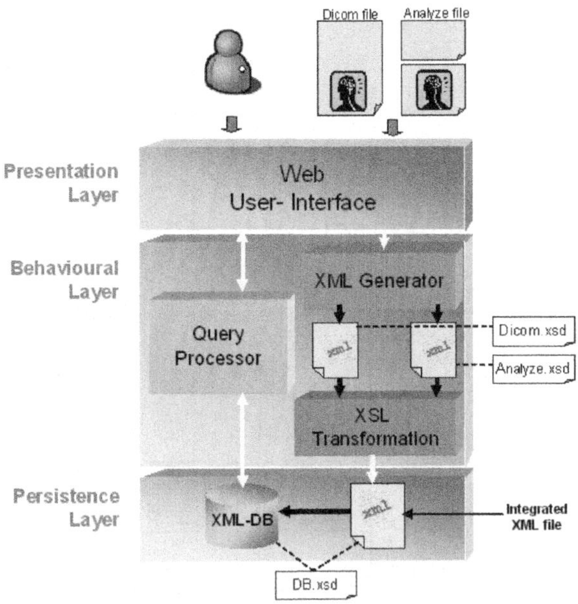

Fig. 2. Web Information System Layered Architecture

- **XML Generator:** This component, developed in Java, takes as inputs DICOM or Analyze files and transform them into XML documents. The structure of these intermediate files is described by the XML Schemas Dicom.xsd and Analyze.xsd depending on the input file. In figure 3 we can see the XML schemas, in UML notation, of the intermediate files used to store the extracted data from DICOM and Analyze files.
  The structure of the DICOM intermediate XML document (see figure 3 (a)) is based on the DICOM header structure. Thus, the Data Set is represented as follow: a root element called *Header* with attributes that describe the DICOM source file (Path, Format, Size, etc). Internally the Data Elements are organized in groups, the attribute *Number* of the *DICOMGroupType* represents the DICOM Group number of the data element (first number of the DICOM data element tag). The *DICOMElement* contains the rest of the Data Element attibutes: *Number*(second number of the DICOM data element tag) , *Value Field* and *VR*.
  The structure of the Analyze intermediate XML document (see figure 3 (b)) has been obtained from the Analyze data model.
- **XSL Transformation:** This component, developed using XSLT [30], takes as inputs the intermediate XML files generated by the XML Generator component and transform them in a different XML document conform with the database XML Schema.
  For modularity and portability reasons, it is necessary to obtain an intermediate representation of the DICOM and Analyze files, before inserting them

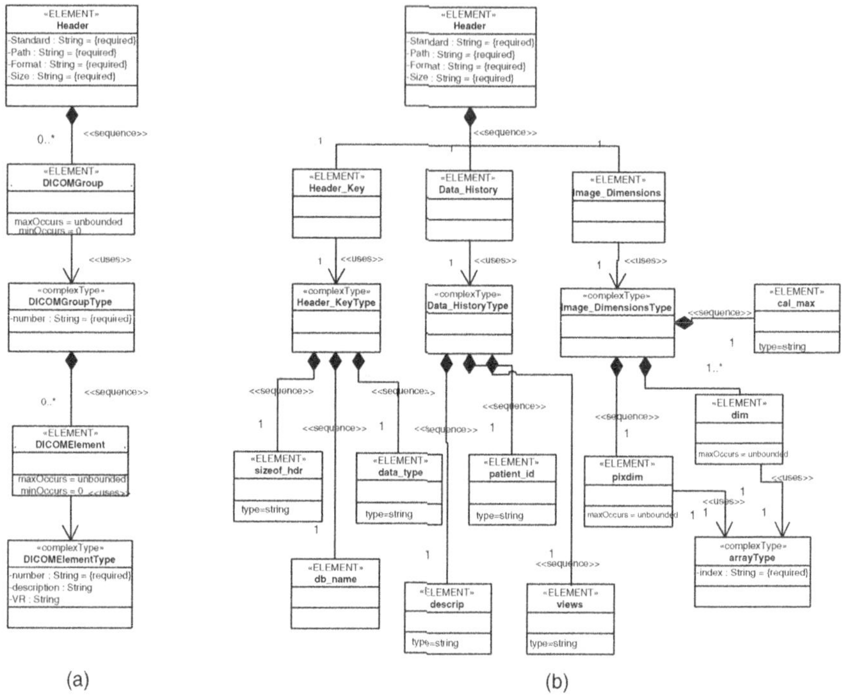

Fig. 3. XML Schema of the DICOM and Analyze intermediate files

into the database. DICOM is a continuously evolving standard, therefore if the way in which the information is represented changes, these modifications will affect only to the *XML Generator* component. This component encapsulates the DICOM and Analyze files treatment. Similarly, if the database schema must be modified or the database management system changed, only the *XSL Transformation* component must be modified or replaced without affecting the remaining components.

- **Query Processor:** This component is responsible for building the user queries in order to execute them on the DBMS, and showing, in a right way, the result of the queries through the Web-user interface. To make the queries, the user enters data in the Web application forms, then this component transforms the data into query expressions in XPath [4], which is the Oracle XML DB language to access XML documents.

3.3 XML Database Schema

At the moment, most of the applications use XML merely as a mean to transport data generated by a database or a file system. However, there are many benefits to storing XML Schema compliant data in a database system that manages directly XML documents, including: a) better queryability, optimized updates and stronger validation [19], b) great saving of resources when the information is interchanged among applications, the source application must translate the data to an XML document and the destiny application must "shred" the XML document to import it, generally, to a relational database [22], c) avoid the semantics lost between the XML document structure and the relational database schema, that could happen when the XML document is stored in a conventional database.

There exists different solutions for the XML documents storage, which could be roughly categorized according to common terminology into two main groups: *native* XML databases [7] like Tamino [23], X-Hive/DB [29], eXcelon XIS [6]; and XML database *extensions* enabling the storage of XML documents within conventional, usually relational or object-relational DBMSs like Oracle XML DB [9], IBM DB2 XML Extender [10] or Microsoft SQLXML [17]. The notion of a *native* XML database solution is still cloudy and there exists no widely accepted definition [28].

Although, at first glance, the *native* XML databases could be seen as the most intuitive solution, the XML database *extensions* are based on long established traditional database technology. Consequently, they can benefit from the mature implementations of classic DBMS functionality of the underlying DBMSs. Moreover, it has been a trend in the recent years to make traditional DBMS more extensible with new functionality and index structures. As XML database extensions can directly exploit these extension mechanisms for their own purposes, they are also strong with respect to extensibility.

In [28] an exhaustive analysis of XML database solution for the management of MPEG Media Description, is presented. Due to our Web application must also manage the images associated to DICOM and Analyze files, we were based in [28] to choose the most adecuate DBMS. Thus, Oracle XML DB it seems to be the best adapted solution according to the requirements of the developed WIS, providing, among others, the following features: Versioning, Fine-grained access, Path Index Structures,Access Optimization, Fine-grained updates and Typed Access

Another reason for choosing an Oracle solution is that in the last years, we have been working with Oracle databases. So, for example we have developed UML extensions to model object-relational databases, based on the SQL:1999 object-relational model and in Oracle8i as an example of product [12, 11].

To develop the XML database Schema, we have followed the next steps:

1. We have obtained the DICOM and Analyze conceptual data models. After analysing both models, we conclude that all concepts defined by Analyze are included in the DICOM data model. Therefore, as a result, we have obtained an unified conceptual model, which integrates both kind of files.
2. Starting from the integrated conceptual model, obtained in the previous step, we have derived the XML database schema by following MIDAS, a methodology for the development of Web Information System, and specifically using the Web Database Development aspect [26, 13, 14, 25]. Finally we have obtained the database XML Schema. We have modelled the XML

Schemas using the UML extensions proposed in [25]; the figure 5 represents the database XML Schema.

The complete data conceptual model of the WIS is presented in figure 4.

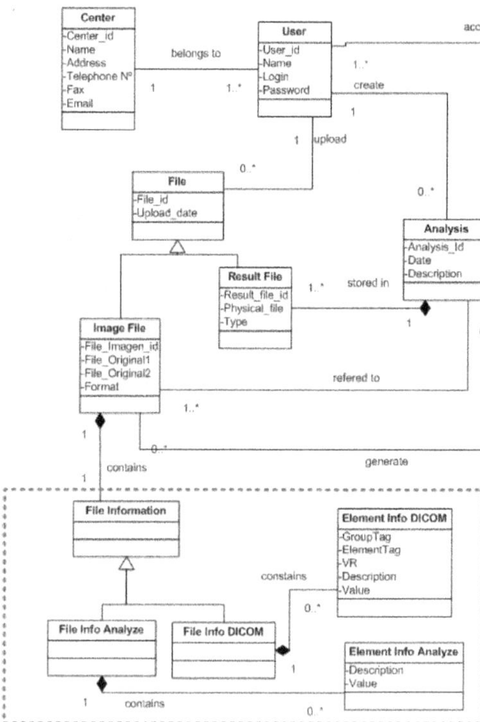

Fig. 4. Data Conceptual Model of the WIS

The part remarked with a dotted line is the part of the conceptual data model that corresponds to the DICOM and Anlyze attributes representation. As it's been said before, the DICOM and Analyze data organization is close to XML. This part or the data conceptual model was represented in the logical model using an XML schema, to obtain it we has followed the guidelines the XML Schema of a XML database from Data Conceptual model proposed in [26]. The obtained XML Schema is depicted in figure 5.

The rest of the diagram (see figure 4) include all the necessary classes to manage the DICOM and Analyze files, as well as the studies and analysis. This part was implemented by mean of object-relational database elements.

3.4 Web-User Interface

Except for diagnostic workstations, the medical desktop application for different purposes such as image analysis and viewing, are widely used in medical area.

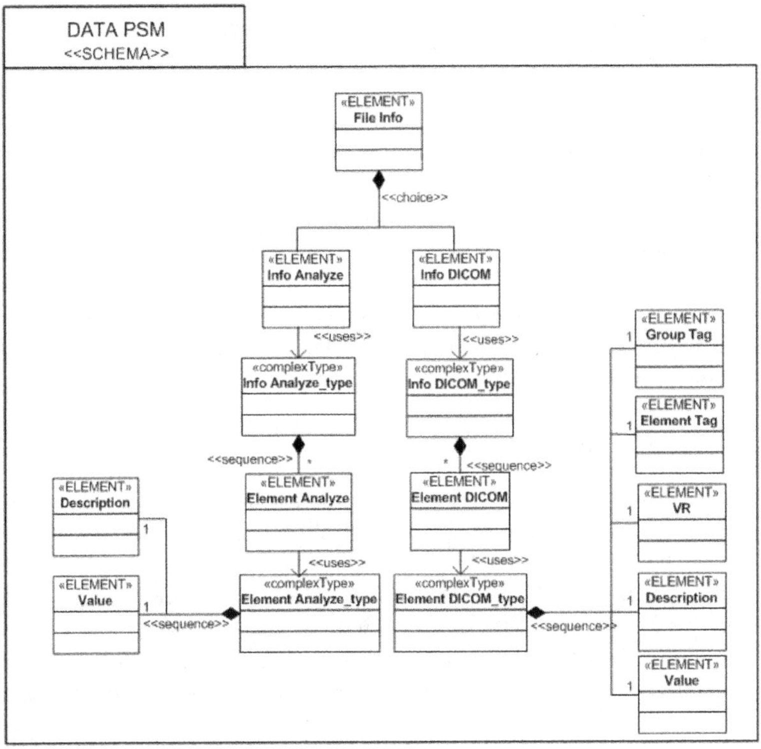

Fig. 5. DICOM and Analyze XML Schema

Low cost image delivery and display are needed in most networked hospitals. A a Web-based user interface for medical image systems are the most effective solution for these purposes. To use web browsers to deliver and access medical images are more universal and convenient than DICOM and professional medical display workstations in intranet and Internet environments.

For this WIS we have developed a user-friendly Web Interface for its implementation we have used ASP.Net.

4 Conclusions and Future Work

DICOM is the most accepted standard for the medical image information interchange and representation. However, the way in which the information is represented, enables an effective interchange only between medical imaging equipment and specific applications; for this reason, there are serious limitations when a more extended integration and interchange of medical information is required. Moreover, the medical information contained in DICOM files can only be managed through specific tools called PACSs, which are generally developed by different suppliers and use proprietary structures and format to store the information, making even more difficult the integration.

This paper has showed a Web Information System which allows to get the XML representation of DICOM and Analyze files improving, in this way, the interchange and integration of medical images information in a broader context. This application uses an XML database system to manage the information obtained from DICOM and Analyze files. Using a XML database instead of a relational one, the XML documents translation to a relational structure is avoided, also preventing the semantics lost during the translation process.

At the moment we are studying the integration of other medical images standards and formats. As main future work we considered the development of an architecture for the integration of multiple Web applications that manage different digital archives. The showed application, will be used as starting point for the definition of the integration architecture.

Acknowledgement

We would like to thank Marcos López for his intervention in the implementation of the showed WIS. This research is partially granted by the projects: EDAD (07T/0056/2003 1) financed by Autonomous Community of Madrid; DAWIS (TIC 2002-04050-C02-01), financed by the Ministry of Science and Technology of Spain ; Statistic reconstruction of tomographic images by positron emission, based on high performance computing technics (TIC2001-0175-C03-03) financed by the Ministry of Science and Technology of Spain and Thematic network of cooperative research on molecular and multimodality medical image of the Carlos III Health Institute.

References

1. Ahn C., Nah Y., Park S. and Kim J. *An Integrated Medical Information System Using XML*,W. Kim et al. (Eds.): Human Society Internet 2001, LNCS 2105, pp. 307-322, 2001.
2. ACR-NEMA, *The DICOM Standard*, Retrieved from http://medical.nema.org/, 2003.
3. Bray T. et al. *Extensible Markup Language (XML) 1.0 (Second Edition)*, W3C Recommendation. Retrieved from: http://www.w3.org/TR/2000/REC-xml-20001006/, 2003.
4. Clark J. and DeRose S., *XML Path Language (XPath) Version 1.0*, W3C Recommendation, Retrieved from: http://www.w3.org/TR/xpath, 2004.
5. DICOM Strategic Working Group *DICOM Structured Reporting (SR) object and XML, HL7 V3.0 RIM, HL7 Clinical Document Architecture*, Retrieved from: http://medical.nema.org, 2004.
6. eXcelon Corp., *Managing DXE. System Documentation Release 3.5.*, eXcelon Corp. Burlington, Web site: www.excelon.corp.com, 2003.
7. Fiebig T. et al. *Anatomy of a native XML base management system*, VLDB J., Vol. 11, No 4, pp. 292-314, 2002.
8. Harding P., Li Q. and Moon B. *XISS/R: XML Indexing and Storage System Using RDBMS*, Proceedings of the 29th VLDB Conference, Berlín, Germany, 2003.
9. Higgins S. et al. *Oracle 9i XML Database Developer's Guide - Oracle XML DB. System documentation Release 2*, Oracle Corp. 2002.

10. IBM Corp. *IBM DB2 Universal Database - XML Extender Administration and Programming*, Product Documentation Version 7. IBM Corporation, 2000.
11. Marcos E., Vela B. y Cavero J.M. *Extending UML for Object-Relational Database Design.* Fourth International Conference on the Unified Modeling Language, UML 2001, Springer Verlag LNCS-2185, pp. 225-239, 2001.
12. Marcos E., Vela B. y Cavero J.M. *Aggregation and composition in object-relational database design.* Advanced Databases and Information Systems. Communications of the 5th East-European Conference, 2001.
13. Marcos E. et al. *MIDAS/BD: a Methodological Framework for Web Database Design.*, Conceptual Modeling for New Information Systems Technologies, Ed.: H. Arisawa, Y. Kambayashi, V. Kumar, H. C. Mayr, and I. Hunt, Springer Verlag LNCS-2465, pp. 227-238, 2002.
14. Marcos E., Vela B. and Cavero J.M. *Methodological Approach for Object-Relational Database Design using UML*, Journal on Software and System Modeling (SoSyM), Vol. 2, pp.59-72, 2003.
15. Mayo Clinic, *Analyze Software*, Retrieved from: http://www.mayo.edu/bir/Software/Analyze /Analyze.html, 2004.
16. Microsoft Corp., *Microsoft .NET*, Retrieved from: http://www.microsoft.com/net/, 2004.
17. Microsoft Corp. *Microsoft SQL Server - SQLXML 2.0*, System Documentation. Microsoft Corporation, 2000.
18. Moreno R. and Furuie S., *Integration of Heterogeneous Systems via DICOM and the Clinical Image Access Service*, IEEE Computers in Cardiology, 2002.
19. Murthy R. and Banerjee S. *XML Schemas in Oracle XML DB*, Proceeding of the 29 th VLDB Conference, Berlin, Germany, 2003.
20. Oosterwijk H, *Dicom Basics (2nd Ed.)*, O Tech Ed., 2002.
21. Oosterwijk H., *The DICOM Standard, Overview and Characteristics*, Retrieved from http://www.otechimg.com/ publications/articles/pdf/mri-1.pdf, 2003.
22. Silberschatz A. et al. *Database System Concepts (4th Ed.)*, McGraw-Hill, 2002.
23. Software AG, *Tamino X-Query. System Documentation Version 3.1.1.*, Software AG, Darmstadt, Germany. Web site: www.softwareag.com,2001
24. Sun Microsystems, *Java 2 Platform Enterprise Edition (J2EE)*, Retrieved from: http://java.sun.com/j2ee/, 2004.
25. Vela B. and Marcos E. *Extending UML to represent XML Schemas*, The 15th Conference On Advanced Information Systems Engineering, CAISE'03 FORUM. Ed.: J. Eder and T. Welzer, 2003.
26. Vela, B., Acuña C. y Marcos E. *A Model Driven Approach for XML Database Development.* 23rd International Conference on Conceptual Modeling (ER2004) Shanghai, China. (Accepted for publication)
27. W3C XML Schema Working Group. *XML Schema Parts 0-2: Primer, Structures, Datatypes. W3C Recommendation.* Retrieved from: http://www.w3.org/TR/xmlschema-0/, http://www.w3.org/TR/xmlschema-1/ and http://www.w3.org/TR/xmlschema-2/, 2003.
28. Westermann U. and Klas W. *An Analysis of XML Database Solutions for the Management of MPEG-7 Media Descriptions*, ACM Computing Surveys, Vol. 35, No 4, pp. 331-373, 2003.
29. X-Hive Corp., *X-Hive/DB 2.0-Manual. System Documentation Release 2.0.2.*, X-Hive Corp., Rotherdam, The Neatherlands. Web site: www.x-hive.com.,2002
30. *XSL Transformation (Version 1.0)*, Retrieved from: http://www.w3c.org/TR/xslt, 2004.

Reliable Space Leaping Using Distance Template

Sukhyun Lim and Byeong-Seok Shin

Inha University, Department of Computer Science and Information Engineering
253 Yonghyeon-Dong, Nam-Gu, Inchon, 402-751, Korea
Phone number : +82-32-860-7452
g2011498@inhavision.inha.ac.kr, bsshin@inha.ac.kr

Abstract. Several optimization techniques for direct volume rendering have been proposed since its rendering speed is too slow. An acceleration method using min-max map requires a little preprocessing and additional data structures while preserving image quality. However, we have to calculate accurate distance from current point to the boundary of a min-max block to skip over empty space. Unfortunately the cost for evaluating the distance is so expensive. In this paper, we propose reliable space leaping method to jump to the boundary of current block using pre-calculated distance template. A template can be reused for entire volume since it is independent on viewing conditions. Our algorithm reduced rendering time in comparison to conventional min-max map based volume ray casting.

Keywords: volume ray casting, space leaping, min-max map, distance template
Paper domain: Biological and medical data visualization

1 Introduction

Volume ray casting is the most famous software-based volume rendering algorithm. Although it produces high-quality perspective images, it takes a long time to make an image. Several acceleration methods have been proposed to speedup [1-7]. They have concentrated mainly on skipping over transparent regions using coherent data structures such as *k*-d trees [1], octrees [2] and run-length encoded volume [4]. Min-max map is a structure that stores minimum and maximum voxel values for the region called min-max block that is covered by each node [8-12]. It can effectively skip transparent voxels since a ray jumps over the current min-max block when minimum and maximum values of current block are not confined within a threshold of non-transparent voxels. However the cost to determine the distance to boundary is mathematically expensive [8-10],[12]. So the method using constant distance instead of accurate calculation was commonly used [2],[11]. When the thickness of an object is smaller than the constant distance, it may skip over those regions. Also it has to jump back to previous point when a ray enters into a min-max block which has a value of nontransparent region.

In this paper, we propose reliable space leaping method using *distance template* to determine distance to the boundary of a min-max block. When a ray enters empty region, it jumps as the amount of distance value stored in the distance template. If the ray enters into the nontransparent block, it performs conventional ray traversal. Since the distance template is independent on the viewing conditions, we can reuse this structure for entire volume.

J.M. Barreiro et al. (Eds.): ISBMDA 2004, LNCS 3337, pp. 60–66, 2004.

2 Problems of Conventional Ray-Traversal Using Min-Max Map

Fig. 1 shows an example of constructing min-max structure from a volume data set.

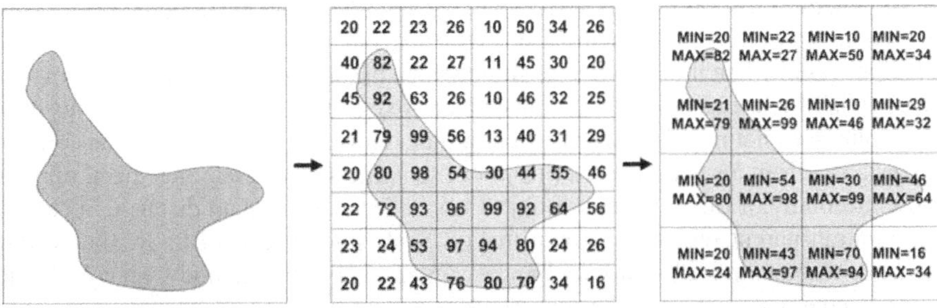

Fig. 1. An example of constructing min-max map. For simplicity, the volume data is represented as a 2D array of min-max blocks. Volume size is 8×8 and block size is 2×2

When a ray skips over transparent regions using min-max map, it has to calculate an accurate distance from current point to the boundary of a block. At first, a ray is fired from each pixel on the image plane and encounters a min-max block. And it determines whether skips the transparent blocks or not based on the value of min-max block. When minimum and maximum values of current block are not confined within a threshold of nontransparent voxels, the ray jumps to the boundary of the block by computing accurate distance. If the ray meets the non-transparent blocks, it starts to perform conventional ray traversal.

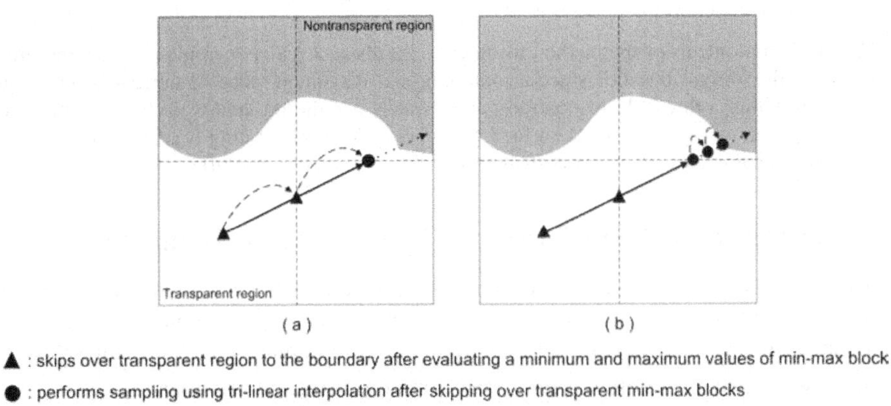

Fig. 2. Ideal procedure of ray traversal using mathematical distance computation : a ray can jump over transparent region by means of distance to the boundary of the block since this block is entirely transparent (a). the ray moves toward surface by applying conventional ray-casting (b)

This method takes a lot of time since it computes the intersections between a ray and boundary of a min-max block. When a transparent region is so narrow and a ray meets with several min-max blocks, a traversal speed in transparent region becomes slower. For this reason, the method using constant distance was exploited as shown Fig. 3. A ray jumps to the next point with the value of uniform distance when minimum and maximum values of current block are not surrounded by a threshold of nontransparent voxels. If the ray encounters the nontransparent region, it should jump back to the previous point since it is possible to excess actual surface.

In general, this approach is faster than the method using accurate distance. However it has two problems as shown in Fig. 3. At first, a ray should jump back to the previous point when it enters into position which has a minimum and maximum value surrounded by a threshold of nontransparent voxels. The cost for returning to previous point does not require long processing time. However when the previous position keeps apart from a surface, it requires more samplings, and rendering speed might be slow. Secondly, if the thickness of object is smaller than constant distance, it can skip the nontransparent region as shown in Fig. 3 (d) since it cannot know the accurate distance to boundary of min-max block. Consequently, the method which efficiently jumps to the boundary of a min-max block is required.

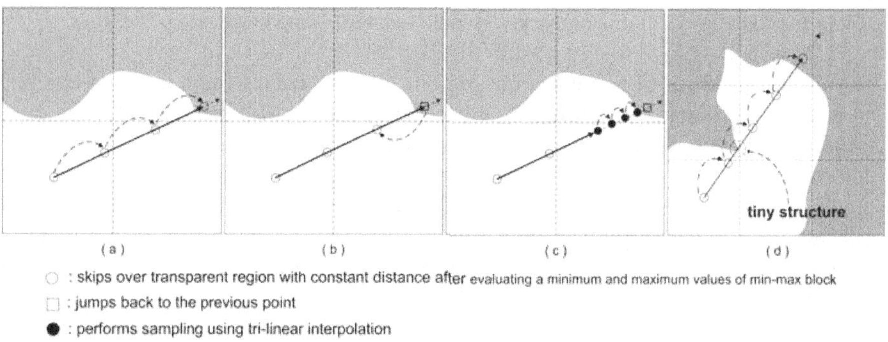

Fig. 3. Two problems of the method using constant distance : a ray can jump over transparent region with constant distance since a minimum and maximum value of current block is not confined within a threshold of nontransparent voxels (a). the ray jumps back to the previous point (b). it moves toward object surface with conventional ray-casting (c). fine details can be lost when the thickness of object is smaller than the constant distance (d)

3 Acceleration of Ray-Traversal Using Distance Template

Space-leaping is a well-known acceleration technique which skips over empty space using distance-map. This method accelerates the ray casting by avoiding unnecessary sampling for empty space. Distance template is a pre-computed distance-map that has the size of $(d+2)^3$, where d is the dimension of each axis in min-max block.

With an estimated distance such as city-block, chess-board and chamfer distance, only approximated evaluation is possible with less computation effort [13]. On the other hand, a tighter bound like Euclidian distance leads better speedup. Since it is generated in preprocessing step, we use Euclidian distance transform approximated by 10, 14 and 17 integers according to directions [13]. Fig. 4 shows an example of distance template.

Fig. 5 illustrates the ray traversal using the distance template. While conventional method with constant distance takes identical distance when a ray is jumped, our algorithm uses different distance depending on the distance template. At first, a ray determines whether leaps the transparent blocks or not by referencing the value of

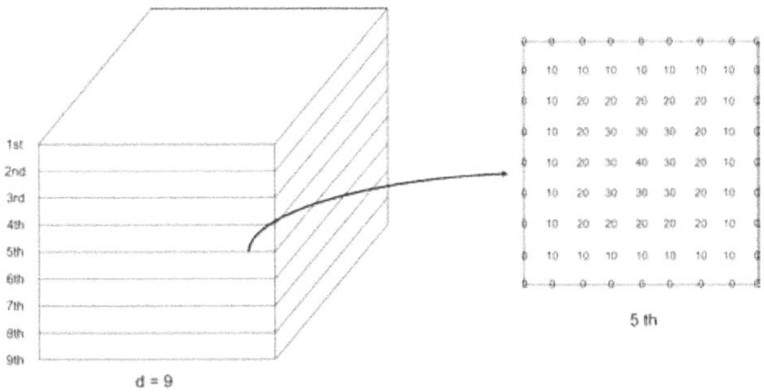

Fig. 4. An example of distance template based on Euclidian distance transform of which the size is $9 \times 9 \times 9$

min-max block. In the case of Fig. 5 (b), the ray can jump over current block based on the value stored on distance template since minimum and maximum values of current block are not confined within a threshold of nontransparent voxels. This procedure iterates until the ray meets the min-max block which is confined within a threshold of nontransparent voxels. Then the ray moves as the conventional ray-casting. Fig. 5 (d) shows a ray traversal with distance template when a situation of Fig. 3 (d) is applied.

As a result, our method can directly access to the boundary of min-max block. Also skipping region does not exact even small structure since distance template provides a reliable distance.

4 Experimental Results

We compare the rendering time and image quality of conventional ray-casting, constant distance method and our method. We use min-max block of which the size is $7 \times 7 \times 7$. All of these methods are implemented on a PC equipped with Pentium IV 3.06GHz CPU, 2GB main memory, and ATI Radeon9800 graphics accelerator. Volume dataset is obtained by scanning a human abdomen with a multi-detector CT of which the resolution is $512 \times 512 \times 541$.

We measure the rendering time in colon cavity under fixed viewing conditions. Table 1 shows the rendering time to get a final image. Rendering speed of our method is 142% faster than the method using constant distance and 320% faster than conventional ray-casting.

Table 1. Comparison of rendering time. Min-max block size is 7 x 7 x 7 and image size is 256 x 256

Method	Rendering time (sec)
Conventional ray-casting	4.91
Constant distance method	2.18
Distance template method	1.53

Fig. 6 shows the quality of images produced by using conventional ray-casting and our distance template structure under fixed viewing condition. It is very hard to recognize the difference between images from the three methods. Therefore we conclude that our method normally renders volumetric scene without loss of image quality.

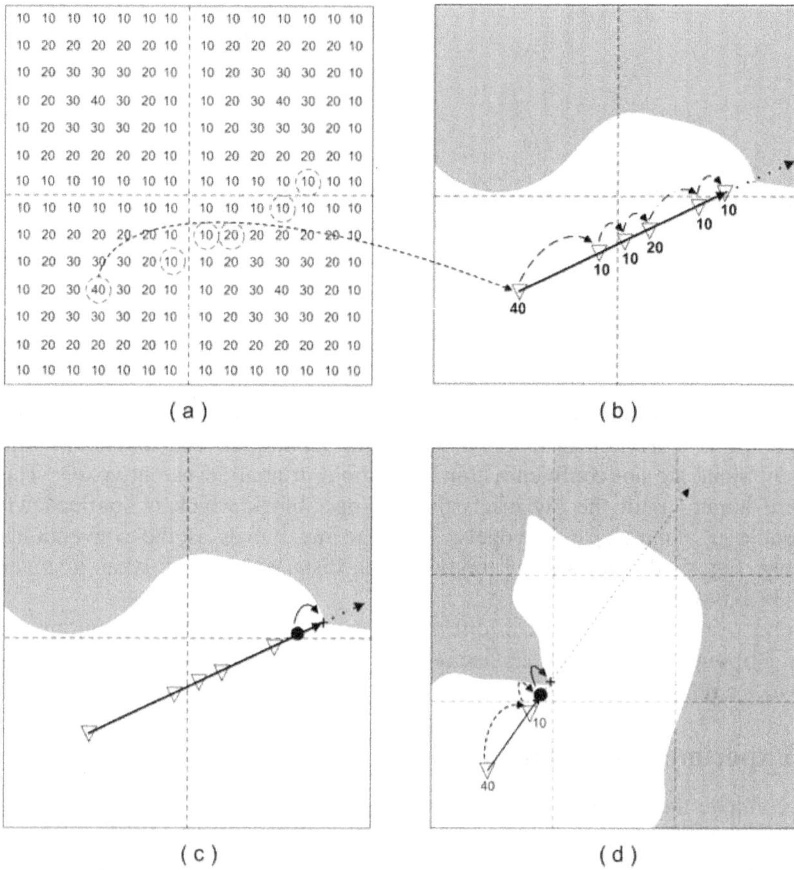

▽ : skips over transparent region with distinct distance to the boundary after evaluating a minimum and maximum values of min-max block

● : performs sampling using tri-linear interpolation

Fig. 5. A modified procedure of ray traversal using distance template : a distance template structure (a). a ray jumps by referencing distance stored on distance template when a minimum and maximum value of current block is not confined within a threshold of nontransparent voxels (b). the ray moves forward with conventional ray-casting (c). fine details can be reached even though the thickness of object is smaller than constant distance (d)

Fig. 7 shows problems when we use constant distance. As you can see, rendering images using conventional ray-casting method (Fig. 7 left) and our method (Fig. 7 right) show ordinary result without image quality deterioration. However the method with constant distance shows unexpected result. This means that distance template provides a reliable distance value.

5 Conclusion

The most important issue in volume visualization is to produce high quality images in real time. We propose a distance template that reduces the rendering time in compari-

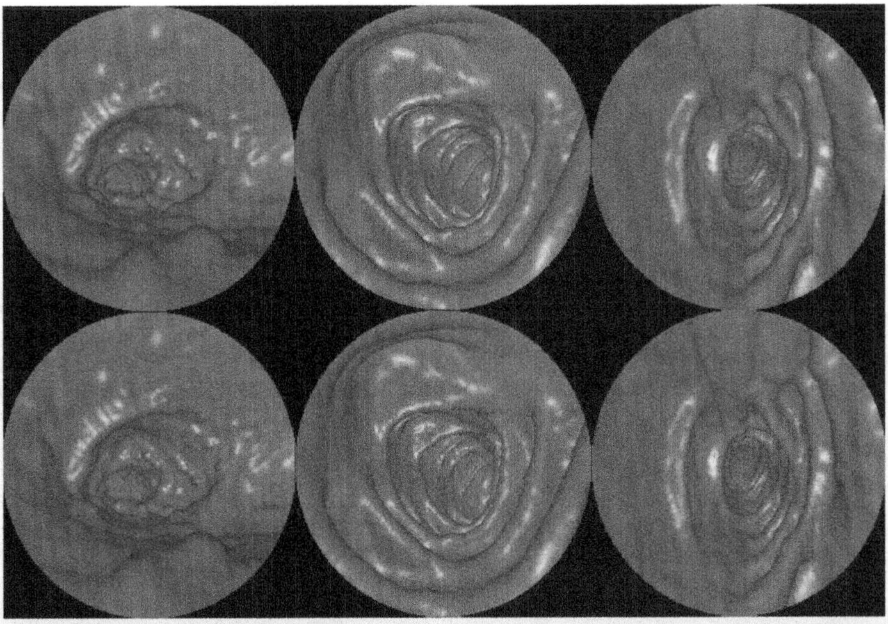

Fig. 6. A comparison of image quality of virtual colonoscopy in several different areas: Upper row shows images using conventional ray-casting and bottom row depicts images obtained by our distance template method

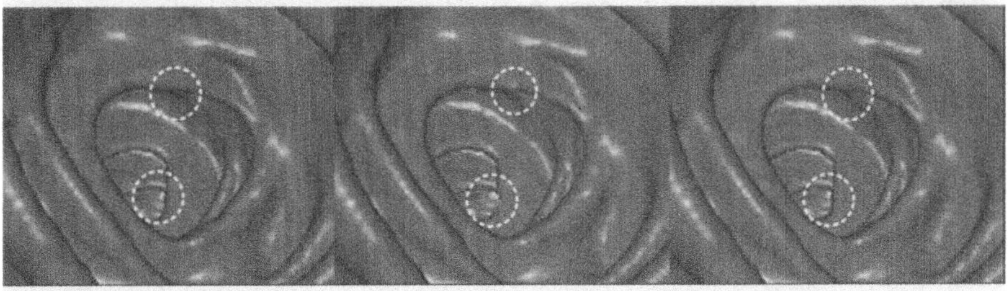

Fig. 7. Images are produced by conventional ray-casting, constant distance method and our method from left to right. Several artifacts occur on middle image

son to the method using accurate distance and constant distance in any situation without loss of image quality. Using pre-computed distance template, it can directly access to the boundary of min-max block. Since our structure is independent on the viewing conditions, we can reuse this structure entire volume space. It can be applied to generate endoscopic image for any kind of tubular-shaped organs. Experimental result shows that it normally produces high-quality images as in ray casting and takes less time for rendering.

Acknowledgment

This research was supported by University IT Research Center Project.

References

1. Subramanian, K., Fussell, D.: Applying Space Subdivision Techniques to Volume Rendering. IEEE Visualization '90. San Francisco, CA (1990) 150–159
2. Levoy, M. : Efficient Ray Tracing of Volume Data. ACM Transactions on Graphics Vol. 9. (1990) 245-261
3. Yagel, R., Kaufman, A.: Template-based Volume Viewing. Computer Graphics Forum (Eurographics 92 Proceedings). Cambridge, UK (1992) 153-167
4. Avila, R., Sobierajski, L., Kaufman, A.: Towareds a Comprehensive Volume Visualization System. IEEE Visualization (1992) 13-20
5. Lacroute, P., Levoy, M.: Fast Volume Rendering Using a Shear-Warp Factorization of the Viewing Transformation. Computer Graphics (SIGGRAPH 94 Proceedings), Orlando, Florida (1994) 451-458
6. Cohen, D., Sheffer, Z.: Proximity Clouds, An Acceleration Technique for 3D Grid Traversal. The Visual Computer Vol. 11, No. 1 (1994) 27-28
7. Westermann, R., Eart, T.: Efficiently Using Graphics Hardware in Volume Rendering Applications. Computer Graphics (1998) 167-177
8. Laur, D., Hanrahan, P.: Hierarchical Splatting-A Progressive Refinement Algorithm for Volume Rendering. Computer Graphics SIGGRAPH`91 (1991) 285-288
9. Danskin, J., Hanrahan, P.: Fast Algorithms for Volume Ray Tracing. Proceedings of 1992 Workshop on Volume Visualization. Boston (1992) 91–105
10. Wilhelms, J., Van Gelder, A.: Octrees for Faster Isosurface Generation. ACM Transactions On Graphics (1992) 201-227
11. Choi, J.J., Shin, B.S., Shin, Y.G., Cleary, K.: Efficient Volumetric Raycasting for Isosurface Rendering. Computers & Graphics (2000) 661-670
12. Krueger, J., Westermann, R.: Acceleration Techniques for GPU-based Volume Rendering, In Proceedings of Visualization 2003 (2003)
13. Sramek, M., Kaufman, A.: Fast Ray-Tracing of Rectilinear Volume Data Using Distance Transforms. IEEE Trans. on Visualization and Computer graphics, Vol 6 (2000) 236-252

A Rule-Based Knowledge System for Diagnosis of Mental Retardation

R. Sánchez-Morgado[1], Luis M. Laita[1], Eugenio Roanes-Lozano[2], Luis de Ledesma[1], and L. Laita[3]

[1] Universidad Politécnica de Madrid, Depto. de Inteligencia Artificial, Campus de Montegancedo, Boadilla del Monte, 28660-Madrid, Spain
morgado@mi.madritel.es, {laita,ledesma}@fi.upm.es
[2] Universidad Complutense de Madrid, Depto. de Algebra, c/ Rector Royo Villanova s/n, 28040-Madrid, Spain
eroanes@mat.ucm.es
[3] Universidad Complutense de Madrid, Escuela Universitaria de Enfermería, Ciudad Universitaria, 28040-Madrid, Spain

Abstract. We present in this paper a Rule-Based Knowledge System that both verifies the consistency of the knowledge explicitly provided by experts in mental retardation, and automatically extracts consequences (in this case: diagnoses) from that knowledge.
Expert knowledge is translated into symbolic expressions, which are written in CoCoA (a Computer Algebra language). The program, using a theory developed by this research team, outputs diagnoses from the different inputs that describe each patient.

Keywords: Medical Diagnosis, Mental Retardation, Rule-Based Knowledge Systems, Computer Algebra

1 Introduction

The design of a Rule-Based Knowledge System, hereinafter denoted as RBKS, requires building a "knowledge base" (to be denoted KB) an "inference engine" (to be denoted IE) and a "user interface" (to be denoted GUI). The first well known work following this approach in Medicine was Buchanan's and Shortliffe's [1].

The KB contains the experts' knowledge in form of condensed expressions (logical expressions in our case). Apart from literature on the topic [2–5], two human experts were consulted.

The IE is a procedure to verify both consistency of the KB and to extract automatically consequences from the information contained in the KB. Our IE is implemented in the Computer Algebra language CoCoA[6, 7][1].

[1] CoCoA, a system for doing Computations in Commutative Algebra. Authors: A. Capani, G. Niesi, L. Robbiano. Available via anonymous ftp from: `cocoa.dima.unige.it`

J.M. Barreiro et al. (Eds.): ISBMDA 2004, LNCS 3337, pp. 67–78, 2004.

The GUI helps users not specialist in the theoretical constructs on which the system is built, to visualize its final results, in our case a diagnosis.

We believe that Rule-Based Knowledge Systems in medicine cannot, so far, substitute a specialist or a team of specialists. Accordingly, our system has been designed to be only a helpful tool for family doctors and sanitary personnel not specialized in mental retardation, who may match their own opinion about a patient against the outputs of the system, before deciding whether sending the patient to a specialist or not.

2 Some Basic Ideas About RBKS

Our KBs consist of logical formulae (which are are called "production rules") like:

$$\neg x[1] \wedge x[2] \rightarrow a[2]$$

and "potential facts". The formula above is read as follows: "IF (not-$x[1]$ AND $x[2]$) hold, THEN $a[2]$ holds".

The symbols "$\neg$", "$\wedge$", "$\vee$" and "$\rightarrow$" translate, respectively, "no", "and", "or" and "implies". The symbols of the form $x[1]$ and their negations, $\neg x[1]$, are called "literals".

The set of all literals that appear on the left-hand side of any production rule and such that neither it nor its contrary appear in in any right-hand side (say, $x[1]$ is the contrary of $\neg x[1]$ and conversely) is called "the set of potential facts".

The users of the RBKS should choose, when studying a patient, a subset of facts from the set of potential facts. This set shouldn't contain simultaneously two contrary literals, in order to avoid contradictions (such sets are called "consistent set of facts").

Moreover, the user can choose exactly one literal from each pair of contrary literals in the list of potential facts. Those subsets are called "maximal consistent set of facts"; and each of them describes a patient.

We shall briefly describe in some detail the construction of the KB and the IE of the first subsystem because the procedure to built the other two is the same. In the second and third subsystems we shall only mention which ones are the perinatal and postnatal factors, respectively.

The combinations of the outputs of the three subsystems will provide a diagnosis, represented by the variable "q", for each patient

Between the construction of the KB and the CoCoA program we shall provide as intuitively as possible, the logical and mathematical results on which the IE is based.

3 Our RBKS

Two kinds of factors may cause mental retardation, the genetic (intrinsic factors) and the ambiental (extrinsic factors); we next deal only with the ambiental, which we have subdivided into "PRENATAL", "PERINATAL" and "POSTNATAL" factors. Accordingly, our system is built up from three subsystems. Each of them gives an output to be denoted by (sets of variables) x, y and w, which in their turn shall give, by combining them, diagnoses represented by "q".

3.1 First Subsystem: Prenatal Factors

During pregnancy, mothers may have suffered prenatal negative factors that may produce mental retardation to their sons. They are: infections, endocrinometabolopathies and intoxications.

- The following literals refer to infections
  - $x[1]$ Rubella
  - $x[2]$ Herpes
- The following literals refer to endocrinometabolopathies
  - $x[3]$ Thyroid disturbances
  - $x[4]$ Diabetes
  - $x[5]$ Nutrition deficit
- The following literals refer to intoxications
  - $x[6]$ Alcohol, tobacco, chemicals (pharmaceutical), drugs
  - $x[7]$ Radiations, poisonous gases.
- The following factors must also be taken into account (for instance pregnancy ages <16 or >40 may represent a danger for the son).
  - $x[8]$ Age < 16
  - $x[9]$ Age > 40
  - $x[30]$ $16 \leq Age \leq 40$
  - $x[10]$ Familiar antecedents of mental retardation.

Table 1 combines the factors "infections" (together with their negations) assigning to these combinations a high, medium or null value to the influence of these kind of factors. $a[1]$ means "high", $a[2]$ means "medium", $a[3]$ means "null". It is important to remark that all values assigned below, represented by the variables a, b, c, d and z, as well as all the other variables that will appear in the second and third subsystems, are assigned after consultation with the expert (another expert could assign different values).

Table 1. Values assigned to infections

	$x[1]$	$\neg x[1]$
$x[2]$	$a[1]$	$a[2]$
$\neg x[2]$	$a[2]$	$a[3]$

From Table 1 one can write the following production rules:

$R1 = x[1] \wedge x[2] \rightarrow a[1]$
$R2 = \neg x[1] \wedge x[2] \rightarrow a[2]$
$R3 = x[1] \wedge \neg x[2] \rightarrow a[2]$
$R4 = \neg x[1] \wedge \neg x[2] \rightarrow a[3]$

Table 2. Values assigned to endocrinometabolopathies

	$x[3] \wedge x[4]$	$x[3] \wedge \neg x[4]$	$\neg x[3] \wedge x[4]$	$\neg x[3] \wedge \neg x[4]$
$x[5]$	$b[1]$	$b[1]$	$b[1]$	$b[2]$
$\neg x[5]$	$b[1]$	$b[2]$	$b[2]$	$b[3]$

For instance, R2 says that "IF rubella = no AND herpes = yes, THEN the value a for infections is medium".

A similar table (Table 2) can be drawn for endocrinometabolopathies:

Seven production rules follow from Table 2. Known logical properties allow simplifications. For instance, as in the second column the same $b[1]$ appears, it means that $x[5]$ has no influence here, resulting the production rule:

$R5 = x[3] \wedge x[4] \rightarrow b[1]$

$R5$ says: IF Thyroid disturbances = yes AND Diabetes = yes, THEN the value b for infections is high.

The table for intoxications is similar and gives rise to three production rules, being now "c" the variable that refer to their values $c[1]$ and $c[2]$.

The variables a, b and c can be combined as Table 3 shows, giving rise to a "supervalue" d ($d[1]$, $d[2]$, $d[3]$ and $d[4]$ meaning, respectively, severe, high-medium, low and null (super)values).

Table 3. "Supervalues" assigned to the three previous values

	$a[1]$			$a[2]$			$a[3]$		
	$b[1]$	$b[2]$	$b[3]$	$b[1]$	$b[2]$	$b[3]$	$b[1]$	$b[2]$	$b[3]$
$c[1]$	$d[1]$	$d[1]$	$d[1]$	$d[1]$	$d[2]$	$d[2]$	$d[1]$	$d[2]$	$d[2]$
$c[2]$	$d[1]$	$d[2]$	$d[3]$	$d[2]$	$d[3]$	$d[3]$	$d[3]$	$d[3]$	$d[4]$

Table 3 gives rise to 16 rules; for the sake of space we only mention three.

R17, for instance, says that "IF the value a for infections if high AND the value b for endocrinometabolopathies is medium AND the value c for intoxication is high, THEN the "supervalue" d (or outline) of these values is high.

$R17 = a[1] \wedge b[2] \wedge c[2] \rightarrow d[2]$
$R21 = a[2] \wedge b[2] \wedge c[1] \rightarrow d[2]$
$R30 = a[3] \wedge b[3] \wedge c[2] \rightarrow d[4]$

The variables "d" must be combined in three different tables with the variables $x[8]$, $x[9]$ and $x[30]$ (ages) because age influence the results "d".

For instance $x[8]$ combined with the "d's" gives Table 4 and the corresponding production rules, of which only two are detailed.

R33=$x[8] \wedge d[3] \wedge x[10] \rightarrow z[3]$
R36=$x[8] \wedge d[4] \wedge \neg x[10] \rightarrow z[4]$

Table 4. Values assigned to age

	$x[8]$			
	$d[1]$	$d[2]$	$d[3]$	$d[4]$
$x[10]$	$z[1]$	$z[2]$	$z[3]$	$z[3]$
$\neg x[10]$	$z[1]$	$z[2]$	$z[4]$	$z[4]$

The variables "z" reflect the final output of the first subsystem of our RBKS regarding the global value or influence of "prenatal factors" ($z[1]$, $z[2]$, $z[3]$ and $z[4]$ meaning, respectively, severe, high-medium, low and null negative influence of prenatal factors).

By doing the same for ages $x[9]$ and $x[30]$, the KB of our first subsystem (influence of prenatal factors) results to be formed by a total of 50 production rules.

3.2 Second and Third Subsystems: Perinatal and Postnatal Factors

As advanced by the end of Section 2, we only provide here the variables that correspond to the perinatal and postnatal factors. The tables and the resulting production rules are built as for prenatal factors. In the same way that the variables "z" were the final outputs of the first subsystem, the variables "y" ($y[1]$ severe, $y[2]$ high-medium, $y[3]$ low, $y[4]$ null) and "w" ($w[1]$ severe, $w[2]$ high-medium, $w[3]$ low, $w[4]$ null) are the final outputs of the second and third subsystems, respectively.

Perinatal Factors: These are the factors which may may produce mental retardation if present during childbirth.

- The following literals refer to metabolopathies
  - $x[11]$ Jaundice
  - $x[12]$ Hypoglycemy
  - $x[13]$ Acidosis
- The following literals refer to cerebral suffering syndrome (CSS).
  - $x[14]$ Placenta previa
  - $x[15]$ Obstetric Trauma
  - $x[16]$ Hypoxia
- The following literals refer to infections
  - $x[17]$ Meningitis
  - $x[18]$ Encephalitis
  - $x[19]$ Virus
- and the literal $x[20]$ refers to premature birth

Our second subsystem (influence of perinatal factors) results to be formed by a total of 93 production rules.

Postnatal Factors: These are the factors which may may produce mental retardation if present after childbirth (we consider those which may last up to five years, which is somewhat arbitrary).

- The following literals refer to infections.
  - $x[21]$ Meningitis
  - $x[22]$ Encephalitis
  - $x[23]$ Rubella
- The following literals refer to endocrinometabolopathies.
  - $x[24]$ Hypoglycemy
  - $x[25]$ Hyperthyroidism
  - $x[26]$ Hypercalcemia
- Other factors.
  - $x[27]$ Intoxications
  - $x[28]$ Hypoxia

Our third subsystem (influence of perinatal factors) results to be formed by a total of 80 production rules.

3.3 Diagnoses

Variables "y", "z" and "w", are combined for constructing the production rules that end in the variables "q", which are the final diagnoses as Table 5 shows. We add a variable $x[29]$ corresponding to other "external factors".

There exists 6 degrees for diagnoses:

- $q[1]$ No mental retardation
- $q[2]$ Mental retardation = low
- $q[3]$ Mental retardation = moderate
- $q[4]$ Mental retardation = severe
- $q[5]$ Mental retardation = profound
- $q[6]$ Mental retardation = death risk

Table 5. Final diagnoses

		$z[1]$				$z[2]$				$z[3]$				$z[4]$			
		$y[1]$	$y[2]$	$y[3]$	$y[4]$	$y[1]$	$y[2]$	$y[3]$	$y[4]$	$y[1]$	$y[2]$	$y[3]$	$y[4]$	$y[1]$	$y[2]$	$y[3]$	$y[4]$
$x[29]$	$w[1]$	$q[6]$	$q[6]$	$q[6]$	$q[6]$	$q[6]$	$q[6]$	$q[5]$	$q[5]$	$q[6]$	$q[5]$	$q[4]$	$q[4]$	$q[6]$	$q[4]$	$q[4]$	$q[4]$
$x[29]$	$w[2]$	$q[6]$	$q[6]$	$q[5]$	$q[5]$	$q[6]$	$q[5]$	$q[5]$	$q[4]$	$q[5]$	$q[5]$	$q[3]$	$q[3]$	$q[5]$	$q[3]$	$q[3]$	$q[2]$
$x[29]$	$w[3]$	$q[6]$	$q[5]$	$q[5]$	$q[4]$	$q[5]$	$q[5]$	$q[4]$	$q[3]$	$q[5]$	$q[4]$	$q[3]$	$q[2]$	$q[5]$	$q[3]$	$q[2]$	$q[1]$
$x[29]$	$w[4]$	$q[5]$	$q[5]$	$q[4]$	$q[4]$	$q[5]$	$q[4]$	$q[4]$	$q[3]$	$q[4]$	$q[3]$	$q[2]$	$q[2]$	$q[3]$	$q[3]$	$q[2]$	$q[1]$
$\neg x[29]$	$w[1]$	$q[6]$	$q[6]$	$q[6]$	$q[6]$	$q[6]$	$q[6]$	$q[5]$	$q[5]$	$q[6]$	$q[5]$	$q[4]$	$q[4]$	$q[5]$	$q[4]$	$q[3]$	$q[3]$
$\neg x[29]$	$w[2]$	$q[6]$	$q[6]$	$q[5]$	$q[5]$	$q[6]$	$q[5]$	$q[5]$	$q[4]$	$q[5]$	$q[4]$	$q[3]$	$q[3]$	$q[4]$	$q[3]$	$q[2]$	$q[2]$
$\neg x[29]$	$w[3]$	$q[6]$	$q[5]$	$q[5]$	$q[4]$	$q[5]$	$q[5]$	$q[4]$	$q[3]$	$q[4]$	$q[3]$	$q[2]$	$q[2]$	$q[4]$	$q[2]$	$q[2]$	$q[1]$
$\neg x[29]$	$w[4]$	$q[5]$	$q[5]$	$q[4]$	$q[4]$	$q[5]$	$q[4]$	$q[3]$	$q[2]$	$q[3]$	$q[3]$	$q[2]$	$q[2]$	$q[3]$	$q[2]$	$q[1]$	$q[1]$

Table 5 gives rise to 128 production rules. For instance, the first one is:

$R529 = z[1] \wedge y[1] \wedge x[29] \wedge w[1] \rightarrow q[6]$

4 Outline of the Theory on Which the IE of Our System Is Based

A logical formula A_0 is a "tautological consequence" of the formulae A_1, A_2,..., A_m if and only if whenever A_1, A_2, ..., A_m are true then A_0 is true.

We all remember that polynomials can be summed and multiplied. The set of polynomials with, e.g., integer coefficients, form a structure called "ring". Some peculiar subsets of a polynomial ring are called "ideals". An ideal is generated by a set of polynomials of the polynomial ring.

Now, logical expressions (both production rules and potential facts of a KB are examples of such expressions) can be translated into polynomials. The polynomial translations of the four basic bivalued logical formulae (those corresponding to the symbols $\neg$ (no), $\vee$ (or), $\wedge$ (and) and $\rightarrow$ (implies) are provided next. The uppercase letters represent the propositional variables that stand in the production rules and the lowercase letters represent their corresponding polynomial variables:

- $\neg X_1$ is translated into the polynomial $1 + x_1$
- $X_1 \vee X_2$ is translated into the polynomial $x_1 \cdot x_2 + x_1 + x_2$
- $X_1 \wedge X_2$ is translated into the polynomial $x_1 \cdot x_2$
- $X_1 \rightarrow X_2$ is translated into the polynomial $x_1 \cdot x_2 + x_1 + 1$.

These translations allow to translate, using CoCoA, any logical formula into a polynomial; the coefficients of these polynomials are just 0 and 1, and the maximum power of variables is 1.

Theorem 1. *A formula A_0 is a tautological consequence of the formulae in the union of the two sets $\{A_1, A_2, ..., A_m\} \cup \{B_1, B_2, ..., B_k\}$ that represent, respectively, a subset of the set of potential facts (that characterizes a patient in this paper) and the set of all production rules of the RBKS if and only if the polynomial translation of the negation of A_0 belongs to the sum of the three ideals $I + K + J$ generated, respectively, by the polynomials $x_1^2 - x_1, x_2^2 - x_2, ..., x_n^2 - x_n$, by the polynomial translation of the negations of $A_1, A_2, ..., A_m$ and by the polynomial translation of the negations of $B_1, B_2, ..., B_k$.*

That A_0 is a consequence of the formulae in $\{A_1, A_2, ..., A_m\} \cup \{B_1, B_2, ..., B_k\}$, can be checked in CoCoA by typing:

```
NF(NEG(A[0]),I+K+J);
```

where "NF" means "Normal Form". If the output is 0, the answer is "yes"; if the output is different from 0, the answer is "no".

The theorem also allows to check that the system is consistent (not contradictory). This condition can be checked by just typing the CoCoA command:

```
GBasis(I+J+K);
```

where "GBasis" means "Gröbner basis" , if the output is 1 (it appears as `[1]` on the screen) the RBKS is inconsistent; otherwise (it may be a large set of polynomials) the RBKS is consistent.

Our description along the last lines has been very informal. The whole theory, founded on "Gröbner bases" and "Normal Forms" [8–10], is quite complex. Its logic and mathematical ideas are based on the works of Moisil [11], Kapur-Narendran, Hsiang and Chazarain et al. [12–14] and our prior work on the application of Gröbner bases to automated deduction [15, 16], which we applied, to the study of medical appropriateness criteria [17], to the diagnosis of anorexia [18] and to other fields like railway interlocking systems [19]. Its CoCoA implementation was successively improved with substantial changes in the basic programs (not in the theory) to end in the implementation provided in this article.

5 CoCoA Implementation of the Inference Engine of the First Subsystem

Section 4 has outlined the theory on which this implementation is based. We only outline afterwards the CoCoA implementation of the first subsystem: the implementations of the two other subsystems are similar.

First Steps: The commands are written in `''typewriter''` font, while the explanations are written in normal font.

The polynomial ring A with coefficients in $Z/2Z$ (that is, allowing only coefficients 0 and 1) and variables $x_1, ..., x_{10}, x_{30}$, $z_1, ...z_4$, $a_1, ..., a_3$, $b_1, ..., b_3$, $c_1, ..., c_2$, $d_1, ..., d_4$ and the ideal I are declared as follows (I is generated by the binomials of the form $v^2 - v$ where v is a polynomial variable and has the effect of reducing all exponents of the polynomials into 1, thus simplifying computations).

```
A::=Z/(2)[x[1..10],x[30],z[1..4],a[1..3],b[1..3],c[1..2],d[1..4]];

I:=Ideal(x[1]^2-x[1],...,x[10]^2-x[10],x[30]^2-x[30],
         z[1]^2-z[1],...,z[4]^2-z[4],a[1]^2-a[1],...,a[3]^2-a[3],
         b[1]^2-b[1],...,b[3]^2-b[3],c[1]^2-c[1],c[2]^2-c[2],
         d[1]^2-d[1],...,d[4]^2-d[4]);
```

(note that "`..`" is an abbreviation accepted by CoCoA, unlike "`,...,`" that is used here to save space and is not acceptable code).

The following commands (see Section 4) produce the polynomial translation of bivalued logical formulae. CoCoA requires that logical formulae be written in prefix form. `NEG`, `OR1`, `AND1`, `IMP` denote $\neg$, $\vee$, $\wedge$, $\rightarrow$, respectively.

```
NEG(M):=NF(1+M,I);
OR1(M,N):=NF(M+N+M*N,I);
AND1(M,N):=NF(M*N,I);
IMP(M,N):=NF(1+M+M*N,I);
```

Entering the KB: All 50 production rules of the first subsystem should be entered first. As said above, CoCoA requires that formulae are written in prefix form. Therefore, production rule such as, for instance, R5: $R5 = x[3] \wedge x[4] \rightarrow b[1]$, must be rewritten this way:

```
R5:=NF(IMP(AND1(x[3],x[4]),b[1]),I);
```

The set of potential facts is entered next. Each patient is characterized by the factors and symptoms that form a maximal consistent subset of the whole set of potential facts (see Section 2).

```
F1:=x[1];                  F1N:=NEG(x[1]);
F2:=x[2];                  F2N:=NEG(x[2]);
......                     ......
F8:=x[8];                  F8N:=NEG(x[8]);
F9:=x[9];                  F9N:=NEG(x[9]);
F10:=x[10];                F10N:=NEG(x[10]);
F30:=x[30];                F30N:=NEG(x[30]);
```

(note that of triple $x[8]$, $x[9]$, $x[30]$ exactly one should be affirmed and two should be negated).

The ideal J, generated by the 50 production rules of the subsystems is:

```
J:=Ideal(NEG(R1),NEG(R2),NEG(R3),...,NEG(R49),NEG(R50));
```

(recall that Theorem 1 implies the need of entering NEG before the rules).

Let us consider, as illustration, the following ideal K that characterizes a patient by factors:

$\neg x[1]$ (Rubella = no)
$x[2]$ (Herpes = yes)
$\neg x[3]$ (Thyroid disturbances = no)
$x[4]$ (Diabetes = yes)
$x[5]$ (Nutritional Deficit = yes)
$\neg x[6]$ (alcohol, drugs,... = no)
$x[7]$ (radiations, poisonous gases... = yes)
$\neg x[8]$ ($age < 16$, no)
$\neg x[9]$ ($40 < age$, no)
$\neg x[10]$ (familiar antecedents = no)
$x[30]$ ($16 \leq age \leq 40$, yes).

```
K:=Ideal(NEG(F1N),NEG(F2),NEG(F3N),NEG(F4),NEG(F5),NEG(F6N),
         NEG(F7),NEG(F8N),NEG(F9N),NEG(F10N),NEG(F30));
```

Let us remember that Theorem 1 implies that all formulae are preceded by `NEG`. So, if the negation of a fact is stated, e.g. F3, something like `NEG(F3N)` will be included in the ideal.

Checking for Consistency: Once the whole set of rules and potential facts has been introduced, it is necessary to check its consistency. Recall that consistency is checked by using command `GBasis` (see Section 4).

```
GBasis(I+K+J);
```

No inconsistency was found (`[1]` was not returned). The same happens with many patients we have tested, and also no inconsistency was found in the other two subsystems. In the way the set of production rules have been built here, with only one literal as consequent, it is not probable to find inconsistencies other that those resulting from misprints.

Extraction of Consequences: Let us consider, as illustration, the ideal K defined above. Let us ask what value of prenatal factors $z[i]$ ($i = 1, ..., 5$) may occur to the patient characterized by the ideal K. The following commands (see Section 4):

```
NF(NEG(z[1]),I+K+J);
NF(NEG(z[2]),I+K+J);
NF(NEG(z[3]),I+K+J);
NF(NEG(z[4]),I+K+J);
```

give, as output, 0, 1, 1, 1, respectively. It means that this patient has a high (negative) ($z[1]$) influence of prenatal factors.

6 Conclusions

We have presented a prototype of a RBKS for the study of mental retardation. At the present state, the RBKS is able to produce automatically a diagnosis of the illness in less than a minute.

Obviously the goal is not to substitute the specialist. There are two possible uses: first, to help in the evaluation of the illness by non-specialists (that must send the patient to a specialist!) and, second, to allow the specialist to compare his diagnosis with the one suggested by the system.

Its KB could be improved, detailed or updated without modifying substantially its inference engine.

Appendix I: Example of Screenshot of the GUI

The screenshot in Fig. 1, refers to triggering factors. The user selects the keys corresponding to the patient, that are translated into literals. The GUI is in Spanish, but the English terms are similar.

References

1. B. Buchanan and E.H. Shortliffe (eds.), *Rule Based Expert Systems: the MYCIN Experiments of the Stanford Heuristic Programming Project* (Addison Wesley, New York, 1984).
2. C.N.R.E.E., *El alumno con retraso mental en la escuela ordinaria* (Ministry of Education, Madrid, 1991 and 1994).

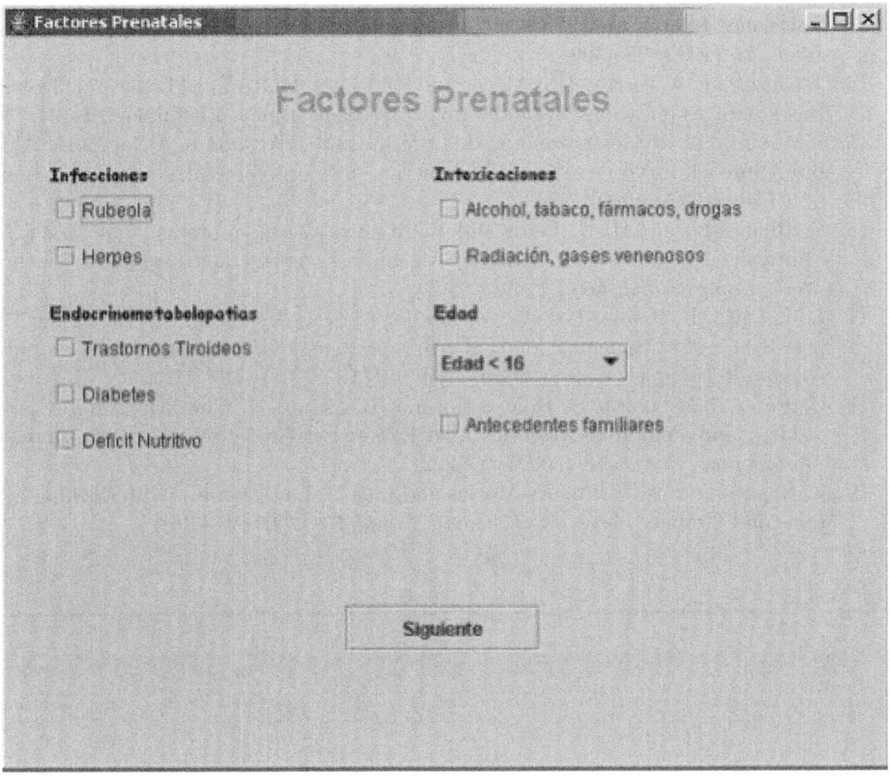

Fig. 1. Screenshot of the GUI of the RBKS

3. S. Molina García, *Deficiencia mental, aspectos psicoevolutivos y educativos* (Ediciones Aljibe, Málaga, 1994).
4. A.P.A. (American Psychiatric Association): D.S.M. IV (A.P.A., 1995). URL: `http://www.appi.org/dsm.cfx`
5. M. A. Verdugo, El cambio de paradigma en la concepción de retraso mental: la nueva definición de A. A. M. R., *Siglo Cero*, **25/3** (1995) 5–22.
6. A. Capani and G. Niesi, *CoCoA User's Manual v. 3.0b* (Dept. of Mathematics, University of Genova, Genova, 1996).
7. D. Perkinson, *CoCoA 4.0 Online Help* (electronic file acompanying CoCoA v.4.0, 2000).
8. W.W. Adams and P. Loustaunau, *An Introduction to Gröbner Bases* (Graduate Studies in Mathematics, American Mathematical Society, Providence, RI, 1994).
9. T. Becker and V. Weisspfenning, *Gröbner bases* (Springer, New York, 1993).
10. F. Winkler, *Polynomial Algorithms in Computer Algebra* (Springer-Verlag, Vienna, 1996).
11. G. C. Moisil, *The Algebraic Theory of Switching Circuits* (Pergamon Press, Oxford, 1969).
12. D. Kapur and P. Narendran, *An Equational Approach to Theorem Proving in First-Order Predicate Calculus* (General Electric Corporate Research and Development Report 84CRD296, Schenectady, NY, March 1984, rev. December 1984). Also in: *Proceedings of IJCAI-85* (1985) 1146-1153.

13. J. Hsiang, Refutational Theorem Proving using Term-Rewriting Systems, *Artif. Intell.* **25** (1985) 255-300.
14. J. Chazarain, A. Riscos, J.A. Alonso and E. Briales, Multivalued Logic and Gröbner Bases with Applications to Modal Logic, *J. Symb. Comp.* **11** (1991) 181-194.
15. L.M. Laita, E. Roanes-Lozano, L. de Ledesma and J. A. Alonso, A Computer Algebra Approach to Verification and Deduction in Many-Valued Knowledge Systems, *Soft Comp.* **3/1** (1999) 7-19.
16. E. Roanes-Lozano, L.M. Laita and E. Roanes-Macías, A Polynomial Model for Multivalued Logics with a Touch of Algebraic Geometry and Computer Algebra, *Math. Comp. Simul.* **45/1** (1998) 83-99.
17. L.M. Laita, E. Roanes-Lozano, V. Maojo, L. de Ledesma, and L. Laita, An Expert System for Managing Medical Appropriateness Criteria Based on Computer Algebra Techniques, *Comp. Math. Appl.* **42/12** (2001) 1505-1522.
18. C. Pérez. L.M. Laita, E. Roanes-Lozano, L. Lázaro, J. González and L. Laita, A Logic and Computer Algebra-Based Expert System for Diagnosis of Anorexia, *Math. Comp. Simul.* **58** (2002) 183-202.
19. E. Roanes-Lozano, E. Roanes-Macías and Luis M. Laita, Railway Interlocking Systems and Gröbner bases, *Math. Comp. Simul.* **51** (2000) 473-481.

Case-Based Diagnosis of Dysmorphic Syndromes

Tina Waligora and Rainer Schmidt

Institute for Medical Informatics and Biometry, University of Rostock, Universität Rostock
Rembrandtstr. 16 / 17, D-18055 Rostock, Germany
Phone: +49.381.494.7307
{tina.waligora,rainer.schmidt}@medizin.uni-rostock.de

Abstract. Since diagnosis of dysmorphic syndromes is a domain with incomplete knowledge where even experts have seen only few syndromes themselves during their lifetime, documentation of cases and the use of case-oriented techniques are popular. In dysmorphic systems, diagnosis usually is performed as a classification task, where a prototypicality measure is applied to determine the most probable syndrome. Our approach additionally applies adaptation rules. These rules do not only consider single symptoms but combinations of them, which indicate high or low probabilities of specific syndromes.

Keywords: Dysmorphic Syndromes, Case-Based Reasoning,, Prototypicality measures, Adaptation
Paper domain: Decision support systems

1 Introduction

When a child is born with dysmorphic features or with multiple congenital malformations or if mental retardation is observed at a later stage, finding the right diagnosis is extremely important. Knowledge of the nature and the etiology of the disease enables the pediatrician to predict the patient's future course. An initial goal for medical specialists is to diagnose a patient to a recognised syndrome. Genetic counselling and subsequently a course of treatments may be established.

A dysmorphic syndrome describes a morphological disorder and it is characterised by a combination of various symptoms, which form a pattern of morphologic defects. An example is Down Syndrome which can be described in terms of characteristic clinical and radiographic manifestations such as mental retardation, sloping forehead, a flat nose, short broad hands and generally dwarfed physique [1].

The main problems of diagnosing dysmorphic syndromes are as follows [2]:

- more the 200 syndromes are known,
- many cases remain undiagnosed with respect to known syndromes,
- usually many symptoms are used to describe a case (between 40 and 130),
- every dysmorphic syndrome is characterised by nearly as many symptoms.

Furthermore, knowledge about dysmorphic disorders is continuously modified, new cases are observed that cannot be diagnosed (it exist even a journal that only publishes reports of observed interesting cases [3]), and sometimes even new syndromes are discovered. Usually, even experts of paediatric genetics only see a small count of dysmorphic syndromes during their lifetime.

So, we have developed a diagnostic system that uses a large case base. Starting point to build the case base was a case collection of the paediatric genetics of the

J.M. Barreiro et al. (Eds.): ISBMDA 2004, LNCS 3337, pp. 79–84, 2004.

University of Munich, which consists of nearly 2.000 cases and 229 prototypes. A prototype (prototypical case) represents a dysmorphic syndrome by its typical symptoms. Many of the dysmorphic syndromes are already known and have been defined in literature. And nearly one third of our entire case base has been determined by semiautomatic knowledge acquisition, where an expert selected cases that should belong to the same syndrome and subsequently a prototype, characterised by the most frequent symptoms of his cases, was generated. To this database we have added cases from "clinical dysmorphology" [3] and syndromes from the London dysmorphic database [4], which contains only rare dysmorphic syndromes.

1.1 Diagnostic Systems for Dysmorphic Syndromes

Systems to support diagnosis of dysmorphic syndromes have already been developed in the early 80th. The simple ones perform just information retrieval for rare syndromes, namely the London dysmorphic database [3], where syndromes are described by symptoms, and the Australian POSSUM, where syndromes are visualised [5]. Diagnosis by classification is done in a system developed by Wiener and Anneren [6]. They use more than 200 syndromes as database and apply Bayesian probability to determine the most probable syndromes. Another diagnostic system, which uses data from the London dysmorphic database was developed by Evans [7]. Though he claims to apply Case-Based Reasoning, in fact it is again just a classification, this time performed by Tversky's measure of dissimilarity [8].

In our system the user can chose between two measures of dissimilarities between concepts, namely a measure developed by Tversky [8] and a measure pruposed by Rosch and Mervis [9]. However, the novelty of our approach is that we do not only perform classification but subsequently apply adaptation rules. These rules do not only consider single symptoms but specific combinations of them, which indicate high or low probabilities of specific syndromes.

1.2 Case-Based Reasoning and Prototypicality Measures

Since the idea of Case-Based Reasoning (CBR) is to use former, already solved solutions (represented in form of cases) for current problems [10], CBR seems to be appropriate for diagnosis of dysmorphic syndromes. CBR consists of two main tasks [10], namely retrieval, that means searching for similar cases, and adaptation, that means adapting solutions of similar cases to the query case. For retrieval, usually an explicit similarity measure or, especially for large case bases, faster retrieval algorithms like Nearest Neighbour Matching [11] are applied. For adaptation only few general techniques exist [12], usually domain specific adaptation rules have to be acquired.

For dysmorphic syndromes it is unreasonable to search for single similar patients (and of course none of the systems mentioned above does so) but for more general prototypes that contain the typical features of a syndrome. Prototypes are generalisations from single cases. They fill the knowledge gap between the specificity of single cases and abstract knowledge in form of rules. Though the use of prototypes had been early introduced in the CBR community [13], their use is still rather seldom. However, since doctors reason with typical cases anyway, in medical CBR systems prototypes are a rather common knowledge form (e.g. for antibiotics therapy advice [14], for diabetes [15], and for eating disorders [16]).

So, to determine the most similar prototype for a given query patient a prototypicality measure is required instead of a similarity measure. For prototypes the list of symptoms usually is much shorter than for single cases. Since many syndromes are very similar and usually further investigation is required to distinguish between them, the result should not be just the one and only most similar prototype, but a list of them – sorted according to their similarity. So, the usual CBR methods like indexing or nearest neighbour search are inappropriate. Instead, rather old measures for dissimilarities between concepts [8, 9] are applied and explained in the next section.

2 Diagnosis of Dysmorphic Syndromes

Our system consists of four steps (fig.1). At first the user has to select the symptoms that characterise a new patient. This selection is long and very time consuming, because more than 800 symptoms are considered. However, diagnosis of dysmorphic syndromes is not a task where the result is very urgent, but it usually requires thorough reasoning, afterwards a long-term therapy has to be started.

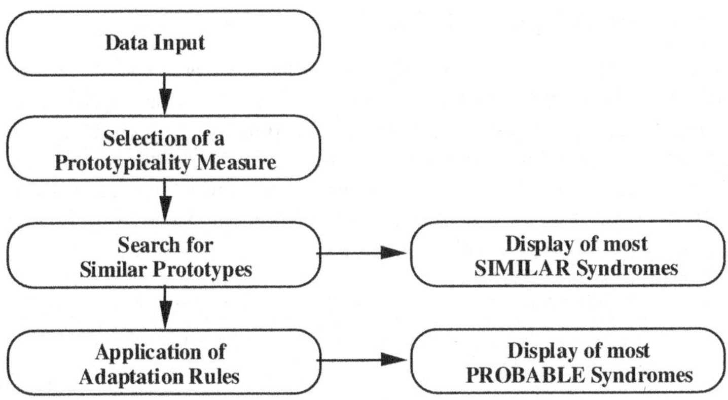

Fig. 1. Steps to diagnose dysmorphic syndromes

Since our system is still in the evaluation phase, secondly the user can select a prototypicality measure. In routine use, this step shall be dropped and instead the measure with best evaluation results shall be used automatically. At present there are three choices. As humans look upon cases as more typical for a query case as more features they have in common [9], distances between prototypes and cases usually mainly consider the shared features. The first, rather simple measure just counts the number of matching symptoms of the query patient (X) and a prototype (Y) and normalises the result by dividing it by the number of symptoms characterising the syndrome. This normalisation is done, because the lengths of the lists of symptoms of the prototypes vary very much. It is performed by the two other measures too.

$$D(X,Y) = \frac{f(X+Y)}{f(Y)}$$

The second measure was developed by Tversky [8]. In contrast to the first measure, additionally two values are subtracted from the number of matching symptoms.

Firstly, the number of symptoms that are observed for the patient but are not used to characterise the prototype (X-Y), and secondly the number of symptoms used for the prototype but are not observed for the patient (Y-X) is subtracted.

$$D(X,Y) = \frac{f(X+Y) - f(X-Y) - f(Y-X)}{f(Y)}$$

The third prototypicality measure was proposed by Rosch and Mervis [9]. It differs from Tversky's measure only in one point: the factor X-Y is not considered:

$$D(X,Y) = \frac{f(X+Y) - f(Y-X)}{f(Y)}$$

In the third step, the chosen measure is sequentially applied on all prototypes (syndromes). Since the syndrome with maximal similarity is not always the right diagnosis, the 20 syndromes with best similarities are listed in a menu.

2.1 Application of Adaptation Rules

In the final step, the user can optionally choose to apply adaptation rules on the syndromes (the result is depicted in figure 2). These rules state that specific combinations of symptoms favour or disfavour specific dysmorphic syndromes. Unfortunately, the acquisition of these adaptation rules is very difficult, because they cannot be found in textbooks but have to be defined by experts of paediatric genetics. So far, we have got only 10 of them. It is not possible that a syndrome can be favoured by one adaptation rule and disfavoured by another one at the same time.

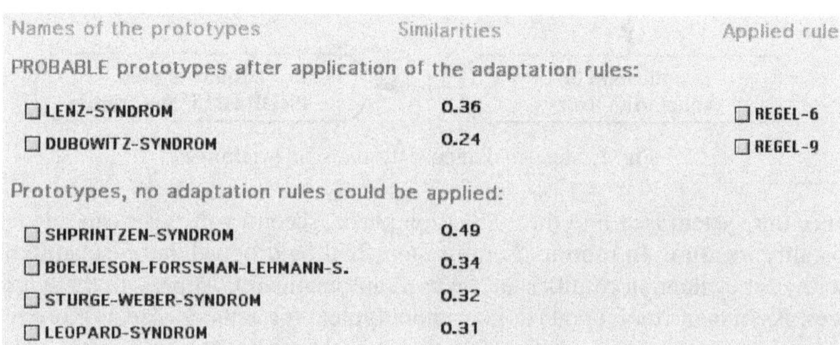

Fig. 2. Top part of the listed prototypes after application of adaptation rules

How shall adaptation rules alter the results? Our first idea was that adaptation rules should increase or decrease the similarity scores for favoured and disfavoured syndromes. But the question is how. Of course no medical expert can determine values to manipulate the similarities by adaptation rules and any general value for favoured or disfavoured syndromes would be arbitrary. So, instead we present a menu containing up to three lists (fig.2). On top the favoured syndromes are depicted, then those neither favoured nor disfavoured, and at the bottom the disfavoured ones. Additionally, the user can get information about the specific rules that have been applied on a particular syndrome (e.g. fig. 3).

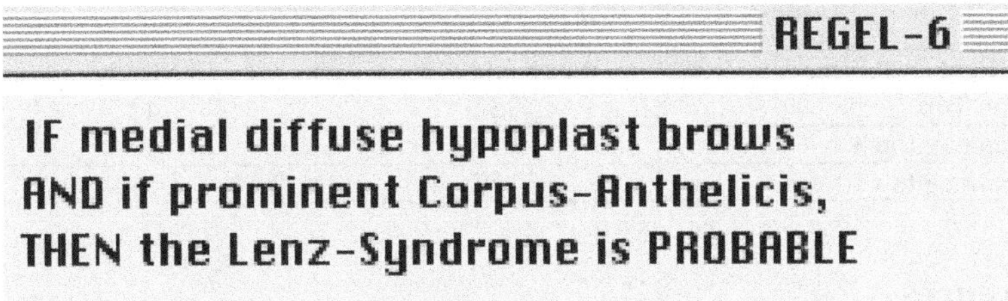

Fig. 3. Presented information about an applied rule

In this example, the right diagnosis is Lenz-syndrome. By application of the prototypicality measure of Rosch and Mervis Lenz-syndrome was the most similar but one syndrome (here Tversky's measure provides a similar result, only the differences between the similarities are smaller). After application of adaptation rules, the ranking is not obvious. Two syndromes have been favoured, the more similar one is the right one. However, Dubowitz-syndrome is favoured too (by a completely different rule), because a specific combination of symptoms makes it probable too, while other observed symptoms indicate a rather low similarity.

3 Results

Cases are difficult to diagnose when patients suffer from very rare dymorphic syndromes for which neither detailed information can be found in literature nor many cases are stored in our case base. This makes evaluation difficult. If test cases are randomly chosen, frequently observed cases resp. syndromes are frequently selected and the results will probably be fine, because these syndromes are well-known. However, the main idea of the system is especially to support diagnosis of rare syndromes. So, we have chosen our test cases randomly but under the condition that every syndrome can be chosen only once. For 100 cases we have compared the results obtained by both prototypicality measures (table 1).

Table 1. Comparison of prototypicality measures

Right Syndrome	Rosch and Mervis	Tversky
on Top	29	40
among top 3	57	57
among top 10	76	69

The results may seem to be rather poor. However, diagnosis of dysmorphic syndromes is very difficult and usually needs further investigation, because often a couple of syndromes are nearly indistinguishable. The intention is to provide information about probable syndromes, so that the doctor gets an idea which further investigations are appropriate. That means, the right diagnoses among the three most probable syndromes already is a good result. Since the number of acquired rules is rather limited, the improvement depends on the question how many syndromes involved by adaptation rules are among the test set. In our experiment just 5 of the right syndromes were favoured by adaptation rules. Since some syndromes had been already diagnosed correctly without adaptation, the improvement is slight (table 2).

Table 2. Results after the application of adaptation rules

Right Syndrome	Rosch and Mervis	Tversky
on Top	32	42
among top 3	59	59
among top 10	77	71

References

1. Taybi, H., Lachman, R.S.: Radiology of Syndromes, Metabolic Disorders, and Skeletal Dysplasia. Year Book Medical Publishers, Chicago (1990)
2. Gierl, L., Stengel-Rutkowski, S.: Integrating Consultation and Semi-automatic Knowledge Acquisition in a Prototype-based Architecture: Experiences with Dysmorphic Syndromes. Artif Intell Med 6 (1994) 29-49
3. Clinical Dysmorphology. www.clindysmorphol.com
4. Winter, R.M., Baraitser, M., Douglas, J.M.: A computerised data base for the diagnosis of rare dysmorphic syndromes. Journal of medical genetics 21 (2) (1984) 121-123
5. Stromme, P.: The diagnosis of syndromes by use of a dysmorphology database. Acta Paeditr Scand 80 (1) (1991) 106-109
6. Weiner, F., Anneren, G.: PC-based system for classifying dysmorphic syndromes in children. Computer Methods and Programs in Biomedicine 28 (1989) 111-117
7. Evans, C.D.: A case-based assistant for diagnosis and analysis of dysmorphic syndromes. Int J Med Inf 20 (1995) 121-131
8. Tversky, A.: Features of Similarity. Psychological Review 84 (4) (1977) 327-352
9. Rosch, E., Mervis, C.B.: Family Resemblance: Studies in the Internal Structures of Categories. Cognitive Psychology 7 (1975) 573-605
10. Kolodner J: Case-Based Reasoning. Morgan Kaufmann, San Mateo (1993)
11. Broder, A.: Strategies for efficient incremental nearest neighbor search. Pattern Recognition 23 (1990) 171-178
12. Wilke, W., Smyth, B., Cunningham, P.: Using configuration techniques for adaptation. In: Lenz, M. et al. (eds.): Case-Based Reasoning technology, from foundations to applications. Springer, Berlin (1998) 139-168
13. Bareiss, R.: Exemplar-based knowledge acquisition. Academic Press, San Diego (1989)
14. Schmidt R, Gierl L: Case-based Reasoning for antibiotics therapy advice: an investigation of retrieval algorithms and prototypes. Artif Intell Med 23 (2001) 171-186
15. Bellazzi, R, Montani, S., Portinale, L.: Retrieval in a prototype-based case library: a case study in diabetes therapy revision. In: Smyth, B., Cunningham, P. (eds.): Proc European Workshop on Case-Based Reasoning, Springer, Berlin (1998) 64-75
16. Bichindaritz, I.: From cases to classes: focusing on abstraction in case-based reasoning. In: Burkhard, H.-D., Lenz, M. (eds.): Proc German Workshop on Case-Based Reasoning, University Press, Berlin (1996) 62-69

Bayesian Prediction of Down Syndrome Based on Maternal Age and Four Serum Markers

Raquel Montes Diez, Juan M. Marin, and David Rios Insua

Computer Science, Statistics and Telematics Department
Rey Juan Carlos University, Madrid 28933, Spain

Abstract. Screening tests have been designed to identify women at increased risk of having a Down syndrome pregnancy. These tests have no risks of miscarriage, but they are not able to determine with certainty whether a fetus is affected. Diagnostic tests such as amniocentesis, on the other hand, are extremely accurate at identifying abnormalities in the fetus, but carry some risk of miscarriage, making it inappropriate to examine every pregnancy in this way. Muller et al.(1999), compares six software packages that calculate Ds risk, concluding that substantial variations are observed among them. In this paper, we provide a Bayesian reanalysis of the current quadruple screening test, based on maternal age and four serum markers (afp, uE3, hCG and DIA), which suggests the need to reevaluate more carefully actual recomendations.

1 Motivation

Prenatal screening can provide important information about potential risks for pregnancy. Screening tests have been designed to identify women at increased risk of having a Down syndrome pregnancy. These tests have no risks of miscarriage, but they are not able to determine with certainty whether a fetus is affected. Diagnostic tests such as amniocentesis, on the other hand, are extremely accurate at identifying certain abnormalities in the fetus, but carry some risk of miscarriage, making it inappropriate to examine every pregnancy in this way.

In the past, screening tests were based on selecting women of advance age (usually older than 35 years old) for diagnostic amniocentesis. Later, some biochemical markers were shown to be associated with DS affected pregnancies, so that information on both maternal age and these serum marker levels could be combined to select women at high risk of having a DS pregnancy. A state–of–the–art review may be seen in Wald et al. (1998, 2003).

In this paper, we extend the work by Marin et.al. (2003) and investigate prenatal screening performed on the basis of four of these maternal serum markers

J.M. Barreiro et al. (Eds.): ISBMDA 2004, LNCS 3337, pp. 85–95, 2004.

namely α-fetoproteine (AFP), unconjugated oestriol (uE3), human chorionic gonadotrophin (hCG) and dimeric inhibin–A (DIA), at 14-20 weeks gestation (second trimester). Markers are usually expressed in units called MoM, the specific multiple of the median to each marker in each week of pregnancy. For instance, for the four considered serum markers, 1.0 MoM is the multiple of the median counted in unaffected pregnancies for every whole pregnancy week. Whereas AFP and uE3 levels tend to be lower in Down pregnancies, with medians of approximately 0.70 MoM, hCG and DIA levels have been shown to be about twice as high in affected pregnancies as in healthy ones.

The analysis presented here is motivated by the work of Muller et al. (1999), in which six software packages (Prenatal Interpretive Software, Prisca, DIANASoft, T21, PrenatScreen and MultiCalc) that calculate the risk of a pregnancy being Down affected, were compared. The authors concluded that substantial variations are observed between these packages. For instance, in a population of 100,000 patients, including 143 cases of DS, the least sensitive software will detect 78 cases of DS through 2400 amniocenteses, as opposed to the most sensitive, which will detect 95 cases through 6800 amniocenteses. These differences could undoubtedly have an impact on public health policy and this lead us to look into the problem from a fully Bayesian point of view.

Here, we estimate the risk related to having a pregnancy resulting in the birth of an infant with Down's syndrome in the absence of antenatal diagnosis and therapeutic abortion. We shall reanalyse some of the available data sets to conclude essentially that further care should be taken when providing a protocol to handle Down syndrome.

2 Background

2.1 Maternal Age and DS Pregnancies

Screening on the basis of selecting women of advanced maternal age for amniocentesis was gradually introduced into medical practice, since Valenti (1968) made the first antenatal diagnosis of Down's syndrome. In the prenatal screening literature, DS-risk is expressed as an odds ratio $1 : u$, where u is the number of unaffected births that occur for each DS birth. The usual screening limit which determines a high DS–risk is then denoted by $1 : 250$. This is the cut-off point associated with 35–years–old mothers (Wald et al. (1998)). Such screening, based on maternal age, identified about 30% of DS affected pregnancies.

Let T be a binary performance variable, defining the presence ($T = 1$) or absence ($T = 0$) of DS so that, when using maternal age (J) as the screening variable,

$$\begin{aligned} P(T = 1 \mid J = j) &= p_j, \\ P(T = 0 \mid J = j) &= 1 - p_j. \end{aligned}$$

where p_j is the probability of DS associated with a mother aged j. The maternal age–specific–risk associated to a j–years–old mother will be then denoted by $1 : u_j$ where

$$u_j = \frac{1 - p_j}{p_j}. \tag{1}$$

Cuckle et al (1987) use combined data of eight large surveys from British Columbia (1961-70), Massachusetts (1958-65), New York (1968-74), Ohio (1970-79), Sweden (1968-70), South Australia (1960-77), South Belgium (1971-78) and South Wales (1968-76) to estimate the probability p_j as

$$p_j = 0.000627 + \exp(-16.2395 + 0.286j)$$

a model we consider has some probabilistic inconsistency, as it may lead to probability values greater that 1.

Following a Bayesian approach, Marin et al (2003) propose a binomial distribution to model the number of DS pregnancies,

$$d_{ij} \sim Bin(n_{ij}, p_{ij})$$

where $i = 1, \ldots, 8$ represents each one of the eight surveys presented in Cuckle et al. (1984), n_{ij} is the total number of pregnant women aged j in survey i and p_{ij} is the corresponding probability of DS, modelled by a quadratic logistic equation

$$logit(p_{ij}) = a_i + b_i \cdot j + c_i \cdot j^2 \tag{2}$$

with common priors $a_i \sim N(\mu_a, \sigma_a^2)$, $b_i \sim N(\mu_b, \sigma_b^2)$, $c_i \sim N(\mu_c, \sigma_c^2)$ and non–informative priors for the hiperparameters μ_a, μ_b, μ_c, σ_a^2, σ_b^2, σ_c^2.

2.2 Serum Markers and DS Pregnancies

Maternal age screening was improved by incorporating information about α-fetoproteine (AFP) levels, a maternal serum marker whose concentration had been founded to be about 25% lower in Ds pregnancies than in unaffected ones (see Merkatz et al. (1984) and Cuckle et. al. (1984)). This new method of screening identified about 35% of DS pregnancies, a 5% greater detection rate than maternal age alone. In 1987 Bogart et al show that levels of maternal serum hCG were about twice as high in DS pregnancies as in unaffected pregnancies. Reports followed (Canick et al (1988), Wald et al (1988)) showing that levels of uE3 were about 25% lower in DS pregnancies. Other serum markers were subsequently identified and incorporated in the design of screening test, including the free units of hCG (α and β) and in 1996 dimeric inhibit–A was shown to increase the detection rate to 76% when used in combination with AFP, uE3 and total hCG (see Wald et. al. (1996, 1997)).

Marin et al (2003) reanalyzed the effect of maternal age and AFP serum marker on prenatal risks of Down syndrome, using a totally Bayesian framework for first time in the Down syndrome literature. Here, we follow their Bayesian approach, and extend their work by incorporating the effect of three other markers, uE3, hCG and DIA, reanalysing this way the currently used quadruple screening test that combines maternal age information as well as four serum markers levels.

3 Method

We are now interested in the development of an antenatal screening procedure on the basis of the serum markers AFP, uE3, hCG and DIA as well as maternal age.

We define a multivariate screening variable $\boldsymbol{X}$ as the log_{10}–value of the concentrations of the four different markers AFP, hCG, uE3, and DIA expressed in MoM, that is $\boldsymbol{X} = (X_1, X_2, X_3, X_4)$ where

$$\begin{aligned} X_1 &= log_{10}(AFP) \\ X_2 &= log_{10}(uE3) \\ X_3 &= log_{10}(hCG) \\ X_4 &= log_{10}(DIA) \end{aligned}$$

so that the probability of a j years old woman having a DS–pregnancy may be expressed as a function of the screening value $\boldsymbol{X}$, i.e. $P(T = 1 \mid J, \boldsymbol{X}) = p_j(\boldsymbol{x})$. We are interested in the associated risk $1 : u_j(\boldsymbol{x})$ which is, after simple computations,

$$\begin{aligned} u_j(\boldsymbol{x}) &= \frac{P(T=0 \mid J, \boldsymbol{X})}{P(T=1 \mid J, \boldsymbol{X})} \\ &= \frac{p(\boldsymbol{x} \mid T=0)P(T=0 \mid J)}{p(\boldsymbol{x} \mid T=1)P(T=1 \mid J)}. \end{aligned}$$

Therefore, we can express the risk factor of interest in terms of

$$u_j(\boldsymbol{x}) = cf(\boldsymbol{x}) \cdot u_j$$

where $cf(\boldsymbol{x})$ is a correction factor summarising the effect of the AFP serum marker

$$cf(\boldsymbol{x}) = \frac{p(\boldsymbol{x} \mid T=0)}{p(\boldsymbol{x} \mid T=1)}$$

and u_j is the age specific relative risk given by (1), estimated here by following the hierarchical Bayesian approach presented in Marin et.al (2003).

It is generally accepted, see Wald et al. (1998), that the distribution of the screening variable $\boldsymbol{X}$ is well specified as a multivariate normal distribution, in each population of interest (DS and non–DS affected fetuses), that is,

$$\boldsymbol{X} \mid T = i, \boldsymbol{\mu}_i, \boldsymbol{\Sigma}_i \sim N(\boldsymbol{\mu}_i, \boldsymbol{\Sigma}_i), \tag{3}$$

with unknown mean vector and covariance matrix $(\boldsymbol{\mu}_i, \boldsymbol{\Sigma}_i)$ for $i = 0, 1$, respectively.

Let the prior knowledge about the parameters $\mu_i, \boldsymbol{\Sigma}_i$ be summarised by the prior distributions $\pi(\mu_i, \boldsymbol{\Sigma}_i)$ for $i = 0, 1$. We shall use independent non–informative prior distributions

$$\pi(\mu_i, \boldsymbol{\Sigma}_i) \propto |\boldsymbol{\Sigma}_i|^{5/2}.$$

Recall that this prior may be seen as the non–informative version of the $NIW(\boldsymbol{A}_i, d_i, \boldsymbol{a}_i, c_i)$ distribution for which $d_i \to -1$, $c_i \to 0$, $\boldsymbol{A}_i \to -1$. By developing a conjugate Bayesian approach, it leads to NIW posterior distributions with parameters,

$$\begin{aligned} \boldsymbol{A}_i^* &= (n_i - 1)\boldsymbol{S}_i \\ d_i^* &= d_i + n_i \\ \boldsymbol{a}_i^* &= \overline{\boldsymbol{x}}_i \\ c_i^* &= n_i. \end{aligned}$$

Furthermore, by assuming those non–informative priors, the predictive posteriors of $\boldsymbol{X} \mid T = i$ are found to be multivariate $Student-t$ distributions with $\nu_i = n_i - 4$ degrees of freedom and parameters $\boldsymbol{m}_i = \bar{\boldsymbol{x}}_i$ and $\boldsymbol{W}_i = \frac{(n_i+1)}{n_i(n_i-4)}\boldsymbol{A}_i^*$, where $\bar{\boldsymbol{x}}_i$, $\boldsymbol{S}_i$ are the usual sample statistics and n_i are the number of observations.

The four serum markers effect correction factor may thus be given by the following expression

$$cf(\boldsymbol{x}) = \frac{\frac{\Gamma(\frac{n_0}{2})/\Gamma(\frac{n_0-4}{2})}{(n_0-4)^2}\,|\boldsymbol{W}_0|^{-1/2}\left\{1 + \frac{(\boldsymbol{x}-\bar{\boldsymbol{x}}_0)^T\boldsymbol{W}_0^{-1}(\boldsymbol{x}-\bar{\boldsymbol{x}}_0)}{(n_0-4)}\right\}^{-n_0/2}}{\frac{\Gamma(\frac{n_1}{2})/\Gamma(\frac{n_1-4}{2})}{(n_1-4)^2}\,|\boldsymbol{W}_1|^{-1/2}\left\{1 + \frac{(\boldsymbol{x}-\bar{\boldsymbol{x}}_1)^T\boldsymbol{W}_1^{-1}(\boldsymbol{x}-\bar{\boldsymbol{x}}_1)}{(n_1-4)}\right\}^{-n_1/2}}.$$

The relationship between DS risk and the serum markers AFP, uE3, hCG and DIA is analytically derived from summary statistics published by Wald et. al. (2003) for $n_1 = 101$ DS and $n_0 = 43712$ unaffected pregnancies, as follow,

- Mean of log_{10}–serum markers values as

  $$\bar{\boldsymbol{x}}_1 = (-0.1308, -0.1549, 0.3118, 0.3384)$$

  in Down syndrome pregnancies and

  $$\bar{\boldsymbol{x}}_0 = (0.0000, 0.0000, 0.0000, 0.0000)$$

  in unaffected pregnancies.
- Covariance matrices between markers as

  $$\boldsymbol{S}_1 = \begin{pmatrix} 0.0224 & 0.0000 & 0.0077 & 0.0081 \\ 0.0000 & 0.0190 & -0.0127 & -0.0112 \\ 0.0077 & -0.0127 & 0.0588 & 0.0284 \\ 0.0081 & -0.0112 & 0.0284 & 0.0741 \end{pmatrix}$$

  and

  $$\boldsymbol{S}_0 = \begin{pmatrix} 0.0224 & 0.0050 & 0.0062 & 0.0073 \\ 0.0050 & 0.0167 & -0.0025 & -0.0024 \\ 0.0062 & -0.0025 & 0.0532 & 0.0217 \\ 0.0073 & -0.0024 & 0.0217 & 0.0456 \end{pmatrix}$$

4 Results

In order to show the performance of the proposed Bayesian method and the importance of presenting results in terms of probability intervals, which indicate the uncertainty in our estimations, rather than point estimates, we consider two different hypothetical values for each one of the four serum markers considered.

Figures 1 to 5 show 95% high probability intervals of risk of having a Down syndrome pregnancy for maternal ages between 35 and 39 and for the different combinations of the serum marker levels. Classical point estimates as calculated by classical methods, and by using Wald et al (2003) summary statitics, are also displayed.

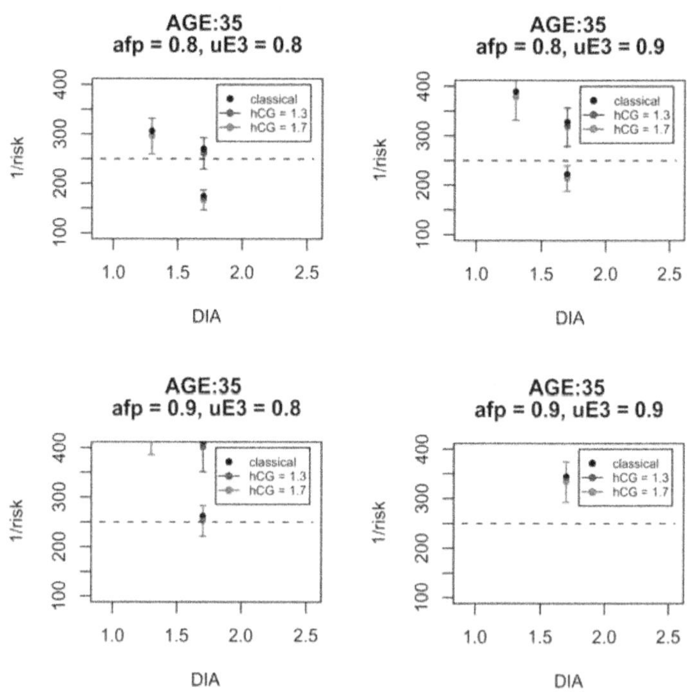

Figure 1: Down Syndrome risk for women aged 35 in combination with several levels of four serum markers (AFP, uE3, hCG and DIA)

As an example, Figure 1 corresponds to a maternal age of 35 years old. The four plots displayed show DIA levels (1.3 and 1.7) against risk of having a DS pregnancy for

- afp levels of 0.8 (two top plots) and 0.9 (two bottom plots),
- uE3 levels of 0.8 (two left plots) and 0.9 (two right plots) and
- hCG levels of 1.3 (blue) and 1.7 (red).

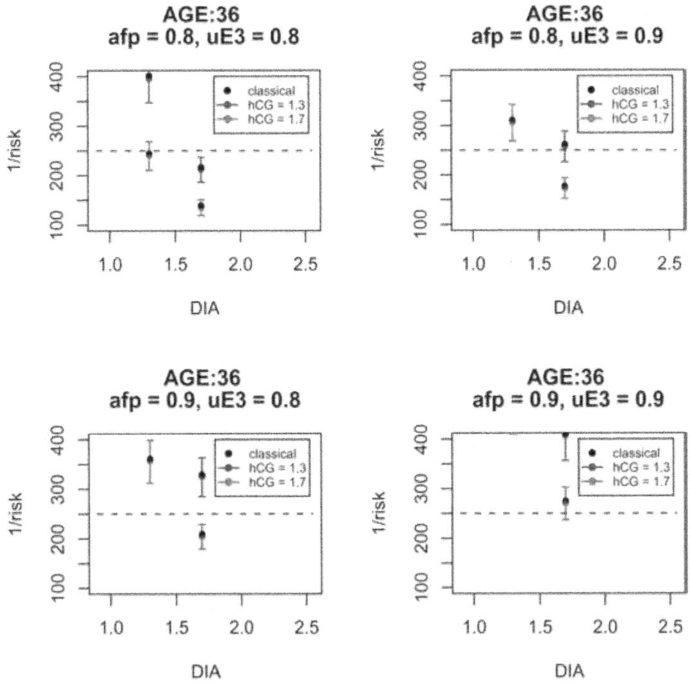

Figure 2: Down Syndrome risk for women aged 36 in combination with several levels of four serum markers (AFP, uE3, hCG and DIA)

Note that AFP and uE3 effects can be appreciated by comparing plots within the same maternal age vertically and horizontally, respectively and hCG effect can be observed by comparing different color probability intervals.

Most importantly, it should be highlighted that by considering probability intervals of the estimated DS risk, instead of point estimates, we can appreciate how much uncertainty it remains in the results of a screening test. Figures 1 to 5 show that some cases that would be negatively screened using the classical screening procedure, would be positively screened by the Bayesian methods developed in this study. Whereas our method would suggest the performance of amniocentesis, no further diagnostic test would be suggested by Wald et al. (2003). Similarly, for some cases where the classic method suggests amniocentesis, there is a reasonable doubt that there is a need for it.

For instance, let us consider two hypothetical cases of two pregnant women, both aged 37 for which blood tests report serum marker levels of $\boldsymbol{x} = (0.8, 0.9, 1.7, 1.3)$ and $\boldsymbol{x}' = (0.9, 0.8, 1.3, 1.7)$ MoM, respectively. The first case would be positively screened for amniocentesis when using classical policy given that their estimate risk (1:245) is higher than the usual cut–off $1:250$. The second case would not be considered for any further diagnostic test as its DS risk is estimated as $1:260$, lower than $1:250$.

4 Results

In order to show the performance of the proposed Bayesian method and the importance of presenting results in terms of probability intervals, which indicate the uncertainty in our estimations, rather than point estimates, we consider two different hypothetical values for each one of the four serum markers considered.

Figures 1 to 5 show 95% high probability intervals of risk of having a Down syndrome pregnancy for maternal ages between 35 and 39 and for the different combinations of the serum marker levels. Classical point estimates as calculated by classical methods, and by using Wald et al (2003) summary statitics, are also displayed.

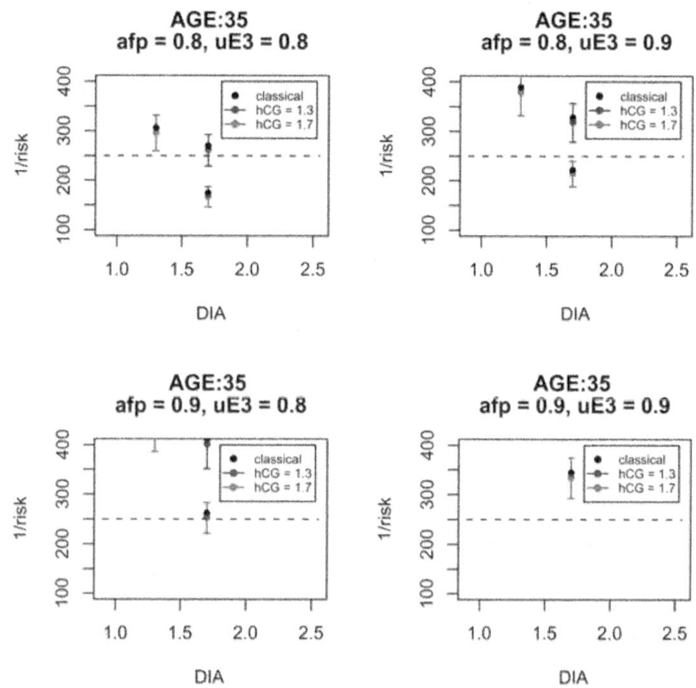

Figure 1: Down Syndrome risk for women aged 35 in combination with several levels of four serum markers (AFP, uE3, hCG and DIA)

As an example, Figure 1 corresponds to a maternal age of 35 years old. The four plots displayed show DIA levels (1.3 and 1.7) against risk of having a DS pregnancy for

- afp levels of 0.8 (two top plots) and 0.9 (two bottom plots),
- uE3 levels of 0.8 (two left plots) and 0.9 (two right plots) and
- hCG levels of 1.3 (blue) and 1.7 (red).

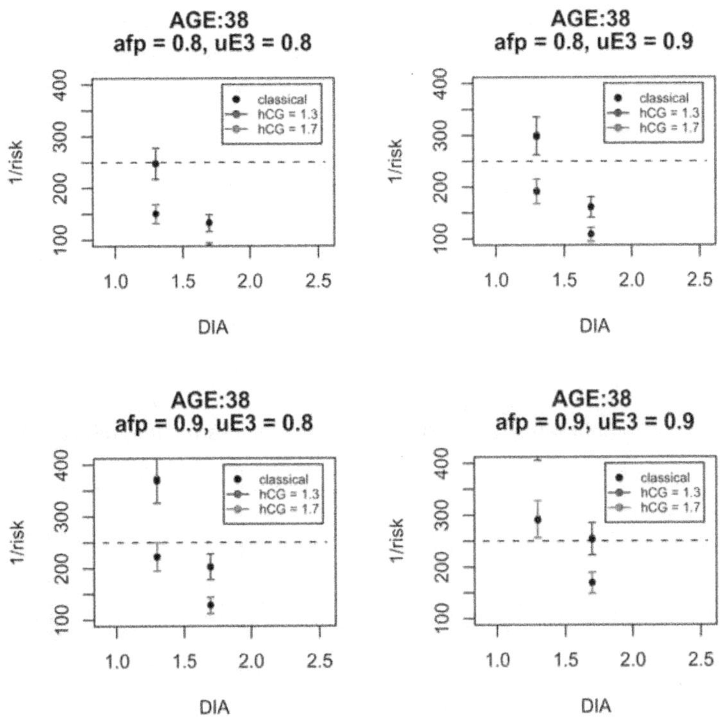

Figure 4: Down Syndrome risk for women aged 38 in combination with several levels of four serum markers (AFP, uE3, hCG and DIA)

exists that could call into doubt the reliability of the DS screening protocol currently used. This is confirmed by software discrepancies as reported by Muller et al. (1999).

We are interested in improving this research by incorporating into the model several factors that have an influence on serum marker levels (gestational age, mother's weight, smoking, ethnic origin, diabetic status, etc.).

Most importantly, we would like to investigate the screening cut–off point which differentiates between low/high–risk pregnancies (and thus which determines the decision of whether or not to perform amniocentesis). The limit was estimated as 1:250 by equating its value to the risk that a miscarriage took place as a consequence of amniocentesis. DS–screening is an area of medical research, constantly being improved with new discoveries. It has come to our attention the fact that such a critical cut-off level has not changed since the very early stages of prenatal screening. Moreover, we are interested in developing a decision analysis and screening procedure which, under the Bayesian framework, allow the antenatal diagnosis of the Down's syndrome.

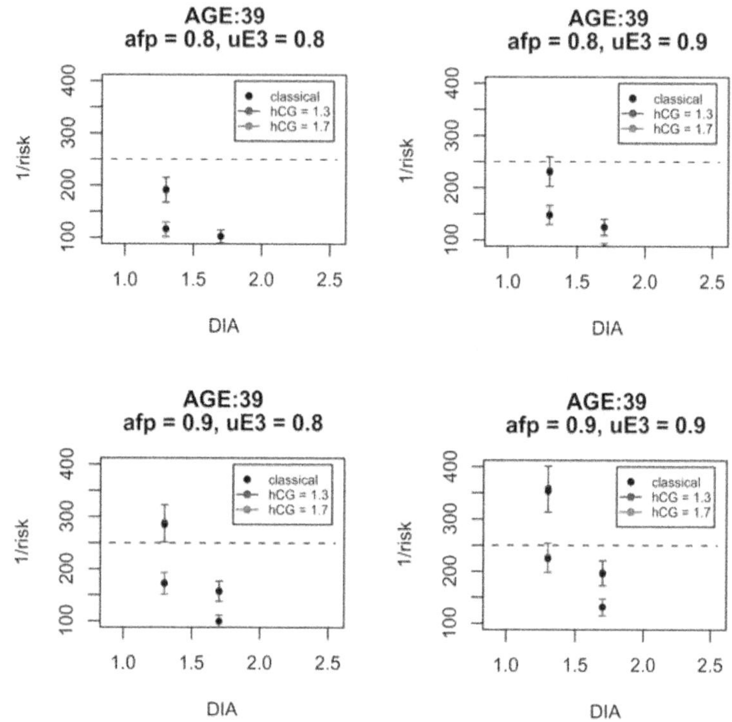

Figure 5: Down Syndrome risk for women aged 39 in combination with several levels of four serum markers (AFP, uE3, hCG and DIA)

Acknowledgments

This research was supported by grants from URJC, CAM and MCYT. The authors would like to thank Dr. Mancheño, head of the Biochemical department of the Gregorio Marañon Hospital of Madrid for pointing out this problem.

References

Canick, J., Knight, G.J., Palomaki, G.E., Haddow, J.E., Cuckle, H.S., Wald, N.J. (1988). Low second trimester maternal serum unconjugate oestriol in pregnancies with Down's syndrome. *British Journal of Obstetrics and Gynaecology*, **95**, 330–333.

Cuckle, H.S., Wald, N.J. and Lindenbaum, R.H. (1984). Maternal serum alpha-fetoprotein measurement: a screening test for Down syndrome. *Lancet* **i**, 926–9.

Cuckle, H.S., Wald, N.J. and Thompson, S.G. (1987). Estimating a woman's risk of having a pregnancy associated with Down's syndrome using her age and serum alpha–fetoprotein level. *British Journal of Obstetrics and Gynaecology*, **94**, 387–402.

Marin,J.M., Montes Diez, R. and Ríos Insua, D. (2003). Some Models for Down's syndrome risk prediction. *Case Studies in Bayesian Statistics*, **6**, 303–312. Springer–Verlag

Merkatz, I.R., Nitowsky, H.M., Macri, J.N. and Johnson, W.E. (1984) An association between low maternal serum alpha-fetoprotein and fetal chromosomal abnormalities. *Am J Obstet Gynecol*, **148**, 886–94.

Muller F., Aegerter, P., Ngo, S., Fort, A., Beauchet, A., Giraudet, P. and Dommergues, M.(1999). Software for Prenatal Down Syndrome Risk Calculation: A Comparative Study of Six Software Packages. *Clinical Chemistry*, **45**, 8, 1278–1280.

Valenti, C., Schutta, E.J. and Kenathy T. Prenatal diagnosis of Down's syndrome. (1968) *Lancet* **ii** 220.

Wald, N.J., Cuckle, H.S., Densem, J.W., Nanchahal, K., Canick, J., Haddow, J.E., et. al. (1988). Maternal serum unconjugated oestriol as an antenatal screening test for Down's syndrome. *British Journal of Obstetrics and Gynaecology*, **95**, 334–341.

Wald, N.J., Densem, J.W., George, L., Muttukrishana, S. Knight, P.G. (1996). Prenatal screening for Down's syndrome using inhibin–A as a serum unconjugated marker. *Prenat Diagn*, **16**, 143–153.

Wald, N.J., Densem, J.W., George, L., Muttukrishana, S. Knight, P.G., Watt, H. et. al. (1997). Inhibin–A in Down's syndrome pregnancies: revised estimate of standard deviation.*Prenat Diagn*, **17**, 285–290.

Wald, N.J., Kennard, A. Hackshaw, A. and McGuire, A. (1998). Antenatal screening for Down's syndrome. *Health Technology Assessment*, **2**, 1.

Wald, N.J., Rodeck, C., Hackshaw, A.K., Walters, J. Chitty, L. and Mackinson, A.M. (2003). First and second trimestre antenatal screening for Down's syndrome: the results of the Serum, Urine and Ultrasound Screening Study (SURUSS). *Health Technology Assessment*, **7**, 11.

SOC: A Distributed Decision Support Architecture for Clinical Diagnosis

Javier Vicente[1,*], Juan M. Garcia-Gomez[1], César Vidal[1], Luís Marti-Bonmati[2], Aurora del Arco[3], and Montserrat Robles[1]

[1] BET, Informática Médica. Universidad Politécnica de Valencia. Spain
[2] Servicio de Radiología. Hospital U. Dr. Peset. Valencia. Spain
[3] Servicio de Hematología. Hospital U. Dr. Peset. Valencia. Spain

Abstract. In this paper we introduce SOC (*Sistema de Orientación Clínica*, Clinic Orientation System), a novel distributed decision support system for clinical diagnosis. The decision support systems are based on pattern recognition engines which solve different and specific classification problems.
SOC is based on a distributed architecture with three specialized nodes: 1) Information System where the remote data is stored, 2) Decision Support Webservices which contains the developed pattern recognition engines and 3) Visual Interface, the clinicians' point of access to local and remote data, statistical anasysis tools and distributed information.
A location-independent and multi-platform system has been developed to bring together hospitals and institutions to research useful tools in clinical and laboratory environments. The nodes maintenance and upgrade are automatically controlled by the architecture.
Two examples of the application of SOC are presented. The first example is the Soft Tissue Tumors (STT) diagnosis. The decision support systems are based on pattern recognition engines to classify between benign/malignant character and histological groups with good estimated efficiency. In the second example we present clinical support for Microcytic Anemia (MA) diagnosis. For this task, the decision support systems are based, too, on pattern recognition engines to classify between normal, ferropenic anemia and thalassemia.
This tool will be useful for several puposes: to assist the radiologist/hematologist decision in a new case and help the education of new radiologist/hematologist without expertise in STT or MA diagnosis.

Keywords: Clinical Decision Support Systems, Health Informatics, Medical Information Systems, Distributed Systems, Web Services, Soft Tissue Tumor, Thalassemia, Pattern Recognition.

1 Introduction

Decision Support Systems (DSS) are interactive computer based systems that assist decision makers to use data, models, solvers, and user interfaces to solve semi-structured and /or unstructured problems [1]. In this framework, a clinical decision support system (CDSS) is defined to be any software (DSS) designed to directly aid

---

* Address for correspondence, Javier Vicente Robledo, Dpto. Física Aplicada., Universidad Politécnica de Valencia, Camino de Vera s/n, 46022, Valencia, Spain, javirob@upvnet.upv.es, Telf: +34 963877000, Ext. 75278

J.M. Barreiro et al. (Eds.): ISBMDA 2004, LNCS 3337, pp. 96–104, 2004.

clinical decision making, whereby through the use of specific CDSS, useful characteristics of the patient are made available to clinicians for considerations [2].

The three main features that a CDSS integrates are: medical knowledge which solves the disease cases, patient data with specific biomedical information of each patient, and specific advice for each case based on the medical knowledge and the patient data [3].

CDSS does not make decisions but supports diagnostic decisions of doctors. CDSS is viewed as information technology, defined as mechanisms to implement desired information handling in the organisation [4]. Thus CDSS also supports work procedures and organisational goals. Some CDSS incorporates fuzzy logic to overcome restrictions of diagnostic programs. Pathophysiologic reasoning has also been used to represent temporal evaluation of single and multiple disease process [5].

The conclusion drawn by a review done by Hunt et al. [2] over a twenty-five years period showed that the CDSS improve health practitioners' performances, but however, less frequently, improve the patients outcome.

In this paper, section two describes the software requirements of the CDSS, the architecture selected and the chosen technology for its implementation. Section three exposes the CDSS visual interface developed and two real examples of application in a hospital. Discussion takes place in section four. This is followed by the conclusions, future works and the acknowledgments.

2 Materials and Methods

2.1 Software Requirements

There are different methods to design CDSS using the artificial intelligence approach. In this study an inductive strategy, more commonly named *pattern recognition* (PR) strategy, was applied. The conclusions made by the *clinical decision support system* were inferred by the knowledge captured from a group of samples representing the problem.

The most difficult problem in decision support developing is to compile enough patients' data to infer good PR models. Due to the need of increasing the available data for improving the PR models, a distribute architecture has been chosen. Thus, maintenance and upgrading of PR models could be done in a transparent way to the user.

A location independent and multi-platform system is required. It is also needs the connection to local databases and Hospital Information System.

2.2 Distributed Decision Support Architecture

Independent nodes compose the SOC (*Sistema de Orientación Clínica*, Clinic Orientation System) architecture. The nodes are specialized in three main groups and a web server infrastructure (see figure 1):

Visual Interface

Provide the only access point to the system. From here, clinicians can obtain decision support and statistical information about soft tissue tumors registers or hematological cases.

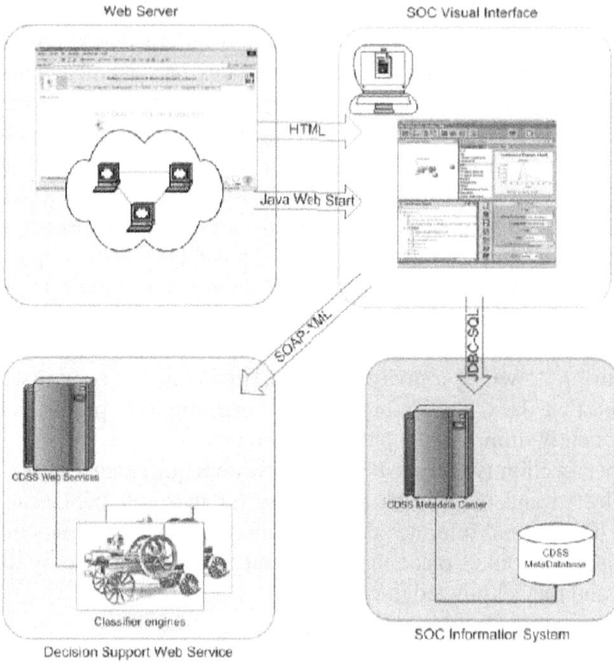

Fig. 1. SOC distributed architecture

Information System
It contains the patients' registers with the variables and diagnosis already accomplished. It incorporates variables meta-information to allow statistical analysis. It also provides secure access to its contents. Modular design allows upgrading the system to connect a general Hospital Information System.

Decision Support Web-Services
Web services provide STT and hematological classifiers engines developed with pattern recognition technology. It can be distributed around Internet and incorporate different PR techniques.

The Visual Interface can connect to local or distributed registers to analyze saved patients or incorporate new data. It also can show statistical information processed locally, or invoke the decision support web-services to take diagnosis decision support for the selected task (STT or hematological studies). Connections between nodes will be secure and nodes will identify itself at each moment.

Maintenance and upgrade process of Visual Interface nodes will be automatically controlled by the Web based system of the SOC architecture.

2.3 Used Technology

One of the main requirements is to develop a location independent and multi-platform system. With Java Web Start technology, clinicians can obtain the latest version of SOC available in a transparent way.

On the other hand, it is desirable to allow an automatic improvement and upgrading of the PR engines. For this purposes, the Decision Support Web Service is located remotely containing the PR classifier engines. Petitions of use and detailed information of engines are sending via XML documents between SOC and web services. This exchange information with XML documents can be easily done with SOAP technology.

3 Results

3.1 Visual Interface Functionalities

The user access to the SOC is achieved using a Visual Interface. This application contains four windows that offer the main system functionalities areas:

Access to Database Registers
It is the access point to local or distributed Information System that contains the features to study (see figure 2). New data can be imported from MSAccess formatted files or other databases.

Statistical Analysis
It shows a statistical report of the data set being used, including graphical charts. It also provides evaluation information like a uni-variable study of the sample distribution per class, frequency of discrete variables or the approximation of a continuous variable to the normal distribution. Finally, it contains a toolkit for extracting probability distributions per class, correlation studies and ROC curves (see figure 3).

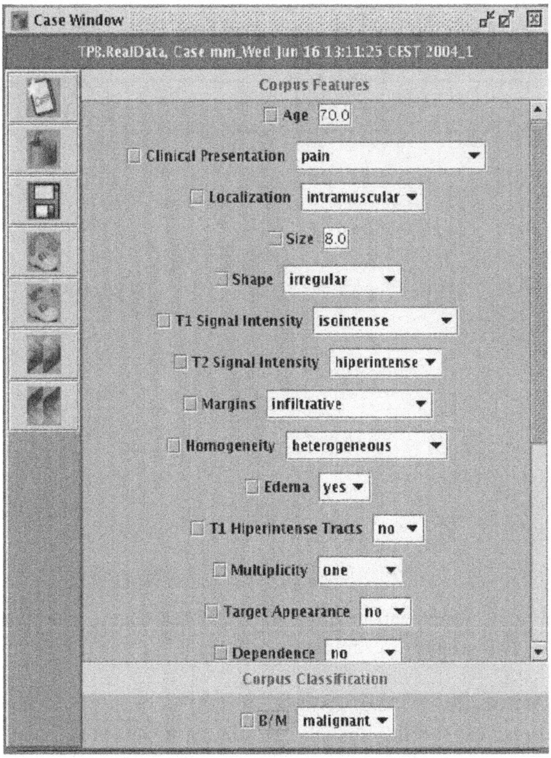

Fig. 2. Database Window aspect in SOC Visual Interface, real patient for Soft Tissue Tumors diagnosis are shown

Graphical Representation of Data
It provides an intuitive graphical representation of features from the selected data set. A 3D representation can be done by selecting three parameters manually or leaving the system to select them automatically (autoselection of features). It also provides a module which can generate PCA and other similar transformations (see figure 4).

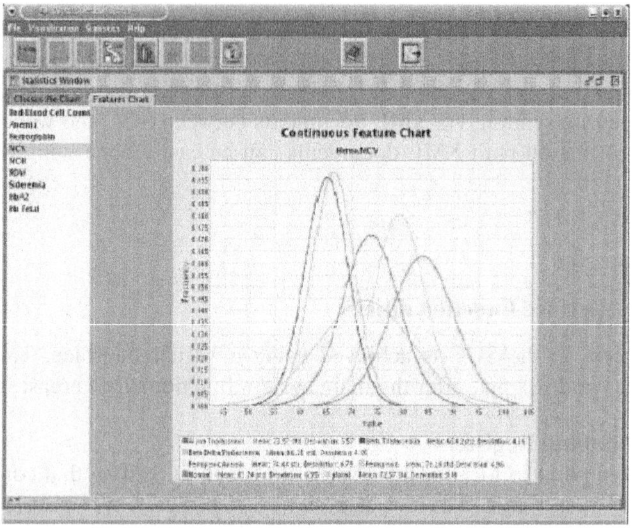

Fig. 3. Statistical window, real continuous distribution of a Microcytic Anemia data set

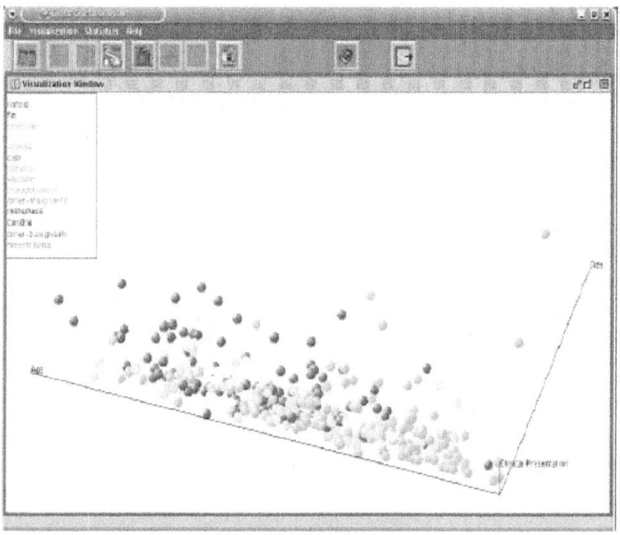

Fig. 4. Visualization window, 3 selected features for real values representation of STT histological groups discrimination

Automatic Classification

It access to the distributed decision support web-services, developed with pattern recognition technology. Each engine located in the PR server contains a scientific report with details of the training process and corpus, evaluation methods, results and audit statistics which enables its reproducibility. XML visualization details are shown at figure 5.

Information exchange between the PR server and SOC is done via XML documents. This allows an efficient communication for sending request and showing results. It also makes easy the upgrading of classifiers which is transparent for the user (see figure 1 at previous subsection).

As a result, the global aspect of the SOC Visual Interface is shown in figure 6.

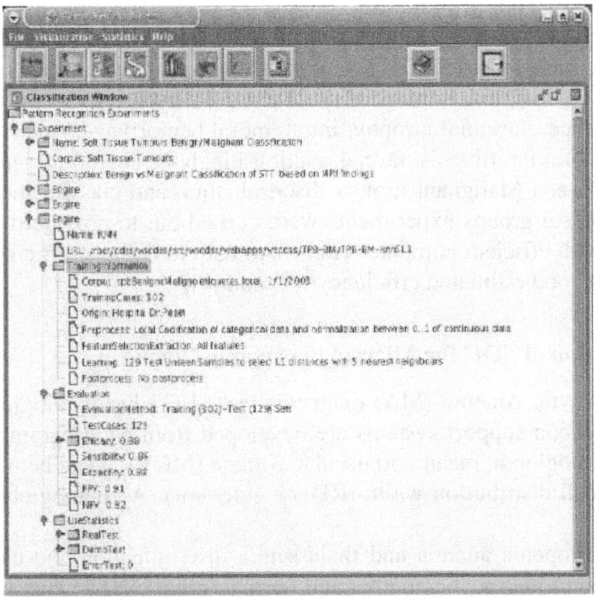

Fig. 5. XML report of a PR engine for STT Benign/Malignant discrimination

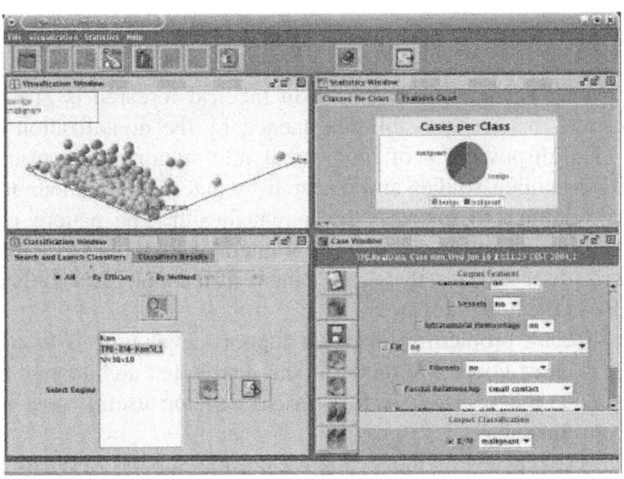

Fig. 6. SOC Visual Interface aspect

3.2 Application of SOC for Soft Tissue Tumors Diagnosis

Two real examples of the application of SOC will be exposed.

In both examples, experiments were developed using consolidated PR techniques as artificial neural networks (ANN), support vector machines (SVM), decision trees

(DT), multinomial (MN) parametric classify and k nearest neighbors (KNN) [6]. Efficiency and other reliability parameters were measured from the classifiers using unseen patient registers.

The first task exposed is the Soft Tissue Tumors (STT) diagnosis. The decision support system uses the following Magnetic Resonance image findings obtained from the radiological examination [7]: age, clinical presentation, localization, size, shape, signal intensity, margins, homogeneity, edema, T1-hyperintense tracts, multiplicity, target appearance, muscular atrophy, intratumoral hemorrhage, calcification, dependence, intratumoral fat, fibrosis, fascial relationship, bone alterations and vessels.

Benign between Malignant tumors discrimination and classification between different histological groups experiments were carried out to provide the decision support system with efficient computer engines to help radiologist. The generated classifiers obtained good estimated efficiency ([7] and [8]).

3.3 Application of SOC for Microcytic Anemia Diagnosis

For the Microcytic Anemia (MA) diagnosis task, 1233 haematological studies were used. The decision support systems are developed from eight parameters: red blood cell count, hemoglobin, mean corpuscular volume (MCV), mean hemoglobin volume (MHV), red cell distribution width (RDW), sideremia, A2 hemoglobin and fetal hemoglobin.

Normal, ferropenic anemia and thalassemia discrimination and classification between 5 different microcytic anemia and normal group experiments were carried out to provide clinical orientation to help hematologist [9].

4 Discussion

The use of pattern recognition approach in medical research is growing more and more, because of the new possibilities opened by the digitalization of biomedical information. The disposability of biomedical information in electronic repositories enables the data mining studies and research by automatic methods to get new and interesting correlations to improve the human health. The pattern recognition approach can help the search of biomedical pointers of important diseases (like tumors or degenerative diseases) and the development of technological tools applied to the clinical and basic medicine research.

The most difficult problem in decision support developing is to compile enough patients' data to infer good PR models. The distributed architecture of SOC, bring together hospitals and research institutions to develop useful tools in clinical and laboratory environments.

Consensus between several independent Decision Support Services could improve individual results of PR engines or experts. A future functionality will show distributed decisions, extracting more confident conclusions.

5 Conclusion

This system could help radiologist with novel and powerful methods in soft tissue tumours diagnosis as well as orientate haematologists on the thalassemia and other microcytyc anemia diagnosis. It provides access to distributed data, statistical analysis, graphical representation and pattern recognition classification.

SOC is a Decision Support System which can supply help on different diagnosis tasks. This tool will be useful for several puposes: to assist the radiologist/hematologist decision in a new case and help the education of new radiologist/hematologist without expertise in STT or MA diagnosis.

The introduced architecture enables experts to audit and upgrade pattern recognition engines and improve together the diagnosis decision tasks.

6 Future Works

SOC is currently being tested and validated in the respective services of Hematology and Radiology of Hospital Universitario Dr. Peset (Valencia, Spain). The main objective of this validation is checking the use that clinicians will do of the CDSS. The feedback obtained from the experience of real final users will allow the SOC visual interface to be retouch or improve according to clinicians' needs and comments.

Finally, one of the future works to be done is adding GRID technology for SOC. It will incorporate more standardized, confident and powered communications to the SOC distributed decision support system allowing several PR engines servers and encrypted communication between SOC and remote servers. It also will provide an authentication system and other important security aspects.

Acknowledgments

The authors thank the involved hospitals in the project (Hospital Universitario San Juan de Alicante, Hospital Universitario Dr Peset de Valencia, Hospital Cruces de Baracaldo, Hospital Juan Canalejo de La Coruña and Hôpital Universitaire de Toulouse) for their recruiting support, ADIRM (Asociación para el Desarrollo y la Investigación en Resonancia Magnética) for their members' scientific advice, Ministerio de Sanidad y Consumo supporting grant INBIOMED, and Universidad Politécnica de Valencia for its supporting grant 20010690.

References

1. Sprague, R. H. (1980), "A Framework for the Development of DSS", MIS Quarterly.
2. Hunt DL, Haynes RB, Hanna SE, Smith K., "Effects of computer based clinical decision support systems on physician performance and patient outcomes: a systematic review", Journal of the American Medical Assoc. (JAMA), 1998; 280: pp.1339-1346.
3. Van der Lei J, Talmon JL (1997) "Clinical decision-support systems". In: van Bemmel, J.H., & Musen, M.A., (eds) (1997) Handbook of medical informatics. pp. 261276. Springer.
4. Avgerou C. and Cornford T., 1993, *Developing Information Systems:Concepts, Issues and Practise,* Basingstroke, UK: Macmillan.
5. Mazoue J. G., 1990, *The Journal of Medicine and Philosophy*, "Diagnosis without doctors", Vol. 15, pp. 559579.
6. Duda R O, Hart Peter E, Stork David G (2001) "Pattern Classification", Wiley- Interscience.
7. Garcia-Gomez, César Vidal, Luis Martí-Bonmatí, Joaquín Galant, Nicolas Sans, Montserrat Robles, Francisco Casacuberta, (2003). "Benign/Malignant Classifier of Soft Tissue Tumours using MR-Imaging". Magma (Accepted, not published yet).

8. García-Gómez J M., Vidal C, Juan A, Martí-Bonmatí L, Galant J, Robles M, (2002) "Pattern classification techniques applied to Soft Tissue Tumours using MR and epidemiological data". Proceedings 19th annual meeting of the European Society for Magnetic Resonance in Medicine and Biology. pp 274-275.
9. Vicente J, del Arco A, García-Gómez J M, Vidal C, Robles M, (2003) "Automatic Classification of thalassemias and other microcytic and hypochrome anemia" (actual text in spanish) Congreso Anual de la Sociedad Española de Ingeniería Biomédica 2003, pp 6369.

Decision Support Server Architecture for Mobile Medical Applications

Marek Kurzynski[1] and Jerzy Sas[2]

[1] Wroclaw University of Technology, Faculty of Electronics, Division of Medical Informatics, Wyb. Wyspianskiego 27, 50-370 Wroclaw, Poland
Marek.Kurzynski@pwr.wroc.pl

[2] Wroclaw University of Technology, Faculty of Computer Science and Management, Division of Computer Science, Wyb. Wyspianskiego 27, 50-370 Wroclaw, Poland
Jerzy.Sas@pwr.wroc.pl

Abstract. In the paper, the architecture for a mobile medical decision support and its exemplary application to medicines prescribing is presented. The aim of the architecture is to provide the decision algorithms and database support for thin client applications running on low cost palmtop computers. We consider the wide class of medical applications, where decision making is equivalent to typical pattern recognition problem. The decision support consists in ordering the decisions by their degree of belief in the context, in which the decision is being made, and presenting them in such order to the user. The role of the palmtop computer is to organize the dialog with the user, while the role of decision support server consists in decision algorithm executing, and delivering the results to a mobile application. Providing the ordered decision list to the palmtop application not only aids the user in making right decision, but also significantly simplifies the user interaction with the keyboard-less palmtop device. The relation between these two topics is shown and the method of user interface dynamic configuration is proposed.

1 Introduction

The mobile access to patient data offers many advantages to physicians. The most important of them are: instant and immediate access to diagnostic and treatment up-to-date information at the point of care, immediate availability of treatment decisions made by other physicians, reduced risk of mistakes introduced on the path from medical decision maker to its execution point, reduction of rework and in result - reduction of healthcare costs. Constantly decreasing prices of handheld computers and the tendency to equip the devices with built-in wireless communication hardware (wireless LAN or Bluetooth) make mobile medical data access systems popular and widely available to hospitals and other healthcare institutions. Mobile devices are typically used as wireless terminals of stationary hospital information systems. Increasing performance of handhelds - currently comparable to typical desktop PC - enables however their usage not only as front-end terminals ([9]) but as fully functional processing units with instant access to database servers maintaining broad range of clinical data. In turn, it makes palmtops effective platform for many medical decision support applications. We will consider the class of medical problems, where decision making consists in selecting the one from the finite set of possible options. Decision support (DS) consists in presenting the ordered set of decisions with the highest belief factor evaluated in the current context influencing the decision process.

J.M. Barreiro et al. (Eds.): ISBMDA 2004, LNCS 3337, pp. 105–116, 2004.

Decisions made in an environment of medical information systems usually concern the patient treatment. Typical examples of such decisions are: decisions concerning medicine orders, application of medical procedures, diagnostic or laboratory test orders etc. Each of them requires entering some data into the computer system using the palmtop interface. Unfortunately, entering data via palmtop is not as comfortable as when using a desktop computer, due to lack of full size keyboard and due to limited size of the palmtop display. Therefore, particular attention has to be paid to careful design of convenient palmtop application user interface (UI). The problem of decision support seems to be strictly related to the problem of making DS palmtop application easy and comfortable in use. Consider for example the problem of drugs prescribing. Using the wireless device, a physician can make decision about drugs administering directly at the patient's bed on the ward. Drug prescribing consists in making the sequence of mutually related decisions, each of them requires some interactions with the palmtop: selecting the medicine from the large set of items, then determining and entering the dosage, specifying the daily repetition count and finally entering the data about administering period. As far as keyboard-less palmtops are concerned the traditional method of data entering using virtual keyboard is troublesome. For this reason the palmtop applications tend rather to use selection list implemented as typical combo box controls. If the lists contain many items then searching the appropriate one also may be inconvenient. If the possible decisions presented on the selection lists will be ordered by their belief factors provided by decision support algorithm, then there is great chance that the decision intended by the user will be close to the top of the list. If so, then it can be easily entered to the computer system just by single tap on the palmtop display.

While the computational power of modern palmtop is sufficient to perform quite complex data processing and calculations, the access to large amount o up-to-date information necessary for decision support is still the problem. Storing the large database on the palmtop side is in many cases impossible due to lack of true mass storage devices. On the other hand, downloading these data from the stationary part of the system, each time the decision is being made, would overload the wireless transmission media. In case of using the communication methods where the transmission cost depends either on the connection time or the volume of transferred data – e.g. with the usage of public cellular phone network - it would cause unacceptable growth of the system operating costs.

Instead of executing the decision algorithms within the palmtop computer, it can be delegated to the stationary part of the medical information system, where large volumes of necessary data can be easily and efficiently retrieved from database server. The application running on the palmtop platform merely prepares the data describing the context of the decision being made, sends it to the stationary part of the system, where the decision is elaborated and finally presents the result to the user. It leads to the concept of back-end Decision Support Server (DSS). DSS is a process running constantly in the stationary part of the medical information system, which executes the decision algorithms on clients requests. In order to assure DSS ability to support various decision problems it must be easily configurable. A special protocol for data exchange between palmtop applications and DSS must also be elaborated.

In this paper, the architecture and exemplary application of a DSS system is described. Chapter 2 contains the formal definition of decision problems class supported by DSS architecture. Particular attention is paid to the relation between decision support and application ease of use aspect. DSS architecture and some design considerations are described in Chapter 3. The exemplary application of the DSS concept in the hospital drug prescription mobile system is presented in Chapter 4. Chapter 5 contains some conclusions and remarks concerning future works.

2 Medical Decision Support and Optimization of Palmtop User Interface

2.1 Preliminaries and the Problem Statement

Let us consider the computer program which makes possible to perform a set of n independent operations:

$$o = \{O_1, O_2, ..., O_n\} . \tag{1}$$

For example, in a medical information system such operations can have the following meaning:

- displaying results of laboratory examinations for given patient for given period,
- prescribing the medicines for a patient,
- ordering the laboratory test, etc.

Operation O_i (i=1,2,...,n) contains a sequence of $m(i)$ data entry actions (DEA):

$$\mathcal{D}_i = (d_{i,1}, d_{i,2}, ..., d_{i,m(i)}) , \tag{2}$$

which sense depends on the meaning of operation (e.g. selection of the patient, selection of the medicine, determining the unit dose, determining how many times per day the medicine should be administered, determining the period of application, etc.).

The jth action for the ith operation $d_{i,j}$ is not any, but it comes from the set of $n(ij)$ admissible possibilities:

$$\mathcal{D}_{i,j} = \{d_{i,j}^{(1)}, d_{i,j}^{(2)}, ..., d_{i,j}^{n(ij)}\} , \; i = 1,2,...,n, \; j = 1,2,..., m(i) . \tag{3}$$

Since the DEA $d_{i,j}$ consists in choice of one element from (3), hence the DEA will be treated as a decision problem with discrete set of outcomes.

As it was mentioned, the proper arrangement of elements of the set (3) on the palmtop screen can significantly simplify user's manual actions and therefore the task of automatic configuration of the UI is important from the practical point of view. On the other hand, such an arrangement can be considerd as a form of decision support presentation.

We propose to solve this problem using concept of soft classifier [1]. Let suppose, that for DEA $d_{i,j}$ the following data (features) are available:

$x \in \mathcal{X}$ - vector of atributes (clinical data) of the patient being under care,

$\overline{d}_{i,j} = (d_{i,1}^{(k_1)}, d_{i,2}^{(k_2)}, ..., d_{i,j-1}^{(k_{j-1})})$ - sequence of previously undertaken DEA (for operation O_i).

The mapping:

$$\psi_{i,j} : \mathcal{X} \times \mathcal{D}_{i,1} \times \mathcal{D}_{i,2} \times ... \times \mathcal{D}_{i,j-1} \rightarrow [0,1]^{n(ij)} . \tag{4}$$

is a soft classifier for DEA $d_{i,j}$ (i = 1, 2, …, n, j = 1, 2, …, $m(i)$).

The components of its output

$$q_{i,j} = (q_{i,j}^{(1)}, q_{i,j}^{(2)}, ..., q_{i,j}^{n(ij)}) \tag{5}$$

can be regarded as "support" given by classifier $\psi_{i,j}$ for the hypothesis that user wants to execute action $d_{i,j}^{(k)}$. It makes possible to arrange decisions (3) on the palmtop screen according to diminishing values of "degree of belief" $q_{i,j}^{(k)}$. The sense of values (5) depends on the adopted mathematical model of classification task. For example, in the probabilistic model, (5) denote appropriate *a posteriori* probabilities and the classifier (4) leads to the randomized decision rule [3]. In the fuzzy approach, however, (5) mean membership function values of the fuzzy set: "user wants to execute DEA".

Let suppose that vector of patient's attributes x and user's decision $d_{i,j}^{(k)}$ are observed values of a couple of random variables ($\boldsymbol{X}, \boldsymbol{d_{i,j}}$). Let next

$$L_{i,j}(q_{i,j}, d_{i,j}^{(k)}) \tag{6}$$

be the user's discomfort factor concerning the sequence of manual actions which the user has to do, when its decision is $d_{i,j}^{(k)}$ and the screen is ordered according to the algorithm output $q_{i,j}$. Values of factor (6) have subjective character and can be chosen according to the user's individual feeling. Some propositions are given in Chapter 4.

Now our purpose is to determine classifiers (4) which minimize expected values of (6), namely:

$$\psi_{i,j}^{*}: \quad E[L_{i,j}(\psi_{i,j}^{*} = q_{i,j}, d_{i,j}^{(k)})] = \min_{\psi_{i,j}} E[L_{i,j}(\psi_{i,j} = q_{i,j}, d_{i,j}^{(k)})]\,. \tag{7}$$

Some propositions of soft classifiers (4) with regard to criterion (7) will be given in the next section.

2.2 Decision Support Algorithms

In the real world usually it is assumed that available information on the decision problem to be considered is contained in a numerical data (learning set), i.e. set of observed features and correct decisions. In the problem under the question such a set for operation O_i ($i = 1,2,...,n$) has the following form:

$$S_i = \{(x_1, d_{i,1}^{(k_{1,1})}, d_{i,2}^{(k_{1,2})}, ..., d_{i,m(i)}^{(k_{1,m(i)})}), (x_2, d_{i,1}^{(k_{2,1})}, d_{i,2}^{(k_{22})}, ..., d_{i,m(i)}^{(k_{2,m(i)})}), ...,$$
$$(x_m, d_{i,1}^{(k_{m,1})}, d_{i,2}^{(k_{m,2})}, ..., d_{i,n(i)}^{(k_{m,m(i)})})\}, \quad x_j \in \mathcal{X}, \ d_{i,j}^{(k)} \in \mathcal{D}_{i,j}, \ j = 1,2,...,m(i)\,. \tag{8}$$

A single sequence in the learning set denotes a single-patient case that comprises attribute vector x and sequence of data entry actions made by a physician.

Empirical knowledge denotes that instead theoretical criterion (7) we will minimize the empirical one, which leads to the following propositions of Decision Support Algorithms (DSA).

The Soft Empirical Bayes Algorithm

Now $q_{i,j}^{(k)}$ ($k = 1,2,...,n(ij)$) in (5) denotes empirical *a posteriori* probability of decision $d_{i,j}^{(k)}$ which can be calculated from (8) according to the Bayes formula:

$$q_{i,j}^{(k)} = P(d_{i,j}^{(k)} / x, \overline{d}_{i,j}) = \frac{\frac{N_k(\overline{d}_{i,j})}{N(\overline{d}_{i,j})} f(x / \overline{d}_{i,j}, d_{i,j}^{(k)})}{\sum_{k=1}^{n(ij)} \frac{N_k(\overline{d}_{i,j})}{N(\overline{d}_{i,j})} f(x / \overline{d}_{i,j}, d_{i,j}^{(k)})}, \tag{9}$$

where

$N(\overline{d}_{i,j})$ - the number of elements in S_i in which sequence $\overline{d}_{i,j}$ has appeared

$N_k(\overline{d}_{i,j})$ - as previously and additionally $d_{i,j}^{(k_{l,j})} = d_{i,j}^{(k)}$

$f(x / \overline{d}_{i,j}, d_{i,j}^{(k)})$ - empirical conditional probability density functions of x (e.g. calculated using histogram or Parzen estimator [3]).

The Soft K-Nearest Neighbours (K-NN) Decision Rule

The K-NN decision rule is very well known and investigated nonparametric pattern recognition technique [2,3]. Using this concept to our decision problem we get:

$$q_{i,j}^{(k)} = \frac{K_k(x, \overline{d}_{i,j})}{\sum_{k=1}^{n(ij)} K_k(x, \overline{d}_{i,j})}, \tag{10}$$

where $K_k(x, \overline{d}_{i,j})$ denotes the number of learning patterns from among the K ones, nearest to the point x (in the attribute space $\mathcal{X}$), in which the sequence ($\overline{d}_{i,j}, d_{i,j}^{(k)}$) has appeared.

The Fuzzy Algorithm

Fuzzy approach to decision problem under the question denotes, that now outputs of algorithm (4) have sense of membership function values, viz.

$$q_{i,j}^{(k)} = \mu_{B_{i,j}}(d_{i,j}^{(k)}). \tag{11}$$

Support of fuzzy set $B_{i,j}$ covers the entire discrete set $\mathcal{D}_{i,j}$ (see (3)), whereas values of its membership function (11) denote degree of truth (in the fuzzy logic) of the sentence: "the user wants to execute data entry action $d_{i,j}^{(k)}$".

In order to receive vector of soft decisions (5) we can use Mamadani fuzzy inference system [4,5] (without defuzzification stage) with procedure of fuzzy rules generating from set (8) based on Wang and Mendel method [6] or genetic algorithm optimization technique [7].

3 Decision Support Server System Architecture

Data constituting the learning set (8) come actually from the medical information system database. The algorithms described in Section 2.2. require extensive access to the learning set data. For the reasons described in Chapter 1, execution of DSA on the palmtop platform is impractical. This task is therefore delegated to the stationary part of the medical information system, where the database server resides and can be efficiently accessed. It leads to the concept of the two-level client-server architecture. In the client layer we have a number of palmtops running user mobile applications. The server layer consists of the specialized process called decision support server (DSS) and the database server. DSS executes decision support algorithms in favour of thin client applications. The database used by DSS is usually the database of the medical information system with appropriate perspectives defined for extracting some data as a learning set. It this chapter, the proposal of the DSS system architecture is presented. The architecture has been implemented and successfully used in the hospital information system with medicines prescribing function available on the mobile palmtop terminals.

Our aim was to design and implement a flexible tool, which makes it possible to define and efficiently execute various DSA algorithms based on learning set usage, including these ones described in Section 2.2. The main functions of the tool are:

- extracting and maintaining data used as learning sets,
- making it available to mobile clients,
- remotely performing DSA algorithms and supplying the results to mobile clients using defined information exchange protocol,
- downloading selected learning sets to mobile clients in packed format.

In the architecture described here, these functions are being done by DSS. DSS constantly runs in the stationary part of the system. It receives the requests from the mobile clients, executes requested DSA algorithm and sends results back to requesters. The result is the degree of belief vector (5) for given decision support task. DSS must be able to support various tasks occurring when performing various operations from the set (1). To achieve it, the server maintains a set of DS problems descriptors. DS problem descriptor consists of features specification, decision set definition, rules determining how to extract the learning set from database and the DSA algorithm type which should be applied. DS problem definition is explained in detail later.

In some circumstances, where direct on-line connection between client and server is temporarily unavailable, it may be desirable to execute DSA algorithm on palmtop platform. It requires the learning set copy to be downloaded to the palmtop. Due to palmtop limitations described in Chapter 1, the complete learning sat available to DSS usually cannot be copied into the palmtop. At the expense of slight DSA performance deterioration, the learning set can be reduced to the size allowing to store it in palmtop memory. DSS role in this procedure is to prepare the reduced version of the learning set for given DS problem and to send it to requesting mobile client.

The following assumptions were considered in DSS design:

1. Database is accessible through the DBMS SQL server located in the stationary part of the system.
2. Clients should be able to work off-line if direct connection to the database is temporarily not available, expensive or slow.
3. The system should be able to process learning sets consisting of hundreds thousands of elements.
4. Processing time for single decision elaboration should be short enough to allow interactive usage.
5. The server should concurrently support many DS problems.

It is also assumed that the data used as a learning set come from general purpose database designed for a medical information system, and maintained by it. The conceptual model of data stored in the database not necessarily is designed taking into account specific decision support needs. We deal with two views (perspectives) of the same data: natural perspective corresponding to the model of medical data flow, for which the database was originally created, and DS perspective – allowing to perceive the selected data as the unified learning set structure. The DS perspective presents the data as a set of pairs <*y*, *j*>, where *j* is the decision, and *y* is the features vector. In the case of the learning set structure (8), all but the last elements of the sequence $(x_m, d_{i,1}^{(k_{m,1})}, d_{i,2}^{(k_{m,2})}, \ldots, d_{i,m(i)}^{(k_{m,m(i)})})$ constitute the features vector. The last element is the decision. DS perspective is defined by a mapping translating natural perspective into DS perspective.

In order to create such perspective, the mapping between domain specific view and DSP view is defined and used by the server. The mapping is a part of DS problem descriptor. DS problem descriptor is a script in simple formal language consisting of the following elements:

- data source localization - the unambiguous identifier of the database containing domain-specific data (usually: ODBC data source name),
- count of features,
- for each feature - its identifier and domain,
- domain of decisions - given either explicitly or by SQL select statement,
- for each nonnumeric domain - its mapping to numbers given either explicitly or by SQL select statement,
- for each numeric domain - its range,
- SQL statement selecting the learning set from the database,
- type of DSA to be used as the classifier for this problem.

The features can be numeric or textual. To define the numeric distance between objects for each nonnumeric value of the feature, the numeric counterpart must be determined. In the descriptor, the numeric counterpart of textual feature value is defined either explicitly in the script, or by giving the SQL statement selecting single numeric value for given textual value of the feature. Similarly, the range of each feature can be given explicitly or by providing the SQL statement selecting two numeric values: minimum and maximum. Each DS problem descriptor must be registered by the server, before the server is able to support the problem. The problem can be registered by issuing appropriate request to the server.

For each registered problem, the server creates binary data structure, and fills it with the data extracted from the database, according to SQL statements contained in the problem description. The binary data in own server structures created for a problem are being refreshed periodically or on an explicit request from the client. Hence, DSS is a kind of data warehouse. When executing requests concerning given problem, the server utilizes created binary data structure optimized for the supported data access algorithms.

The server receives requests from clients, executes them and sends results to requesting clients. The following request types are served:

- REGISTER a problem descriptor,
- DELETE a problem descriptor,
- REFRESH problem binary data,
- EXPORT problem binary packed data reduced to specified size,
- EXECUTE DSA algorithm - return single decision index,
- EXECUTE DSA algorithm - return indices of n decisions with highest degree of belief,
- FETCH k nearest neighbors of the object.

The application program on the mobile computer communicates with DSS through a driver. The driver is an API library. The library can work in two modes: remote or local. In the remote mode, all requests are being sent to the central DSS. In the local mode, the library uses local copy of problem binary data and executes DSA algorithm locally. Working in local mode is possible only if the problem binary data were earlier exported by the server and downloaded to the mobile device.

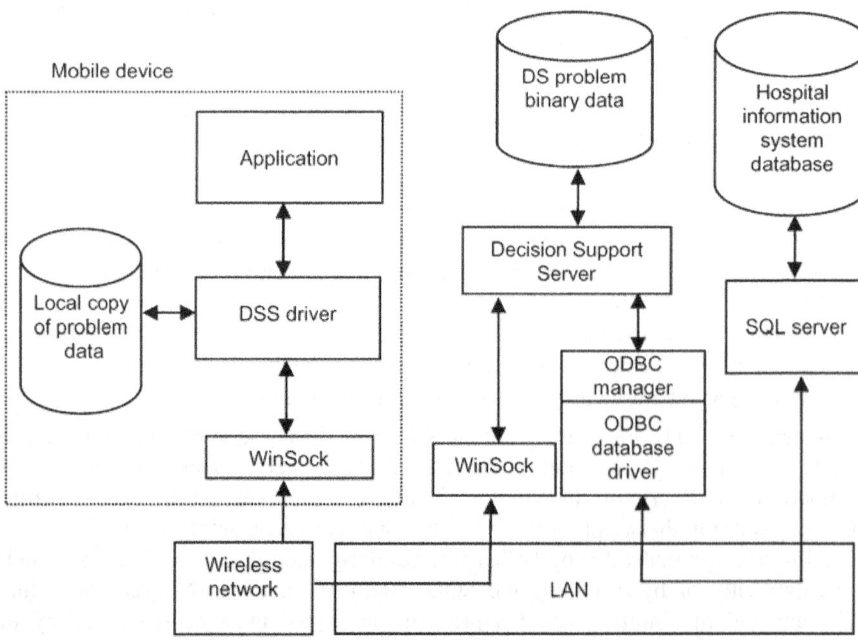

Fig. 1. Pattern recognition server access architecture

The described architecture has been implemented and integrated with the database of certain typical hospital information system. The mobile clients communicate with DSS through TCP/IP protocol, sockets mechanism and wireless communication media. DSS server communicates with the SQL server using ODBC interface. Fig. 1. shows implemented DSS system architecture.

4 Decision Support Server Application in Mobile Medicines Prescribing

The architecture described in the previous chapter has been applied and tested in the drug administration module of a mobile hospital information system. The system consists of two parts:

- stationary part consisting of central database server and the number of clients running in the local area network,
- mobile part containing a number of mobile clients running on palmtop computers.

One of the mobile system functions is physician's support in the process of medicines prescribing. Using the mobile device, a physician is able to prescribe the drug directly at the patient's bed (e.g. during a ward round). The prescription is immediately stored in the main system database and automatically inserted into the ward drug administration schedule.

The soft K-NN algorithm is used in the mobile application running on keyboard-less palmtop computers in order to support the decision about medicine selection and dosage, and to simplify the physician's interaction with the mobile application. The applied methods and its implementation are described in detail in [8]. Here we present only the main concept and implementation based DSS architecture.

Medicine prescribing is a decision process consisting of four stages: medicine selection, determining the unit dose, determining the daily repetition and specifying the dosage period. After the selection of the patient, to whom the drug is to be administered, the program analyses most important patient features: age, sex, weight, main disease, and suggests the most suitable medicines. The most suitable medicines are selected by analyzing the similar cases of prescriptions stored in the database using K-NN algorithm. At the next stage of prescribing process, the dosage is established. Again, the program uses K-NN algorithm to select the most similar cases in the learning set. Now the active substance of the selected medicine is used as an additional feature for similar cases selection.

The mobile application UI is mainly based on combo boxes usage. Due to lack of physical keyboard in the palmtop device, the entered data are rather selected from lists than textually entered by typing. The cases most probable in current context are loaded into the combo boxes lists in the decreased order of approximated degrees of belief. In this way the most probable selection is the default.

The mobile applications access and process data stored in the complex hospital information system database in the stationary part of the system. The learning sets for the K-NN algorithm are supported by DSS running at the dedicated PC and having constant access to the hospital information system database. Four DS problems are defined, which correspond to the four stages of medicine prescribing process. The mobile application can connect to the database either via wireless LAN or using

GPRS transmission in cellular phone network. When running in WLAN, it queries DSS each time, a decision is to be made. When running in GPRS mode however, it uses the local copy of reduced learning sets. In this way, transmission costs are reduced and the system response time is decreased significantly. In the latter case however, the palmtop computer must be equipped with more RAM. In the system being described here 64 MB of RAM is recommended for the mobile terminals. The local copy of the learning set can be downloaded to the palmtop terminal through direct cable connection.

As noted earlier, the side effect of decision support by appropriately arranging application UI controls is the user interaction simplification. The efficiency of the applied method can be assessed by the degree, in which the average number of basic UI actions necessary to make the decision is reduced. We consider the palmtop application built using typical UI controls supported by the mobile computer operating system: combo boxes (data entered by selection from the popup list or with the virtual keyboard), edit fields (data entered only by typing on the virtual keyboard), action buttons, check boxes and radio buttons. The following basic UI actions can be distinguished:

- click on the combo box to display selection list,
- selection list scroll by dragging the slider,
- click on the desired element in the selection list,
- click to open the virtual keyboard,
- click on a key on the virtual keyboard,
- click to close the virtual keyboard
- click to set focus on the edit field,
- click to change the state of radio or combo box,
- click on an action button.

Making four-stage decision about medicine prescription requires doing a series of basic UI actions. The number of actions necessary to make and enter the decision depends on current arrangement of UI controls, in particular on the order in which the possible decisions are placed in combo box selection lists. The result of soft classifier in the form of degree of belief sequence (6) is used to order the selection lists. Let us assume that each of the operations listed above is equally troublesome for the user. Hence the total discomfort factor $L_{i,j}(q_{i,j}, d_{i,j}^{(k)})$ can be calculated as the count of basic UI actions necessary to make the decision $d_{i,j}^{(k)}$, while the UI arrangement is determined by $q_{i,j}$. The efficiency of the method can be assessed by comparing the average count of UI operations necessary to make and enter decision with and without the UI arrangement.

In the series of experiments, DSS efficiency and DSA algorithm performance were tested using the real hospital information system database contents. The database contained 2745 patient records, 6790 records in the medicines catalogue and 8709 prescription records. For various learning set sizes the average system response time was measured. Leave-one-out method was applied to generate test cases. The total time of all four decision support process stages was measured. The experiment was performed for two operation modes: local (leatning set downloaded to the palmtop memory) and remote (DSA algorithm executed by DSS). As mobile terminals, HP iPAQ h4150 palmtop computers equipped with 64 MB RAM and Intel XScale 400

MHz processor were used. DSS was running on a PC with 1.4 GHz Pentium 4 processor. The results are presented in the Table 1.

Table 1. Experiment results

Learning set size	Average response time, remote mode [sec]	Average response time, local mode [sec]	Average basic UI operations count reduction factor
2000	2.75	0.25	1.10
4000	2.81	0.40	1.58
6000	2.81	0.45	1.72
8709	2.87	0.52	1.97

In both cases of operation mode (remote and local) the execution times are short enough to be considered as sufficient for interactive usage. It should be taken into account that the timings presented above concern four subsequent UI operations corresponding to four stages of prescribing process. Hence, the response time per single operation is about 0.7 sec in the case of remote K-NN execution and about 0.15 sec in case of local operation. The response time in case of remote K-NN execution is almost independent of the learning set size. It means, that most of response time is spent on transmitting queries and results between the server and the client. The average basic UI operations count is reduced almost twice, if large enough learning set is used.

5 Conclusions

In the paper, the methods and implementation of a decision support server for mobile medical decision making has been described. The presented solutions were applied in practice in the hospital information system, where selected functionalities are available on the mobile devices. The system was positively evaluated by its users. In particular, significant improvement in the system ease of use was appreciated. The methods presented here can be applied not only for pure decision making support, but also in the mobile medical teleconsultation systems. In future, using HL7 messages as DSS protocol basis will be investigated. Utilizing the distributed HIS databases as the source of learning set data will be also considered.

References

1. L.I. Kuncheva, Using measures of similarity and inclusion for multiple classifier fusion by decision templates, Fuzzy Sets and Systems, 122 (3), 2001, pp.401-407
2. L. Devroye, P. Gyorfi, G. Lugosi, A Probabilistic Theory of Pattern Recognition, Springer Verlag, New York, 1996
3. R. Duda, P. Hart, D. Stork, Pattern Classification, John Wiley & Sons, 2001
4. D. Dubois, H. Prade, Fuzzy Sets and Systems: Theory and Applications, Academic Press, NY 1980
5. M. Kurzynski, Fuzzy Inference Systems for Multistage Diagnosis of Acute Renal Failure in Children, 4th Int. Symp. Medical Data Analysis, ISMDA2003, Springer Verlag, LNCS 2868, Berlin 2003, pp. 99-108
6. L-X Wang, J.M. Mendel, Generating Fuzzy Rules by Learning from Examples, IEEE Trans. on SMC, vol.22, pp. 1414-1427, 1992

7. M. Kurzyński, Multistage Diagnosis of Myocardial Infraction Using a Fuzzy Relation, 7th Int. Conf. on Artificial Intelligence and Soft Computing, ICAISC 2004, Springer Verlag, LNAI 3070, Zakopane (Poland) 2004, pp. 1014 – 1019.
8. P. Radlinski, J. Sas, User interaction simplification method for healthcare mobile applications, Journal of Medical Informatics and Technologies, University of Silesia (Poland), Vol. 4. (2002) 111-117
9. P. Radlinski, J. Sas, Handheld Based Hospital Information System for Fast Data Access at Patient's Bed, Journal of Medical Informatics and Technologies, University of Silesia (Poland), Vol. 2. (2001) 15-19

Ordered Time-Independent CIG Learning

David Riaño

Department of Computer Sciences and Mathematics
Universitat Rovira i Virgili, Tarragona, Spain

Abstract. Clinical practice guidelines are medical and surgical statements to assist practitioners in the therapy procedure. Recently, the concept computer-interpretable guideline (CIG) has been introduced to describe formal descriptions of clinical practice guidelines. *Ordered time-independent one-visit CIGs* are a sort of CIG wich are able to cope with the description and use of real therapies. Here, this representation model and a machine learning algorithm to construct such CIGs from the hospital databases or from predefined CIGs are introduced and tested within the domain of *attrial fibrillation*.

1 Introduction

Knowledge Management (KM) is becoming one of the cornerstones of modern organizations and industries. In the context of health-care, in the last years, there has been an increasing interest in the development of guidelines as a means of representing the clinical knowledge about some medical practices as diagnosis, therapy, and prognosis. More concretely, Clinical Practice Guidelines (CPGs) are defined as systematically developed statements to assist practitioner and patient decisions about appropriate health care for specific clinical circumstances. In the evidence-based medicine community there is a widely accepted opinion that the representation of medical practices as CPGs will have a direct and positive impact on several relevant tasks as clinical decision support, workflow management, quality assurance, and resource-requirement estimates [18].

The way CPGs are represented (knowledge representation), the way they are constructed from hospital databases (machine learning), and the way they are used by the physicians (decision support systems) are the main topics of this paper. As far as *knowledge representation* is concerned, there has been a first generation of guidelines that have been represented as textual descriptions of medical procedures. This approach has been promoted by some international organizations as the HSTAT in the USA, the SIGN and the SIGNet in Scotland, or the NZGG in New Zealand with the purpose of gathering all the available medical knowledge about particular medical practices, regardless whether the final CPG could be used by some computer-based application or not. In the last few years, the new term Computer-Interpretable Guideline (CIG) [20, 12] has been coined to denotate the CPGs that are described by means of some formal representation system that range from formal knowledge representation languages as Arden [5] or Asbru [17] to flowchart-based graphical representation

J.M. Barreiro et al. (Eds.): ISBMDA 2004, LNCS 3337, pp. 117–128, 2004.

systems as EON [10], GLIF [11], GUIDE [13], PRODIGY [19] or PRO*forma* [4], passing through some other Artificial Intelligence models as rules, ontologies, or decision trees [14, 15, 7].

Despite the above alternatives, there is a global agreement that any CIG representation model must comply with some requirements inherited from the CPGs [12]: branching, asserting, unfolding, and state representation. *Branching* means that there can be points in the CIG where a selection from a set of alternatives must be taken based on some predefined criterion; for example, "only if the patient is not responding, defibrillation is applied". *Asserting* is the way that a guideline indicates that some medical actions must be applied in a particular point of the treatment; for example, prescribe some medicines or ask for some medical or surgical procedure or analysis. *Unfolding* is when some parts of the guideline recommend a shift to another guideline; for example, when some additional graver disease is detected a change of treatment could be required. Finally, *state representation* is used to describe specific scenarios of the clinical status of the patient in the context of a particular point of the guideline. Moreover, there are some other more specific CPG features that enlarge the number of requirements of a CIG representation system. For example, the rules in a rule-based CIG can be ordered or disordered [2], a CIG can represent whole treatments or one-visit treatments [1], CIGs can manage temporal assertions (*time-dependence*) or contain exceptions, etc.

Once the CIG representation model has been selected (or created), experts can use it to construct CPGs as a result of a guideline engineering process [3]. Then, the CIGs can be incorporated as knowledge components of a *decision support system* (DSS) that could help physicians in some important tasks as therapy assignment, consultation or treatment verification once the CIG has been validated by some expert.

Similarly to the first generation of Expert System, this manual construction of CIGs represents a first generation approach to CIG-based DSS that will be replaced in the forthcoming years with a second generation approach that will incorporate *machine learning* techniques to mine hospital databases in order to obtain the implicit CPG knowledge.

This paper introduces a CIG representation model that is complemented with a new machine learning process which is able to induce CIGs from hospital databases or combine predefined CIGs as a first step towards the aforementioned second generation of CIG-based DSS. Particularly, the algorithm produces *ordered time-independent one-visit CIGs*, and extends the previous works [14] and [16].

The paper is organised in five sections. In section 2, the properties of the CIGs that the learning process generates are described in detail. In section 3, the learning process is introduced, and tested in section 4. Final conclusions are supplied in section 5.

2 The Structure of CIGs

Computer-Interpretable Guidelines (CIGs) are described as formal representations of CPGs that are capable of being automatically or semi-automatically

Table 1. Grammar for rule-based CIGs

```
CIG         ::= CIG-id CIG-body
CIG-body    ::= [state-rep][asserting][branching] | unfolding
branching   ::= IF condition THEN t-conclusion ELSE f-conclusion
asserting   ::= { medical-acts }
unfolding   ::= CIG-id
state-rep   ::= " state-description "
```

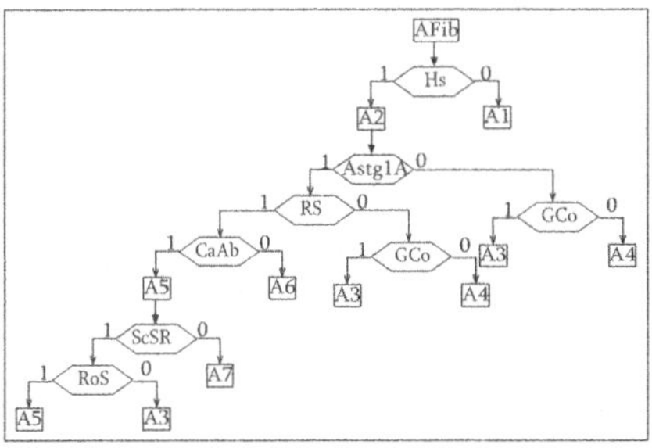

Hs	Hemodynamic stable
Astg1A	Afib < 48h, anticoagulation > 3w or not trombos
GCo	Good control of the cardiac rate and symptoms
RS	Sinus Rhythm goal
CaAb	Cardiopatia absence
ScSR	Spontaneous Conversion to Sinus Rhythm
RoS	Recurrent or very symptomatic
A1	Electrical cardioversion, heparine
A2	Control cardiac rate and prophylaxis TE
A3	Hospital discharge
A4	Hospital Admitter
A5	Flecainida or propafenona (300 mg/600mg)
A6	Electrical cardioversion and evaluate amodarona
A7	Electrical cardioversion (in < 48 hours)

Fig. 1. Atrial Fibrillation CIG_1

interpreted [20, 12]. CIGs contain a representation of the medical knowledge involved in the medical practice for which the CIG was generated.

Any system used to represent CIGs must be able to incorporate branching, asserting, unfolding, and state representation constructors [12]. In rule-based CIGs, these constructors are as the grammar in table 1 depicts. For example, the CIG body `"not responsive"` {`apply-defibrillator`} `IF breathing THEN` {`place-in- recovery-position`} `ELSE` CIG_1 represents a clinical act related to the patients that arrive to a health-care institution in a "not responsive" state. The first clinical action is to apply the defibrillator and then, if the patient is breathing, he or she is placed in recovery position. Otherwise, the guideline CIG_1 shown in figure 1, is unfold.

The way IF-THEN rules are combined defines whether the CIGs are ordered or non-ordered. *Non ordered rule-based CIGs* are considered in [16] as sets of IF-THEN rules (i.e. branching components) whose order is irrelevant during the reasoning process. These rules are represented following the grammar in table 1, where `t-conclusion` and `f-conclusion` are CIG-bodies without branching.

On the contrary, *ordered CIGs* represent a CPG as a single IF-THEN rule where both THEN and ELSE conclusions are again ordered (sub-)CIGs. These rules are written following the grammar in table 1, where `t-conclusion` and `f-conclusion` are CIG-bodies. For example, figure 2 shows the ordered CIG that figure 1 represents as a tree.

Another important feature of CIGs is whether they are able to represent the temporal aspects of the CPGs. Although in the field of medicine time is relevant, the approach described in this paper only considers time-independent CIGs, and leave the construction of time-dependent CIGs for future consideration.

```
IF Hs
THEN {A2}
     IF AstgIA
     THEN IF RS
          THEN IF CaAB
               THEN {A5}
                    IF ScSR
                    THEN IF RoS
                         THEN {A5}
                         ELSE {A3}
                    ELSE {A7}
               ELSE {A6}
           ELSE IF GCo
                THEN {A3}
                ELSE {A4}
     ELSE IF GCo
          THEN {A3}
          ELSE {A4}
ELSE {A1}
```

Fig. 2. Ordered rule-based CIG for Atrial Fibrillation

Finally, CIGs can represent one-visit or whole-treatment CPGs. In the first case, all the stages of a medical episode are independent inputs in the CIGs. As a result of that, complex patients with multi-stage treatments have to pass several times through the CIG before the treatment finishes, in opposition to whole-treatment CPGs in which the patient enters somewhere in the CIG at the begining of the treatment and leaves the CIG at the discharge moment.

2.1 Ordered Time-Independent One-Visit CIGs

In this paper, only *ordered time-independent one-visit CIGs* are considered. This decision arises from the difficulties of generating less restricted CIGs which is the goal pursued by a longer research work which includes this one. Here, CIGs are halfway between the simplest non-ordered time-independent one-visit CIGs [14, 16] and the most complex ordered time-dependent whole-treatment CIGs which will be developed in the future.

On the one hand, ordered time-independent one-visit CIGs have some drawbacks that cause some limitations in the sort of CPGs that can be represented: medical decision cannot be based on temporal aspects, the degree of illnesses is internal to the CIG because it is one-visit, etc. On the other hand, these CIGs have some clear advantages with respect to other sort of CIGs: there is a method to transform these CIGs into decision trees, it is possible to reconstruct the data of the original treatments that was used to generate the CIGs, the troubles caused by the loops in the CPG are avoided because CIGs are defined one-visit, etc.

2.2 The Defactorising Process

As a consequence of the time-independent property of the CIGs, the assertions that appear in intermediate positions of a particular CIG can be moved down the branches of the tree to the leaves, transforming the original CIG into a decision tree where classes are sets of medical assertions. For example, after the defactorizing process, the CIG in figure 2 becomes the decision tree shown in figure 3. Observe that some individual assertion can appear several times in a final assertion class at the bottom of the decision tree, meaning for instance that a particular drug has been prescribed several times or that a medical analysis has been repeated. For example, in figure 3, A5 (i.e. *flecainida or propafenona*) appears two times in the first assertion set.

```
IF Hs
THEN IF AstgIA
     THEN IF RS
          THEN IF CaAB
               THEN IF ScSR
                    THEN IF RoS
                         THEN {A2 A5 A5}
                         ELSE {A2 A5 A3}
                    ELSE {A2 A5 A7}
               ELSE {A2 A6}
           ELSE IF GCo
                THEN {A2 A3}
                ELSE {A2 A4}
     ELSE IF GCo
          THEN {A2 A3}
          ELSE {A2 A4}
ELSE {A1}
```

Fig. 3. Defactorised CIG or Decision Tree for Atrial Fibrillation

The opposite process is called *factorizing* and consists in moving the individual assertions as higher as possible to the top of the tree. Finally, observe that factorizing a defactorized CIG results in the same CIG only if the original CIG is initially completely factorized. The assumption that original CIGs are completely factorized seems absolutely natural for time-independent CIGs where medical actions must be taken as soon as possible. Moreover, it is more realistic to apply medical actions before branching the CIG if such actions are to be taken either if the patient satisfies the branching condition or not. For example, it is more natural to describe a therapy as "prescribe flecainida and then if the patient is hemodynamically stable control the cardiac rate or, otherwise, apply electrical cardioversion" than as "if the patient is hemodynamically stable then prescribe flecainida and control the cardiac rate or, otherwise, prescribe flecainida as well and apply electrical cardioversion". Observe that this statement is not so when dealing with time-dependent CIGs where the moment a medical

Table 2. Data Matrix for Atrial Fibrillation

Hs	AstgIA	RS	CaAB	ScSR	RoS	GCo	Class
1	1	1	1	1	1	*	C_1
1	1	1	1	1	0	*	C_2
1	1	1	1	0	*	*	C_3
1	1	1	0	*	*	*	C_4
1	1	0	*	*	*	1	C_5
1	1	0	*	*	*	0	C_6
1	0	*	*	*	*	1	C_5
1	0	*	*	*	*	0	C_6
0	*	*	*	*	*	*	C_7

action is taken is decisive. Another justification for having CIGs as completely factorized decision trees is that if a medical act is not applied as soon as possible, and therefore as close to the tree root as possible, that is because some condition must be checked or satisfied before. This fact may delay the application of medical acts, and the delaying condition must appear explicitly in the CIG as a branching point where only the "then" branch must contain the medical act. Since the "else" branch do not contain it, factorization is not possible.

2.3 The Flattening Process

After defactorising a CIG, each one of the leaves represent an assertion class. Some of these classes, as {`A2 A3`} or {`A2 A4`}, can be repeated in different leaves of the tree, representing all of them the same medical action. So, the decision tree in figure 3 has seven different assertion classes, i.e. C_i, $i = 1..7$, which stand for {`A2 A5 A5`}, {`A2 A5 A3`}, {`A2 A5 A7`}, {`A2 A6`}, {`A2 A3`}, {`A2 A4`}, and {`A1`}, respectively.

Starting from a defactorised CIG or decision tree, the *flattening process* consists in the construction of a data matrix containing a training set which is sound with the decision tree. The process defines a column for each one of the different conditions in the decision tree and one last column to contain the assertion class. Then, all the possible combinations of values of the condition columns are considered, and the respective assertion class is determined according to the decision tree. For example, table 2 contains a data set generated from de decision tree shown in figure 3. In the data matrix, the symbol * indicates that either the value 1 or 0 drives the reasoning process to the same assertion. For example, the first row of table 2 indicates that regardless of whether the value for `GCo` (i.e. *good control of cardiac rate*) is 0 or 1, if the rest of the features are 1, the assertion class is C_1 (i.e. {`A2, A5, A2, A5`}).

Every row of a data matrix representing a defactorised flattened CIG is called a *single medical act* and symbolizes a cause-effect knowledge $x \rightarrow y$, where x stands for the patient description in terms of the condition columns, and y stands for the assertion class. For example, $(Hs = 1)\&(Astg1A = 0)\&(GCo = 0) \rightarrow$ {`A2 A4`} is the eighth single medical act of the data matrix in the table 2.

The opposite process is called *unflattering* and it is equivalent to the induction of a decision tree form a supervised data matrix. It can be proved that flattening and unflattering a decision tree ends up in the same decision tree only if the order of the conditions in the source tree is maintained. Otherwise, a different CIG can be obtained in which only the sort and number of assertions (but not their respective order in the tree) remain the same, for all the possible uses of the tree (i.e. CIG alternatives).

3 Learning CIGs

CPGs can be learned from the activities of the physicians in a hospital with respect to the patients diagnosed of a particular disease (e.g. *atrial fibrillation*), but also from the integration of CPGs published by health-care organizations.

In the first case, the activities of the physicians can be represented as single medical acts where causes represent the conditions that justify the effects. For example, if a doctor decides to supply *flecainide* because the patient is not hemodynamically stable, the single medical act $(Hs = 0) \rightarrow \{\texttt{A5}\}$ can be represented as the data matrix row `(0 * * * * * {A5})` that is in contradiction or complementing the knowledge that the data matrix in table 2 contains. In the second case, predefined CPGs can be directly represented as data matrices after applying the defactorising and flattening processes.

If learning CIGs is defined as the process of integrating new knowledge in the form of single medical acts to a possibly-empty CIG, the same learning process can be applied to learn CIGs from both patient treatments and CPGs represented as CIGs.

3.1 Distance Between Single Medical Acts

A distance function has been defined to evaluate how close two single medical acts $s_i \equiv x_i \rightarrow y_i$ $(i = 1, 2)$ are one to the other. The function is defined by equation 1 as the weighted contribution of the distance between the left hand side of two single medical acts ($dist_1$), and the distance between the right hand side of the same single medical acts ($dist_2$), with α a weighted factor between 0 and 1 measuring the importance of the left hand side of the medical act with respect to the right hand side.

$$distance(s_1, s_2) = \alpha \cdot dist_1(x_1, x_2) + (1 - \alpha) \cdot dist_2(y_1, y_2) \tag{1}$$

$$dist_1(x_1, x_2) = \sum_{i=1}^{n} diff(x_{1i}, x_{2i}) \tag{2}$$

$$dist_2(y_1, y_2) = \frac{y_1 \triangle y_2}{y_1 \nabla y_1} \tag{3}$$

$$diff(v_1, v_2) = \begin{cases} 0 \text{ if } v_1 = v_2 \\ \frac{1}{2} \text{ if } v_1 = * \text{ or } v_2 = * \\ 1 \text{ otherwise} \end{cases} \tag{4}$$

Table 3. Basic Rules of Integration

	guideline	*patient*	*output guideline*
subsumption	$A[*] \rightarrow B$	$A \rightarrow B$	$A[*] \rightarrow B$
1-complementarity	$Aa[*] \rightarrow B$	$A\bar{a} \rightarrow B$	$A[*] \rightarrow B$
N-complementarity	$AA'[*] \rightarrow B$	$AA'' \rightarrow B$	$AA'[*] \rightarrow B$ $AA''[*] \rightarrow B$
Extension	$AA'[*] \rightarrow B$	$A \rightarrow B$	$A[*] \rightarrow B$

Since y_1 and y_2 can contain repeated assertions, $dist_2$ is defined as the quotient of the operations $\triangle$ and ∇. Both operations are based on the one-to-one connection of equal elements in the operands. Then, $y_1 \triangle y_2$ represents the number of one-to-one connections, and $y_1 \nabla y_2$ the number of one-to-one connections plus the number of elements in y_1 and y_2 that could not be connected. For example, if the connections are indicated by subindexes, $\{a_1\, a_2\, b_1\, c_1\, c_2\} \triangle \{a_1\, b_1\, b_2\, c_1\, c_2\} = \#\{a_1\, b_1\, c_1\, c_2\} = 4$ and $\{a_1\, a_2\, b_1\, c_1\, c_2\} \nabla \{a_1\, b_1\, b_2\, c_1\, c_2\} = \#\{a_1\, b_1\, c_1\, c_2\, a_2\} = 5$.

3.2 Rules of Knowledge Integration

According to the left hand side, a single medical act can subsume, 1-complement, n-complement, or extend any other single medical act. Specifically, if m is the number of condition columns in the CIG and s_i represents the single medical act $(p_1 = v_{i1})\&...\&(p_m = v_{im}) \rightarrow y_i$ with $v_{ij} \in \{0, 1, *\}$, $(j = 1..m)$, we say that (a) s_1 *subsumes* s_2 if and only if for all p_k, $v_{1k} = v_{2k}$ or $v_{1k} = *$; (b) s_1 *1-complements* s_2 if and only if there is only one p_j such that $v_{2j} = 1 - v_{1j}$, and $v_{2k} = v_{1k}$ for $k \neq j$; (c) s_1 *n-complements* s_2 if and only if there are some, but not all p_j such that $v_{2j} \neq v_{1j}$, and (d) s_1 *extends* s_2 if and only if for all p_k, $v_{2k} \neq * \Rightarrow v_{1k} = v_{2k}$.

According to the right hand side, a single medical act can be consistent or contradictory with other single medical acts. Specifically, s_1 is consistent with s_2 if and only if $y_1 = y_2$, and s_1 contradicts s_2, otherwise.

Tables 3 and 4 contain the rules used to integrate knowledge in the form of consistent and contradictory single medical acts, respectively. Knowledge integration is based on the incremental incorporation of the knowledge about the treatment of single patients into the guideline that is being constructed. The columns of the above mentioned tables contain the name of the rule, the medical action that is being modified in the guideline , the patient medical action that is modifying the guideline, and the medical actions of the guideline after the modification. Table 4 distinguishes between three alternative modifications, representing three working modes: avoid, restrict, and accept. *Avoid* mode rejects new knowledge if it is contradictory with the previous knowledge. *Restrict* mode reduces the assertion classes in the right hand side of the output single medical act to contain only the coincident assertions. Finally, *accept* mode admits all the assertions in the right hand sides of the single medical acts and adds them to the final assertions as many times as the maximum number of times they appear.

Table 4. Basic Rules of Integration of Contradiction

			output guideline		
	guideline	*patient*	*avoid*	*restrict*	*accept*
subsumption	$A[*] \to BB'$	$A \to BB''$	$A[*] \to BB'$	$A[*] \to B$	$A[*] \to BB'B''$
1-complement	$Aa[*] \to BB'$	$A\bar{a} \to BB''$	$Aa[*] \to BB'$	$A[*] \to B$	$A[*] \to BB'B''$
N-complement	$AA'[*] \to BB'$	$AA'' \to BB''$	$AA'[*] \to BB'$	$AA'[*] \to B$ $AA''[*] \to B$	$AA'[*] \to BB'B''$ $AA''[*] \to BB'B''$
Extension	$AA'[*] \to BB'$	$A \to BB''$	$AA'[*] \to BB'$	$A[*] \to B$	$A[*] \to BB'B''$

```
algorithm Make_Guideline (CIG1, CIG2, mode)
  for all the single medical acts s2 in CIG2
    find the closest to s2 single medical act s1 in CIG1
    if s1 is in contradiction with s2 then apply rules in table 3
    else apply rules in table 4 according to the working mode
```

Fig. 4. Algorithm to learn CIGs

In the rules, each symbol A, A' or A'' represents one or more fixed single conditions, a and $\bar{a}$ are one single condition and its opposite, [*] is an undefined number of conditions, and B, B' and B'' one or more fixed single assertions. For example, if $A = \{HsGCo\}$, $a = AstgIA$, and $B = C_5$, the fifth medical action in table 2 fits the expression $Aa[*] \to B$ (with $[*]=\{\overline{RS}\}$), the eight one the expression $A\bar{a} \to B$, and the *1-complementarity* rule in table 3 is applicable.

3.3 The Learning Process

The learning process is defined as the incremental incorporation of the knowledge of a single medical act in a CIG. If two CIGs have to be combined, one of them acts as CIG, and the other one is interpreted as a set of single medical acts that have to be incorporated in the previous one. All the CIGs involved in the process must be defactorised and flattened before the algorithm in figure 4 is used.

4 Tests and Results

In order to analyze the algorithm of the previous section, we have tested our implementation with the cardiac disease of *atrial fibrillation* that is the most common sustained arrhythmia encountered in clinical practice. The three CPGs depicted in figures 1, 5 and 6 were introduced as CIG_1, CIG_2 and CIG_3.

All the possible combinations of two different CIGs were used to evaluate the three working modes (i.e. avoid, restrict, and accept) in order to find out which one produces best final CIGs. After every integration of two CIGs (CIG_i and CIG_j) a new CIG (CIG_{ij}) was obtained. Then, with the n different variables that are used in the conditions of CIG_i and CIG_j and using their three possible values in the data matrix (i.e. 0, 1, and *), the 3^n possible combinations were generated. Each combination was transformed into a medical act by adding as right hand side an empty assertion class representing a patient that has still not been treated

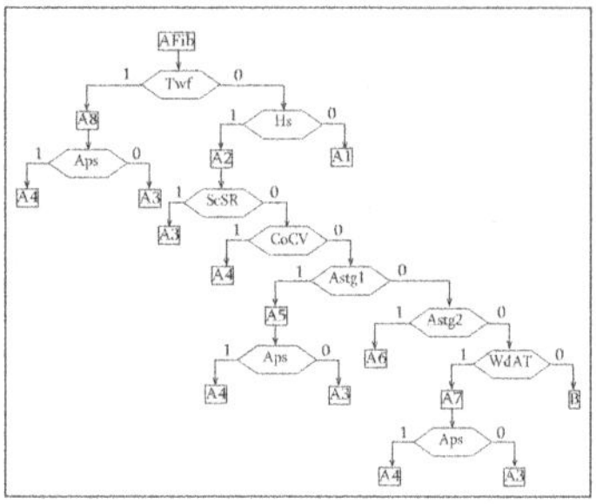

PWCI	Patient treated w/o compelling indications
ScS	Is secondary cause suspected
RiskA	Risk group A
RiskB	Risk group B
RiskC	Risk group C
Stage0	BP High-normal(Systolic 130-139/Diastolic 85-89)
Stage1	Systolic BP 140-159/Diastolic BP 90-99
Stage2	Systolic BP > 160/Diastolic BP > 100
Bpg	Not goal blood pressure
RHyp	Resistant hypertension
A1	Complete initial assessment
A2	Order additional work-up, considerer referral
A3	LifeStyle modifications
A4	LifeStyle modification (up to 12 mo)
A5	LifeStyle plus drug therapy
A6	LifeStyle modification (up to 6 mo)
A7	Change ttmt: increase init agent, add agent of a different class, substitute new agent
A8	Hypertension consult
A9	Hypertension continuing care
B	Not Applicable

Fig. 5. Attrial Fibrillation CIG_2

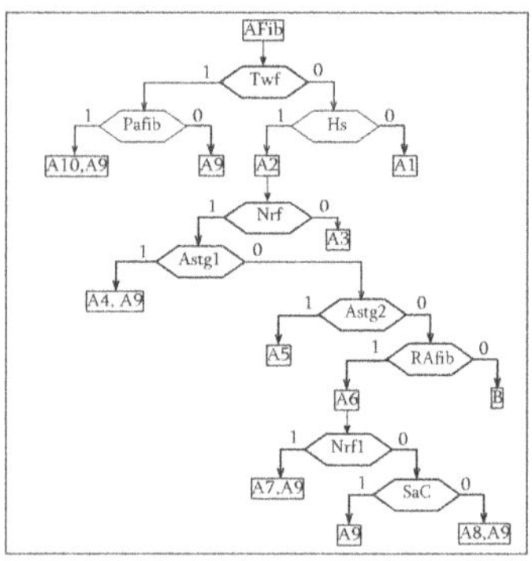

Twf	Patient treated with werfarin (Astg2)
Hs	Hemodynamic stable
Nrf	Not Risk Factors
Astg1	Afrib < 48 hours
Astg2	Afib > 48 hours or unknown duration
RaFib	Recurrent Afib
Nrf1	Not Risk Factors in recurrent fibrillation
SaC	Symptoms adequately controlled
Pafib	Afib persist
A1	Emergent electrical cardioversion
A2	Establish adequate rate control
A3	Procedures for control risk
A4	Observed or treated with electrical cardioversion
A5	Anticoagulation (INR >= 2.0)for 3 weeks
A6	Chronic rate control
A7	Chronic anticoagulation
A8	Intermittent cardioversion, antiarrhythmic agent
A9	Patient education
A10	Electrical cardioversion or use of antiarrhythmics
B	No applicable

Fig. 6. Atrial Fibrillation CIG_3

for atrial fibrillation. The two original CIGs were used to propose the therapy actions for all 3^n medical acts. Each proposal was compared with the therapy actions proposed by CIG_{ij}. The distance function $dist_2$ was used to evaluate this comparison. The distances obtained from the comparison of the proposals supplied by CIG_{ij} with any of the two original CIGs were accumulated in two separated counters (i.e. $C_k = \sum_p dist_2(CIG_k(p), CIG_{ij}(p))$). These counters are in the third and forth columns of the table 5, for the CIG_i and the CIG_j indicated in the first two columns. The mean value of those two counters is depicted in the fifth column. The last two columns show the fifth and the third columns normalized to the number of cases that have been accumulated (i.e. 3^n).

The results show that there is not a clear advantage of using the avoid or the restrict working modes, since all the values are close to 37%. However, they show that the accept mode is not as efficient as the previous ones. The reason is that the accept mode produces single medical acts that contain all the assertions that appear in the original medical acts and, after combining all the single medical acts in a CIG, the number of assertions of the final CIG have increased more than if other mode was used.

Table 5. Results of the CIG learning in *atrial fibrillation*

	CIG_i	CIG_j	C_i	C_j	$\frac{C_i+C_j}{2}$	$\%_1$	$\%_2$
	CIG_1	CIG_2	47628	307449	177538,5	33,41%	8,96%
avoid	CIG_1	CIG_3	118098	3472227	1795162,5	37,53%	2,47%
	CIG_2	CIG_3	6534	1244322	625428,0	39,23%	0,41%
	CIG_1	CIG_2	158031	200880	179455,5	33,76%	29,73%
restrict	CIG_1	CIG_3	757431	2950992	1854211,5	38,76%	15,83%
	CIG_2	CIG_3	454329	794367	624348,0	39,16%	28,49%
	CIG_1	CIG_2	306099	264276	285187,0	53,66%	57,60%
accept	CIG_1	CIG_3	7445520	7457427	7451473,5	155,79%	155,67%
	CIG_2	CIG_3	1346040	1506294	1426167,0	89,45%	84,42%

The last column shows a clear advantage of the avoid mode with respect to the other two alternatives. The reason is that this column shows the average distance per patient with respect to the CIG that has incorporated the knowledge of the other CIG. Since avoid is the mode that rejects the new knowledge that contradicts the one already present in the CIG, it seems natural that this working mode obtains the bests results.

5 Conclusions

Generating computer-interpretable guidelines is a complex new task that will become of great relevance in the next years. This paper describes a representation model and a new machine learning process which is able to induce CIGs from hospital databases or to combine predefined CIGs. The work is integrated in an ongoing research towards the construction of more expressive CIGs that could capture some medical practice aspects as temporal restrictions, repetitive sub-treatments, exceptions, etc. Therefore the results must be taken as provisional and improvable as the algorithm will evolve. Here, the current machine learning process has been tested with real CIGs that represent the treatment of *atrial fibrillation*, showing that permissive policies as the accept mode do not achieve the same degree of success as other less permissive working modes.

References

1. J. A. Bohada, D. Riaño, A CPG-based CBR model to offer the best available medical therapy. (submitted to) STAIRS 2004, Valencia, Spain, 2004.
2. P. Clark, T. Niblett, The CN2 induction algorithm. ML 3 (1989): 261–283.
3. Council of Europe. Developing a methodology for drawing up guidelines on best medical practice. Recomendation Rec(2001)13 and explanatory memorandum. Strasburg, Council of Europe Publishing 2002.
4. J. Fox, A. Rahmanzadeh, Disseminating Medical Knowledge: the PROforma Approach, Artificial Intelligence in Medicine 14: 157-181, 1998.
5. G. Hripcsak, P. Ludemann, T.A. Pruor, O.B. Wigertz, P.B. Clayton, Rationale for the Arden Syntax, Computers in Biomedical Research 27(4): 291–324, 1994.

6. M. Kukar, Transductive reliability estimation for medical diagnosis, Artificial Intelligence in Medicine **29** (2003) 81–106.
7. A. Kumar, B. Smith, D. Pisanelli, et al., An ontological framework for the implementation of CPG in health care organisations. EuroMISE 2004, 122.
8. N. Lavrac, E. Keravnou, B. Zupan, Intelligent Data Analysis in Medicine, In Encyclopedia of Computer Science and Technology, **42** (2000) 113-157.
9. N. Lavrac, DM in medicine: selected Tech. and Appl., AIMED **16** (1): 3-23, 1999.
10. M.A. Musen, S.W. Tu, A.K. Das, Y. Shahar,EON: A component-based approach to automation of protocol-directed therapy, JAMIA 3(6): 367-388, 1996.
11. M. Peleg A. Boxwala O. Ogunyemi, GLIF3: The Evolution of a Guideline Representation Format, Proceedings of the AMIA Fall Symposium, 2000.
12. M. Peleg, S. Tu, J. Bury, P. Ciccarese, et al. Comparing Computer-Interpretable Guideline Models: A Case-Study Approach, JAMIA 10(1): 52-68, 2003.
13. S. Quaglini, M. Stefanelli, M. Lanzola, et al., Flexible Guideline-Based Patient Careflow Systems, Artificial Intelligence in Medicine 22: 65–80, 2001.
14. D. Riaño, Guideline Composition from Minimum Basic Data Set, The 16th IEEE Symposium on Computer-Based Medical Systems, 231-35, NY, 2003.
15. D. Riaño, J. A. Bohada, T. Welzer, The DTP Model: Integration of intelligent techniques for the decision support in Healthcare Assistance, Eng. Int. Syst. (2004).
16. D. Riaño, Time-Independent Rule-Based Guideline Induction, ECAI 2004.
17. Y. Shahar, S. Miksch, P. Johnson, The Asgaard Project: A Task-Specific Framework for the Application and Critiquing of Time-Oriented Clinical Guidelines, Artificial Intelligence in Medicine 14: 29–51, 1998.
18. Proc. of the Symposium on Computerized Guidelines and Protocols (CGP 2004). K. Kaiser, S. Miksch, S.W. Tu (Eds.) 2004.
19. M. Veloso, J. Carbonell A. Pérez, et al., Integrating planning and learning, Journal of Experimental and Theoretical Artificial Intelligence 7(1), 1995.
20. D. Wang, M. Peleg, S.W. Tu, A.A. Boxwala, et al. Representation primitives, process models and patient data in CIGs. Int J. Med Info **68** (1-3): 59-70, 2002.

SINCO: Intelligent System in Disease Prevention and Control. An Architectural Approach

Carolina González[1,2], Juan C. Burguillo[1], Juan C. Vidal[2], and Martin Llamas[1]

[1] Departamento de Ingeniería Telemática, Universidad de Vigo
Vigo 36200, Spain
{cgonzals,jrial,martin}@det.uvigo.es
[2] Departamento de Sistemas, Universidad del Cauca, Colombia
{cgonzals,jcvidal}@unicauca.edu.co

Abstract. SINCO is a research effort to develop a software environment that contributes to the prevention and control of infectious diseases. This paper describes the system architecture already implemented where four important elements interact: (a) expert system (b) geographical information system (c) simulation component, and (d) training component. This architecture is itself a scalable, interoperable and modular approach. The system is being currently used in several health establishments as part of its validation process.

1 Introduction

The PanAmerican Health Organization (PAHO) [1] is an international public health agency that works to improve health and living standards of the people from the Americas. Its principal objective is the prevention and control of diseases. The high incidence of diseases signals the need to intensify prevention and control activities. The problem is growing exponentially, and a new approach to program management must be adopted to address solutions for this public health problem.

The New Generation of Programs for Prevention and Control operates under the aegis of health promotion, since health is a collective social good. The paradigm for promotion is centered on the principle that health is the greatest resource for social, economic, and personal development, as well as an important dimension of the quality of life. It also recognizes that political, economic, social, cultural, environmental, behavioral and biological factors can improve people health as much they can damage it. The solution lies in this holistic vision of promotion. It is essential to promote behavioural changes not only in the community, but also in the development and organization of prevention and control programs. The current interventions in the countries are not working at all. They have not been successful or sustainable over the years because of their very costly vertical structure, and because they use community participation and health education only in epidemics and emergencies.

J.M. Barreiro et al. (Eds.): ISBMDA 2004, LNCS 3337, pp. 129–140, 2004.

In the last years an increasing number of new, emerging, and reemerging infectious diseases have been identified in several nations. These diseases threaten to increase in the near future. They include Acquired Immnunodeficiency Virus (AIDS), which emerged in the 1980s and now affects about 16 million people worldwide; and cholera, which returned for the first time this century in 1991 and has caused more than 1 million cases and 9,000 deaths in the Americas. Other infectious diseases like the Tuberculosis declared for the World Health Organization (WHO) in 1993 a global emergency, describing 8 million new cases and 2,500 deaths every year. The elimination of a communicable disease is not feasible, requires new strategies of prevention and control.

The problematic described above, presents a series of questions that can be solved with our project, in order to contribute to the improvement of the efficiency and effectiveness concerning health services delivery. How to obtain reliable information about medical conditions and treatments to accomplish a diagnostic evaluation and a intensive supervision of the diseases? How to predict and validate specific hypothesis diseases diffusion? and, how to guarantee that health professionals (doctors and nurses) receive the adequate education and capacitating about critical problems within the Public Health domain?

Our principal objective is to develop a technological solution that contributes in the fulfillment of the goals established by the Public Health Organizations within of the Prevention and Control Diseases Programs. These programs include: (1) clinical characterization of the diseases of high prevalence, (2) diagnosis, (3) treatment/control and (4) health education. Our approach integrates a set of components that interoperate allowing the interchange information and reuse. The expert component on the base objected oriented allows easily update and adapt the system for any type of disease. The simulator and geographical components are analysis tools for contribute to the monitoring and evaluation of the interventions in health. The ITS for health education improvement the learning and the making-decisions process, by means of the use of personalized tutoring and the case-based reasoning paradigm. Besides, it can incorporate complex medical knowledge, and the adaptation to new teaching strategies or modifications according to the study disease. This architecture is validated within the SINCO-TB project (Intelligent System for prevention and control of Tuberculosis), a system developed at the University of Cauca in Colombia funded by the National System of Science and Technology (Colciencias) [2] and the Departmental Direction of Health [1](DDSC) [3].

This paper is organized as follows. Section 2 describes the antecedents of intelligent systems in health domain. The general architecture of the system is presented in section 3. In section 4 a case of study is exposed. Finally, in the section 5 some conclusions and future work are presented.

[1] The government institution responsible of manage the public health at regional level. To supervise the aplication of the Health Ministery Norms.

2 Antedecedents

2.1 Expert Systems (ES)

Expert systems are programs employed for solving problems and for giving advice within a specialized area of knowledge [4]. An expert system that is well designed and contains an extensive knowledge base, the facts and rules that experts use for making judgments and decisions, can rival the performance of a human specialist in any discipline. Several expert systems have been developed in medicine for medical diagnosis but a small number of ES to help in the decision-making process during the treatment of infectious diseases.

PERFEX [5] is a system based in clinical knowledge to interpret information in 3D of myocardium. This system uses production rules obtained by means of analysis of real clinical cases with the collaborating experts. Murmur Clinic [6] is an expert system supporting in decision-making in the cardiac auscultation process. Prodigy [7] aims to offer an expert system based on high quality medical knowledge.

Our system allows to generate information for patients affected with infectious diseases and to make a careful pursuit of evolution for each patient. In addition considers possible collateral effects that the patient can present with the provision of prescribed treatment.

2.2 Geographical Information Systems (GIS)

GIS are exciting new technologies that combine geography, computing, natural resource management and spatial decision making. The application of geographical information systems to public health problems constitutes a tool of great potential for health research and management. The spatial modelling capacity offered by GIS is directly applicable to understanding the spatial variation of the disease, and allows to establishing relationship with environmental factors and the health care system. Recent advances in geographic information have created new opportunities in health domain [8].

Our GIS contribute to the strengthening of the capacity for epidemiological analysis of the health workers, providing an efficient tool that facilitates such analysis tasks. This computer-based tool will permit the health situation analysis, the monitoring and the evaluation of the effectiveness of interventions that are required for the decision-making and the planning in health. The integration of GIS with the components of the Intelligent System is important for predicting the behaviour of the disease and for visualizing the information spatially facilitating the making-decision process.

2.3 Modelling and Agent-Based Simulation

Nowadays, component-oriented simulation systems belong to the state of the art into the field of public health domain. These systems are not agent-based, are usually dominated by the classical paradigms of technical simulation. Besides, these simulation systems generally neglect the very important impact of human decision making. When the human factor is considered, it is reduced to a status at which human beings are simply seen as passive work pieces.

Our solution to integrate agent-based approaches into classical simulation systems. This allow (1)to construct simulation systems that are able to cope with influences stemming from individual decisions and actions of human beings (2)to design complex simulation models and (3)to improve the quality of results that can be obtained by simulation models that have to deal with human influences in some sense.

2.4 Intelligent Tutoring Systems (ITSs)

Students who receive personalized instruction perform better than students who receive traditional instruction [9]. Realizing that a human teacher cannot possibly provide personalized instruction to every student, the application of technology to contribute to the personally learning seems to be a good idea. Intelligent Tutoring Systems (ITS) provide a way to do just that. For the last twenty years, ITSs have been a focus of research and development of applications in Artificial Intelligence (AI) for education. There has been much development in this area, so it may be safe to claim the field has somewhat matured, and it is time to look in new directions for AI and education.

An ITS consists of four major components: (1)the expert model (2) the student model(3)the pedagogical model and (4)the user interface.

The early applications of technology in education were in computer-aided instruction (CAI) and computer-based instruction (CBI). The late 1980s and early 1990s generated a lot of research into ITSs and their application to individualized instruction. Basic design requirements became well defined. At the same time, changes were occurring in learning and education, and researchers started to look at including these changes in a new generation of intelligent teaching tools. This ITS of the future would need to be transportable, would have to know what to teach, how to teach, and who is being taught.

In the health domain a variety of systems have been developed. Of these, the GUIDON project [10] is most directly relevant. GUIDON used 200 tutorial rules and MYCIN's [11] 400 domain rules to teach medical students to learn to identify the more probable cause in cases of infectious meningitis and bacteremia. However in these systems the scope of domain knowledge was quite small and, the feedback was only relevant to a very small part of the domain. Other ITSs have been developed for diagnosis in radiology as: RAD-TUTOR [12], VIA-RAD [13], and others.

3 The Proposed Architecture

Due to the changes in the health sector, solutions to support decision-making and more complex interventions are required. Our approach, show up as a solution that integrates a set of components. They contribute to the epidemiologic

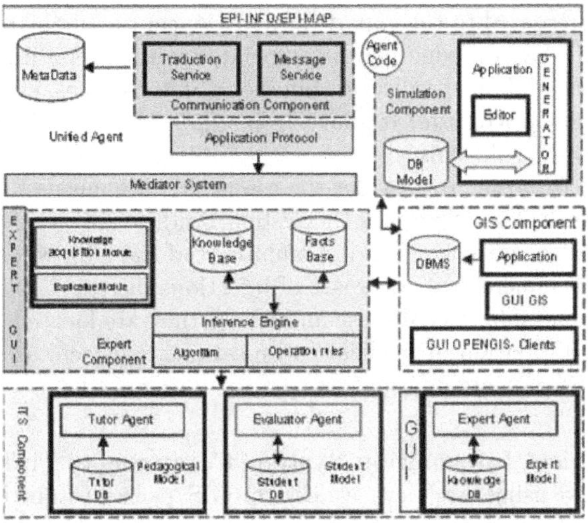

Fig. 1. General System Architecture

analysis, the design and the evaluation of strategies for the prevention and control of infectious diseases. The proposed architecture is depicted in Figure 1. The components of the proposed system are:

a. Expert Component: This component is used in real clinical environments by several users. It supports four roles: expert doctor, general doctor, nurse, and system administrator. We choose Java as the programming language for the development of this program due to their robustness and portability. The main classes of the expert system are implemented as JavaBeans (BeanTreatment, BeanGroupPatient, and BeanRepository). For the handling information stored in XML, we use JDOM an API to read, to create and to manipulate the XML documents. Finally, Mandarax is used for deduction rules because it is object oriented and uses reasoning in Prolog which uses a backward chaining style of reasoning. The following is a brief description of each one of modules that integrate the expert component:

•*Expert GUI:* Provides different Graphic User Interfaces (GUI) to interact with the system. These interfaces allow the user provides useful information of patients to Expert System like weight, age, treatment time, other diseases, etc.

•*Expert Module:* This module includes the representation, handling and processing (querying) of the knowledge base.

•*Knowledge Acquisition Module:* It allows knowledge base editing. Its designed by experts in the domain. The aim of this module is to provide a non-technical view of domain to the expert. The rules, facts and other objects of the domain are represented like sentences of natural language and sequences of words. At this way, a friendly graphical interface for the maintenance of knowledge base is presented to the expert doctor. Conceptually, the concept of repository is added. A knowledge base is associated with a repository that contains meta-information about predicates, functions, data sources, etc.

• ***Explanatory Module:*** It allows to justify and to explain the problem and to propose several solutions.

• ***Control Module:*** It provides the essential mechanisms to exchange information among the components of the system. Additionally, this module provides patients information to the generic simulator and the GIS, whose objectives are to determine the increase or decrease of infectious disease identifying the population group that suffer the disease and where they are located. Furthermore, it handles the information of medical consultations and facilitates the storage in the database of patients information.

b. Geographical Information System Component: This component has been developed using ArcView, a desktop GIS package from Esri [14]. GIS is easy to use and integrates charts, maps, tables and graphics. It has exceptional analysis capabilities and dynamic data updating. It uses the ArcView Spatial Analysis Extension that allows to create, query, map, and analyze cell-based raster data and to perform integrated vector-raster analysis. The information is stored and management using a relational database to assure persistence.

c. Disease Diffusion Simulator Component: The principal objective of the simulation component is to predict the behavior and the diffusion dynamics of the infectious diseases according to socio-economic factors of the environment. By means of the simulator, its possible to validate hypothesis of diffusion of diseases. Besides, the integration with the GIS allows to obtain and to generate scenes of simulation with real data of the survey region. We utilize the multi-agent paradigm in order to obtain reliable information of the regions of high prevalence of infectious diseases. A model based in individuals is created. This model allows: (1) to manage heterogeneous individuals in a community, (2) to let the interaction of each one of the individuals with the environment, (3) to create realistic environment (4) to visualize the simulated phenomenon in a GIS. The Swarm software was used for the multi-agent simulation.

d. Intelligent Tutoring System (ITS): The ITS considers the MASCommonKADS methodology, which proposes seven models for the definition of the multi-agent system (agents, tasks, experience, coordination, communication, organization and design). The system is developed under a multi-agent approach compatible with the FIPA standards [15]. In the ITS development we use Java, JavaScript and XML. The ITS modules are distributed and divided in smaller parts called agents. These agents work like autonomous entities, and act rationally in accordance with its environment perceptions and knowledge status. Moreover, the agents exchange information with one another, providing modularity and interoperability. Next a brief description of each one of modules that integrate the ITS:

• ***Expert Agent:*** It is responsible for guiding and controlling the tutoring process. The expert agent includes expert knowledge concerning teaching, learning and evaluation. Besides it is responsible for directing the execution of the tutoring process according to the data introduced by the student.

• ***Evaluator Agent:*** This agent to evaluate the student behavior. According to the student evolution during the instructional plan, the evaluator agent modifies the student profile or, requests to the tutor agent the instructional plan reform.

• ***Tutor Agent:*** It is responsible for reasoning about student behavior. Its objective is to generate the instructional plan adapted to the student needs. This agent works with the case-base reasoning (CBR) learning paradigm [16], derived from Artificial Intelligence, to teach abstract knowledge based on problem classes. This paradigm exhibit two kinds of learning: learning from memorisation and learning from their own experiences. The basic idea of CBR is solve new problems by adapting successful solutions that were used previously. The tutor agent will modify the teaching strategy according to the information given by the evaluator agent.

• ***Student Database:*** It is used for storing information about student profile, characteristics, student record, and student knowledge.

• ***Knowledge Database:*** It contains the information domain. This information is essential in order to decide the students tasks according to the learning objectives.

• ***Tutor Database:*** It contains the information about the learning-teaching process.

• ***Agents Communication:*** In order to provide agent communication, we use the set of KQML performatives [17]. In the communication model, the expert agent checks the student profile and sends the information to the agent tutor in order to generate the teaching strategy. The agent tutor compares the student actions with the teaching strategy and communicates the results to the evaluator agent. It updates the student profile and notifies the changes to the expert agent. The expert agent accomplishes the adaptations to continue the learning process.

• ***Communication Component:*** This component is scalable and robust. It provides multiple interfaces for connecting with other systems. It manages messages between the components due to the necessity of systems interoperability. It consists of three modules: Metadata Repository, Message Service and Traduction Service. XML Schemas are used for metadata generation. The communication between components is accomplished through SOAP - Simple Object Access Protocol specially used for the interchange information in a distributed environment.

4 SINCO-TB: An Approach for the Prevention and Control of Tuberculosis

The Tuberculosis (TB) is an infectious disease. In Colombia the TB constitutes a critical problem in public health. The largest number of cases occurs due to neglect in the Prevention and Control Programs, inefficient anti-tuberculosis practices, the lethal combination HIV-TB, the increase demographic population, etc. In this section, the particularities about the specific task for diagnosis, treatment/control and training in tuberculosis together with the solutions proposed and implemented in the SINCO-TB prototype are discussed.

For the system development we have taken the following information: (a) medical patient record (b) Individual Patient Card (c) Health National Norm (d) medications (e) medical reports (f) population classified by: stratus, district and communes, (g) organization processes provided by the DDSC, and (h) cartography of the study regions. Initially the study regions are the cities of Popayán, Santander de Quilichao and Silvia located in the department of Cauca (Colombia).

The diagnosis, treatment and control process has three main phases: (1) classification of the patient in one of the categories (patients affected by pulmonary tuberculosis, or extra-pulmonary tuberculosis), (2) evaluation of the specific diagnosis and provition the adequate treatment, and (3) accomplishment the tracking and patient control.

(1) the distinction between the two types of tuberculosis is important because the treatment and control in each category is different. The pulmonary tuberculosis is a contagious disease, each person with active TB disease will infect on average between 10 and 15 people every year. The patients with pulmonary tuberculosis require a strict treatment. When patients do not take all their medicines regularly for the required period, these patients become drug-resistant. The bacilli in their lungs may develop resistance to anti-TB medicines. The people they infect will have the same drug-resistant strain. While drug-resistant TB is generally treatable, it requires extensive chemotherapy that is often prohibitively expensive and is also more toxic for the patients. The extra-pulmonary tuberculosis patients are usually not infectious. The diagnostic guidelines are less specific and include strong clinical evidence made by a clinician for treat with anti-TB chemotherapy.

(2) Once the system identifies the type of tuberculosis affecting the patient, the expert component of SINCO-TB lets to register the patients information. For each patient, the doctor introduces the following information:(a)basic data: name, weight and age of the patient (b) scheme: it identifies the type of patient (new, chronic case,etc) (c) special situations: it allows specifying if the patient suffers other diseases such as diabetes mellitus and fails renal, among others, and (d) test of sensitivity: it establishes sensitivity or resistance to medicines. Once introduced the data above mentioned, the system chooses a base treatment. In this selection only considers the characteristic of the patient from which its possible to obtain a general treatment. In this process a knowledge base with the rules necessary is loaded to generate the treatment and some recommendations. This treatment is obtained from the database as a XML document which is turned to serializables java objects. Once generated the base treatment, the system loads a new specific knowledge base which contains the rules necessary to generate modifications that are applied to the base treatment to generate the final treatment. The treatment is visualized in the GUITreatment as is depicted in the Figure 2. Besides for the monitoring and tracking of therapy for patients in treatment, the system to generate alerts when patients can not be carried out the treatment regimens. Finally the medical prescription is printed and the medical reports are generated. These reports store the results of this intensive process and are delivery to the DDSC and the Health Ministery.

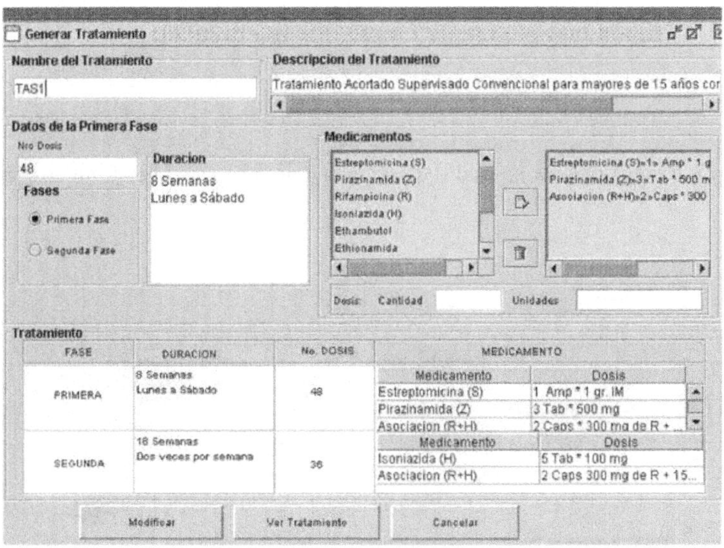

Fig. 2. GUITreatment

(3) In the control process, the geographical component obtains the patients information through the communication with the expert component. The GIS store the spatial data and non-spatial or attribute data in an information infrastructure. This infrastructure includes a single database system for managing spatial data, and a data structure that is independent of the application. The benefits of this approach include (1) better data management for spatial data (2) spatial data are stored in Database Management Systems (DBMS), and (3) decrease the complexity of system management by eliminating the hybrid architecture of GIS data models.

As soon as GIS is used as disease management system, patients location is displayed on the map. It solve the problem of data visualization, moreover, we can query patient spatial data from attribute data or vice versa. This is depicted in the Figure 3.

The GIS is enabled (1) to locate high prevalence areas and populations at risk (2) to classify by type of patient (3) to identify areas in need of resources, and (4) to make decisions on resource allocation. In the figure 4 are depicted some functions about it.

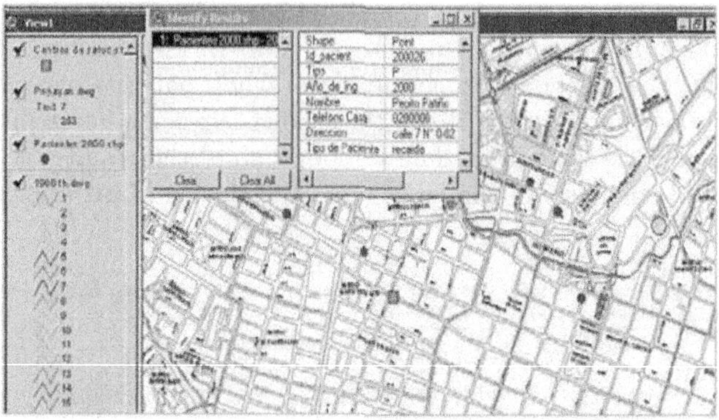

Fig. 3. Query patient spatial data or query patient attribute from spatial data

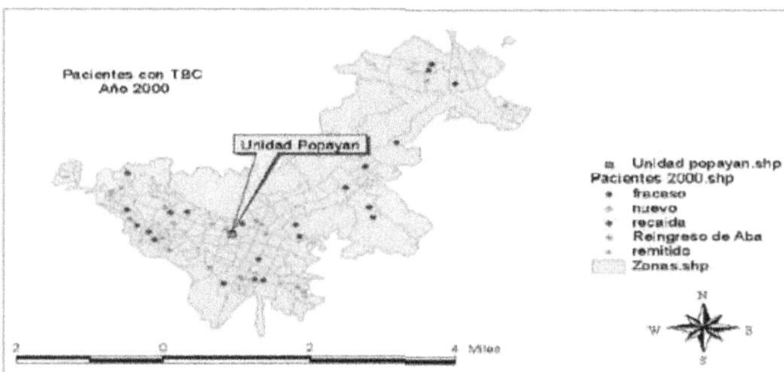

Fig. 4. Determination of critical zones and ubication of type of patients

Finally, the multi-agent simulator gets information of the GIS to process and to visualize graphically a future scene of the prevalence of tuberculosis in different groups of ages. This component to allow (1) to identify the group more affected, and (2) to provide information that suggest to the health professionals the elaboration of preventive strategies in specific zones and oriented to specific groups. The GIS generates information in a compatible format with Epi-Info and Epi-Map. These systems allow generate analysis statistical and geographical treatment respectly.

In the training process the development of the Intelligent Tutoring System will contribute to the formation at clinic, epidemiological and operative level. The system takes the information of real cases provided by the expert component. Afterwards the traduction service of the system structures the information guarantying its privacy. The students interact with the system, which is composed of different agents, filtering, processing and evaluating the learning information. The ITS is the last component built and is under testing by medical students and professionals.

5 Conclusions and Future Work

The aim of this paper was to show the use of information technology to improve (1) the medical data analysis (2) the making decisions process and, (3) the health education processes. In the presented research we employed several Artificial Intelligence techniques as Expert Systems, Intelligent Tutoring Systems and Machine Learning, together with Decision Support Systems as GIS and simulation models.

The SINCO-TB system is being used in the DDSC and several health establishments with the purpose of validating and measuring its real benefits. The effect of SINCO-TB has been analyzed with a experimental set of infectious patients composed by 40 patients, 30 of them with pulmonary tuberculosis and the rest with extra-pulmonary tuberculosis.

The health professionals that were in charge of using SINCO-TB in their establishments provided a set of medical reports [18] about patient evolution. These reports determined the decrease in cases and also in anti-TB drugs patients.

A evaluation survey [18] on the effectiveness of SINCO-TB has also been performed. The results obtained shown that SINCO-TB has been considered a huge profit because it allowed: (1) to manage better the patients information (2) to provide a quick and adequate diagnostic (3) to contribute in the taking of decisions related with the patient treatment (4) to accomplish strict controls, and (5) to predict and validate hypothesis concerning the diffusion of the diseases. Besides, the system provided opportunities for environmental epidemiologists to study associations between environmental exposure and the spatial distribution of infectious diseases.

This encouraging results have been obtained due to the contributions of SINCO-TB to track the Directly Observed Treatment Strategy (DOTS) and the efficient application of Health National Norm.

Finally, we observed that SINCO approach can be easily used to manage other infectious diseases such as: dengue, cholera, malaria, etc. As future work, we plan to extend its functionality to manage more types of infectious diseases.

References

1. Alleyne, George. : Health in the Americas II Edition. http://www.paho.org, 2002.
2. Instituto Colombiano para el Desarrollo de la Ciencia y la Tecnología "Francisco José de Caldas" COLCIENCIAS. http://www.colciencias.gov.co, 2003.
3. Dirección Departamental de Salud del Cauca. http://www.ddsc.gov.co, 2004.
4. Park, John, Stanley Y. W.An integrated approach to heterogeneous expert systems. *Proceedings of the third international conference and engineering applications of artificial intelligence and expert systems,* 2:53-592. ACM Press. Charleston South Carolina, United States, 1990.
5. N.F. Exquerra, R. Mullick, E. V. Gracia, C. D. Cooke., and E. Kanchouska. PERFEX: An Expert System for interpreting 3D Myocardial Perfusion. *Expert Systems with Applications.* Pergamon Press, 1992.

6. Leong, T. Y. Murmur Clinic:A diagnostic expert system for auscultation. *In Proceedings of the 11th Annual Symposium on Computer Applications in Medical Care,* pages 166-170. IEEE, 1987.
7. Etzioni O. and Minton S. Why EBL produces overly-specific knowledge: A critique of the Prodigy approaches. *In International Conference on Machine Learning,* pages 137-143. Aberdeen, Scotland.Morgan Kaufmann, 1992.
8. Noon, E. Charles. Spatial Data Visualization in HealthCare. *In Proceedings of the International Conference on System Sciences.* IEEE, 2001.
9. Bloom, B. S. The 2-sigma problem. The search for methods of group instruction as effective as one-to-one tutoring. *Educational Researcher,* Vol 13, pages 3-16, 1984.
10. Clancey, WJ. Overview de GUIDON. *Journal of Computer-Based Instruction,* 10:8-15, 1982.
11. Davis, R., Buchanan B. and Shortliffe, E. Production Rules as a Representation for Knowledge-Based Consultation Programs. *Readings in Medical Artificial Intelligence: The First Decade,* pages 98-130. Addison Wesley, 1984.
12. Azevedo, R. and Lajoie, SP. The cognitive basis for the design of a mammography interpretation tutor. *International Journal of Artificial Intelligence in Education,* 9:32-34, 1998.
13. Rogers, E. VIA-RAD: a blackboard-based system for diagnostic radiology. *Journal of Artificial Intelligence in Medicine,* 7(4):343-60, 1995.
14. Geographic Information Systems and Mapping. ESRI. USA. http://www.esri.com/company/copyright.html, 2004.
15. Nicol, R. and O'brien. FIPA-Towards a Standard for Software Agents. http://www.bt.com/bttj/vol16no3/06.pdf, 2004.
16. Aamodt, A. Explanation-Driven case based reasoning. *In S. Wess, K Althoff, M. Ritcher. (eds.): Topics en Case-based reasoning,* pages 274-288. Springer Verlag, 1994.
17. May, J., Labrou, Y. and T, Finin. Evaluating KQML as an agent communication language. *Intelligent Agents II, Lecture Notes in Artificial Intelligence 1039,* pages 347-360, Berlin, Germany Springer, 1996.
18. Vidal, J. C. Intelligent System for the Control of Tuberculosis. Project Research Report. *SINCO-TB Project, code 1103-04-13015, contract 523-2002. Colciencias,* University of Cauca. Colombia.

Could a Computer Based System for Evaluating Patients with Suspected Myocardial Infarction Improve Ambulance Allocation?

Martin Gellerstedt, Angela Bång, and Johan Herlitz

Sahlgrenska University Hospital, Göteborg, Sweden
martin.gellerstedt@htu.se

Keywords: acute myocardial infarction, logistic regression, ambulance allocation, decision support

1 Introduction

The very early handling of patients with suspected acute myocardial infarction (AMI) is crucial for the outcome. In Gothenburg approximately two-third of all patients with AMI dial the emergency number for ambulance transport (reference). Gothenburg has a two different types of ambulances; special ambulances with paramedics and a nurse onboard and standard ambulances (personnel with 7 weeks of medical education). The dispatchers are instructed to call for a special ambulance if the case history implies an AMI or other life-threatening diseases, whereas the standard ambulance is to be used in less alarming cases. However, statistics shows that a disappointingly high proportion of AMI patients were transported by the standard ambulance and not the mobile coronary art unit, i.e. the special ambulance (referens). The evaluation of a telephone interview is not an easy task. The information left by the patient and relatives is often limited and symptoms like for instance chest pain could arise for various reasons other than ischaemic heart disease. The judgment made by the dispatcher is subjective and based on vague information. In order to learn more about allocation and outcome for patients a prospective survey was performed including 503 consecutive patients who dialed the emergency number and complained about chest pain. We have earlier reported (referens) that there was a direct relationship between the dispatcher's initial suspicion of AMI and the subsequent diagnosis. However, the early mortality rate was similar in patients with at least a strong suspicion of AMI and those with only a moderate, vague or no suspicion. Therefore it is important to identify methods for better delineate patients with a life-threatening condition already at the dispatch centre. In an earlier study (Baxt 1991), including patients presenting to an emergency department with chest pain, it is reported that a neural network may be a valuable aid to the clinical diagnosis of AMI. To evaluate a patient's condition based on a short telephone interview is a difficult task. Since the interview contains a number of questions which must be considered mutually, the judgment must be considered as a multivariable task. It is therefore interesting to evaluate the use of a multivariate model as a support for such a judgment.

The aim with the present study is to evaluate if a computer based decision support system, including a multivariate model, could be useful for identifying patients with AMI or life-threatening conditions and thereby improving ambulance allocation.

J.M. Barreiro et al. (Eds.): ISBMDA 2004, LNCS 3337, pp. 141–147, 2004.

2 Patients and Methods

Studied Population

The municipality of Gothenburg had at the time of the study 434 000 inhabitants. All patients who called the emergency number from an address within the municipality and who were assessed by the dispatchers as having acute chest pain were included in the study.

Variables and Definitions

For each enrolled patient a specific case record form was used. This includes a standardized set of questions regarding: duration of pain, intensity (severe/vague) and presence of the following symptoms: dyspnoea, cold sweat, nausea, vertigo and syncope. Patients were also generally asked about age but not about previous history. In the end of the telephone interview, the dispatcher used a five graded scale for judging suspicion of AMI, based on the answers during the interview. The five grades were: 1=no suspicion, 2=vague suspicion, 3=moderate suspicion, 4=strong suspicion, 5=convincing AMI. According to established routines the were three levels of dispatch based on the suspected severity: (1) highest priority and call for special ambulance, (2) highest priority but don't call for special ambulance and (3) not highest priority and don't call for special ambulance.

At the hospital a final diagnosis was set. For confirmed AMI at least two of the following had to be fulfilled: chest pain with a duration of at least 15 min; elevated serum enzyme activity of the MB form of creatine kinase (CK-MB) at least twice above the upper normal limit; or development of Q-waves in at least two leads in a 12-lead standard electrocardiogram (ECG).

Retrospectively, each call was classified as life-threatening (LT) or not. To be judged as LT, one of the following must be fulfilled: death before discharge; a final diagnosis of AMI or ischaemia, pulmonary embolism, aortic aneurysm or pneumothorax; or any of the following either prior to hospital admission or during hospitalization – ventricular fibrillation, ventricular tachycardia, asystole or pulseless electrical activity.

Organization

All ambulances were dispatched by one centre. For each call assessed as priority 1 with a need for a special ambulance, a mobile care unit, if available, and the nearest standard ambulance were simultaneously dispatched. There were two mobile coronary care units working on a full-time basis. There were 11 standard ambulances located at six fire departments, situated in a way that 50% of patients will be reached within 5 min and 97% within 10 min after a call being received. A nurse was onboard the mobile coronary care unit from 8 a.m. to 5 p.m., furthermore two paramedics, with 39 weeks medical training, were always onboard. The personnel in the standard ambulances had 7 weeks medical training. The dispatchers had all received two weeks medical training (repeated 3 days every year), emphasizing on identifying relevant symptoms via telephone interviews.

The coronary care unit crew was delegated to intubate, and part of the crew were delegated to give intravenous medication. Thrombolytic agents were not given in the prehospital phase and there were no facilities for external pacing. All standard ambulances were equipped with semi-automatic defibrillators.

Statistical Methods

The primary variables in this study were final diagnosis of AMI and if a patient were retrospectively classified as a patient with life-threatening condition (LTC) or not. Univariate analyses of gender and symptoms in relationship to AMI/LTC are analyzed by chi-square test. Possible differences in age between patients with or without AMI/LTC are analyzed by a standard t-test. For multivariate analyses regarding the relationship between patient characteristics (according to case record form used during the interview) and the dichotomous response variables (AMI/LTC), logistic regression was used (one model for AMI and one model for LTC). For each patient a probability of AMI/LTC was calculated based on these models. These probabilities could be regarded as comprehensive index, including the multivariable characteristics of the patient, which indicate the severity of the patients' condition and could therefore be used for allocating ambulances. Assuming that this estimated model was available at the start of the study, we use the probabilities retrospectively for a fictive allocation of ambulances. This model allocation is then compared with the true allocation made by the dispatchers. The allocation based on the model simply uses the estimated probabilities, and for each patient the allocation of an ambulance follows the simple rule:

If probability of AMI > threshold value ,
then use special ambulance otherwise use standard ambulance

The same rule is also applied in the second model with LTC as a target. The choice of threshold value affects the sensitivity and specificity of the allocation, i.e. in this case sensitivity represents the probability that a patient with AMI/LTC is transported with special ambulance, specificity is the probability that a patient without AMI/LTC gets the standard ambulance. The choice of a threshold value is arbitrary, but for being able to make a fair comparison we identified the threshold value which gave 381 transportations with special ambulance and 122 with the standard ambulance, which is identical with the true allocation made by the dispatchers. Thus, with the same distribution between special and standard ambulances we have the possibility to evaluate possible benefits, e.g. decreased medical risk – defined as an AMI patient transported in standard ambulance.

In the basic model for AMI and LTC we used all variables included in the interview except duration of pain (due to missing values). Furthermore the dispatcher's initial suspicion of AMI was not included in the models, since we wanted to evaluate a model without subjective judgments from the dispatchers. However, in an explorative analysis we added this variable to the model. In an explorative manner we also evaluated models with other variables included which not were included in the case record forms but which in the future could be added.

Possible differences between dispatcher allocation and allocation based on logistic regression probabilities were analyzed with the McNemars test.

Since this study, is of an explorative nature and since there are many tests performed, no formal level of significance is stated and p-values should be interpreted with care, i.e. a low p-value should be regarded more as an indicator than a formal confirmation.

Table 1. Age, gender and symptomprofile, by AMI

		AMI			
		No	**Yes**	**Total**	**p-value**
	N	398	105	503	
	%	79.1	20.9	100	
Age	Mean	70.1	73.7	70.8	0.008
	Median	73.0	77.0	74.0	
	SD	14.7	11.5	14.2	
Gender	% Male	49.5	60.0	51.7	0.055
Pain	% Strong	65.1	81.9	68.6	0.001
Dyspnoea	% Yes	19.6	23.8	20.5	>0.20
Cold sweat	% Yes	15.6	23.8	17.3	0.047
Nausea	% Yes	33.9	36.2	34.4	>0.20
Vertigo	% Yes	8.5	3.8	7.6	0.103
Syncope	% Yes	4.8	3.8	4.6	>0.20

Table 2. Age, gender and symptomprofile, by LT

		LTC			
		No	**Yes**	**Total**	**p-value**
	N	273	220	493	
	%	55.4	44.6	100	
Age	Mean	68.4	74.3	71.0	0.000
	Median	72.0	76.0	74.0	
	SD	15.5	11.1	14.0	
Gender	% Male	49.1	54.1	51.3	>0.20
Pain	% Strong	65.6	72.3	68.6	0.111
Dyspnoea	% Yes	20.5	20.0	20.3	>0.20
Cold sweat	% Yes	15.8	19.1	17.2	>0.20
Nausea	% Yes	33.7	35.5	34.5	>0.20
Vertigo	% Yes	9.5	5.5	7.7	0.092
Syncope	% Yes	5.1	3.6	4.5	>0.20

3 Results

Demographics

During this three months long period 503 patients calling about chest pain were enrolled, all patients received a diagnosis and for 493 patients it was possible to retrospectively classify the condition as LT or not. In this study we focus on the characteristics found during the interview, and basic differences between patients with and without AMI/LTC is found in tables 1 and 2. A more detailed description about patient demographics, medical history, status during hospitalization, prior medication, etc is found in earlier studies (reference). Naturally, we want to identify variables that could discriminate patients with vs. without AMI/LTC. Regarding AMI, age and pain (vague/strong) are significantly different; gender and cold sweat are also possible discriminating variables, while other symptoms are less likely to contribute significantly in the separation of patients. Regarding LTC, there is no sharp difference in profiles, but age and possibly pain and vertigo may contribute to separate patients with and without LTC. Regarding the initial suspicion of AMI made by the dispatchers there is a direct relationship to the diagnosis of AMI (and LTC) as described in earlier study (ibid). The relationship is also presented in table 3. With consecutive higher degree of initially suspected AMI a consecutively increased prevalence of AMI/LTC is followed.

Table 3. Relationship between dispatchers initial suspicion of AMI and prevalence of AMI and LTC

Suspicion of AMI	% AMI (N=484)	% LTC (N=474)
No	**7.7**	**35.9**
Vague	**17.3**	**36.7**
Moderate	**17.6**	**42.4**
Strong	**26.6**	**51.9**
Convincing	**50**	**61.1**
% Tot	**20.9**	**44.5**

Table 4. AMI by ambulance allocation a comparison: Dispatchers vs. Model

			Ambulance – Dispatchers allocation		Ambulance – Model allocation	
			Standard	**Special**	**Standard**	**Special**
	No	n	107	291	114	284
	N=398 (79%)	%	26.9	73.1	28.6	71.4
AMI	**Yes**	n	15	90	8	97
	N=105 (21%)	%	14.3	**85.7**	7.6	**92.4**
Total	N=503	n	122	381	122	381

p-value=0.167, regarding sensitivity (McNemar)

Allocation in Relation to AMI

In table 4 the relationship between patients with and without AMI and the choice of ambulance is illustrated. The true allocation made by the dispatchers is compared with the fictive allocation based on the logistic regression model. As we earlier mentioned the threshold value is chosen on a level which gives exactly the same distribution between standard ambulances and special ambulances as the distribution made by the dispatchers. The sensitivity, i.e. the proportion of AMI patients transported by special ambulance was 85.7% regarding the true allocation made by the dispatchers. The corresponding sensitivity regarding allocation made by the model was 92.4% (p-value=0.167). The specificity is also slightly higher for the model allocation than dispatchers' allocation. Thus, we can see that the fictive allocation decreased the number of AMI patients erroneous allocated a standard ambulance, without increasing the use of a special ambulance.

Allocation in Relation to LTC

Naturally, we want to allocate the special ambulance for all patients in a severe condition and not only AMI patients. Therefore, evaluation of allocation in relationship to the retrospectively classification of patients as patients with a life-threatening condition or not, may be more relevant. In table 5 we can see that the proportion of patients with LTC was 0.45. Allocation made by dispatchers gives a sensitivity of 80.9% and corresponding sensitivity for allocation made by the model is 86.4%, p-value 0.149. The allocation made by dispatchers includes 42 patients with LTC transported with standard ambulance. This must be considered as an error related to a medical risk and the corresponding figure for allocation based on the model is 30 (29% decrease). At the same time, the specificity is slightly higher for allocation based on the model.

Table 5. LTC by ambulance allocation a comparison: Dispatcher vs Model

			Ambulance – Dispatchers allocation		**Ambulance – Model allocation**	
			Standard	**Special**	**Standard**	**Special**
	No	n	75	198	87	186
	N=273(55%)	%	27.5	72.5	31.9	68.1
LTC	**Yes**	n	42	178	30	190
	N=220(45%)	%	19.1	**80.9**	13.6	**86.4**
Total	N=493	n	117	376	117	376

p-value=0.149, regarding sensitivity (McNemar)

4 Discussion

We have pointed out that the fictive allocation based on the model decreased the number of AMI patients erroneous allocated a standard ambulance, without increasing the use of a special ambulance. It is also interesting to evaluate if we could decrease the use of special ambulance without declining the medical quality. We changed the threshold level and decreased the proportion of special ambulances used, but without exceeding 15 AMI patients transported with standard ambulance. We found that by using allocation according to the model the use of special ambulance could be decreased 31 times (around 8% decrease) during this period without increasing the medical risk (15 AMI patients in standard ambulance).

A patient with AMI transported with a standard ambulance is an incorrect allocation and the dispatchers had 15 such cases while the model allocation had 8 cases (47% decrease). It is interesting to note that within these eight patients there are only two of them which belong to the 15 cases wrongly allocated by the dispatchers. Allocations seams to be based on different sources. We analyzed the 15 patients with AMI who were allocated a standard ambulance by the dispatchers and 9 died (8 during and 1 after hospitalization). The corresponding figures among the 8 patients with AMI allocated a standard ambulance by the model, only 1 patient died (in hospital), p-value=0.021. Generally, there were in total 46 cases of death (1 prior to hospital, 32 in hospital and 13 after hospitalization) and out of these patients the dispatchers used the standard ambulance in 14 cases while the model (based on high probability of AMI) allocated the standard ambulance in only 4 cases, p-value 0.013.

We also elaborated with a lot of different models, where we for instance added the initial suspicion of AMI, if patient had an earlier AMI etc. We found that the allocation could be slightly improved by adding these variables and the number of incorrect allocations could be decreased even more, i.e. two fewer erroneous allocations (AMI in standard ambulance).

We found it interesting that the erroneous allocation done by the model mainly were on other patients than the patients wrongly allocated by the dispatchers. Unfortunately the sample size is to little to find any convincing patterns, but among the 15 patients with AMI allocated a standard ambulance by dispatchers, two-third of these were females (compared to 48% females of all patients), and among these ten females 6 had weak pain.

The logistic regression model we have used could of course be implemented in computer software and a computer based decision support system (CBDSS)could be built. Then it would be possible for the dispatchers to enter answers during the interview and to get a suggested allocation according to the model. Of course the dispatchers may receive other information during the interview more than just the answers, for instance an anxious voice etc, and based on experience the dispatchers may evaluate the patient different than the model. However, it is possible to include the dispatchers preferred ambulance as a variable in the model. In that way the softer information and dispatchers experience could be taken into account. As we noticed in our explorative analyses, adding the dispatchers initial suspicion of AMI actually improved the allocation, even if all questions asked was included as well. In the explorative analyses we also found other variables which could improve allocation if they were added to the interview. For instance information about earlier AMI was essential.

Furthermore, it may be possible to improve the allocation by making questions clearer. For instance, whether pain is vague or strong may be a subjective question and answers may differ due to age, gender, etc.

As we have noticed in our database, allocation made by dispatcher is subjective, two patients with similar profiles could actually receive different care, i.e. one could be allocated a standard ambulance and the other the special ambulance. If a CBDSS is used the allocation would be standardized and objective.

5 Validity of the Study

Since our model is applied on the same data set as it is estimated up on, allocation performance may be overestimated. Furthermore, the threshold level was not predefined and even if our choice of level intended to get a fair comparison it is an advantage to be able to retrospectively choose a level and this could also imply over optimistic performance of the model. It would be good if the performance is confirmed by applying the model on a new independent data set. However, in an reliability check, we divided the data set in two parts and developed a model and a threshold level with one part and applied it on the second part, and the results from that cross-validation is consistent with the results in this study.

Moreover, the dataset has been used in a number of courses in statistics and data mining as an assignment and even in a student thesis (reference). In these courses regression models have been compared with other analysis techniques such as neural networks and a lot of different models have been evaluated. Generally, the results from these assignments are that a model could improve allocation.

6 Conclusion

In summary, we believe that a computer based decision support system including a regression model would be a valuable tool for allocating ambulances. Such a system may also be valuable in similar settings were the severity of a patients condition must be judged rapidly. However, the case record form used for the interview can be refined and a model based on a larger sample and confirmed in prospectively studies is recommended.

On the Robustness of Feature Selection with Absent and Non-observed Features

Petra Geenen[1], Linda C. van der Gaag[1], Willie Loeffen[2], and Armin Elbers[2]

[1] Institute of Information and Computing Sciences, Utrecht University
P.O. Box 80.089, 3508 TB Utrecht, The Netherlands
{petrag,linda}@cs.uu.nl
[2] Central Institute For Animal Disease Control, Wageningen UR
P.O. Box 2004, 8203 AA Lelystad, The Netherlands
{willie.loeffen,armin.elbers}@wur.nl

Abstract. To improve upon early detection of Classical Swine Fever, we are learning selective Naive Bayesian classifiers from data that were collected during an outbreak of the disease in the Netherlands. The available dataset exhibits a lack of distinction between absence of a clinical symptom and the symptom not having been addressed or observed. Such a lack of distinction is not uncommonly found in biomedical datasets. In this paper, we study the effect that not distinguishing between absent and non-observed features may have on the subset of features that is selected upon learning a selective classifier. We show that while the results from the filter approach to feature selection are quite robust, the results from the wrapper approach are not.

1 Introduction

Naive Bayesian classifiers have proven to be powerful tools for solving classification problems in a variety of domains. A Naive Bayesian classifier in essence is a model of a joint probability distribution over a set of stochastic variables. It is composed of a single class variable, modelling the possible outcomes or classes for the problem under study, and a set of feature variables, modelling the features that provide for distinguishing between the various classes. In the model, the feature variables are assumed to be mutually independent given the class variable [5]. Instances of the classification problem under study are represented as value assignments to the various feature variables. For a given problem instance, the classifier returns a probability distribution over the class variable. Naive Bayesian classifiers have been successfully applied in the medical domain where they are being used for solving diagnostic problems.

Bayesian classifiers are typically learned from data. Learning a Naive Bayesian classifier amounts to establishing the prior probabilities of the classes discerned and estimating the conditional probabilities of the various features given each of the classes. A real-life dataset often includes more features of the problem's instances than are strictly necessary for the classification task at hand. When constructing a classifier from the dataset, these more or less redundant

J.M. Barreiro et al. (Eds.): ISBMDA 2004, LNCS 3337, pp. 148–159, 2004.

features may bias the classifier and result in a relatively poor classification accuracy. Now, by constructing it over a carefully selected subset of the features, a less complex classifier is yielded that tends to have a better generalisation performance [6, 9]. The features to be included in such a restrictive classifier can be selected in different ways. Within the filter approach feature selection is performed in a pre-processing step before the actual learning algorithm is applied, while within the wrapper approach the selection of features is merged with the learning algorithm; while different in concept, the two approaches are considered to be comparable in many respects [10]. We would like to note that the subset of features selected by either one of the approaches typically includes the features that are the most discriminative between the different classes and can therefore serve as the basis for further data collection.

In a project in the domain of veterinary medicine, we studied a dataset on Classical Swine Fever for learning various Bayesian classifiers and for selecting an appropriate subset of the available features for further data collection. Classical Swine Fever is a highly infectious viral disease of pigs, which has serious socio-economical consequences. As the disease has a potential for rapid spread, it is imperative that its occurrence is detected in the early stages. The overall aim of our project is to develop a classifier for distinguishing between herds that are infected by Classical Swine Fever and herds that are not, based upon readily observed clinical symptoms. The data that we have at our disposal to this end, were collected during the 1997/1998 Classical Swine Fever epidemic in the Netherlands. The data include the clinical symptoms observed by veterinarians in 490 herds. The collected data had been analysed before using statistical techniques, from which a deterministic classification rule had been derived [2].

During the 1997/1998 Classical Swine Fever epidemic, veterinarians recorded the clinical symptoms that they observed in the herds under their consideration. Upon constructing the dataset, the symptoms recorded by a veterinarian were encoded as '1's for the appropriate variables; symptoms that were not explicitly recorded were assumed to be absent and were encoded as '0's. In the resulting dataset, therefore, the clinical symptoms encoded as '1's indeed are known to have been present in the various herds. Since there is no distinction in our dataset between absence of a symptom and the symptom not having been addressed or observed, however, it is unknown whether the symptoms encoded as '0's were really absent. Such a lack of distinction is not uncommonly found in datasets in veterinary and human medicine. In this paper, we study the effect that not distinguishing between absent and non-observed features may have on the subset of features that is selected upon learning a selective Naive Bayesian classifier. We show that, for our dataset, the results from the filter approach to feature selection are relatively robust in the sense that the results are not strongly affected by the lack of distinction outlined above; the results from the wrapper approach to feature selection, on the other hand, are considerably less robust. Although we studied just a single dataset, our findings suggest that the filter approach may be the preferred approach when performing feature selection on a small to moderately-sized dataset in which no distinction is made between features that are truly absent and features that have not been addressed or observed.

The paper is organised as follows. In Section 2, we briefly review Classical Swine Fever; we further describe the dataset that we have available for our study. In Section 3, the design, the results and some conclusions from our study are presented. The paper ends in Section 4 with our concluding observations and directions of future research.

2 The Domain of Classical Swine Fever

We provide some background knowledge on Classical Swine Fever and describe the dataset that we have available for learning purposes.

2.1 Classical Swine Fever

Classical Swine Fever is a highly infectious viral disease of pigs that has a potential for rapid spread. The virus causing the disease is transmitted mainly by direct contact between infected and non-infected susceptible pigs, although transmission by farmers, veterinarians, equipment or artificial insemination may also occur. When a pig is infected, the virus first invades the lymphatic system and subsequently affects the blood vessels thereby giving rise to bleedings. The virus ultimately affects the internal organs and the pig will die. As a consequence of the infection, a pig will show various disease symptoms, such as fever, reduced food intake, inflammation of the eyes, walking disorders, and haemorrhages of the skin. Classical Swine Fever is quite common in parts of Europe and Africa, and in many countries of Asia, Central and South America [1].

Since an outbreak of Classical Swine Fever has a major impact on international trade of animals and animal products, extensive measures have been taken within the European pig husbandry to prevent the introduction and spread of the disease. Nevertheless, each year several outbreaks occur which have serious socio-economical consequences. In the 1997/1998 epidemic in the Netherlands, for example, 429 herds were infected and 12 million pigs had to be killed. The total costs involved were estimated to be 2.3 billion US dollars. One of the major factors that affects the total costs of an epidemic, is the time between introduction of the virus and first diagnosis of the disease. The longer the disease remains undetected, the longer the virus can circulate without hindrance and the more herds can become infected. In the 1997/1998 epidemic in the Netherlands, for example, it was estimated that the disease remained undetected for six weeks and that, by that time, already 39 herds were infected [3].

Clinical symptoms seen by the farmer or by a veterinarian are usually the first indication of the presence of Classical Swine Fever in a pig herd. When a suspicion of the disease is reported to the ministry, a veterinary expert team visits the farm to inspect the herd. Depending on the clinical symptoms observed, the team decides whether or not the disease indeed is indicated and decides upon the samples to be taken for laboratory diagnosis. The clinical symptoms of Classical Swine Fever, unfortunately, are mainly atypical and may vary from mild to severe, as a consequence of which the disease can remain undetected for weeks.

To improve upon early detection, we are developing a classifier for distinguishing between herds that are infected by Classical Swine Fever and herds that are not, based upon easily observed clinical symptoms.

2.2 The Data

During the 1997/1998 Classical Swine Fever epidemic in the Netherlands, veterinary expert teams visited quite a number of suspected pig herds. The body temperature of the diseased pigs in such a herd were measured. Also, the presence of disease symptoms within the herd were recorded on the investigation form used; if a single pig was observed to suffer from inflammation of the eyes, for example, then this symptom was marked as being present in the herd. Pigs with apparent clinical symptoms were euthanised and submitted to the Animal Health Service for a post-mortem examination. If one or more pigs from such a submission proved to be infected with the virus, then the herd was diagnosed as positive for Classical Swine Fever. If all pigs from the submission were negative upon examination and the herd remained to be so for at least six months after the submission, then the herd was classified as negative for the disease.

For an earlier study [2], a dataset had been constructed from the investigation forms that were available from 245 positive and 245 negative herds. On these forms, 32 distinct clinical symptoms had been recorded. Upon constructing the dataset, the recorded symptoms were encoded as '1's for the appropriate stochastic variables; symptoms that were not explicitly recorded were assumed to be absent and were encoded as '0's. The resulting dataset thus has 15 680 data slots, all of which are filled with either a '1' or a '0'; note that, strictly speaking, there are no missing values. We found that 10.2% of the slots are filled with '1's. The mean number of '1's is 3.5 for positive herds and 3.0 for negative herds; the mean number of '1's is significantly higher in positive herds (Mann Whitney U-test, $p < 0.01$).

3 The Experiment

As a consequence of the way in which clinical symptoms are typically recorded during a disease outbreak, our dataset on Classical Swine Fever exhibits a lack of distinction between absence of a clinical symptom and the symptom not having been addressed or observed. We designed an experiment to investigate the degree to which the results of feature selection from our dataset could be affected by this lack of distinction. Informally speaking, the less affected the set of selected features is, the more useful this set is for further data collection. In this section, we describe the set-up of our experiment; we further present the results that we obtained and discuss the conclusions to be drawn from them.

3.1 The Set-Up of the Experiment

To investigate the robustness of the results of feature selection from our dataset, we decided to construct a number of artificial datasets by changing some of the

'0's to '1's. For this purpose, we looked upon the '0's in our dataset essentially as missing values. For filling in missing values, generally an imputation method is used. We observe that in our dataset we have reliable information about the presence of symptoms that can be used for the purpose of imputation, but we do not have any reliable information about the absence of symptoms. As imputation methods require information about both the absence and the presence of symptoms, these methods cannot be employed for our purposes just like that. Our method of constructing artificial datasets from the available real data now is based upon the assumption that most investigation forms had been filled in with reasonable accuracy and that, for each herd, the veterinarians had not overlooked more symptoms than they had observed. Building upon these assumptions, we replaced all '0's in our dataset by either a '0' or a '1' according to the following two conditional probability distributions:

$$\Pr(\text{feature} = 1 \mid \text{CSF} = \text{yes}) = 0.11$$
$$\Pr(\text{feature} = 1 \mid \text{CSF} = \text{no}) = 0.09$$

using a random number generator. Note that this scheme for replacing the '0's in our dataset shows a close resemblance to imputation. Using our scheme, we constructed ten different artificial datasets.

From the original and artificial datasets, we learned full and selective Naive Bayesian classifiers using ten-fold cross validation, with the Elvira software package [4]. Feature selection was performed with the filter and wrapper methods provided by Elvira. The filter method selects features to be included in the classifier based upon the properties of the data under study. More specifically, the filter method includes the various feature variables in the order of their decreasing mutual information with the class variable. In our experiment, we took the mutual information $I(X,Y)$ of the feature variable X with the class variable Y to be defined as

$$I(X,Y) = \sum_{x,y} p(x,y) \cdot \ln \frac{p(x,y)}{p(x) \cdot p(y)}$$

where the probabilities $p(x)$, $p(y)$ and $p(x,y)$ are established from the frequencies observed in the data. The wrapper method, on the other hand, selects the various features based upon the accuracy of the classifier under construction. The method starts with the empty classifier and iteratively includes a feature variable that improves the accuracy the most. The inclusion of feature variables is pursued until the accuracy can no longer be improved upon [6, 9].

While the wrapper method uses the accuracy of the classifier under construction to decide when to stop including additional features, the filter method does not have associated such a natural stopping criterion. To decide, in our experiment, upon the number of feature variables to be selected with the filter method, we built upon the property that $2 \cdot N \cdot I(X,Y)$ asymptotically follows a $\chi^2_{(r-1)(s-1)}$ distribution, where r is the number of possible values of X and s is the number of values of Y; note that for our datasets we have that $r = s = 2$. We decided to use $\alpha = 0.01$ for the level of significance with the χ^2 distribution to decide upon inclusion of a feature variable X. With this level of significance,

Table 1. Mean accuracy and standard deviation of the full and selective Naive Bayesian classifiers learned from the original dataset and from the ten artificial datasets.

	Naive Bayes	*Filter*	*Wrapper*
original dataset	0.64 ± 0.07	0.63 ± 0.06	0.62 ± 0.06
artificial dataset 1	0.61 ± 0.08	0.59 ± 0.06	0.60 ± 0.08
artificial dataset 2	0.64 ± 0.07	0.63 ± 0.07	0.62 ± 0.08
artificial dataset 3	0.58 ± 0.08	0.62 ± 0.06	0.57 ± 0.08
artificial dataset 4	0.60 ± 0.06	0.56 ± 0.08	0.58 ± 0.08
artificial dataset 5	0.61 ± 0.09	0.64 ± 0.10	0.58 ± 0.05
artificial dataset 6	0.65 ± 0.07	0.62 ± 0.09	0.60 ± 0.06
artificial dataset 7	0.60 ± 0.06	0.59 ± 0.07	0.55 ± 0.06
artificial dataset 8	0.62 ± 0.08	0.59 ± 0.09	0.55 ± 0.07
artificial dataset 9	0.63 ± 0.03	0.62 ± 0.07	0.54 ± 0.04
artificial dataset 10	0.63 ± 0.09	0.62 ± 0.06	0.60 ± 0.06

the filter method is as restrictive as the wrapper method in terms of the number of selected features when averaged over all folds during cross validation for all datasets. With $\alpha = 0.01$, only feature variables X for which $2 \cdot N \cdot I(X, Y) > 6.64$ were included in the classifier under construction.

We compared the full and selective classifiers constructed from the original and artificial datasets, with respect to their accuracy. We further compared the numbers of features included in the selective classifiers. The robustness of the results of feature selection was evaluated by studying the variation of the features selected by the wrapper and filter methods over the folds of the various runs.

3.2 The Results

The accuracies of the full and selective Naive Bayesian classifiers learned from the various datasets are summarised in Table 1. The accuracies shown in the table are averaged over the ten folds during cross validation; the table further shows the standard deviations of the averaged accuracies.

The mean accuracy of the full Naive Bayesian classifiers learned from the original dataset, averaged over ten folds, was 0.64; the mean accuracy of the full classifiers learned from the artificial datasets, averaged over all 100 folds, was 0.62. The mean accuracy of the full classifiers learned from the original dataset was not significantly higher than the mean accuracy averaged over the artificial datasets (Mann Whitney U-test, $p = 0.21$). With the filter method, the mean accuracy of the selective Naive Bayesian classifiers learned from the original dataset was 0.63; the mean accuracy of the classifiers learned from the artificial datasets was 0.61, which was not significantly lower (Mann Whitney U-test, $p = 0.14$). The mean accuracies of the selective classifiers resulting with the filter method, moreover, were not higher than those of the full classifiers. With the wrapper method, the mean accuracy of the selective Naive Bayesian classifiers learned from the original dataset was 0.62, which was significantly higher than the mean accuracy of 0.58 established from the selective classifiers learned from the artificial datasets (Mann Whitney U-test, $p < 0.01$). The mean accuracy of the selective classifiers learned from the artificial datasets with the filter method was higher than that of the selective classifiers learned with the wrapper method (Mann Whitney U-test, $p < 0.05$). The mean accuracy of the selective classifiers resulting from the wrapper method was not higher than the mean accuracy of the full Naive Bayesian classifiers.

Figure 1 summarises the results of applying the filter method for feature selection: Figure 1(a) shows the distribution of the various selected feature variables for the original dataset, taken over the ten folds of cross validation; Figure 1(b) shows the distribution of selected features for the ten artificial datasets, taken over all 100 folds of cross validation. The mean number of feature variables selected with the filter method was 5.4 for the original dataset and 4.7 for the artificial datasets. From both the original dataset and the artificial datasets, the features v5 (not eating) and v12 (walking disorder) were selected in all folds. Other often selected features were v2 (inflammation of the eyes), v7 (respiratory problems) and, for the original dataset, v20 (not reacting to treatment with antibiotics) and v30 (birth of weak and trembling piglets). The number of features that were selected at least once for the original dataset, was 9; for the artificial datasets, this number was 25, which indicates that even when taking the uncertainty of the '0's into consideration, more than 20% of the recorded features were considered not to be discriminative for Classical Swine Fever.

Figure 2 summarises the results of applying the wrapper method for feature selection: Figure 2(a) shows the distribution of the various selected feature variables for the original dataset, taken over the ten folds of cross validation; Figure 2(b) shows the distribution of selected features for the ten artificial datasets, taken over all 100 folds of cross validation. The mean number of feature variables selected with the wrapper method from the original dataset and from the artificial datasets were 8.0 and 5.0, respectively. A striking difference between Figures 1(a) and 2(a) is the number of the features that were selected at least once from the original dataset: while the filter method selected only 9 features, the wrapper method selected almost all features at least once. Upon comparing Figures 1(b) and 2(b), a difference is seen in the number of features that are selected most often. While with the filter method five important feature variables v2, v5, v7, v12 and v20 still stand out, the selection by the wrapper method is less marked. With the wrapper method only the features v5 and v12 stand out, while all other features are selected almost equally often.

We would like to note that the original data were analysed using logistic regression in an earlier study [2]. From the analysis resulted a deterministic classification rule which in essence is a disjunction of clinical symptoms. The symptoms to be included in the rule were established using backward selection, optimising both its sensitivity and specificity. The thus included symptoms are v2 (inflammation of the eye), v5 (not eating), v12 (walking disorder), v20 (not reacting to treatment with antibiotics), and v24 (hard faecal pellets). A comparison against the features that were selected by especially the filter method from the original dataset, reveals a considerable overlap. We observe that, in

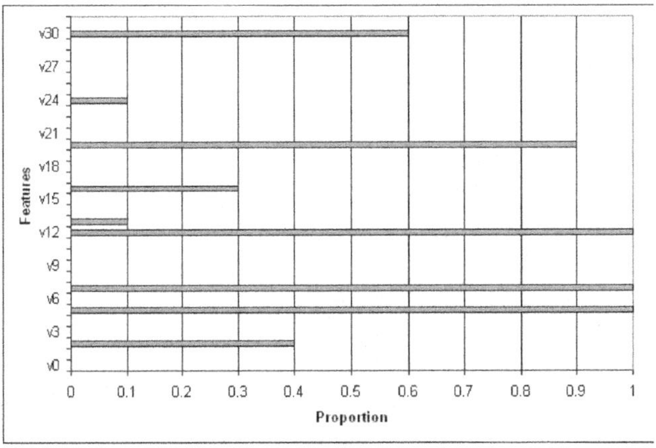

(a)

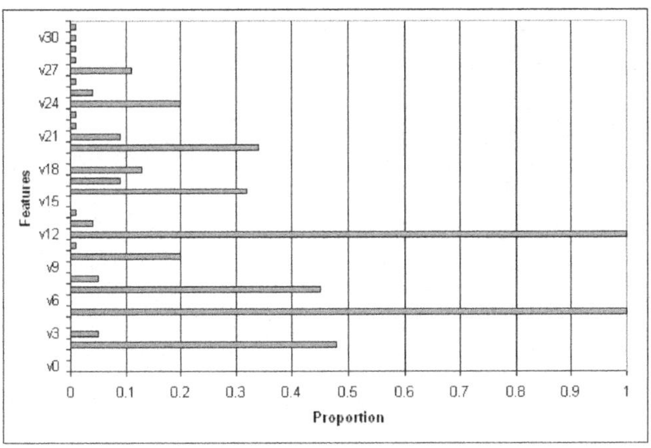

(b)

Fig. 1. The results of applying the filter method for feature selection; the results obtained from the original dataset (a), and from the artificial datasets (b).

contrast with Naive Bayesian classifiers, the disjunctive classification rule did not take into account that a clinical symptom could point to absence of Classical Swine Fever. The symptom v7, as a result, was not selected for the rule, while it features quite prominently in the various constructed classifiers.

3.3 Discussion

In our experiment, we compared the full and selective classifiers learned from the various datasets, with respect to their accuracies. The robustness of the results of

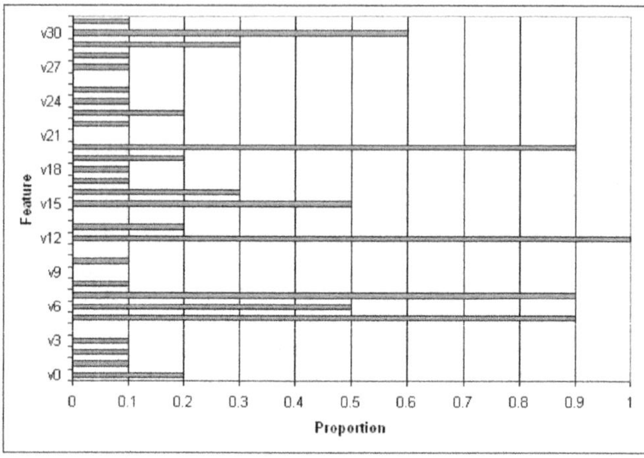

(a)

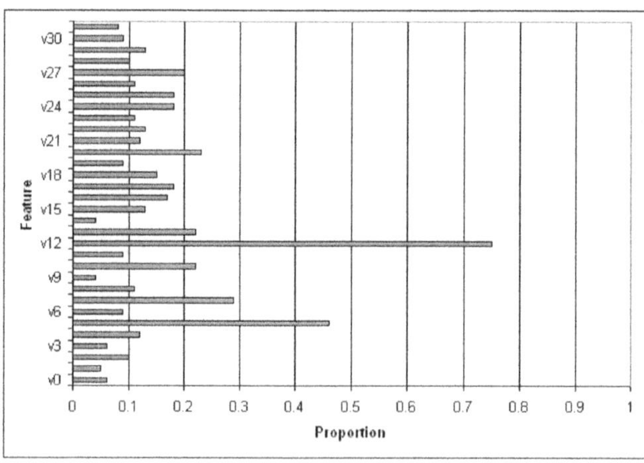

(b)

Fig. 2. The results of applying the wrapper method for feature selection; the results obtained from the original dataset (a), and from the artificial datasets (b).

feature selection was evaluated by studying the variation of the features selected by the wrapper and filter methods over the folds of the various runs.

We found that the mean accuracy of the full Naive Bayesian classifiers learned from the original dataset was not significantly higher than that of the full classifiers learned from the artificial datasets. The parameter probabilities established for the classifiers from the various datasets, therefore, must have been sufficiently similar not to influence their accuracies. We conclude that the learned full classifier is quite insensitive to a 10% variation in the number of '0's in our original dataset. Similar results were found with the filter method for feature selection upon learning selective Naive Bayesian classifiers from the various datasets. With the wrapper method, however, the mean accuracy of the selective classifiers learned from the original dataset was significantly higher than that of the classifiers learned from the artificial datasets. The selective classifiers constructed with the wrapper method thus were found to be more sensitive to a 10% variation in the number of '0's, than those learned with the filter method. This higher sensitivity is also clearly reflected in the distribution of selected features. Figures 1(a) and 1(b) show that, while the variation in the number of '0's in the original dataset introduces some variation in the feature variables that are selected by the filter method, five of the most important features still stand out. Figures 2(a) and 2(b) reveal that the 10% variation in the number of '0's has a much stronger effect on the distribution of selected features with the wrapper method. In fact, only two of the important features stand out, while the other important features are effectively hidden by the more uniform distribution.

To explain the observed difference in sensitivity between the two methods for feature selection, we recall that the filter method chooses the features to be included in a classifier based upon their mutual information with the class variable. For computing the mutual information for a feature variable, in each fold during cross validation some 50 instances per class are available. The probabilities required for establishing the mutual information, therefore, are calculated from a relatively large set of data. Since our artificial datasets differ only in the values of a relatively small number of variables, these differences are likely to have little effect on the mutual information computed for the various feature variables. The results of feature selection with the filter method therefore are expected to be rather insensitive to the 10% variation in the number of '0's. Our experimental results serve to corroborate this expectation. In fact, similar results were also found in a second experiment in which we used $\alpha = 0.05$ for the level of significance with the χ^2 distribution: although now more feature variables were selected by the filter method for inclusion in the classifiers, the distribution of selected features did not reveal a substantially stronger variation.

We further recall that the wrapper method chooses the features to be included based upon the accuracy of the classifier under construction. More specifically, a feature variable is added to the classifier only if it contributes to the accuracy in view of the previously selected variables. The wrapper method thus selects the variables to be included based upon a measure that is discrete in nature. Our experimental results now show a large variation in the features that are selected by the wrapper method in the various folds upon learning selective classifiers from the different datasets. The results therefore reveal a considerable sensitivity to the 10% variation in the number of '0's in our original dataset. After the first few, most discriminative feature variables have been selected, therefore, the remaining variables must have roughly equal contributions to the classifier's accuracy *given* these previously selected features, since only then can minor changes in the data lead to different selections. After a number of variables have been selected, moreover, further inclusion of a *single* feature variable is not likely to increase the classifier's accuracy, even though it may considerably change the probability distributions yielded over the class variable. A combination of additional feature variables might then still serve to increase the accuracy. The decrease in the mean accuracy of the selective classifiers constructed from the artificial datasets thus has its origin in the greedy selection behaviour of the wrapper method.

4 Concluding Observations and Future Research

In this paper, we addressed the robustness of feature selection with datasets that exhibit a lack of distinction between absent and non-observed features. Using a real-life dataset on Classical Swine Fever, we investigated the effect that this lack of distinction may have on the subset of features that are selected upon learning selective classifiers with the filter and wrapper methods. We found that, given a 10% variation in the number of absent features, the results obtained with the filter method were more robust than the results obtained with the wrapper method. We attributed the apparent robustness of the results from the filter method to the observation that this method selects the feature variables to be included based upon proportions computed from the entire dataset under study. The sensitivity of the results from the wrapper method could be attributed to the observation that the method uses a measure that in essence is discrete in nature, to decide upon inclusion of a variable. The lack of distinction between absent and non-observed features is not uncommonly found in biomedical datasets. Although we studied just a single dataset in detail, our findings suggest that, as a consequence of its robustness, the filter approach may be the preferred approach when performing feature selection on small to moderately-sized datasets that are known to exhibit this lack of distinction.

For our overall project aimed at early detection of Classical Swine Fever, the results from our study yielded additional insight into which clinical symptoms are the most discriminative for the disease. Based upon this insight, the investigation forms that are filled in by the veterinary expert teams upon inspecting herds, have been modified. The forms, moreover, have been changed to enforce a more strict data-gathering protocol which should in time result in a new dataset in which absent and non-observed features are more clearly distinguished. Our study of the different approaches to feature selection, unfortunately, did not result in a classifier of sufficiently high performance. We are currently developing a Bayesian network for the diagnosis of Classical Swine Fever with the help of domain experts, that will hopefully improve upon the accuracy of the various Naive Bayesian classifiers.

Acknowledgements

This research has been partly supported by the Netherlands Organisation for Scientific Research (NWO). We would like to thank Rosa Blanco for her help with learning the Naive Bayesian classifiers and performing the feature selection.

References

1. S. Edwards, A. Fukusho, P.C. Lefevre, et al., 2000. Classical Swine Fever: the global situation. Veterinary Microbiology, vol. 73, pp. 103 – 119.
2. A.R.W. Elbers, A. Bouma, J.A. Stegeman (2002). Quantitative assessment of clinical signs for the detection of classical swine fever outbreaks during an epidemic. *Veterinary Microbiology*, vol. 85, pp. 323 – 332.
3. A.R.W. Elbers, J.A. Stegeman, H. Moser, H.M. Ekker, J.A. Smak, F.H. Pluimers, 1999. The classical swine fever epidemic 1997-1998 in The Netherlands: descriptive epidemiology. Prev. Vet. Med. 42, 157-184.
4. Elvira consortium (2002). Elvira: an environment for probabilistic graphical models. In: J. Gómez, A. Salmerón (editors). *Proceedings of the First European Workshop on Probabilistic Graphical Models*, Cuenca, pp. 222 – 230.
5. N. Friedman, D. Geiger, M. Goldszmidt (1997). Bayesian network classifiers. *Machine Learning*, vol. 29, pp. 131 – 163.
6. G.H. John, R. Kohavi, K. Pfleger (1994). Irrelevant features and the subset selection problem. *Machine Learning: Proceeding of the 11th International Conference*, Morgan Kaufmann Publishers, San Francisco, pp. 121 – 129.
7. S.B. Kleiboeker, 2002. Swine fever: classical swine fever and African swine fever. Vet. Clin. Food. Anim. vol. 18, pp. 431 – 451.
8. R. Kohavi, G.H. John (1997). Wrappers for feature subset selection. *Artificial Intelligence Journal*, pp. 273 – 324.
9. P. Langley, S. Sage (1994). Induction of selective Bayesian classifiers. In: *Proceedings of the 10th Conference on Uncertainty in Artificial Intelligence.* pp. 399 – 406.
10. I. Tsamardinos, C. Aliferis (2003). Towards principled feature selection: relevancy, filters and wrappers. *Proceedings of the Ninth International Workshop on Artificial Intelligence and Statistics*, Key West, Florida.

Design of a Neural Network Model as a Decision Making Aid in Renal Transplant

Rafael Magdalena[1], Antonio J. Serrano[1], Agustin Serrano[2], Jorge Muñoz[1], Joan Vila[1], and E. Soria[1]

[1] Electronic Engineering Dpt, University of Valencia, 50 Dr. Moliner Ave, E46100 Burjasot, Spain
{Rafael.Magdalena,Antonio.J.Serrano,Jordi.Munoz,Joan.Vila}@uv.es
[2] Nephrology and Urology Paediatric Service, University Hospital 'La Fe' of Valencia, 21 Campanar Ave., E46009 Valencia, Spain
serrano_agu@gva.es

Abstract. This paper presents the application of this new tool of data processing in the study of the problem that arises when a renal transplant is indicated for a paediatric patient. Its aim is the development and validation of a neural network based model which can predict the success of the transplant over the short, medium and long term, using pre-operative characteristics of the patient (recipient) and implant organ (donor). When compared to results of logistic regression, the results of the proposed model showed better performance. Once the model is obtained, it will be converted into a tool for predicting the efficiency of the transplant protocol in order to optimise the donor-recipient pair and maximize the success of the transplant. The first real use of this application will be as a decision aid tool for helping physicians and surgeons when preparing to perform a transplant.

1 Introduction

The current process of globalisation of economy is compelling the governments of many European countries to increase the efficiency of services provided to its patient population. As a result National Health Agencies are being forced to invest increasing resources in evaluating the quality of services provided. Without doubt, the first consequence of these facts, and the one that generates most uncertainty, is the increasing obligation for health professionals to document and evaluate these services.

This evaluation of services also applies to the field of renal transplant (RT). Moreover, resource optimisation is also required, which in transplant terms means the search for the most suitable kidney-recipient pair. This fact, which is of great relevance for adult patients, is more important indeed in paediatric renal transplant (PRT), due to various factors [1,2]:

1. Terminal Renal Insufficiency (TRI) is an irreversible disease, with serious consequences for the paediatric patient, their family and for the Health Service [3].
2. There is no therapeutic alternative available, because any type of dialysis is simply a maintenance method, and is even less effective in children than in adults. RT is superior to dialysis in terms of economy, mortality and quality of life [3–7].

J.M. Barreiro et al. (Eds.): ISBMDA 2004, LNCS 3337, pp. 160–170, 2004.

3. The limited duration of the kidney graft (survival of graft at 12 months: 80–90 %; at 60 months: 60–70%; at 84 months: 58% [8,9]) means that the patient who receives a renal transplant in childhood will probably have to be re-transplanted at least once during their lifetime.

Since the commencement of transplants in the 1950's [10], all available scientific resources have been utilised in order to identify those factors implicated in transplant failure. This has been carried out using statistical methods, mainly logistic regression (LR) [9, 11, 12].

Nephrology and Paediatric Urology Services at the University Children's Hospital of La Fe in Valencia, Spain, began its Paediatric Renal Transplant Program in April 1979, and is currently the most experienced service in Spain in this field.

In order to identify the key factors in the suitability of the graft-recipient pair, and thus obtain the maximum survival of the graft, they have been compiling and analysing potentially significant data, both from the donor and patient. It is important to emphasise that the optimisation of the graft-recipient pair will help to avoid the performance of transplants with a high probability of failure, and will promote the realization of those with probability of success. In addition, from an economic point of view, the improvement in the suitability of organs will increase the accuracy and efficacy of the treatment in the patient, with a subsequent reduction in costs.

The objective of this paper is the optimisation of the graft-recipient pair using classical techniques, namely logistic regression, and its modern and natural extension, artificial neural networks (ANN). The outline of this article is as follows: first ANNs will be briefly described, followed by discussion of the characteristics of the data sets used in the experiment. Finally results and conclusions will be presented.

2 Artificial Neural Networks

The last few years have seen an exponential increase in the use of ANNs in many different fields (control, signal processing, expert system, temporal series prediction, etc.) [13,15]. This considerable growth can be explained by the wide range of applications of ANNs (Fig. 1).

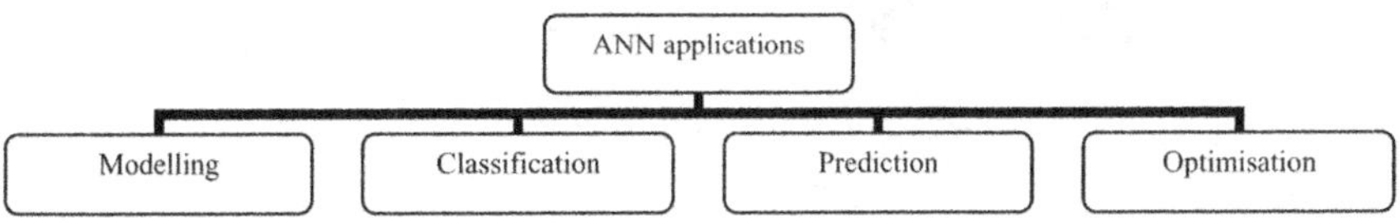

Fig. 1. Artificial Neural Networks application.

ANNs are preferable to other mathematical methods when the problem shows some of the following characteristics:

- It is difficult to find rules that define the target variable from the independent variables considered in the model.

- The data are imprecise or contain statistical noise.
- A considerable number of variables are needed to define the problem.
- The model is non-linear.
- A great amount of data is available.
- The work environment is variable.

The characteristics above are representative of the variability in medical sciences for the following reasons:

- The human body, and its interactions with different elements in the environment, is a very complex system. It is logical, therefore, to consider these relationships as non-linear.
- There are many variables that define the behaviour of a particular problem in health sciences. Consequently, the more the problem is simplified, the more errors will be present in the model.
- Sheets for gathering data on a particular pathology can be incomplete or contain measurement errors.
- Clinical data grow in time, so the best models are those that can adapt themselves with accuracy and reliability, taking new data into account.

ANNs are mathematical models, generally non-linear, consisting of elemental units of calculation called neurons. The network used in this paper is known as multilayer perceptron, and is composed of several neurons with the following structure (Fig. 2):

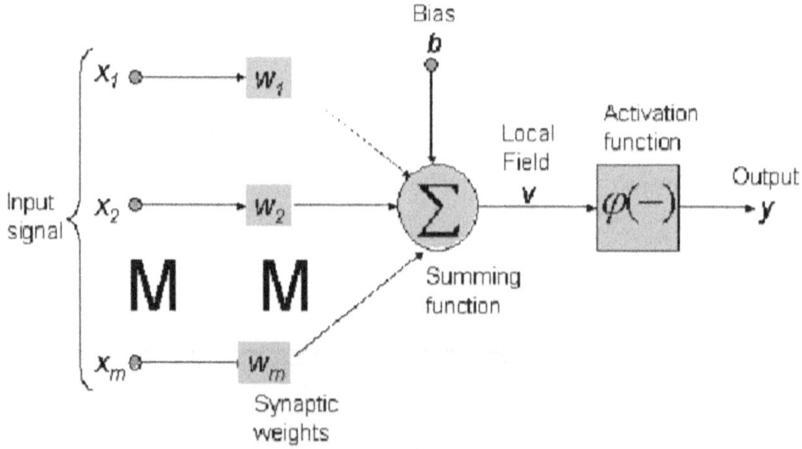

Fig. 2. Structure of an artificial neuron.

The elements that compose the neuron are:

- *Inputs*. These are the data processed by the neuron. They can be the input variables or the output of other neurons.

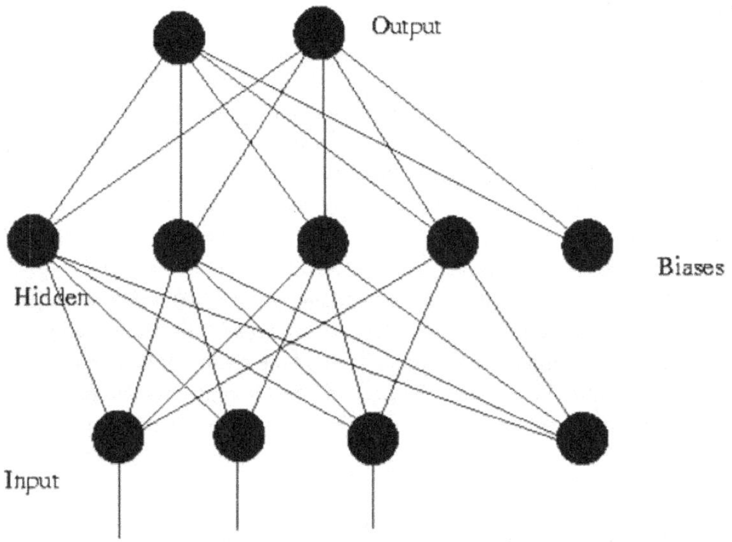

Fig. 3. Structure of Multiplayer perceptron, showing one input layer, one hidden layer and one output layer.

- *Synaptic connections.* These are also called weights in ANN theory. They are multiplicative factors of the inputs to the neuron. There can be an additional weight named threshold with 1 as input. Learning of a network is the process of adapting the values of these weights according to an algorithm.
- *Activation function.* The key element in the neuron. This function gives the neuron a non-linear behaviour, and therefore broadens the field of application of ANNs, as opposed to classical methods of data analysis.

If this neuron structure is combined with the most popular activation function, the sigmoid, a mathematical relation generally used as diagnostic test arises: the logistic regression. When logistic regression is used, it can be interpreted as using a neural network with just one neuron. Obviously, this approach can be improved. Multilayer perceptron extends the capacity of modelling and classification of one neuron by combining several neurons in layers, as shown in Fig. 3.

The structure in Fig. 3 is a universal, very versatile modeller. This versatility can become a problem when the network overfits the model. The adjustment of the synaptic connections is called a learning algorithm, and one of the most frequently used is known as the back propagation (BP) algorithm. This optimises an error function that measures the error made by the network, using an iterative algorithm of minimum local search known as delta rule. The disadvantage of this method is that an incorrect initialisation of synaptic weights can produce models that fall in local minima. The problem can be solved by testing different initial weights from a candidate set.

3 Proposed Problem

This paper presents a retrospective, analytical study of the results of the 271 consecutive renal transplants carried out at the Children's Hospital of La Fe, Valencia from April 1979 to December 2002. Patients were added consecutively and continuously by non-probabilistic sampling. The study included only paediatric patients with TRI of any etiology, who had been subsequently transplanted and their renal function monitored at the Children's Hospital La Fe, until their transfer as adults to a corresponding adult centre. They included transplants with grafts from both live and cadaver donors, as well as first, second and subsequent re-transplants (until fifth). Only those patients with complete data sets available were included in the study. All the data used were obtained from the database of the Paediatric Renal Transplant Team of La Fe Hospital. This has been carefully compiled over the 25 years of the paediatric transplant program, and has been continuously updated whenever changes in the status of the patients or organs appeared.

3.1 Material and Methods

The original database contains 168 variables per transplant. The target variables of the study were selected from these, and made up the definitive database. This was then exported to Excel® format in order to facilitate its use.

A total of 10 variables were chosen from the original database, corresponding to factors from both patient and donor, all of them strictly pre-transplant, and in agreement with those factors considered in the published literature to have the strongest influence. The main references used were the latest articles from NAPRTCS[9,16,17], the most extensive publication in the field of paediatric renal transplant.

From a purely medical point of view, the chosen variables reasonably represent the problem, while at the same time defining a mathematical complexity, which can be managed using ANNs. The same variables were proposed in the hypothesis of the LR model. The chosen variables are shown in Table 1.

The only output variable of the predictive model was the functionality of the graft, measured as functioning or non-functioning, one month after the transplant. A graft is described as 'functioning' if there is no need for dialysis one month after the transplant, and 'non-functioning' if dialysis is required within the first month.

In order to compare the results of the ANNs with a well-established and accepted statistical method, the progress of the transplant was also predicted using logistic regression.

4 Results

Commercial software SPPS® version 10.0 for Windows® was used in the development of the logistic model. The influence of the factors on the hazard rate of graft failure was estimated using the Cox regression, which ranks the variables in order of importance. Multivariant analysis of the factors included in the study was carried out, according to the success of the transplant at a given point in time. The Hosmer Lemeshow test

Table 1. Description of the variables considered in the problem, ordered by dependence on donor or recipient.

Variables:	Type of variable	Units
- Factors depending on donor:		
- Age.	Continuous	years
- Type of donor.	Binary	1= alive related 0= dead
- Factors depending on recipient:		
Age.	Continuous	years
Presence of cytotoxic ab. (grouped by titre into: <5, 5–50, >50).	Categorical	0= <5 1= 5–50 2= >50
Main pathological cause of renal failure, according to ERA-EDTA (grouped into: glomerulopathies, metabolopathies and others).	Categorical	1= glomerulopathies 2= metabolopathies 3= others
Number of transplant for recipient.	Continuous	1, 2, 3, 4, 5.
Time in pre-transplant dialysis.	Continuous	Months
Number of pre-transplant blood transfusions	Continuous	
- Factors depending on donor and recipient:		
Number of HLA compatibilities (A/B/DR).	Categorical	0, 1, 2, 3, 4.
- Time of cold ischemia of the organ.	Continuous	Hours

was applied in order to determine the homogeneity of the trial. The predictive capacity of the logistic model was represented by the receiver operating characteristic (ROC) curve. The areas under the curve and the optimal intersection point were also calculated. This point determined the sensitivity (Se), specificity (Sp), positive and negative predictive values (PPV and NPV) and the verisimilitude ratio of positive (PVR) and negative (NVR) tests.

With regard to the training of the neural network, a self-designed code in Matlab® environment was used. All the parameters of the network and learning algorithm were scanned (architecture of the network, weight initialisation and learning constant). The end of the training was determined by the cross validation technique, in order to avoid overfitting of the network to the training data. This overfitting simply means that the network learns the whole data, so new inferences are not possible. The data were randomly split into two sets, 66%:33%; the larger set was used for training while the remaining data was used for network validation. Training stops when the error at the network reaches a minimum.

In this study, networks were programmed and trained on a personal computer (AMD® Athlon XP 1500 microprocessor, 1.5 GB RAM, OS Linux 2.4.19 and Matlab® 5.1 and Matcom® compiler).

The criteria for choosing the best network was the confusion matrix. Models with Sp and Se values less than 70% are considered inadequate as a medical decision aid. The network with the highest values in the sum of Sp and Se in both training and validation gives the best model.

The comparison between ANN and LR results was carried out by calculating and comparing the area under the ROC curves. These areas were measured with SPSS® and Matlab® software, and compared using the Hanley and McNeil method [18]. In order to determine the importance of the pre-transplant variables, the concept of "physical sensitivity" was used. Once the network is definitively trained and verified, the sensitivity of the final algebraic formula for every variable is calculated. [19]

Logistic Regression Model

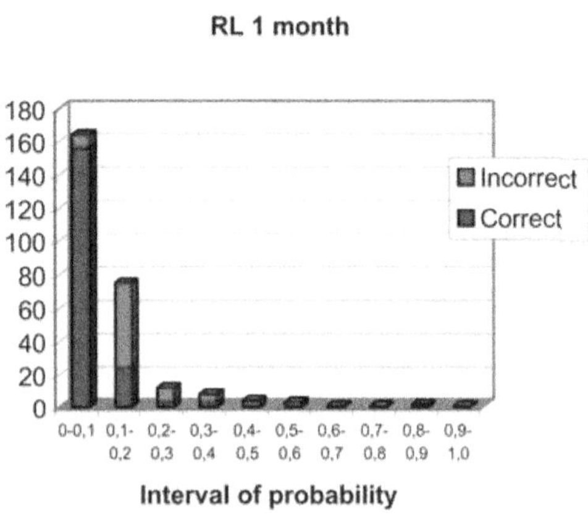

Fig. 4. Histogram for LR predictions.

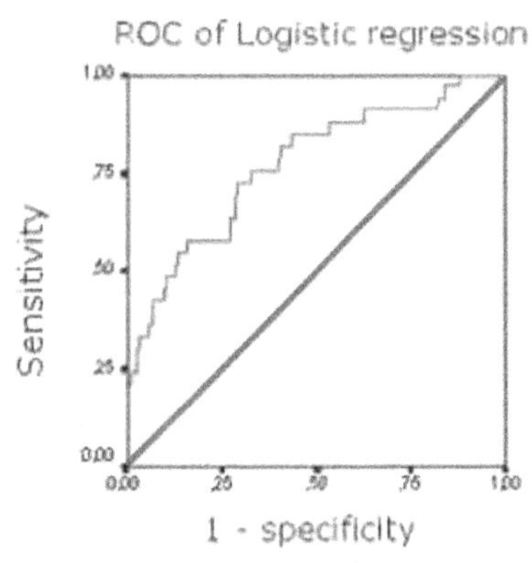

Fig. 5. Receiver Operating Characteristic (ROC) Curve

Table 2. Results for Logistic Regression.

	LR Results	CI 95%
Se	72.7%	55.8% to 84.9%
Sp	71.4%	65.4% to 76.8%
PPV	26.1%	18.2% to 35.9%
NPV	95.0%	90.7% to 97.3%
PVR	2.55	1.90 to 3.40
NVR	0.38	0.22 to 0.68
Correct	71.6%	65.9% to 76.6%
AUC	0.771	0.679 to 0.862
Intersec.point	0.108	

Neural Network Structure

Input layer	Hidden layer	Output layer
12	8	1

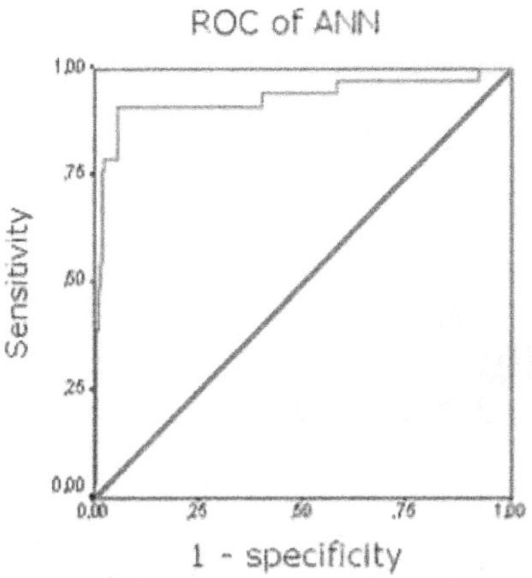

Fig. 6. ROC curve of Artificial Neural Network.

Table 3. Table of resuts for neuronal model.

	RN	IC 95%
Se	90.8 %	89.4% to 93.8%
Sp	93.9 %	80.4% to 98.3%
PPV	99.1 %	96.7% to 99.7%
NPV	58.5 %	45.1% to 70.7%
PVR	14.97	3.91 to 57.41
NVR	0.10	0.07 to 0.15
Correct	91.1 %	87.2% to 94.0%
AUC	0.928	0.862 to 0.994
Intersec. point	0.502 8	

Comparison

Comparison of ROC

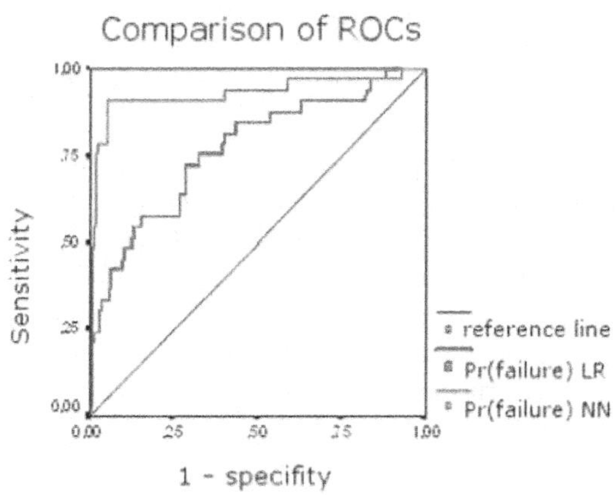

Fig. 7. ROC curves for ANN and LR models.

Importance of variables for LR according to the expression
@ = -2.541 - 2.375 Diagnostic (2= metabolopathies) + 0.667 Diagnostic (1= glomerulopathies) + 0.582 number of graft + 3.105 Cytotoxic Ab. (2= more than 50) + 0.769 Cytotoxic Ab. (1= from 5 to 50) - 0.079 recipient age

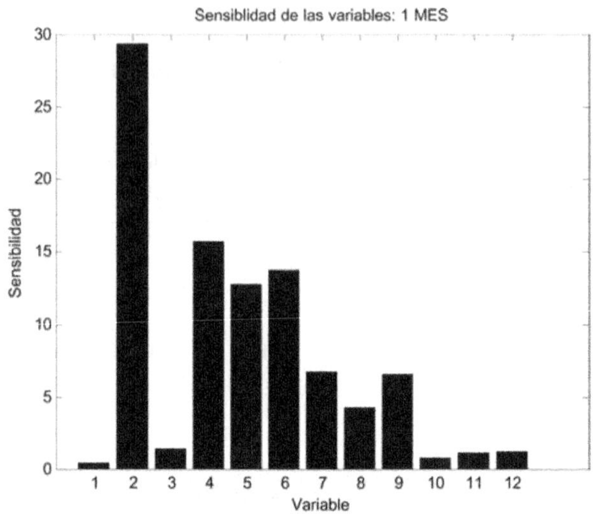

Fig. 8. Importance of the variables in ANN (1= donor age; 2= type of donor; 3= age of recipient; 4= Cytotoxic Antibody; 5= EDTA diagnostic 1; 6= EDTA diagnostic 2; 7= EDTA diagnostic 3; 8= compatibility; 9= number of graft for recipient; 10= time at dialysis; 11= number of transfusions; 12= time of cold ischemia).

5 Conclusions

Artificial Neural Networks are a powerful tool when applied to the problem of paediatric renal transplant. Their implementation, based on pre-transplant variables, offers good predictability in monitoring the short-term progress of the transplant, and can present results in terms of probability.

The use of logistic regression as a classical reference method for comparison with neural networks in paediatric renal transplant is suitable in this case, as it presents results in a way similar to ANNs (a numerical value of probability), thus allowing comparison between methods. The area under the ROC curves proves to be a valuable parameter for evaluation and comparison of the two methods.

The predictive capability of ANNs is always superior to that of LR. Statistical conclusions can be drawn by comparing the two methods: independent of the evolving time considered, ANNs appear to be a strong alternative to LR in this field of work.

This outstanding performance of ANN against LR in paediatric renal transplant points to the existence of complex, non-linear relations amongst the variables of the study which logistic regression cannot model. It has been shown that the variables selected in this study are valid for successful neural network modelling.

Variables such as *initialisation of renal function post-transplant* and *episodes of acute rejection* can increase the predictive capacity of the model. However, this data is not available at the time of surgery and only information available pre-transplant was used in this study.

Neural networks are also able to rank problem variables according to their order of importance (sensitivity). This ranking is consistent with medical and scientific studies.

According to ANNs, the *type of donor* is the most important variable in successful paediatric renal transplant. This 'favours' the practice of this type of graft.

The use of ANNs as a user-friendly interface presents a decision aid in the suitability of the donor-recipient pair. The ability to increase the capacity of ANNs to handle precise information about various events in the rejection of the graft, before they happen, will make it possible to design different strategies for the predicted event, thus minimising the risk of failure. It will be possible, therefore, to dedicate more attention to the prevention, rather than the resolution, of complications. In this way the intervention will allow, at least potentially, an increase in survival of the graft and therefore the quality of life of the patient.

Given that ANNs constitute a useful decision aid in paediatric renal transplant, we recommend their use in other types of organ transplant.

References

1. Schurman S, Mcenery PT. Factors influencing short-term and long-term pediatric renal transplant survival. J Pediatr. (1997). 130(3): p. 455–62.
2. Lewy JE. Treatment of children in the U.S. with end-stage renal disease (ESRD). Med Arh, (2001). 55(4): p. 201–2.
3. Warady B, Alexander SR, Watkins S, Kohaut E, Harmon WE. Optimal care of the pediatric end-stage renal disease patients on dialysis. Am J Kidney Dis (1999). 33(3): p. 567–83.
4. National Institutes of Health NIDDK/CKUHD. Excerpts from the United States Renal Data System's 2003 Annual Data Report: Atlas of end-stage renal disease in the United States. Am J Kid Dis (2003). 42(6, Suppl 5): p. S115–S128.
5. Davis ID, Bunchman TE, Grimm PC, Benfield MR, Briscoe DM, Harmon WE, Alexander SR, Avner ED, Pediatric renal transplantation: indications and special considerations. Pediatr Transplantation (1998). 2(2): p. 117–29.
6. Edwards E, Bennett LE, Cecka JM. Effect of HLA matching on the relative risk of mortality for kidney recipients: a comparison of the mortality risk after transplant to the mortality risk of remaining on the waiting list. Transplantation (1997). 64(9): p. 1274–7.
7. Schnuelle P, Lorenz D, Trede M, Van Der Woude FJ. Impact of renal cadaveric transplantation on survival in end-stage renal failure: evidence for reduced mortality risk compared with hemodialysis during long-term follow-up. J Am Soc Nephrol (1998). 9(11): p. 2135–41.
8. Tejani A, Sullivan EK, Harmon WE, Fine RN, Kohaut E, Emmett L, Alexander SR. Pediatric renal transplantation - The NAPRTCS experience, en Clinical Transplantation, J. Cheka, Terasaki PI, Ed. (1997). UCLA Tissue Typing Laboratory: Los Angeles, California. p. 87—100.
9. Seikaly M, Ho PL, Emmett L, Tejani A. The 12th Annual Report of the North American Pediatric Renal Transplant Cooperative Study: renal transplantation from 1987 through 1998. Pediatr Transplant (2001). 5(3): p. 215–31.
10. Merril JP, Murray JE, Harrison JH. Succesful homotransplantation of the human kidney. JAMA (1956). 160: p. 277–282.
11. Ojogho O, Sahney S.Cutler D, Abdelhalim F, Hasan M, Baron P, Concepcion W. Superior long-term results of renal transplantation in children under 5 years of age. Am Surg (2002). 68(12): p. 1115–9.
12. McEnery PT, Stablein DM, Arbus G, Tejani A. Renal transplantation in children. A report of the North American Pediatric Renal Transplant Cooperative Study. N Engl J Med (1992). 326(26): p. 1727–32.

13. Haykin S. Back propagation. En: Haykin S, editor. Neural Networks. A comprehensive foundation. Englewood Cliffs, New Jersey: McMillan College Publishing Comany Inc. (1994).
14. Ripley BD. Pattern recognition and neural networks. Cambridge: Cambridge University Press (1996).
15. Bishop CM. Neural Networks for Pattern Recognition. (1996), Oxford: Clarendon Press.
16. Tejani A, Sullivan EK, Alexander SR, Fine RN, Harmon WE, Kohaut EC. Predictive factors for delayed graft function and its impact on renal graft survival in children: a report of the North American Pediatric Renal Transplant Cooperative Study (NAPRTCS). Pediatr Transplantation, (1999). 3(4): p. 293–300.
17. Benfield M, McDonald R, Sullivan EK, Stablein DM, Tejani A. The 1997 annual renal transplantation in children report of the North American Pediatric Renal Transplant Cooperative Study (NAPRTCS). Pediatr Transplantation (1999). 3(2): p. 152–67.
18. Smith J, Ho PL, McDonald RA. Renal transplant outcomes in adolescents: a report of the North American Pediatric Renal Transplant Cooperative Study. Pediatr Transplant (2002);6(6):493–9.
19. Engelbretch, AP, Cloete, I, Zurada, JM. Determining the significance of input parametersusing sensitivity analisys. International Workshop on Artificial Neural Networks. Torremolinos, Spain. Lecture Notes in Computer Science (1995) 930: p. 382–388.

Learning the Dose Adjustment for the Oral Anticoagulation Treatment

Giacomo Gamberoni[1], Evelina Lamma[1], Paola Mello[2], Piercamillo Pavesi[3], Sergio Storari[1], and Giuseppe Trocino[4]

[1] Dipartimento di Ingegneria, University of Ferrara, Via saragat 1, 44100 Ferrara, Italy
{ggamberoni,elamma,sstorari}@ing.unife.it

[2] DEIS, University of Bologna, Viale Risorgimento 2, 40136 Bologna, Italy
pmello@deis.unibo.it

[3] Divisione di Cardiologia, Ospedale Maggiore, largo bartolo nigrisoli 2, 40133 Bologna, Italy
piercamillo.pavesi@ausl.bologna.it

[4] Divisione di Cardiologia, Ospedale San Gerardo, via doninzetti 106, 20052 Monza, Italy
g.trocino@hsgerardo.org

Abstract. Several attempts have been recently provided to define Oral Anticoagulant (OA) guidelines. These guidelines include indications for oral anticoagulation and suggested arrangements for the management of an oral anticoagulant service. They aim to take care of the current practical difficulties involved in the safe monitoring of the rapidly expanding numbers of patients on long-term anticoagulant therapy. Nowadays, a number of computer-based systems exist for supporting hematologists in the oral anticoagulation therapy. Nonetheless, computer-based support improves the quality of the Oral Anticoagulant Therapy (OAT) and also possibly reduces the number of scheduled laboratory controls. In this paper, we discuss an approach based on statistical methods for learning both the optimal dose adjustment for OA and the time date required for the next laboratory control. This approach has been integrated in DNTAO-SE, an expert system for supporting hematologists in the definition of OAT prescriptions. In the paper, besides discussing the approach, we also present experimental results obtained by running DNTAO-SE on a database containing more than 4500 OAT prescriptions, collected from a hematological laboratory for the period December 2003 – February 2004.

1 Introduction

The number of patients in therapy with Oral Anticoagulant (OA) drugs has increased in recent decades, due to the increasing number of cardiovascular diseases which need to be treated by OA drugs. Several attempts have been provided recently to define guidelines for the correct management of Oral Anticoagulant Therapy (OAT). These guidelines include indications for oral anticoagulation and suggested arrangements for the management of an oral anticoagulant service. They aim to take care of the current practical difficulties involved in the safe monitoring of the rapidly expanding numbers of patients on long-term oral anticoagulant therapy.

The International Normalized Ratio (INR) is the recommended method for reporting prothrombin time results for control of blood anticoagulation. Since the adoption of the INR system, the usual practice has been to adjust the dose of Warfarin, or other

J.M. Barreiro et al. (Eds.): ISBMDA 2004, LNCS 3337, pp. 171–181, 2004.

oral vitamin K antagonist, to maintain the INR within a therapeutic range. Usually, for each kind of cardiac disease, guidelines report indications of the target INR, expressed as a range. Long-term OAT patients are then subjected to periodic controls, and at each control, on the basis of the measured INR, the dose of OA drugs are adjusted to maintain the INR in the therapeutic range (we refer this dose as the maintenance dose, since it aims at maintaining the patient's INR in the therapeutic range). The date for the next INR control is also assigned.

Nowadays, a number of computer-based systems exist (see [3,5,6] for instance) for supporting haematologists in OAT management. Nonetheless, computer-based support improves the OAT quality and also possibly reduces the number of scheduled laboratory controls.

For 20 years, it is known that mathematical models, usually derived by regression analysis of prothrombin times against time following the loading dose of OA drug, can be adopted to determine the maintenance dose, and these models were implemented in PARMA [5].

In this paper, we refine this approach and discuss how statistical methods, and regression in particular, can be exploited to learn the optimal OA dose adjustment model. This approach has been integrated in DNTAO-SE, an expert system for supporting hematologists in the definition of OAT prescriptions.

In the paper, we also present experimental results obtained by running DNTAO-SE on a database containing more than 4500 OAT prescriptions, collected from a hematological laboratory for the period December 2003 – February 2004.

The paper is organized as follows. In Sect. 2 we briefly introduce OAT and its phases. Sect. 3 describes DNTAO-SE objectives and architecture. Sect. 4 describes the experiments conducted for learning the regression model for automatic dose suggestion. Sect. 5 describes a test conducted in order to evaluate DNATO-SE suggestion reliability. Sect. 6 presents some related works. Finally Sect. 7 concludes and presents future work.

2 Oral Anticoagulant Therapy

The Oral Anticoagulant Therapy (OAT) is an important treatment to prevent and treat thrombotic events, either venous or arterial.

In the last few years these kind of pathologies have been increased and, as a consequence, also the number of patients being treated with OA is growing: at this moment, patients being treated with OA in Italy are about 400000. In some clinical circumstances (stroke, atrial fibrillation, venous thrombosis etc.), the OA treatment has a determined period. In other pathologies, which are the greatest part of indications (mechanical prosthetic heart valve, recurrence of arterial thromboembolism, inherited thrombophilia), the treatments last the patient's entire life. In this case, treatment looks like a therapy for a chronic disease for patients of every age. It is necessary to keep the same decoagulation level of the blood to prevent occlusion, because in high-risk cases it can be fatal to the patient. This is the reason why patients under OAT are continuously under surveillance. This kind of surveillance consists in monitoring the INR level (a variable that measures the coagulation level of the blood), therapy prescriptions, medical consults, and evaluations about pharmacological interactions and other clinical situations.

A patient's INR indicates to the doctor how the therapy has to be adjusted, trying to keep the INR in a fixed range of values, called therapeutic range. The objective is to maintain this value near to the centre (target) of this range, which is considered as the optimal result. Therapeutic range is different from patient to patient and is determinate on the therapeutic indication of the patient.

There are many anticoagulation substances and they work in different ways to inhibit homeostatic system. Sintrom and Warfarin are the most used drugs in OAT.

Once therapeutic range has been determined, therapy can start. Therapy is based on three main phases: stabilization phase, maintenance phase, management of the INR excesses. The first objective of the therapy is to stabilize the patient's INR into the therapeutic range and then find the right dose of Warfarin needed on the second phase (maintenance phase) to keep INR in the range. The process of stabilization is very delicate and if it is badly managed, serious hemorrhagic events can occur. In this phase, the INR level must be checked daily and the next dose must be calibrated at every coagulation test, until the INR is stable. This objective is usually achieved within a week.

Once stabilization is reached is necessary to find the maintenance dose: this dose is the one capable to keep the INR stable inside the range (when there are no other clinic complications that can modify the coagulation level). In this phase, control frequency can be reduced from daily to weekly and in some cases to monthly (if the patient shows a high grade of stability).

If INR value gets off the therapeutic range more than the 25% of the range amplitude, specific dose adjustments are necessary.

3 DNTAO-SE

DNTAO-SE, described in details in [2], is an expert system developed in order to improve DNTAO [4], an OAT data management system, by introducing as new functionality the automatic suggestion of the most suitable OAT prescription (dose and next control date).

The development of DNTAO-SE has been based on several considerations about the different steps followed by OA patients, nurses and haematologists for the execution of an OAT control. In the first step, a patient goes to the OAT control centre, where a nurse makes questions about the therapy status and other related events (Checklist) occurred after the last therapy prescription. In the second step, a blood sample is taken, and then is sent to a lab to be analyzed by an automatic device. The blood sample test is needed to measure the INR level. In the third step, a haematologist evaluates the checklist, the INR level, the patient clinical history (formerly INR levels and assigned doses in the previous prescriptions) and other relevant clinical information in order to define the next therapy.

DNTAO-SE supports the haematologist in the third step, automatically retrieving all the information previously described and applying a knowledge base and an inference engine to propose the most suitable next therapy. The architecture of the DNTAO-SE prototype can be seen in Fig. 1.

DNTAO-SE uses its knowledge base to subdivide patients in four categories: high risk patients; medium risk patients; low risk patients who need little therapy adjustment; low risk patients who do not need a therapy change. For each patient category,

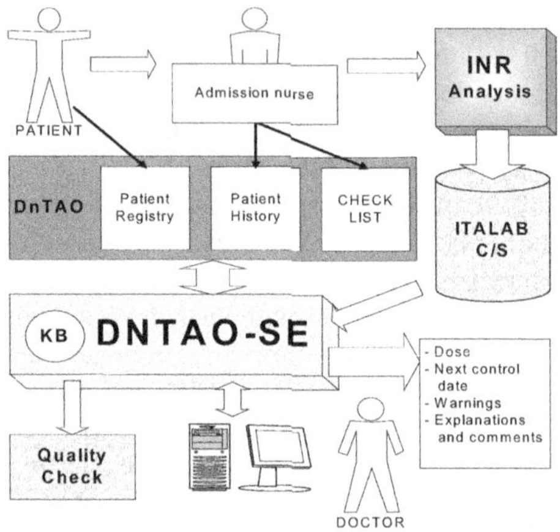

Fig. 1. Prototype architecture

there is a different methodology to define both the therapeutic anticoagulant dose and the time before the next control.

For low risk patient, DNTAO-SE usually confirms the dose and the therapy time length given at previous control. If the INR level is inside the therapeutic range, but the INR trend of previous controls indicates a hypothetical next value outside the range, then DNTAO-SE confirms the previous dose but automatically suggests a small dose adjustment for the next two days. DNTAO-SE computes the most frequent AOT prescription time length for low risk patients, and sets the next control date within this time value (usually about four weeks).

For medium risk patients, DNTAO-SE is able to automatically suggest the dose adjustment hypothetically needed to bring the INR into the therapeutic range. DNTAO-SE performs this crucial task (this is the most numerous category) by using a regression model, learned starting from a dataset of previous OAT prescriptions as described in Sect. 4. DNTAO-SE computes the most frequent AOT prescription time length for medium risk patients, and sets the next control date within this time value (usually about two weeks).

Referring to high risk patients, the ability to manage this cases is one of the more distinguishing DNTAO-SE feature because the other systems, presented in Sect. 5, leave haematologists without support. DNTAO-SE uses a part of its knowledge base, which considers international guidelines, to identify different subcategories of high-risk patients, suggesting for each one a different therapy management. DNTAO-SE sets the next control date within a week.

4 Models for Automatic Dose Prescription

As described in Sect. 3, one of the main objectives of DNTAO-SE is to efficiently manage medium risk patients. To reach this objective, we decided to use regression models learned from dataset of OAT prescriptions. In this section, organized in three subsections, we describe the criteria followed and experiments conducted in order to develop the most suitable and performing model.

In the first subsection (Sect. 4.1), we describe the available dataset and the meaningful observations which can be used as parameters to learn the regression models. In the second (Sect. 4.2), we briefly describe how to learn a regression models and how to evaluate its performance. Then in Sect. 4.3 we illustrate the experiments made and the model integrated in DNTAO-SE.

4.1 Dataset Preparation

The first fundamental step for developing a model is to identify the set of useful observation between the set of the available ones. In our experiments, the observations are composed by parameters which express the linkage between the prescribed anticoagulant dose and the induced INR.

The initial available dataset was composed by more than 40000 OAT prescriptions (INR, OA drug dose and next control date) performed in four years at the "Maggiore" hospital in Bologna (Italy) on more than 1000 patients. Following the indications of some haematologists, we identified the target of the model (i.e. the parameter which has to be described) and the set of OAT parameters to be used as model variables.

The target is the dose variation percentage, that represents the percentage of weekly dose variation between the new prescription and the previous one.

The most interesting OAT parameters to be considered are: the starting dose (the weekly anticoagulant dose (in mg) assumed since the previous AOT), referred as dose_iniz; the dose variation percentage (percentage of dose variation between the starting dose and the one assigned in the prescription), referred as delta_dose_perc; the INR variation percentage (percentage of INR variation induced by the dose variation), referred as delta_INR_perc; the therapeutic range assigned to the patient; the patient's age; the patient's sex; the main therapeutic indication (the diagnosis that have led the patient to start the OAT).

Table 1. Collection of patient prescriptions

Row number	Patient ID	Prescription date	INR	Proposed dose
1	5600010009	07/03/2001	2.3	15
2	5600010009	04/04/2001	3.5	12.5
3	5600010009	26/04/2001	3.1	13.75
4	5600010009	24/05/2001	4	12.5

Given the AOT database, we grouped the ones associated to the same patient as pointed out in Tab. 1. Starting from this group of prescriptions, we decided to exclude some of them, considered unsuccessful. The exclusion criterion establishes that if the INR value found during the AOT control at time T, and induced by dose variation proposed during the AOT control at time T-1, is out of patient therapeutic range, then the prescription made by the haematologist at time T-1 is assumed to be unsuccessful and the relative prescription has not to be taken into account for regression model learning. Let us consider, for example, the observations reported in Table 1 which refer to a patient with a therapeutic range between 2.5 and 3.5:

- the observation number 1 is characterized by an induced INR value of 3.5: this value is inside the therapeutic range, so this observation is considered successful.

- the observation number 2 is characterized by an induced INR value of 4: such value is external to the therapeutic range, so this observation is considered unsuccessful.

For the observation number 1, delta_dose_perc and delta_INR_perc are computed as follows:

$$delta\_dose\_perc = \frac{dose_2 - dose_1}{dose_1} * 100 = \frac{3.5 - 2.3}{2.3} * 100 = 52.17$$

$$delta\_INR\_perc = \frac{INR_3 - INR_2}{INR_2} * 100 = \frac{13.75 - 12.5}{12.5} * 100 = 10$$

where the dose variation ($dose_2 - dose_1$) induced the INR variation ($INR_3 - INR_2$).

We also excluded from the original dataset, the observations with a starting dose value and a starting INR value of 0, because their relative percentage variations would be infinite. We also consider only the prescription relative to the Warfarin drug because the DNATO-SE knowledge base contains only rules about its management.

The dataset obtained applying all the exclusion criteria, is the one used to learn the regression model.

4.2 Regression Model Learning and Performance Evaluation

Given a parameter y, called dependent variable, we suppose that its value depends, according to an unknown mathematic law, on a set of k parameters $x_1, ..., x_k$ called regressors, linearly independent each others.

Given a dataset of n observations and under particular hypotheses, generally verified in natural systems, it is possible to use the least squares method [1] to extract a mathematic regression model capable to describe y as a function of the set of regressors $x_1, ..., x_k$.

In order to evaluate the performance of a regression model the literature introduces three parameters: the total deviance (SST), the dispersion deviance (SSE) and the regression deviance (SSR). The total deviance (SST) is defined as the sum of the dispersion deviance (SSE) and the regression deviance (SSR) as shown in Form. (1). In this formula we use the following notations: y_i is the i-th value of the observed y; avg(y) is average of the observed values of y; $\hat{y}_i$ represents the value of y obtained by using the regression model and assigning to the regressors the parameters of the i-th observation; n represents the number of dataset observations.

$$\underbrace{\sum_{i=1}^{n}(y_i - avg(y))^2}_{\text{SST}} = \underbrace{\sum_{i=1}^{n}(y_i - \hat{y}_i)^2}_{\text{SSE}} + \underbrace{\sum_{i=1}^{n}(\hat{y}_i - avg(y))^2}_{\text{SSR}} \qquad (1)$$

SST, SSE are then aggregated to compute, thanks to Form. (2), the linear determination coefficient R^2, that gives the evaluation of the performance of a regression model:

- $R^2 = 1$, means that the regression model perfectly forecast the y values;
- $R^2 = 0$, means that the regression model has a forecast accuracy level equal to that of the average of y;
- $R^2 < 0$, means that the model is even worse than the average of y.

$$R^2 = 1 - \frac{SSE}{SST} \tag{2}$$

$$R^2_{adj} = 1 - \left[\left(1 - R^2\right) \frac{n-1}{n-k-1} \right] \tag{3}$$

R^2_{adj} (referred in the tables as R^2-AG), computed thanks to Form. (3), is called adjusted linear determination coefficient and is used to consider in the performance evaluation also the number of regressors used in the model.

4.3 Development of the DNTAO-SE Regression Model

The starting point of our experiments was the regression model adopted by PARMA [5] (briefly described in Sect. 6). This model uses the following function:

delta_dose_perc = f (dose_iniz * delta_INR_perc, delta_INR_perc)

in which the regressors are the same parameters described in Sect. 4.1.

Given this model (referred as general-DNTAO), we tried to develop a new model capable to achieve a significant improvement. The experiments was conducted in three steps: in the first, described in Sect. 4.3.1, we modified the model function; in the second, described in Sect. 4.3.2, we identified group of affine prescriptions, which requires a specific model; in the third, described in Sect. 4.3.3, we combined the results achieved in the previous steps and built the final set of models used by DNTAO-SE.

The dataset was composed by 43523 OAT prescriptions performed by "Maggiore" hospital in Bologna (Italy) from November 1999 to October 2003. Applying the exclusion criteria described in Sect. 4.1, the number of prescriptions suitable for building a regression model was reduced to 23192: this set of prescriptions is referred in the paper as whole dataset (WD).

4.3.1 Experimenting Different Model Functions

Starting from general-DNTAO and the whole dataset (WD), we tried to achieve significant model improvements thanks to these criteria:

- Adding new regressors to the model function;
- Increasing the degree of existing regressors.

Some results achieved adding new regressors and/or increasing the degree of the existing regressors, are shown in Tab. 2.

The best results were produced raising the degree of dose_iniz. Considering only dose_iniz as extra regressor and gradually increasing its degree (up to the 4-th degree in order to avoid to develop an excessively complex model), the best performing model is the number 8. Comparing its performance with the general-DNTAO one:

general-DNTAO:	$R^2 = R^2_{adj} = 0.0477$
model 8:	$R^2 = R^2_{adj} = 0.0827$

we observe a performance improvement of about **3.5%.**

Table 2. Models learned on the whole dataset

1	delta_dose_perc = f (dose_iniz*delta_INR_perc, delta_INR_perc)	SSE = $1.9436 * 10^7$ (PARMA)
2	delta_dose_perc = f (dose_iniz, dose_iniz*delta_INR_perc, delta_INR_perc)	SSE = $1.9386 * 10^7$
3	delta_dose_perc = f (dose_iniz, dose_iniz*delta_INR_perc, delta_INR_perc, range_min, range_max)	SSE = $1.9384 * 10^7$
4	delta_dose_perc = f (dose_iniz, dose_iniz*delta_INR_perc, delta_INR_perc, delta_INR_perc^2, range_min, range_max)	SSE = $1.9378 * 10^7$
5	delta_dose_perc = f (dose_iniz, dose_iniz*delta_INR_perc, delta_INR_perc, delta_INR_perc^2, range_min, range_max, eta)	SSE = $9.9870 * 10^{10}$
6	delta_dose_perc = f (dose_iniz, dose_iniz^2, dose_iniz*delta_INR_perc, delta_INR_perc, delta_INR_perc^2, range_min, range_max)	SSE = $1.9244 * 10^7$
7	delta_dose_perc = f (dose_iniz, dose_iniz^2, dose_iniz^3, dose_iniz*delta_INR_perc, delta_INR_perc)	SSE = $1.9040 * 10^7$
8	delta_dose_perc = f (dose_iniz, dose_iniz^2, dose_iniz^3, dose_iniz^4, dose_iniz*delta_INR_perc, delta_INR_perc)	SSE = $1.8719 * 10^7$

4.3.2 Models Learned on Dataset Partitions

Alternatively to the criteria described in Sect. 4.3.1, we tried to obtain model improvements, dividing the dataset into affinity groups and learning a model for each group.

First of all, we restricted the dataset only to prescriptions with a starting dose within 5 and 50 mg/week, obtaining a dataset of 22322 elements (referred as reduced dataset or RD). Then we evaluated the general-DNTAO performance on RD:

$$R^2 = R^2_{adj} = 0.2386$$

an higher value than the one achieved by the same model on WD. Evidently the group of observations characterized by "extreme" dose values, makes general-DNTAO less successful, showing the need for an ad-hoc model. Learning the regression model on RD, the performance of the resulting model (referred as reduced-DNTAO), was:

$$R^2 = R^2_{adj} = 0.2433$$

a slight improvement with respect to general-DNTAO.

In order to further improve the regression model, we decided to divide RD in more affinity groups by using some OAT parameters and to learn for each one a regression model (referred as group model). For each group, we compared the performance achieved by general-DNTAO, reduced-DNTAO and group models on the prescriptions belonging to each group. The parameters used in experiments were: therapeutic indication, extreme dose values, therapeutic range and patient sex.

Using as parameter the therapeutic indication (TI), we learned eight regression models as shown in Tab. 3. The performance achieved by these models are better than the ones achieved by general-DNTAO and reduced-DNTAO. The improvements are evident for the group with therapeutic indication 4 (ischemic cardiopathy) (improvement of 4.46% with respect to reduced-DNTAO and 8.53% with respect to general-DNTAO), and the one with therapeutic indication 8 (valvulopathy) (improvement of 4.09% with respect to reduced-DNTAO, and 7.35% with respect to general-DNTAO).

Another experiment was conducted considering "extreme" dose values, extracting from WD two prescription groups characterized respectively by a starting dose lesser than 5 mg/week and by a starting dose greater than 50 mg/week. The performances of the models learned on each group (shown in Tab. 4) are significantly better than the general-DNTAO ones (37% on high doses group) on the same group.

As regard experiments related to therapeutic range and patient sex, they did not reveal any significant improvement with respect to general-DNTAO.

Table 3. Performance of models learned on prescriptions grouped by therapeutic indication

GROUP	Group model		reduced-DNTAO		general-DNTAO		Number of observations
	R^2	R^2-AG	R^2	R^2-AG	R^2	R^2-AG	
TI1	0.2989	0.2988	0.2947	0.2945	0.2781	0.2780	11759
TI 2	0.6998	0.6776	0.5365	0.5022	0.4356	0.3938	30
TI 3	0.3346	0.3336	0.2989	0.2979	0.3050	0.3041	1471
TI 4	0.3494	0.3488	0.3049	0.3042	0.2642	0.2635	2346
TI 5	0.3937	0.3901	0.3735	0.3697	0.3757	0.3719	387
TI 6	0.2191	0.2186	0.1932	0.1927	0.2022	0.2017	3510
TI 7	0.1601	0.1590	0.1551	0.1540	0.1456	0.1445	1605
TI 8	0.3276	0.3270	0.2868	0.2861	0.2542	0.2535	2084

Table 4. Performance of models learned on prescriptions with extreme doses

GROUP	Group model		General-DNTAO		Number of observations
	R^2	R^2-AG	R^2	R^2-AG	
Starting Dose < 5 mg/week	0.0386	0.0226	-0.0934	-0.1116	123
Starting Dose > 50 mg/week	0.3717	0.3700	-2.8035	-2.8138	747

4.3.3 The DNTAO-SE Regression Model

Considering the results of the previous experiments, we decided to use in DNTAO-SE three models: one for starting dose lesser than 5 mg/week (referred as group1), one for starting dose greater than 50 mg/week (referred as group2) and one for the remaining prescriptions (this set is equal to RD).

For group1 and group2, the regression models use the same function as general-DNTAO but are obtained learning the model on the respective prescriptions (as described in Sect. 4.3.2).

About group3, performing further evaluations on this dataset, we observed that the relation between dose_iniz and the ratio of delta_dose_perc on delta_INR_perc is similar to a logarithmic function. For this reason we introduced a new model referred as ln-DNTAO:

$$\text{delta\_dose\_perc} = f\left(\frac{\text{delta\_INR\_perc}}{\ln(\text{dose\_iniz}/2)}, \text{delta\_INR\_perc}\right)$$

The performances of ln-DNTAO and general-DNTAO (that is the starting model of our experiments) on RD are:

general-DNTAO : $R^2 = R^2_{adj} = 0.2386$
ln-DNTAO-SE : $R^2 = R^2_{adj} = 0.2667$

The improvement achieved is 11.8% and involves the prescriptions in the reduced dataset (RD) that are the 96% of the ones in the whole dataset (WD).

5 DNTAO-SE Testing

In order to evaluate the performance of DNTAO-SE knowledge base and its regression model set (described in Sect. 4.3.3), we used a new dataset of 4616 OAT prescriptions performed by "Maggiore" hospital in Bologna (Italy) from December 2003 to February 2004. DNTAO-SE suggestions were compared with the haematologist's ones and the results are reported in Tab. 5. The central columns of this table report the average of days and doses difference (in percentage) among DNATAO-SE and hematologist suggestions. Analyzing these results, we observe that DNATO-SE works very well on low (7.7% of the dataset prescriptions) and medium (62.1% of the dataset prescriptions) risk patients. The executed test provided many insights to haematologists too (we discovered some mistakes done by them).

A more complex evaluation is needed to understand the system performance on high risk patients. At the moment, haematologists manually prescribe the dose adjustments for this kind of patients usually without taking care of international guidelines for OAT management. The DNTAO-SE knowledge base includes these guidelines and introduces some degrees of flexibility in order to provide the most suitable suggestion. Comparing DNTAO-SE suggestions with the ones provided by hematologists that use those guidelines, we achieved the following results:

- The average difference between the next OAT prescription date is 8.85%;
- About the prescribed dose, the ones provide by DNTAO-SE and hematologists are equal in 48% of the prescriptions.

These results need to be improved, refining the related knowledge base.

Table 5. DNTAO-SE testing results

Patient kind	Average diff. days	Average diff. doses	Number of observations
Low risk	2.16	0.23%	355
Medium risk	4.55	2.21%	2865

6 Related Work

Some computer systems are nowadays used for OAT management. Among the analyzed systems, we briefly describe DAWN AC 6 [3][6] and PARMA [5].

DAWN AC 6 [3] is a intelligent data management system for OAT therapy prescription. It contains an expert system [6] with a extensible and customizable knowledge base. It permits also to plan the activity of the blood drawing center, to execute statistical analyses on therapy trends.

PARMA (Program for Archive, Refertation and Monitoring of Anticoagulated patients) [5] is a product of Instrumentation Laboratory realized in collaboration with many hospitals in Parma (Italy). The basic characteristics of this system are: management of patient records, an algorithm for the automatic suggestion of OAT therapy; automated reporting; statistical analysis.

With respect to that systems, DNTAO-SE offers a more complete support of OAT because is capable to manage not only therapy start and maintaining but also the return to the target range of patient with INR significantly out of it. DNTAO-SE also integrates a more sophisticated regression model which improves the reliability of its suggestions. It is also capable to make hematologists aware of the motivations that had led the reasoning to the proposed conclusions. Another important advantage of

DNTAO-SE is flexibility as it allows rule customization and updating. Other systems, like PARMA for example, do not propose this important feature.

7 Conclusions and Future Work

In this paper we described a system for supporting haematologists in the definition of Oral Anticoagulant Therapy (OAT) prescriptions.

DNTAO-SE provides this support automatically retrieving all the information about the patient clinical history (formerly INR levels and assigned doses in the previous prescriptions) and other relevant clinical information and applying a knowledge base and an inference engine to propose the most suitable next therapy.

During the reasoning, the patient is classified in tree risk levels and for each level, a specific methodology for therapy definition is proposed. Each risk level is strictly related to a specific OAT. With respect to other OAT management systems, DNTAO-SE offers a more complete support to haematologists because is capable to manage not only therapy start and maintaining but also the return to the therapeutic range of patients with an INR level significantly out of it.

The suggestion of the most suitable therapy dose for medium risk patient, is achieved by using a regression model learned on dataset of previous OAT prescriptions. Although this approach has been used also by other systems, the models used in DNTAO-SE are more sophisticated and are capable to guarantee better performances. In the paper we described in details (see Sect. 4) the steps followed to develop these regression models.

The DNTAO-SE performance test, executed on a dataset of prescriptions (see Sect. 5) has shown the reliability of its suggestions. The executed test provided many insights to haematologists too (we discovered some mistakes done by them).

In the future we plan to further improve the reliability of DNTAO-SE knowledge base and regression model, collecting more information about the patient anamnesis (checklist improvement).

Acknowledgements. This work has been partially supported by BMG Consulting Srl under the regional project "Innovative actions in health care" Prot. AIA/PSE/03 n. 25281 del 19/8/03. The authors would like to thank Claudio Coreggioli for his help.

References

1. Anderson, D. R., Sweeney, D. J., Williams, T. A.: Introduction to Statistics concepts and applications, Third Edition, West Publishing Company (1994)
2. Barbieri, B., Gamberoni, G., Lamma, E., Mello, P., Pavesi, P.C., Storari, S., Trovino, G.: Un sistema basato sulla conoscenza per la terapia anticoagulante orale. Intelligenza Artificiale 4, AIIA, (2004)
3. DAWN AC 6, see the web site: http://www.4s-dawn.com
4. Dianoema S.p.A., see the web site: http://www.dianoema.it
5. Mariani, G., Manotti, C., Dettori, A.G.: A computerized regulation of dosage in oral anticoagulant therapy. Ric Clin Lab 20 (1990) 119-25
6. Poller, L., Shiach, C.R., MacCallum, P.K.,. Johansen, A.M, Münster, A.M., Magalhães, A., Jespersen, J.: Multicentre randomised study of computerised anticoagulant dosage. The Lancet 352 (1998) 1505-1509

Thermal Medical Image Retrieval by Moment Invariants

Shao Ying Zhu[1] and Gerald Schaefer[2]

[1] Applied Computing, University of Derby, Derby, UK
S.Y.Zhu@derby.ac.uk
[2] School of Computing and Informatics, Nottingham Trent University
Nottingham, UK
Gerald.Schaefer@ntu.ac.uk

Abstract. Thermal medical imaging provides a valuable method for detecting various diseases such as breast cancer or Raynaud's syndrome. While previous efforts on the automated processing on thermal infrared images were designed for and hence constrained to a certain type of disease we apply the concept of content-based image retrieval (CBIR) as a more generic approach to the problem. CBIR allows the retrieval of similar images based on features extracted directly from image data. Image retrieval for a thermal image that shows symptoms of a certain disease will provide visually similar cases which usually also represent similarities in medical terms. The image features we investigate in this study are a set of combinations of geometric image moments which are invariant to translation, scale, rotation and contrast.

Keywords: Thermal medical images, medical infrared images, content-based image retrieval, moment invariants.

1 Introduction

While image analysis and pattern recognition techniques have been applied to infrared (thermal) images for many years in astronomy and military applications, relatively little work has been conducted on the automatic processing of thermal medical images. Furthermore, those few approaches that have been presented in the literature are all specific to a certain application or disease such as the detection of breast cancer as in [6].

In this paper we consider the application of content-based image retrieval (CBIR) for thermal medical images as a more generic approach for the analysis and interpretation of medical infrared images. CBIR allows the retrieval of visually similar and hence usually relevant images based on a pre-defined similarity measure between image features derived directly from the image data. In terms of medical infrared imaging, images that are similar to a sample exhibiting symptoms of a certain disease or other disorder will be likely to show the same or similar manifestations of the disease. These known cases together with their medical reports should then provide a valuable asset for the diagnosis of the unknown case.

J.M. Barreiro et al. (Eds.): ISBMDA 2004, LNCS 3337, pp. 182–187, 2004.

The rest of the paper is organised as follows. Section 2 provides a brief introduction to the field of thermal medical imaging while Section 3 gives some background on content-based image retrieval. Our proposal of CBIR for thermal medical images is discussed in Section 4 with experimental results provided in Section 5. Section 6 concludes the paper.

2 Thermal Medical Imaging

Advances in camera technologies and reduced equipment costs have lead to an increased interest in the application of infrared imaging in the medical fields [2]. Medical infrared imaging uses a camera with sensitivities in the (near-)infrared to provide a picture of the temperature distribution of the human body or parts thereof. It is a non-invasive, radiation-free technique that is often being used in combination with anatomical investigations based on x-rays and three-dimensional scanning techniques such as CT and MRI and often reveals problems when the anatomy is otherwise normal. It is well known that the radiance from human skin is an exponential function of the surface temperature which in term is influenced by the level of blood perfusion in the skin. Thermal imaging is hence well suited to pick up changes in blood perfusion which might occur due to inflammation, angiogenesis or other causes. Asymmetrical temperature distributions as well as the presence of hot and cold cold are known to be strong indicators of an underlying dysfunction [8]. Computerised image processing and pattern recognition techniques have been used in acquiring and evaluating medical thermal images [5, 9] and proved to be important tools for clinical diagnostics.

3 Content-Based Image Retrieval

Content-based image retrieval has been an active research area for more than a decade. The principal aim is to retrieve digital images based not on textual annotations but on features derived directly from image data. These features are then stored alongside the image and serve as an index. Retrieval is often performed in a query by example fashion where a query image is provided by the user. The retrieval system is then searching through all images in order to find those with the most similar indices which are returned as the candidates most alike to the query.

A large variety of features have been proposed in the CBIR literature [7]. In general, they can be grouped into several categories: color features, texture features, shape features, sketch features, and spatial features. Often one or more feature types are combined in order to improve retrieval performance.

4 Retrieving Thermal Medical Images

In this paper we report on an initial investigation on the use of CBIR for thermal medical images. One main advantage of using this concept is that it represents a generic approach to the automatic processing of such images. Rather than employing specialised techniques which will capture only one kind of disease or defect, image retrieval when supported by a sufficiently large medical image database of both 'healthy' and 'sick' examples will provide those cases that are most similar to a given one. The query by example method is perfectly suited for this task with the thermal image of an 'unknown' case as the query image.

The features we propose to store as an index for each thermal image are invariant combinations of moments of an image. Two-dimensional geometric moments m_{pq} of order $p+q$ of a density distribution function $f(x,y)$ are defined as

$$m_{pq} = \int_{-\infty}^{\infty}\int_{-\infty}^{\infty} x^p y^q f(x,y)dxdy \tag{1}$$

In terms of a digital image $g(x,y)$ of size $N \times M$ the calculation of m_{pq} becomes discretised and the integrals are hence replaced by sums leading to

$$m_{pq} = \sum_{y=0}^{M-1}\sum_{x=0}^{N-1} x^p y^q g(x,y) \tag{2}$$

Rather than m_{pq} often central moments

$$\mu_{pq} = \sum_{y=0}^{M-1}\sum_{x=0}^{N-1} (x-\bar{x})^p (y-\bar{y})^q g(x,y) \tag{3}$$

with

$$\bar{x} = \frac{m_{10}}{m_{00}} \quad \bar{y} = \frac{m_{01}}{m_{00}}$$

are used, i.e. moments where the centre of gravity has been moved to the origin (i.e. $\mu_{10} = \mu_{01} = 0$). Central moments have the advantage of being invariant to translation.

It is well known that a small number of moments can characterise an image fairly well; it is equally known that moments can be used to reconstruct the original image [1]. In order to achieve invariance to common factors and operations such as scale, rotation and contrast, rather than using the moments themselves algebraic combinations thereof known as moment invariants are used that are independent of these transformations. It is a set of such moment invariants that we use for the retrieval of thermal medical images. In particular the descriptors we use are based on Hu's original moment invariants given by [1]

$$\begin{aligned} M_1 &= \mu_{20} + \mu_{02} \\ M_2 &= (\mu_{20} - \mu_{02})^2 + 4\mu_{11}^2 \\ M_3 &= (\mu_{30} - 3\mu_{12})^2 + 3(\mu_{21} + \mu_{03})^2 \\ M_4 &= (\mu_{30} + \mu_{12})^2 + (\mu_{21} + \mu_{03})^2 \\ M_5 &= (\mu_{30} - 3\mu_{12})(\mu_{30} + \mu_{12})[(\mu_{30} + \mu_{12})^2 - 3(\mu_{21} + \mu_{03})^2] + \\ &\quad (3\mu_{21} - \mu_{03})(\mu_{21} + \mu_{03})[3(\mu_{30} + \mu_{12})^2 - (\mu_{21} + \mu_{03})^2] \end{aligned} \tag{4}$$

$$M_6 = (\mu_{20} - \mu_{02})[(\mu_{30} + \mu_{12})^2 - (\mu_{21} + \mu_{03})^2] + 4\mu_{11}(\mu_{30} + \mu_{12})(\mu_{21} + \mu_{03})$$
$$M_7 = (3\mu_{21} - \mu_{03})(\mu_{30} + \mu_{12})[(\mu_{30} + \mu_{12})^2 - 3(\mu_{21} + \mu_{03})^2] + (\mu_{30} - 3\mu_{12})(\mu_{21} + \mu_{03})[3(\mu_{30} + \mu_{12})^2 - (\mu_{21} + \mu_{03})^2]$$

Combinations of Hu's invariants can be found to achieve invariance not only to translation and rotation but also to scale and contrast [4]

$$\beta_1 = \frac{\sqrt{M_2}}{M_1} \tag{5}$$
$$\beta_2 = \frac{M_3\mu_{00}}{M_1M_2}$$
$$\beta_3 = \frac{M_4}{M_3}$$
$$\beta_4 = \frac{\sqrt{M_5}}{M_4}$$
$$\beta_5 = \frac{M_6}{M_1M_4}$$
$$\beta_6 = \frac{M_7}{M_5}$$

Each thermal image is characterised by these six moment invariants $\Phi = \{\beta_i, i = 1...6\}$. Image retrieval is performed by finding those images whose invariants are closest to the ones calculated for a given query image. As a similarity metric or distance measure we use the Mahalanobis norm which takes into account different magnitudes of different components in Φ. The Mahalanobis distance between two invariant vectors $\Phi(I_1)$ and $\Phi(I_2)$ computed from two thermal images I_1 and I_2 is defined as

$$d(I_1, I_2) = \sqrt{(\Phi_1 - \Phi_2)^T C^{-1} (\Phi_1 - \Phi_2)} \tag{6}$$

where C is the covariance matrix of the distribution of Φ.

5 Experimental Results

The moment invariant descriptors described above were used to index an image database of 530 thermal medical images provided by the University of Glamorgan [3]. An example of an image of an arm was used to perform image retrieval on the whole dataset. The result of this query is given in Figure 1 which shows those 20 images that were found to be closest to the query (sorted according to descending similarity from left to right, top to bottom). It can be seen that all retrieved images contain an arm of a subject.

Unfortunately, due to the lack of enough samples of cases of known diseases, such retrieval as outlined earlier cannot be performed at the moment. We are in the processes of collecting a large number of thermograms, both images of 'normal' people [3] and cases of known symptoms of diseases. This documented dataset will then provide a testbed for the evaluating of our method proposed in this paper as well as future approaches.

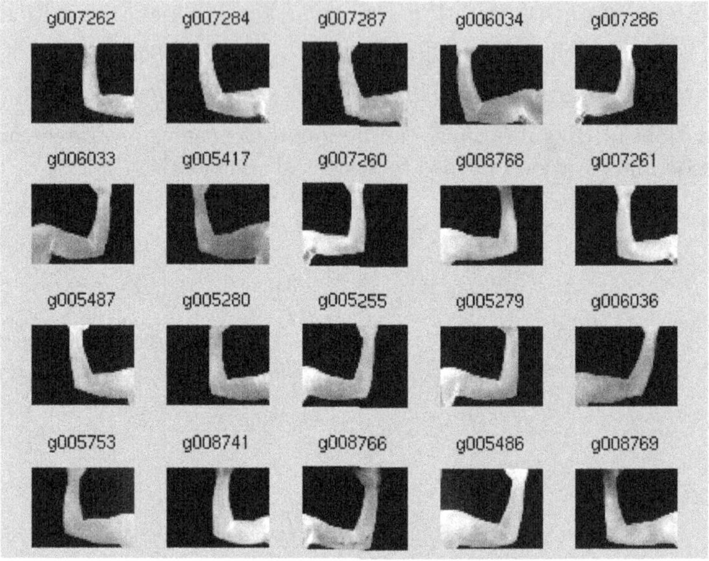

Fig. 1. Example of retrieving thermal images of arms using moment invariants.

6 Conclusions

We have investigated the application of content-based image retrieval to the domain of medical infrared images. Each image is characterised by a set of moment invariants which are independent to translation, scale, rotation and contrast. Retrieval is performed by returning those images whose moments are most similar to the ones of a given query image. Initial results on a dataset of more than 500 infrared images have proved the feasibility and usefulness of the introduced approach.

Acknowledgements

The authors wish to thank the Nuffield Foundation for their support under grant number NAL/00734/G and the Medical Computing Research Group of the University of Glamorgan for providing the test image dataset.

References

1. M.K. Hu. Visual pattern recognition by moment invariants. *IRE Transactions on Information Theory*, 8(2):179–187, February 1962.
2. B.F. Jones. A re-appraisal of infrared thermal image analysis for medicine. *IEEE Trans. Medical Imaging*, 17(6):1019–1027, 1998.
3. B.F. Jones. EPSRC Grant GR/R50134/01 Report, 2001.
4. S. Maitra. Moment invariants. *Proceedings of the IEEE*, 67:697–699, 1979.

5. P. Plassmann and B.F. Jones. An open system for the acquisition and evaluation of medical thermological images. *European Journal on Thermology*, 7(4):216–220, 1997.
6. H. Qi and J. F. Head. Asymmetry analysis using automatic segmentation and classification for breast cancer detection in thermograms. In *23rd Int. Conference IEEE Engineering in Medicine and Biology*, 2001.
7. A.W.M. Smeulders, M. Worring, S. Santini, A. Gupta, and R.C. Jain. Content-based image retrieval at the end of the early years. *IEEE Trans. Pattern Analysis and Machine Intelligence*, 22(12):1349–1380, December 2000.
8. S. Uematsu. Symmetry of skin temperature comparing one side of the body to the other. *Thermology*, 1(1):4–7, 1985.
9. B. Wiecek, S. Zwolenik, A. Jung, and J. Zuber. Advanced thermal, visual and radiological image processing for clinical diagnostics. In *21st Int. Conference IEEE Engineering in Medicine and Biology*, 1999.

Employing Maximum Mutual Information for Bayesian Classification

Marcel van Gerven and Peter Lucas

Institute for Computing and Information Sciences, Radboud University Nijmegen
Toernooiveld 1, 6525 ED Nijmegen, The Netherlands
{marcelge,peterl}@cs.kun.nl

Abstract. In order to employ machine learning in realistic clinical settings we are in need of algorithms which show robust performance, producing results that are intelligible to the physician. In this article, we present a new Bayesian-network learning algorithm which can be deployed as a tool for learning Bayesian networks, aimed at supporting the processes of prognosis or diagnosis. It is based on a maximum (conditional) mutual information criterion. The algorithm is evaluated using a high-quality clinical dataset concerning disorders of the liver and biliary tract, showing a performance which exceeds that of state-of-the-art Bayesian classifiers. Furthermore, the algorithm places less restrictions on classifying Bayesian network structures and therefore allows easier clinical interpretation.

1 Introduction

The problem of representing and reasoning with medical knowledge has attracted considerable attention during the last three decades; in particular, ways of dealing with the *uncertainty* involved in medical decision making has been identified again and again as one of the key issues in this area. *Bayesian networks* are nowadays considered as standard tools for representing and reasoning with uncertain biomedical, in particular clinical knowledge [1]. A Bayesian network consists of a structural part, representing the statistical (in)dependencies among the variables concerned in the underlying domain, and a probabilistic part specifying a joint probability distribution of these variables [2].

Learning a Bayesian network structure is NP hard [3] and manually constructing a Bayesian network for a realistic medical domain is a very laborious and time-consuming task. Bayesian classifiers may be identified as Bayesian networks with a fixed or severely constrained structural part, which are dedicated to the correct classification of a patient into a small set of possible classes based on the available evidence. Examples of such Bayesian classifiers are the naive Bayesian classifier [4], where evidence variables $\mathcal{E} = \{E_1, \ldots, E_n\}$ are assumed to be conditionally independent given the class variable C and the tree-augmented Bayesian classifier [5], where correlations between evidence variables are represented as arcs between evidence variables in the form of a tree. In the following we take the TAN classifier to be the canonical Bayesian classifier.

J.M. Barreiro et al. (Eds.): ISBMDA 2004, LNCS 3337, pp. 188–199, 2004.

Bayesian classifiers have proven to be a valuable tool for automated diagnosis and prognosis, but are lacking in some respects. Firstly, the constraints on classifier structure disallow many dependence statements, such as the encoding of higher-order dependencies, where the *order* of a dependency is the size of the conditioning set $parents(X)$ of the conditional probability $\Pr(X \mid parents(X))$ associated with the dependency [6]. Also, these constraints lead to classifier structures which may be totally unintelligible from the viewpoint of the physician. We feel that intelligible classifier structures will increase the acceptance of the use of Bayesian classifiers in medical practice because of an improved accordance with a physician's perception of the domain of discourse. Classifier performance will also benefit from such an agreement, since the physician may now aid in identifying counter-intuitive dependency statements. Finally, Bayesian classifiers disregard the direction of dependencies, which may lead to suboptimal performance.

In this article, we introduce a new algorithm to construct Bayesian network classifiers which relaxes the structural assumptions and may therefore yield a network structure which is more intuitive from a medical point of view. This so-called *maximum mutual information* (henceforth MMI) algorithm builds a structure which favours those features showing maximum (conditional) mutual information. The structural assumptions it does make, take into account the direction of dependencies, leading to improved classification performance.

Next to the problems arising from constraints on classifier structure, Bayesian classifiers perform poorly in the face of small databases. Dependency statements may have only little support from the database (in terms of number of records) and yet are encoded within the classifier structure. The MMI algorithm incorporates a solution by making use of *non-uniform Dirichlet priors* during structure learning in order to faithfully encode higher-order dependencies induced by multiple evidence variables.

Bayesian network learning algorithms using information-theoretical measures such as mutual information are known as *dependency-analysis* based or *constraint-based* algorithms and have been used extensively [5, 7]. For instance, Cheng at al. devised an information-theoretical algorithm which uses dependency analysis to build a general Bayesian network structure. Three phases are distinguished: *Drafting*, where an initial network is built by computing the mutual information between pairs of vertices. *Thickening*, in which arcs between vertices are added when they are conditionally dependent on some conditioning set. *Thinning*, in which arcs between vertices are removed if the vertices are conditionally independent. In contrast, in our research we do not aim to build general Bayesian network structures, but instead aim to build a structure learning algorithm for Bayesian classifiers that provides a balance between the complexity issues associated with general structure learning algorithms and the highly restrictive structural assumptions of classifier structure learning algorithms.

In order to determine the performance of the MMI algorithm we make use of a clinical dataset of hepatobiliary (liver and biliary) disorders whose reputation has been firmly established. Performance of the algorithm is compared with an existing system for diagnosis of hepatobiliary disorders and other Bayesian classifiers such as the naive Bayesian classifier and the tree-augmented Bayesian classifier.

We feel that this new algorithm presents a solution to a number of problems associated with contemporary Bayesian classifiers. The algorithm is capable of constructing high fidelity Bayesian classifiers and it is hoped that the medical community will benefit from this in its application to decision-support in diagnosis and prognosis.

2 Preliminaries

In this section we present the theory on Bayesian classification and introduce the dataset used in this study.

2.1 Bayesian Classification

The MMI algorithm constructs a Bayesian network with a specific structure which is optimized for classification. A *Bayesian network* $\mathcal{B}$ (also called belief network) is defined as a pair $\mathcal{B} = \langle G, \Pr \rangle$, where G is a directed, acyclic graph $G = \langle V(G), A(G) \rangle$, with a set of vertices $V(G) = \{X_1, \ldots, X_n\}$, representing a set of stochastic variables, and a set of arcs $A(G) \subseteq V(G) \times V(G)$, representing conditional and unconditional stochastic independences among the variables, modelled by the absence of arcs among vertices. Let $\pi_G(X_i)$ denote the conjunction of variables corresponding to the parents of X_i in G. On the variables in $V(G)$ is defined a joint probability distribution $\Pr(X_1, \ldots, X_n)$, for which, as a consequence of the local Markov property, the following decomposition holds: $\Pr(X_1, \ldots, X_n) = \prod_{i=1}^{n} \Pr(X_i \mid \pi_G(X_i))$.

In order to compare the performance of the MMI algorithm with different Bayesian classifiers we introduce the *forest-augmented naive classifier*, or FAN classifier for short (Fig. 1). A FAN classifier is an extension of the naive classifier, where the topology of the resulting graph over the evidence variables $\mathcal{E} = \{E_1, \ldots, E_n\}$ is restricted to a forest of trees [8]. For each evidence variable E_i there is at most one incoming arc allowed from $\mathcal{E} \setminus \{E_i\}$ and exactly one incoming arc from the class variable C.

The algorithm to construct FAN classifiers used in this paper is based on a modification of the algorithm to construct *tree-augmented naive* (TAN) classifiers

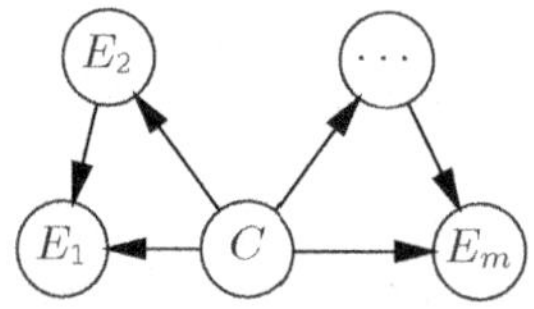

Fig. 1. Forest-augmented naive (FAN) classifier. Notice that both the naive classifier and the tree-augmented naive classifier are limiting cases of the forest-augmented naive classifier.

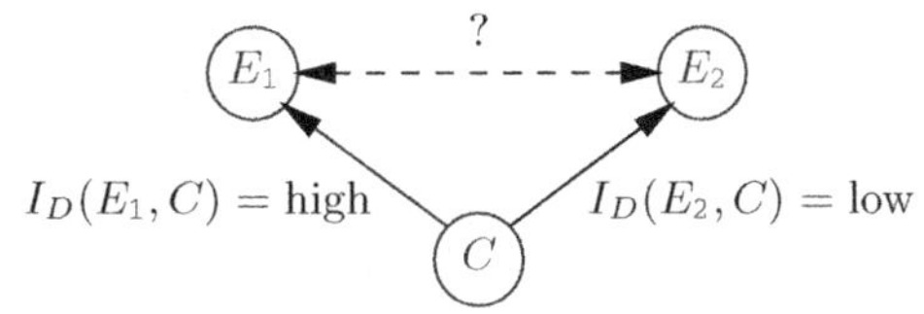

Fig. 2. Choosing E_1 as the root node would encode the conditional probability $\Pr(E_2 \mid C, E_1)$ which has low impact on classification accuracy due to the low mutual information between E_2 and C.

by Friedman et al. [5] as described in [8], where the *class-conditional mutual information*

$$I_D^{cc}(E_i, E_j \mid C) = \sum_{E_i, E_j, C} \Pr(E_i, E_j, C) \log \frac{\Pr(E_i, E_j \mid C)}{\Pr(E_i \mid C)\Pr(E_j \mid C)}, \qquad (1)$$

computed from a database D is used to build a maximum cost spanning tree between evidence variables. Note that the use of a tree which encodes the between evidence dependencies implies that only first-order dependencies of the form $\Pr(E_i \mid C)$ and second-order dependencies of the form $\Pr(E_i \mid C, E_j)$ with $E_i \neq E_j$ can be captured. Furthermore, the root of the tree is chosen arbitrarily, thus neglecting the mutual information as defined in equation (2) between evidence variables and the class variable, as is exemplified by Fig. 2.

The performance of the classifiers was determined by computing *zero-one loss* or *classification accuracy*, where the value c^* of the class variable C with largest probability is taken: $c^* = \arg\max_c \Pr(C = c \mid \mathcal{E})$. 10-fold cross-validation was carried out in order to prevent overfitting artifacts. Apart from looking at classification performance we will also discuss the resulting network structures and their interpretation from a medical point of view.

In this research, the joint probability distributions of the classifiers were learnt from data using Bayesian updating with uniform Dirichlet priors. The conditional probability distribution for each variable V_i was computed as the weighted average of a probability estimate and the Dirichlet prior, as follows:

$$\Pr_D(V_i \mid \pi(V_i)) = \frac{N}{N + N_0} \widehat{\Pr}_D(V_i \mid \pi(V_i)) + \frac{N_0}{N + N_0} \Theta_i$$

where $\widehat{\Pr}_D$ is the probability distribution estimate based on a given dataset D, and Θ_i is the Dirichlet prior. We choose Θ_i to be a uniform probability distribution. Furthermore, N_0 is equal to the number of past cases on which the contribution of Θ_i is based, and N is the size of the dataset. When there were no cases at all in the dataset for any configuration of the variable V_i given a configuration of its parents $\pi(V_i)$, a uniform probability distribution was assumed. We have chosen a small Dirichlet prior of $N_0 = 8$ throughout experimentation.

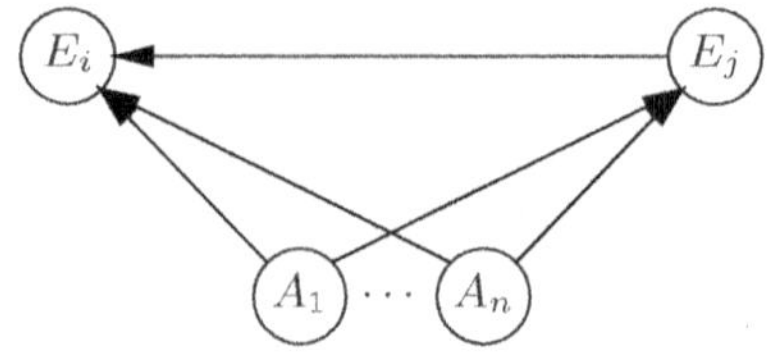

Fig. 3. Network used to compute conditional mutual information, with $A_1 \cdots A_n$ representing a full probability distribution of the type $\Pr(A_1 \mid A_2, \ldots, A_n)$ $\Pr(A_2 \mid A_3, \ldots, A_n) \cdots \Pr(A_n)$.

2.2 The COMIK Dataset

We made use of the COMIK dataset, which was collected by the Copenhagen Computer Icterus (COMIK) group and consists of data on 1002 jaundiced patients. The COMIK group has been working for more than a decade on the development of a system for diagnosing liver and biliary disease which is known as the Copenhagen Pocket Diagnostic Chart [9]. Using a set $\mathcal{E}$ of 21 evidence variables, the system classifies patients into one of four diagnostic categories: *acute non-obstructive*, *chronic non-obstructive*, *benign obstructive* and *malignant obstructive*. The chart offers a compact representation of three logistic regression equations, where the probability of *acute obstructive jaundice*, for instance, is computed as follows: $\Pr(\textit{acute obstructive jaundice} \mid \mathcal{E}) = \Pr(\textit{acute} \mid \mathcal{E}) \cdot \Pr(\textit{obstructive} \mid \mathcal{E})$. The performance of the system has been studied using retrospective patient data and it has been found that the system is able to produce a correct diagnostic conclusion (i.e. in accord with the diagnostic conclusion of expert clinicians) in about $75 - 77\%$ of jaundiced patients [10].

3 The Maximum Mutual Information Algorithm

The maximum mutual information algorithm uses both the computed mutual information between evidence variables and the class-variable, and the computed conditional mutual information between evidence-variables as a basis for constructing a Bayesian classifier. Mutual information (MI) between an evidence variable E and the class-variable C for a database D can be computed using the (conditional) probabilities of Bayesian networks of the type $C \to E$ learnt from the database, such that

$$I_D(E, C) = \sum_{E,C} \Pr(E \mid C) \Pr(C) \log \frac{\Pr(E \mid C)}{\sum_{c \in C} \Pr(E \mid c) \Pr(c)} . \qquad (2)$$

Conditional mutual information between evidence variables is similar to the definition of class-conditional mutual information as defined in equation 1 where the conditional may be an arbitrary set of variables $\mathcal{A} = \{A_1, \ldots, A_n\}$. It may be computed from the Bayesian network depicted in Fig. 3 as follows:

Algorithm 1: MMI construction algorithm

input: G {empty Bayesian network structure}, D {database}, c {class variable}, $\mathcal{E}$ {evidence-variables}, N {number of arcs}

$\mathcal{C} \leftarrow$ a set of elements $\langle c,e \rangle$, with $e \in \mathcal{E}$, sorted by $I_D(c,e)$

$\mathcal{A} \leftarrow \varnothing$, $\mathcal{AO} \leftarrow \varnothing$ {ordering on the attributes}

for $i = 0$ to N **do**

  if $\mathcal{A}$ is empty **or** $I_D(\mathcal{C}_0) > I_D^c(\mathcal{A}_0)$ **then**

    Let e be the evidence variable in $\mathcal{C}_0$

    remove $\mathcal{C}_0$ from $\mathcal{C}$

    add e to the ordering $\mathcal{AO}$

    add $\langle c, e \rangle$ to the arcs of G

    for all $e' \in \mathcal{E} \setminus \mathcal{AO}$ **do**

      add candidate $\langle e', e \rangle$ to $\mathcal{A}$

    end for

    sort($\mathcal{A}$) by $I_D^c(e', e \mid \pi(e))$

  else

    Let e', e be the evidence variables in $\mathcal{A}_0$

    remove $\mathcal{A}_0$ from $\mathcal{A}$

    add $\langle e', e \rangle$ to the arcs of G

    for all pairs $\langle a, e \rangle \in \mathcal{A}$ **do**

      recompute $I_D^c(a, e \mid \pi(e))$

    end for

    sort($\mathcal{A}$)

  end if

end for

return G

$$I_D^c(E_i, E_j \mid \mathcal{A}) = \sum_{E_i, E_j, \mathcal{A}} \Pr(E_i \mid E_j, \mathcal{A}) \Pr(E_j \mid \mathcal{A})$$

$$\Pr(A_1 \mid A_2, \ldots, A_n) \cdots \Pr(A_n) \log \frac{\Pr(E_i \mid E_j, \mathcal{A})}{\sum_{e_j \in E_j} \Pr(E_i \mid e_j, \mathcal{A}) \Pr(e_j \mid \mathcal{A})} . \tag{3}$$

Contrary to naive and TAN classifiers, the MMI algorithm makes no assumptions whatsoever about the initial network structure. The MMI algorithm starts from a fully disconnected graph, whereas the FAN algorithm starts with an independent form model such that $\langle C, E_i \rangle \in A(G)$ for all evidence variables E_i. Since redundant attributes are not encoded, network structures are sparser, at the same time indicating important information on the independence between class and evidence variables. In this sense, the MMI algorithm can be said to resemble *selective Bayesian classifiers* [11].

The algorithm iteratively selects the arc with highest (conditional) mutual information from the set of candidates and adds it to the Bayesian network B with classifier structure G (algorithm 1). It starts by computing $I_D(E_i, C)$ for a list $\mathcal{C}$ of arcs between the class variables C and evidence variables E_i. From this list it selects the candidate having highest MI, say $\langle C, E_i \rangle$, which will be removed from the list and added to the classifier structure. Subsequently, it will construct

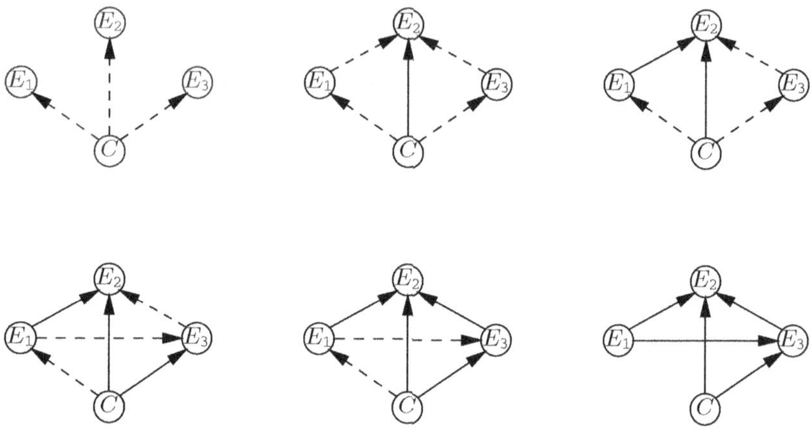

Fig. 4. An example of the MMI algorithm building a Bayesian classifier structure. Dashed arrows represent candidate dependencies. The final structure incorporates feature selection, orientational preference of dependencies and the encoding of a third-order dependency $\Pr(E_2 \mid C, E_1, E_3)$.

all candidates of the form $\langle E_j, E_i \rangle$ where $\langle C, E_j \rangle$ is not yet part of the classifier structure G and add them to the list $\mathcal{A}$. The conditional mutual information $I_D^c(E_i, E_j \mid \pi(E_i))$ is computed for these candidates. Now, the algorithm iteratively selects the candidate of list $\mathcal{C}$ or $\mathcal{A}$ having the highest (conditional) mutual information. If a candidate E_i from $\mathcal{A}$ is chosen, then $I_D^c(E_i, E_j \mid \pi(E_i))$ for all pairs $\langle E_i, E_j \rangle \in \mathcal{A}$ is recomputed since the parent set of E_i has changed. By directing evidence arcs to attributes which show high mutual information with the class variable, we make maximal use of the information contained within the network and enforce the resulting structure to remain an acyclic digraph. Figure 4 shows an example of how the MMI algorithm builds a Bayesian classifier structure.

Looking back at equation (3) a possible complication is identified. Since the parent set $A_1, \ldots, A_n$ may grow indefinitely and the number of parent configurations grows exponentially with n, the network may become victim of its own unrestrainedness in terms of structure. Note also that since one has a finite (and often small) database at ones disposal, this means that the actual conditional probability $\Pr(E_i \mid A_1, \ldots, A_n)$ will become increasingly inaccurate when the number of parents grows; configurations associated with large parent-sets cannot be reliably estimated from moderate size databases, introducing what may be termed *spurious dependencies*. When we compute conditional information over a database consisting of k records, the average number of records providing information about a particular configuration of a parent set of size n containing binary variables will only be $k2^{-n}$ on average. So even for moderate size databases such inaccuracies will arise rather quickly.

In order to prevent the occurrence of spurious dependencies, we make use of non-uniform Dirichlet priors. The probability $\Pr(E_i, E_j \mid \mathcal{A})$ is estimated to be equal to

$$\frac{N^*}{N^* + N_0^c}\mathrm{Pr}_D(E_i, E_j \mid \mathcal{A}) + \frac{N_0^c}{N^* + N_0^c}\mathrm{Pr}_D(E_i \mid \mathcal{A})\mathrm{Pr}_D(E_j \mid \mathcal{A}),$$

where Pr denotes the estimate $\widehat{\mathrm{Pr}}$, regularized by the uniform prior, N^* is the number of times the configuration $A_1, \ldots, A_n$ occurs in D and N_0^c is the setting used during computation of the conditional mutual information. In this manner, both distributions will only marginally differ if the number of times the configuration occurs is small. Note that a uniform distribution will not work, since this *will* make both distributions differ substantially. In the following we will use $N_0^c = 500$ throughout our experiments, unless indicated otherwise.

4 Results

In this section we will demonstrate the usefulness of the N_0^c parameter, compare the classification performance of both the FAN and MMI classifiers on the COMIK dataset and give a medical interpretation of the resulting structures.

4.1 Non-uniform Dirichlet Priors

First we present the results of varying the parameter N_0^c in order to determine whether this has an effect on the classification performance and network structure of our classifiers. To this end, we have determined the classification accuracy and summed squared fan-in of the nodes in the classifier for a network of 30 arcs. Let $\mid \pi_G(X) \mid$ denote the cardinality of the parent set of a vertex X. The summed squared fan-in $\mathrm{F}(\mathcal{B})$ of a Bayesian network $\mathcal{B} = \langle G, \mathrm{Pr} \rangle$ containing vertices $V(G)$ is defined as $\mathrm{F}(\mathcal{B}) = \sum_{X \in V(G)} \mid \pi_G(X) \mid^2$. Table 1 clearly shows that the summed squared fan-in decreases when N_0^c increases; indicating that spurious dependencies are removed. This removal also has a beneficial effect on the classification accuracy of the classifier, which rises from 74.75% for $N_0^c = 1$ to 76.25% for $N_0^c = 660$. We have experimentally proven the validity of the use of non-uniform priors during classifier structure learning. A setting of $N_0^c = 500$ seems reasonable, for which classification accuracy is high and the influence on structural complexity is considerable, but not totally restrictive.

4.2 Classification Performance

We have compared the performance of the MMI algorithm with that of the FAN algorithm. Figure 5 shows that in terms of performance, both algorithms perform

Table 1. Effects of varying parameter N_0^c for a model consisting of 30 arcs.

N_0^c	%	F($\mathcal{B}$)	N_0^c	%	F($\mathcal{B}$)	N_0^c	%	F($\mathcal{B}$)
1	74.75	87	102	75.95	65	800	76.25	59
4	74.75	77	290	75.95	63	900	76.25	59
36	74.85	71	610	75.95	61	2000	76.25	57
56	75.15	67	660	76.25	61			

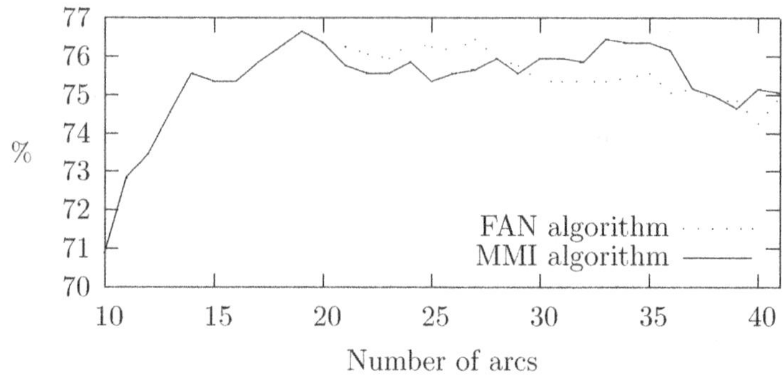

Fig. 5. Classification accuracy for Bayesian classifiers with a varying number of arcs learnt using the FAN algorithm or the MMI algorithm for the COMIK dataset.

comparably and within the bounds of the Copenhagen Pocket Diagnostic Chart. Both the MMI and FAN algorithm show a small performance decrease for very complex network structures, which may be explained in terms of overfitting artifacts. The last arcs added will be arcs having very small mutual information, which can be a database artifact instead of a real dependency within the domain, thus leading to the encoding of spurious dependencies. Best classifier accuracy for the MMI algorithm is 76.65% for a network of 19 arcs versus 76.45% for a network of 27 arcs for the FAN algorithm.

When looking at network structures, one can observe that both algorithms represent similar dependencies, with the difference that those of the MMI algorithm form a subset of those of the FAN algorithm. The best FAN classifier has a structure where there is an arc from the class variable to every evidence variable and the following arcs between evidence variables: *biliary-colics-gallstones* → *upper-abdominal-pain* → *leukaemia-lymphoma* → *gall-bladder*, *history-ge-2-weeks* → *weight-loss*, *ascites* → *liver-surface* and *ASAT* → *clotting-factors*. The MMI algorithm has left *leukaemia-lymphoma,congestive-heart-failure* and *LDH* independent of the class-variable and shows just the dependency *liver-surface* → *ascites* between evidence variables.

The independence of evidence variables demonstrates that the structural assumptions made for FAN classifiers can be overconstrained. Another problem arising with FAN classifiers, which does not arise with MMI classifiers is that the FAN algorithm shows no preference regarding the orientation of arcs between evidence variables; an arbitrary vertex is chosen, which serves as the root of a directed tree (viz. Fig. 2). This implies that even though a variable X may have very high mutual information with the class-variable and a variable Y may have very low mutual information with the class-variable, the FAN classifier may add the arc $X \to Y$, which adds little information in terms of predicting the value of the class-variable. The MMI algorithm in contrast will always select the vertex with lowest mutual information to be the parent vertex such that an arc $Y \to X$ is added. The change in direction of the dependency between *liver-*

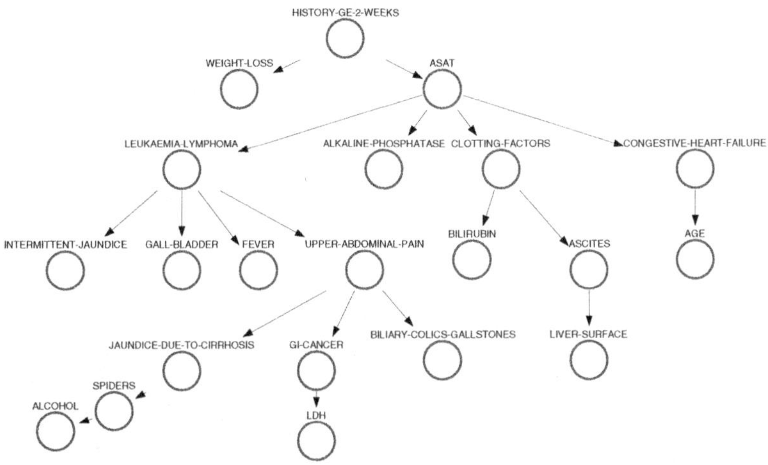

Fig. 6. Dependencies for the COMIK dataset using a FAN classifier containing 41 arcs. The class-variable was fully connected with all evidence variables and is not shown.

surface and *ascites* when comparing the FAN and MMI classifiers illustrates this phenomenon.

4.3 Medical Interpretation of Classifier Structure

Given our aim of learning classifying Bayesian networks that not only display good classification performance, but are comprehensible to medical doctors as well, we have carried out a qualitative comparison between two of the Bayesian networks learnt from the COMIK data: Figure 6 shows a FAN classifier which was learnt using the FAN algorithm described previously [8], whereas Figure 7 shows an MMI network with the same number of arcs. Clearly, the restriction imposed by the FAN algorithm that the arcs between evidence variables form a forest of trees does have implications with regard to the understandability of the resulting networks. Yet, parts of the Bayesian network shown in Figure 6 can be given a clinical interpretation. Similar remarks can be made for the MMI network, although one would hope that giving an interpretation is at least somewhat easier.

If we ignore the arcs between the class vertex and the evidence vertices, there are 20 arcs between evidence vertices in the FAN and 22 arcs between evidence vertices in the MMI network. Ignoring direction of the arcs, 9 of the arcs in the MMI network are shared by the FAN classifier. As the choice of the direction of arcs in the FAN network is arbitrary, it is worth noting that in 4 of these arcs the direction is different; in 2 of these arcs it is medically speaking impossible to establish the right direction of the arcs, as hidden variables are involved, in 1 the arc direction is correct (*congestive-heart-failure* $\rightarrow$ *ASAT*), whereas in the remaining arc (*GI-cancer* $\rightarrow$ *LDH*) the direction is incorrect.

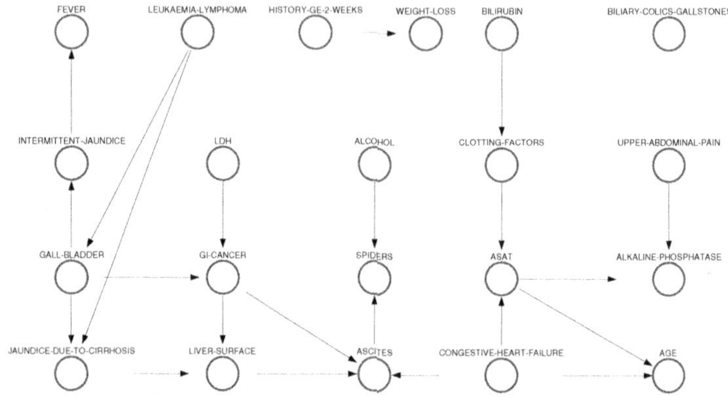

Fig. 7. Dependencies for the COMIK dataset using an MMI classifier containing 41 arcs. The class-variable was fully connected with all evidence variables and is not shown.

Some of the 13 non-shared arcs of the MMI network have a clear clinical interpretation. For example, the arcs *GI-cancer* → *ascites*, *congestive-heart-failure* → *ascites* and *GI-cancer* → *liver-surface* are examples of arcs that can be given a causal interpretation, as gastrointestinal (GI) cancer and right-heart failure do give rise to the accumulation of fluid in the abdomen (i.e. ascites), and there are often liver metastases in that case that may change the liver surface. Observe that the multiple causes of ascites cannot be represented in the FAN network due to its structural restrictions. The path *gallbladder* → *intermittent-jaundice* → *fever* in the MMI network offers a reasonably accurate picture of the course of events of the process giving rise to fever; in contrast, the situation depicted in the FAN, where *leukaemia-lymphoma* acts as a common cause, does not reflect clinical reality. However, the arc from *upper-abdominal-pain* to *biliary-colics-gallstones* in the FAN, which is correct, is missing in the MMI network. Overall, the MMI network seems to reflect clinical reality somewhat better than the FAN, although not perfectly.

Note that in this example, the MMI network is *forced* to contain 41 arcs, while it is more sound to encode just those dependencies that show sufficient (conditional) mutual information. An optimal setting of N_0^c may significantly improve the medical validity of the resulting classifiers.

5 Conclusion

This article contributes to the use of machine learning in medicine by presenting a number of new ideas which can improve both the performance and intelligibility of Bayesian classifiers. The MMI algorithm makes fewer structural assumptions than most contemporary Bayesian classification algorithms, while still remaining tractable. It iteratively builds classifier structures that reflect *existing* higher-order dependencies within the data, taking into account the mutual information between evidence variables and the class variable. The use of non-uniform Dirichlet priors during the estimation of conditional mutual information prevents the construction of overly complex network structures and the introduction of spurious dependencies. As is shown, the number of higher-order dependencies will only increase if this is warranted by sufficient evidence. To the best of our knowledge, this is the first time non-uniform Dirichlet priors are employed during the estimation of (conditional) mutual information. The correlation between the classifier structure generated by the MMI algorithm and the actual dependencies within the domain is in our opinion imperative to improve both the acceptance and quality of machine-learning techniques in medicine.

References

1. Lucas, P.J.F., van der Gaag, L., Abu-Hanna, A.: Bayesian networks in biomedicine and health-care. Artificial Intelligence in Medicine **30** (2004) 201–214
2. Pearl, J.: Probabilistic Reasoning in Intelligent Systems: Networks of Plausible Inference. Morgan Kaufmann Publishers (1988)
3. Chickering, D.M., Geiger, D., Heckerman, D.: Learning Bayesian networks is NP-hard. Technical report, Microsoft Research (1994)
4. Duda, R., Hart, P.: Pattern Classification and Scene Analysis. Wiley (1973)
5. Friedman, N., Geiger, D., Goldszmidt, M.: Bayesian network classifiers. Machine Learning **29** (1997) 131–163
6. van Dijk, S., van der Gaag, L.C., Thierens, D.: A skeleton-based approach to learning Bayesian networks from data. In Lavrac, N., et al, eds.: Proceedings of the Seventh Conference on Principles and Practice of Knowledge Discovery in Databases. Volume 2838 of Lecture Notes in Computer Science., Springer (2003) 132–143
7. Cheng, J., Greiner, R., Kelly, J., Bell, D., Liu, W.: Learning Bayesian networks from data: An information-theory based approach. Artificial Intelligence **137** (2002) 43–90
8. Lucas, P.J.F.: Restricted Bayesian network structure learning. In Gâmez, J., Moral, S., Salmeron, A., eds.: Advances in Bayesian Networks, Studies in Fuzziness and Soft Computing. Volume 146., Springer-Verlag, Berlin (2004) 217–232
9. Malchow-Møller, A., Thomson, C., Matzen, P., et al.: Computer diagnosis in jaundice: Bayes' rule founded on 1002 consecutive cases. J. Hepatol. **3** (1986) 154–163
10. Lindberg, G., Thomson, C., Malchow-Møller, A., Matzen, P., Hilden, J.: Differential diagnosis of jaundice: applicability of the Copenhagen pocket diagnostic chart proven in Stockholm patients. Liver **7** (1987) 43–49
11. Langley, P., Sage, S.: Induction of selective Bayesian classifiers. In: Proceedings of UAI-94. (1994)

Model Selection for Support Vector Classifiers via Genetic Algorithms. An Application to Medical Decision Support

Gilles Cohen[1], Mélanie Hilario[2], and Antoine Geissbuhler[1]

[1] Medical Informatics Service, University Hospital of Geneva,
1211 Geneva, Switzerland
{Gilles.Cohen,Antoine.Geissbuhler}@sim.hcuge.ch
[2] Artificial Intelligence Laboratory, University of Geneva,
1211 Geneva, Switzerland
Melanie.Hilario@cui.unige.ch

Abstract. This paper addresses the problem of tuning hyperparameters in support vector machine modeling. A Genetic Algorithm-based wrapper, which seeks to evolve hyperparameter values using an empirical error estimate as a fitness function, is proposed and experimentally evaluated on a medical dataset. Model selection is then fully automated. Unlike other hyperparameters tuning techniques, genetic algorithms do not require supplementary information making them well suited for practical purposes. This approach was motivated by an application where the number of parameters to adjust is greater than one. This method produces satisfactory results.

1 Introduction

Support vector machines (SVM) are a powerful machine learning method for classification problems. However, to obtain good generalization performance, a necessary condition is to choose an appropriate set of model hyperparameters (i.e regularization parameter C and kernel parameters) based on the data. The choice of SVM model parameters can have a profound affect on the resulting model's generalization performance. Most approaches use trial and error procedures to tune SVM hyperparameters while trying to minimize the training and test errors. Such an approach may not really obtain the best performance while consuming an enormous amount of time. Recently other approaches to parameter tuning have been proposed [1, 3, 13]. These methods use a gradient descent search to optimize a validation error, a leave-one-out (LOO) error or an upper bound on the generalization error [7]. However, gradient descent oriented methods may require restrictive assumptions regarding, e.g., continuity or differentability. Typically criteria such as LOO error are not differentiable, so approaches based on gradient descent are not generally applicable to cross-validation based criteria. Furthermore, they are very sensitive to the choice of starting points; an incorrect choice may yield only local optima.

J.M. Barreiro et al. (Eds.): ISBMDA 2004, LNCS 3337, pp. 200–211, 2004.

In the present work we propose a Genetic Algorithm (GA) approach to tuning SVM hyperparameters and illustrate its effectiveness in classification tasks. The main advantages of a GA based strategy lie in (1) the increased probability of finding the global optimum in a situation where a large number of closely competing local optima may exist; (2) suitability for problems for which it is impossible or difficult to obtain information about the derivatives. We illustrate this approach by applying it to medical decision support.

The paper is organized as follows. In Section 2 a brief introduction to SVM classification is given. In Section 3 different criteria for SVM classification model selection are described. In Section 4 the GA approach to model selection is introduced and its application to the problem of nosocomial infection detection is discussed in Section 5. Experiments conducted to assess this approach as well as results are described in Section 6. Finally, Section 7 draws a general conclusion and previews future work.

2 Support Vector Machines

Support vector machines [15, 5] (SVM) are state of the art learning machines based on the *Structural Risk Minimization principle* (SRM) from statistical learning theory. The SRM principle seeks to minimize an upper bound of the generalization error rather than minimizing the training error (Empirical Risk Minimization (ERM)). This approach results in better generalization than conventional techniques generally based on the ERM principle.

Consider a training set $S = \{(\mathbf{x}_i, y_i)\}_{i=1}^{n}$, $y_i \in \mathcal{Y} : \{-1, +1\}$, $\mathbf{x}_i \in \mathcal{X} \subset \mathbb{R}^d$ drawn independently according to a fixed, unknown probability function $P(\mathbf{x}, y)$ on $\mathcal{X} \times \mathcal{Y}$. SVM maps each data point $\mathbf{x}$ onto a high dimensional space $\mathcal{F}$ by some function ϕ, and searches for a canonical[1] separating hyperplane in this space which maximises the *margin* or distance between the hyperplane and the closest data points belonging to the different classes (hard margin). When nonlinear decision boundaries are not needed $\phi(\mathbf{x})$ is an identity function, otherwise $\phi(.)$ is performed by a non linear function $k(.,.)$, also called a *kernel*, which defines a dot product in $\mathcal{F}$. We can then replace the dot product $\langle\phi(\mathbf{x}), \phi(\mathbf{x}_i)\rangle$ in feature space with the kernel $k(\mathbf{x}, \mathbf{x}_i)$. Conditions for a function to be a kernel are expressed in a theorem by Mercer [2, 6]. Some valid kernel functions are listed in table 1.

For a separable classification task, such an optimal hyperplane $\langle\mathbf{w}.\phi(\mathbf{x})\rangle + b = 0$ exists but very often, the data points will be almost linearly separable in the sense that only a few of the data points cause it to be non linearly separable. Such data points can be accommodated into the theory with the introduction of slack variables that allow particular vectors to be misclassified. The hyperplane margin is then relaxed by penalising the training points misclassified by the system (soft margin). Formally the optimal hyperplane is defined to be the hyperplane which

[1] A hyperplane $H : \{\mathbf{x} \in \mathbb{R}^n : \langle\mathbf{w}, \mathbf{x}\rangle + b = 0,\ \mathbf{w} \in \mathbb{R}^n,\ b \in \mathbb{R}\}$ is called canonical for a given training set if and only if $\mathbf{w}$ and b satisfy $\min_{i=1,\ldots,n} |\langle\mathbf{w}, \mathbf{x}_i\rangle| = 1$, with $\mathbf{w}$ the weight vector and b the bias and where $\langle.,.\rangle$ denotes the dot product.

maximizes the margin and minimizes some functional $\theta(\xi) = \sum_{i=1}^{n} \xi_i^{\sigma}$, where σ is some small positive constant. Usually the values $\sigma = 1$ is used since it is a quadratic programming problem (QP) and the corresponding dual does not involve ξ and therefore offers a simple optimization problem. The optimal separating hyperplane with $\sigma = 1$ is given by the solution to the following minimization problem:

$$L_P(\mathbf{w}, \xi, b) = \frac{1}{2}\|\mathbf{w}\|^2 + C\sum_{i=1}^{n} \xi_i \tag{1}$$

$$\text{subject to} \quad y_i(\langle \mathbf{w}, \phi(\mathbf{x}_i)\rangle + b) \geq 1 - \xi_i, \ \forall i$$
$$\xi_i \geq 0, \ \forall i$$

where $b/|\mathbf{w}\|$ is the distance between origin and hyperplane, ξ_i is a positive slack variable that measures the degree of violation of the constraint. The penalty C is a regularisation parameter that controls the trade-off between maximizing the margin and minimizing the training error. This is a QP, solved by the Karush-Kuhn-Tucker theorem. Let $\boldsymbol{\alpha} = (\alpha_1, \alpha_2, \ldots, \alpha_n)^T$ be the n non negative Lagrange multipliers associated with the constraints, the solution to the problem is equivalent to determining the solution of the *Wolfe dual* [8] problem.

$$L_D(\alpha) = \mathbf{e}^T\boldsymbol{\alpha} - \frac{1}{2}\boldsymbol{\alpha}^T Q\boldsymbol{\alpha}. \tag{2}$$

$$\text{subject to} \quad \boldsymbol{\alpha}\mathbf{y}^T = 0 \text{ and } 0 \leq \alpha_i \leq C \quad i = 1, \ldots, n$$

where $\mathbf{e}$ is a vector of all ones and Q is a $n \times n$ matrix with $Q_{ij} = y_i y_j k(\mathbf{x}_i, \mathbf{x}_j)$. The only difference from the hard margin ($C \rightarrow \infty$) is that the Lagrange multipliers are upper bounded by C. The KKT conditions imply that non-zero slack variables can only occur for $\alpha_i = C$. For the corresponding points the distance from the hyperplane is less than $1/\|\mathbf{w}\|$ as can be seen from the first constraint in (1).

One can show that a $\mathbf{w}$ which minimize (1) can be written as $\mathbf{w} = \sum_{i=1}^{n} y_i \alpha_i \mathbf{x}_i$. This is called the dual representation of $\mathbf{w}$. An $\mathbf{x}_i$ with nonzero α_i is called a support vector. The optimal decision function becomes

$$f(\mathbf{x}) = sign\left(\sum_{i}^{n} \alpha_i k(\mathbf{x}, \mathbf{x}_i) + b\right) \tag{3}$$

2.1 Asymmetrical Soft Margin

The above formulation of the SVM is inappropriate in two common situations : in case of unbalanced distributions, or whenever misclassifications must be penalized more heavily for one class than for the other. In order to adapt the SVM algorithm to these cases [12, 16] the basic idea is to introduce different error weights C^+ and C^- for the positive and the negative class, which results

Table 1. Some valid Kernel functions.

Kernel type	Kernel structure
Linear	$k(\mathbf{x}, \mathbf{z}) = \langle \mathbf{x}, \mathbf{z} \rangle$
Polynomial	$k(\mathbf{x}, \mathbf{z}) = (\langle \mathbf{x}, \mathbf{z} \rangle + 1)^p$
Radial basis function (RBF)	$k(\mathbf{x}, \mathbf{z}) = e^{-\gamma \|\mathbf{x}-\mathbf{z}\|^2}$

in a bias for larger multipliers α_i of the critical class. This induces a decision boundary which is more distant from the smaller class than from the other. This transforms (1) into the following optimization problem:

$$\begin{aligned} minimize \ & \frac{1}{2}\|\mathbf{w}\|^2 + C^- \sum_{i:y_i=-1}^{n} \xi_i + C^+ \sum_{i:y_i=+1}^{n} \xi_i \\ s.t \ & \langle \mathbf{w}, \mathbf{x}_i \rangle + b \geq 1 - \xi_i, \ \forall i : y_i = +1 \\ & \langle \mathbf{w}, \mathbf{x}_i \rangle + b \leq -1 + \xi_i \ \forall i : y_i = -1 \end{aligned} \tag{4}$$

3 SVM Model Selection Criteria

The model selection problem consists in choosing, from a set of candidate models, that which minimizes the real loss over all possible examples drawn from the unknown distribution $\mathcal{P}(\mathbf{x}, y)$. This is the so called *expected risk* defined as

$$R(f_\theta) = \int_{\mathcal{X}\times\mathcal{Y}} \ell(f(\mathbf{x}, y))dP(\mathbf{x}, y) \tag{5}$$

where $\ell : \mathcal{Y}^2 \rightarrow \mathbb{R}$ is an appropriate loss function for classification, e.g. the zero one loss $\ell(f(\mathbf{x}, y)) = \mathbb{I}_{(-yf(\mathbf{x})>0)}$ with $\mathbb{I}_P$ representing the indicator function; equal to 1 if proposition P is true, and 0 otherwise.
As the data distributions $\mathcal{P}$ in real problems are not known in advance, (5) is not computable and one needs some reliable estimates of generalization performance.

There has been some work on efficient methods for estimating generalization performance such as LOO, the $\xi\alpha$ bound [11], the radius margin bound and span bound [3] in SVM classification. A review and a comparative analysis of all these techniques, covering both empirical and theoritical methods, can be found in [7]. Two of the proposed estimators are detailed below.

3.1 *k*-Fold Cross-Validation and Leave-One-Out

Croos-validation (CV) is a popular technique for estimating generalization error. In k- fold cross-validation the original training set S is randomly partitioned into k non-overlapping subsets S_j of approximately equal size. The learning machine is trained on the union of $(k-1)$ subsets; the remaining k-th subset is used as a test set in view of measuring the associated classification performance. This procedure is cycled over all possible k test sets, and the average test error gives an estimate of the expected generalization error. The CV error on a training set $S = \{(\mathbf{x}, y)\}_{i=1}^{n}$ is defined as

$$R_{CV}(S) = \frac{1}{k}\sum_{j=1}^{k}\left(\sum_{i=1}^{|S_j|}\ell(f_{S^{\setminus S_j}}(\mathbf{x}_i), y_i)\right) \tag{6}$$

where $S^{\setminus S_j}$ denotes the dataset obtained by removing the subset S_j from the set S, $f_{S^{\setminus S_j}}$ the corresponding classifier and $|S_j|$ the cardinality of subset S_j.

The LOO can be viewed as an extreme form of k-fold cross-validation in which k is equal to the number of examples. The LOO error on a training set $S = \{(\mathbf{x}, y)\}_{i=1}^{n}$ is defined as

$$R_{loo}(S) = \frac{1}{n}\sum_{i=1}^{n}\ell(f_{S^{\setminus i}}(\mathbf{x}_i), y_i) \tag{7}$$

where f_S denotes the classifier learned from the dataset S, $S^{\setminus i} = S\backslash\{(\mathbf{x}_i, y_i)\}$ the dataset obtained by removing the ith example, and $f_{S^{\setminus i}}$ the corresponding classifier. This measure counts the fraction of examples that are misclassified if we leave them out of learning.

Averaged over datasets this is an almost unbiased estimate of the average test error for our algorithm that is obtained from training sets of $n-1$ examples [14].

$$\mathbb{E}_{S_{n-1}}[R(f_{S_{n-1}})] = \mathbb{E}_{S_n}[R_{loo}(S_n)] \tag{8}$$

where $R(f_{S_{n-1}})$ is the expected risk of a classifier derived from the dataset S_{n-1} and $\mathbb{E}_{S_{n-1}}[R(f_{S_{n-1}})]$ is the actual risk over all choices of training set of size $n-1$. This says nothing about the variance of the estimate; nevertheless, one may hope that R_{loo} is a reasonable estimate for the test error that one wishes to optimize. For large datasets, the computational load for R_{loo} is prohibitive and one is driven to look for cheaper bounds or approximations.

3.2 $\xi\alpha$ Bound

The following estimator has been described by Joachims in [11], where it is also generalized for predicting recall and precision in the context of text classification. This method holds for non-zero bias b, and in the non-separable case (soft margin). This estimator can be computate using α from the the solution of the SVM dual formulation (2) and ξ from the solution of SVM primal formulation (1).

$$\mathbb{E}_{S_n}[R_{loo}(S_n)] \leq \frac{1}{n}\mathbb{E}\left[\sum_{i=1}^{n}\mathbb{I}_{(\rho\alpha_i^* R^2 + \xi_i \geq 1)}\right] = R_{\xi\alpha}(S_n) \tag{9}$$

where $\mathbb{I}_P$ is the indicator variable; equal to 1 if proposition P is true, and 0 otherwise.

3.3 Alternative Performance Measures

In classification tasks, the most commonly used performance metric by far is predictive accuracy. This metric is however close to meaningless in applications with significant class imbalance. To see this, consider a dataset consisting of 5% positive and 95% negatives. The simple rule of assigning a case to the majority class would result in an impressive 95% accuracy whereas the classifier would have failed to recognize a single positive case—an inacceptable situation in medical diagnosis. The reason for this is that the contribution of a class to the overall accuracy rate is a function of its cardinality, with the effect that rare positives have an almost insignificant impact on the performance measure.

To discuss alternative performance criteria we adopt the standard definitions used in binary classification. TP and TN stand for the number of true positives and true negatives respectively, i.e., positive/negative cases recognized as such by the classifier. FP and FN represent respectively the number of misclassified positive and negative cases. In two-class problems, the accuracy rate on the positives, called sensitivity, is defined as $TP/(TP+FN)$, whereas the accuracy rate on the negative class, also known as specificity, is TN/(TN+FP). Classification accuracy is simply $(TP+TN)/N$, where $N = TP+TN+FP+FP$ is the total number of cases.

To overcome the shortcomings of accuracy and put all classes on an equal footing, some have suggested the use of the geometric mean of class accuracies, defined as $gm = \sqrt{\frac{TP}{TP+FN} * \frac{TN}{TN+FP}} = \sqrt{sensitivity * specificity}$. The drawback of the geometric mean is that there is no way of giving higher priority to the rare positive class. In information retrieval, a metric that allows for this is the F-measure $F_\beta = \frac{PR}{\beta P+(1-\beta)R}$, where R (recall) is no other than sensitivity and P (precision) is defined as $P = TP/(TP+FP)$, i.e., the proportion of true positives among all predicted positives. The β parameter, $0 < \beta < 1$, allows the user to assign relative weights to precision and recall, with 0.5 giving them equal importance. However, the F-measure takes no account of performance on the negative class, due to the near impossibility of identifying negatives in information retrieval. In medical diagnosis tasks, however, what is needed is a relative weighting of recall and specificity. To combine the advantages and overcome the drawbacks of the geometric mean accuracy and the F-measure, we propose the mean class-weighted accuracy (CWA), defined formally for the K-class setting as $cwa = \frac{1}{\sum_{i=1}^{k} w_i} \sum_{i=1}^{k} w_i accu_i$, where $w_i \in \aleph$ is the weight assigned to class i and $accu_i$ is the accuracy rate computed over class i. If we normalize the weights such that $0 \leq w_i \leq 1$ and $\sum w\xi\alpha_i = 1$, we get $cwa = \sum_{i=1}^{k} w_i accu_i$ which simplifies to $cwa = w_i * sensitivity + (1 - w_i) * specificity$ in binary classification.

Since cwa is the only acceptable performance measure in driving model selection in case of data imbalance, we propose to generalize the estimators described above to it. This is straightforward for cross-validation, where we simply replace accuracy with cwa. For the $\xi\alpha$ bound one can easily deduce the following generalization

$$R_{cwa-\xi\alpha} = w_i * \left(1 - \frac{FN}{N^+}\right) + (1 - w_i) * \left(1 - \frac{FP}{N^-}\right) \tag{10}$$

where N^+ and N^- represent the number of positive and negative examples respectively, and $FN : R_{\xi\alpha}(S_{N^-})$ and $FP : R_{\xi\alpha}(S_{N^+})$ the number of false negative and false positive leave-one-out errors respectively.

Notice that, since the estimate of an SVM through k-fold cross-validation LOO error or $\xi\alpha$ bound requires the use of the non-differentiable indicator function $\mathbb{I}_P$, a gradient descent approach to minimizing those estimates is not applicable.

4 SVM Model Selection Using Genetic Algorithms

To obtain good performance, some parameters in SVMs have to be selected carefully. These parameters include:

- the regularization parameters C_i, which determine the tradeoff between minimizing model complexity and the training error,
- the parameter vector $\boldsymbol{\theta} = (\theta_1, \ldots, \theta_n)$ of the kernel function, which implicitly defines the non linear mapping to some high-dimensional feature space.

These "higher level" parameters are usually refered as metaparameters or hyperparameters. We propose a GA as a search method for exploring the hyperparameters space steered by selection criteria described in the previous section.

4.1 Genetic Algorithms

Genetic algorithms (GAs) are stochastic global search techniques and optimization methods deeply rooted in the mechanism of evolution and natural genetics. By mimicking biological selection and reproduction, GAs can efficiently search through the solution space of complex problems. In GAs a population of possible solutions called chromosomes is maintained. Each chromosome, which is composed of genes, represents an encoding of a candidate solution of the problem and is associated with a fitness value, representing its ability to solve the optimization problem and evaluated by a fitness function. The goal of GAs is to combine genes to obtain new chromosomes with better fitness, i.e., which are better solutions of the optimization problem. Basically, there are three operators that lead to good results in a genetic algorithm, namely reproduction, crossover, and mutation.

Selection. This is a process in which chromosomes are copied onto the next generation. Chromosomes with a higher fitness value have more chances of making it to the next generation. Different schemes can be used to determine which chromosomes survive into the next generation. A frequently used method is roulette wheel selection, where a roulette wheel is divided in a number of slots, one for each chromosome. The slots are sized according to the fitness of the chromosomes. Hence, when we spin the wheel, the best chromosomes are the most likely to be selected. Another well known method is ranking. Here, the chromosomes are sorted by their fitness value, and each chromosome is assigned an offspring count that is determined solely by its rank.

Crossover. This operation takes two chromosomes, the parents, and produces two new ones, the offspring. Genes are exchanged between the parent chromosomes. The hope is that combining the best of both chromosomes will yield an even better chromosomes after the operation. Many kinds of crossover can be thought of.

Mutation. This is the process of randomly altering the chromosomes. A randomly selected gene in a chromosome takes a new value. The aim of this operator is to introduce new genetic material in the population, or at least prevent its loss. Under mutation, a gene can acquire a value that did not occur in the population before, or that has been lost due to reproduction.

For a more thorough description of genetic algorithms the reader can refer to Goldberg (1989) [9].

4.2 Encodings and Fitness Functions

Generally to achieve a chromosomal representation of a real-valued solution the real-valued variables (i.e. hyperparameters) are encoded in a binary string composed of 0's and 1's with fixed length ℓ. The evolution process takes place at this chromosome level. The string length depends on the field variables and the desired precision. Before the evaluation process, the bit string $\langle b_\ell, b_{\ell-1}, \ldots, b_0 \rangle$ is decoded back to real number by the following formula:

$$\theta_i = \theta_i^{min} + \frac{\theta_i^{max} - \theta_i^{min}}{2^{\ell_i} - 1} \sum_{j=1}^{\ell_i} b_j 2^j$$

where ℓ_i is the string length used to code the i-th variable and θ_i^{min} and θ_i^{max} respectively the lower and upper bound for the i-th variable.
For example, the 8-bit string illustrated below can be explained to exhibit a biological representation of an SVM hyperparameter set having a regularization parameter $C = 10$ and a width kernel parameter $\gamma = 1$.

$$(C, \gamma) = (10, 1)$$
$$(Chromosome) = 1010 \mid 0001$$

Usually only discrete values for hyperparameters need to be considered, e.g. $10^{-3}, \ldots, 10^4$. Instead of directly encoding the hyperparameter we will encode the exponent $\theta_i^{'}$ giving the new decoding formula: $\theta_i = 10^{\theta_i^{'}}$. Only three bits are then necessary to obtain the desired range of hyperparameters values: $[-3, 4]$.
For example, the 6-bit string illustrated below can be explained to exhibit a biological representation of an SVM hyperparameter set having a regularization parameter $C = 0.001$ and a width kernel parameter $\gamma = 100$.

$$(C, \gamma) = (0.001, 100)$$
$$(Chromosome) = 101 \mid 000$$

The fitness function of each individual is evaluated either by using the $\xi\alpha$ bound or by performing cross-validation based on *cwa*.

5 Application to Nosocomial Infection Detection

We tested the performance of SVMs on a medical problem, the detection of nosomial infections. A nosocomial infection (from the Greek word *nosokomeion* for hospital) is an infection that develops during hospitalization whereas it was not present nor incubating at the time of the admission. Usually, a disease is considered a nosocomial infection if it develops 48 hours after admission.

The University Hospital of Geneva (HUG) has been performing yearly prevalence studies to detect and monitor nosocomial infections since 1994 [10]. Their methodology is as follows: the investigators visit every ward of the HUG over a period of approximately three weeks. All patients hospitalized for 48 hours or more at the time of the study are included. Medical records, kardex, X-ray and microbiology reports are reviewed, and additional information is eventually obtained by interviewing nurses or physicians in charge. Collected variables include demographic characteristics, admission date, admission diagnosis, comorbidities, McCabe score, type of admission, provenance, hospitalization ward, functional status, previous surgery, previous intensive care unit (ICU) stay, exposure to antibiotics, antacid and immunosuppressive drugs and invasive devices, laboratory values, temperature, date and site of infection, fulfilled criteria for infection.

The resulting dataset consisted of 688 patient records and 83 variables. With the help of hospital experts on nosocomial infections, we filtered out spurious records as well as irrelevant and redundant variables, reducing the data to 683 cases and 49 variables. The major difficulty inherent in the data (as in many medical diagnostic applications) is the highly skewed class distribution. Out of 683 patients, only 75 (11% of the total) were infected and 608 were not. This application was thus an excellent testbed for assessing the efficacy of the use of genetic algorithms to tune SVM hyperparameters in the presence of class imbalance.

6 Experimentation

6.1 Experimental Setup

The experimental goal was to assess a GA-based optimization method for tuning SVM hyperparameters. To allievate the class imbalance problem, we propose to assign different misclassification costs to the different class dataset. To train our SVM classifiers we use a radial basis kernel (see table 1). Thus the corresponding hyperparameters set to tune is $\boldsymbol{\theta} : (\sigma, C^+, C^-)$. The genetic algorithm parameters used for these experiments are shown in Table 2. The fitness function was evaluated for the CV criterion generalization error by using 5-fold cross-validation based on *cwa* (10-fold cross-validation would have resulted in an extremely small number of infected test cases per fold). The complete dataset was randomly partitioned into five subsets. On each iteration, one subset (comprising 20% of the data samples) was held out as a test set and the remaining four (80% of the data) were concatenated into a training set. The training sets consisted only of non infected patients whereas the test sets contained both infected and non infected

Table 2. Genetic Parameters.

Crossover rate	0.9
Mutation rate	0.002
Chromosomes length	7
Population size	50
Stopping criterion	200 generations

patients according to the original class distribution. Error rates estimated on the test sets were then averaged over the five iterations. The best individual of the last generation gives the performance measures for an optimum set of hyperparameters setting. For the $\xi\alpha$ bound criterion based on *cwa* the fitness function was evaluated by computing the bound without any extra work after the SVM was trained on the whole training data. The optimum set of hyperparameters setting was picked from the best individual of the last generation and then a 5-fold cross-validation was performed.

The regularization parameter C^- and the kernel parameter γ were encoded with three bits giving the following discrete values: $10^4, \ldots, 10^{-3}$. For C^+ since we want $C^+ > C^-$ to obtain an asymmetrical margin in favor of the majority class the third variable represents a weight w and $C^+ = w * C^-$. w was coded with 4 bits with the following field $[1, 50]$.

6.2 Results

Table 3 summarizes performance results for SVMs with symmetrical margins, accuracy rates hover constantly around 82% whereas even the best sensitivity remains barely higher than 30%. This clearly illustrates the inadequacy of the symmetrical soft margin approach as well as the inappropriatness of accuracy as a performance criterion for the nosocomial infection. Table 4 summarizes performance results for SVMs with asymmetrical margins. k-fold cross-validation yielded the best performance. It appears that the $\xi\alpha$ bound is not always tight, in particular for sensitivity. Note that since the margin is pushed towards the majority class only a small number of examples from the minority class will be close to the decision boundary. Only a small number of examples from the minority class are then likely to correspond to LOO errors for any sensible classifier. The resulting highly quantised nature of the LOO error may in part explain the low value of the $\xi\alpha$ for sensitivity with asymmetrical margin.

Table 3. Performance of SVMs for optimum parameters settings using an RBF Gaussian kernel (γ, C) found via GA based method. Bracketed values correspond to $\xi\alpha$ values.

Fitness Function	C	γ	Acc. %	Sens. %	Spec. %	CWA %
CWA-$\xi\alpha$ Bound	10000	0.001	89 [81.7]	48 [29.3]	94 [88.15]	61.92[46.95]
5-cv with CWA	10000	0.01	90.4	46.7	95.9	61.46

Table 4. Performance of SVMs for optimum parameters settings using an RBF Gaussian kernel (γ, C^+, C^-) found via GA based method. Bracketed values correspond to $\xi\alpha$ values.

Fitness Function	C^+	C^-	γ	Acc. %	Sens. %	Spec. %	CWA %
CWA-$\xi\alpha$ Bound	0.4	0.1	0.01	83 [75.9]	73.3 [16]	84.2 [83.4]	76.57[36.1]
5-cv with CWA	14	1	0.001	80	92	78.3	87.9

7 Conclusion and Future Work

We have presented an algorithm based on GAs that can reliably find very good hyperparameter settings for SVMs with RBF kernels in a fully automated way. GAs have proven to be quite successful on a wide number of difficult optimization problems [9]. Model selection based on a genetic algorithm search offers a compromise. Speed of convergence of gradient descent search methods is sacrificed, but the chance of being trapped in a local minimum is greatly reduced. Additionaly, this algorithm might be used to obtain a good starting point for others approaches, which can be sensitive to the initial condition of its search. On the nosocomial dataset, the method also improves on performance obtained in a previous study [4] on the detection of nosocomial infections. In spite of these encouraging results our approach steel needs to be extensively explored on a wide range of machine learning problems. We have also shown that using a LOO error bound instead CV is a viable alternative. An important characteristic of GAs is that they produce a potential solution population. In contrast, all the other methods seek only a single point of the search space. Consequently GA-based techniques can be used for multi-objective optimization. In the near future, we intend to investigate multi-objective GAs for model selection with sensitivity and specificity as two conflicting objectives. Overall we feel that GAs offer a promising approach to the model selection problem.

Acknowledgements

The authors are grateful for the data provided by the infection control team at the University of Geneva Hospitals.

References

1. N. Ayat, M. Cheriet, and C. Suen. Empirical error based optimization of SVM kernels, 2002.
2. C.J.C. Burges. A tutorial on support vector machines for pattern recognition. *Data Mining and Knowledge Discovery*, pages 121–167, 1998.
3. O. Chapelle, V. Vapnik, O. Bousquet, and S. Mukherjee. Choosing multiple parameters for support vector machines. *Machine Learning*, 46(1):131–159, 2002.
4. G. Cohen, M. Hilario, H. Sax, and S. Hugonnet. Asymmetrical margin approach to surveillance of nosocomial infections using support vector classification. In *Intelligent Data Analysis in Medicine and Pharmacology*, 2003.

5. C. Cortes and V. Vapnik. Support vector networks. *Machine Learning*, 20(3):273–297, September 1995.
6. N. Cristianini and Taylor J.S. *An Introduction to Support Vector Machines*. Cambridge University Press, 2000.
7. K. Duan, S.S. Keerthi, and A.N. Poo. Evaluation of simple performance measures for tuning svm hyperparameters. In *Technical Report CD-01-11, Department of Mechanical Engineering, National University of Singapore, Singapore*, 2001.
8. R. Fletcher. *Practical Methods of Optimization*. John Wiley and Sons, 1987.
9. D.E. Goldberg. *Genetic Algorithms in Search, Optimization, and Machine Learning*. Addison-Wesley, Reading, 1989.
10. S. Harbarth, Ch. Ruef, P. Francioli, A. Widmer, D. Pittet, and Swiss-Noso Network. Nosocomial infections in Swiss university hospitals: a multi-centre survey and review of the published experience. *Schweiz Med Wochenschr*, 129:1521–28, 1999.
11. Thorsten Joachims. Estimating the generalization performance of a SVM efficiently. In Pat Langley, editor, *Proceedings of ICML-00, 17th International Conference on Machine Learning*, pages 431–438, Stanford, US, 2000. Morgan Kaufmann Publishers, San Francisco, US.
12. G. Karakoulas and J. Shawe-Taylor. Optimizing classifiers for imbalanced training sets. In *Advances in Neural Information Processing Systems (NIPS-99)*. MIT Press, 1999.
13. S.S. Keerthi. Efficient tuning of svm hyperparameters using radius/margin bound and iterative algorithms. In *IEE Transactions on Neural Networks*, pages 1225–1229, 2003.
14. A. Luntz and V. Brailowsky. On estimation characters obtained in statistical procedure of recognition. *Technicheskaya Kibernetica*, 3, 1969. In russian.
15. V. Vapnik. *Statistical Learning Theory*. Wiley, 1998.
16. K. Veropoulos, N. Cristianini, and C. Campbell. Controlling the sensitivity of support vector machines. In *Proc. International Joint Conference on Artificial Intelligence*, 1999.

Selective Classifiers Can Be Too Restrictive: A Case-Study in Oesophageal Cancer

Rosa Blanco[1], Linda C. van der Gaag[2], Iñaki Inza[1], and Pedro Larrañaga[1]

[1] Department of Computer Science and Artificial Intelligence
University of Basque Country, P.O. Box 649 E-20080 San Sebastián, Spain
{rosa,inza,ccplamup}@si.ehu.es

[2] Institute of Information and Computing Sciences, Utrecht University
P.O. Box 80089, 3508 TB Utrecht, The Netherlands
linda@cs.uu.nl

Abstract. Real-life datasets in biomedicine often include missing values. When learning a Bayesian network classifier from such a dataset, the missing values are typically filled in by means of an imputation method to arrive at a complete dataset. The thus completed dataset then is used for the classifier's construction. When learning a selective classifier, also the selection of appropriate features is based upon the completed data. The resulting classifier, however, is likely to be used in the original real-life setting where it is again confronted with missing values. By means of a real-life dataset in the field of oesophageal cancer that includes a relatively large number of missing values, we argue that especially the wrapper approach to feature selection may result in classifiers that are too selective for such a setting and that, in fact, some redundancy is required to arrive at a reasonable classification accuracy in practice.

1 Introduction

Real-life datasets record instances of every-day problem solving. Especially in the biomedical domain, such datasets tend to include a considerable number of missing values [1]. The presence of missing values has its origin in, for example, the data-gathering protocols used: in the medical domain, a diagnostic test is not performed on a patient if its result is not expected to contribute to the patient's diagnosis. Missing values may also occur as a result of omissions in the data-entry process and as a result of indeterminate or unclear findings. Upon learning Bayesian network classifiers from datasets with missing values, usually an imputation method is used to complete the data. With such a method, the missing values are replaced by plausible values for the appropriate variables [2]. The thus completed dataset then is used for the construction of the classifier.

Real-life datasets also tend to include more variables than are strictly necessary for the classification task at hand. More specifically, a dataset may include variables that are irrelevant to the classification, such as a patient's name, as well as variables that are redundant in the presence of other variables. The presence of such irrelevant and redundant variables tends to decrease the performance

J.M. Barreiro et al. (Eds.): ISBMDA 2004, LNCS 3337, pp. 212–223, 2004.

of a classifier learned from the dataset. Often, therefore, only a subset of the available variables is included in the classifier. The problem of finding the subset of variables that yields the highest classification accuracy is known as the *feature subset selection* problem [3]. The two most commonly used approaches to feature subset selection are the *filter approach*, which decides upon inclusion of specific variables based upon intrinsic characteristics of the data, and the *wrapper approach*, which takes the characteristics of the classifier into account.

Bayesian network classifiers are typically learned from datasets that have been completed, as described above. Also the selection of appropriate variables to be included is performed on the completed dataset. Once constructed, however, the selective classifier is likely to be used in the original real-life setting where it is again confronted with problem instances with missing values. In this paper, we study the effect that feature selection with the completed dataset may have on the performance of Bayesian network classifiers on instances with missing values. We conduct our study in the medical domain of oesophageal cancer. From the Antoni van Leeuwenhoekhuis in the Netherlands, we have available a set of data from real patients suffering from cancer of the oesophagus; these data are relatively sparse, including a large number of missing values. From a fully specified Bayesian network developed for the same domain, we generated a separate, complete dataset. From this latter dataset we constructed various selective classifiers, including Naive Bayes classifiers, tree-augmented network classifiers, and k-dependence Bayes network classifiers. For each of these classifiers, we established its accuracy with the available real data.

Our experimental results suggest that especially the Bayesian network classifiers learned with the wrapper approach to feature selection can be too restrictive. Compared with the classifiers constructed with the filter approach, the wrapper-based classifiers tend to include relatively small numbers of variables. More specifically, these classifiers tend not to allow for any redundancy among their variables. Despite their inclusion of some redundancy, the filter-based classifiers were found to perform significantly better on the real patient data than the classifiers constructed with the wrapper approach to feature selection. Because of the relatively large number of missing values, the wrapper-based classifiers often had too few data at their disposal to establish the correct diagnosis for a patient's cancer. From our experimental results we conclude that, when a classifier is to be used in a real-life setting with missing values, some redundancy among its variables is required to arrive at a reasonable performance.

The paper is organised as follows. In Section 2, we present some preliminaries on Bayesian network classifiers and introduce the filter and wrapper approaches to feature selection. The domain of oesophageal cancer is described in Section 3. The set-up of our study and its results are discussed in Section 4. The paper ends with our conclusions and directions for further research in Section 5.

2 Bayesian Classification Inducers

Supervised learning for a classification task amounts to constructing, from a dataset of labelled instances, a classification model that provides for assigning class labels to new instances. We distinguish a set of *feature variables* $\boldsymbol{x} = (x_1, \ldots, x_n)$, $n \geq 1$, and a designated *class variable* C with the labels $1, \ldots, r_0$, $r_0 \geq 2$. A classification model now in essence is a function $\gamma(\boldsymbol{x})$ that assigns, for each instance $\boldsymbol{x}$ over $x_1, \ldots, x_n$, a unique label to the class variable, c.

A *Bayesian network classifier* builds upon a joint probability distribution $p(x_1, \ldots, x_n, c)$ over the variables involved in the classification task. In essence, it aims at minimising the total misclassification cost through

$$\gamma(\boldsymbol{x}) = \arg\min_k \left(\sum_{c=1}^{r_0} cost(k, c) p(c \mid x_1, \ldots, x_n) \right),$$

where $cost(k, r)$ denotes the cost of assigning the class r to an instance that has k for its true class [4]. For the 0/1 loss function, where the cost associated with an erroneous classification universally equals 1, the Bayesian network classifier assigns the *a posteriori most probable class* to an instance, that is,

$$\gamma(\boldsymbol{x}) = \arg\max_c \, p(c \mid x_1, \ldots, x_n).$$

where the conditional probability distribution $p(c \mid x_1, \ldots, x_n)$ is obtained using Bayes' formula:

$$p(c \mid x_1, \ldots, x_n) = \frac{p(c, x_1, \ldots, x_n)}{p(x_1, \ldots, x_n)} = \frac{p(c) p(x_1, \ldots, x_n \mid c)}{p(x_1, \ldots, x_n)}.$$

Note that under the simplifying assumption of all instances being equiprobable, we have that $p(c \mid x_1, \ldots, x_n) \propto p(c) p(x_1, \ldots, x_n \mid c)$.

Bayesian network classifiers have gained considerable popularity over the last decades, owing to their simplicity and ease of interpretation. As for Bayesian networks in general [5, 6], Bayesian network classifiers include a graphical structure that reflects the probabilistic relationships among the variables of the domain under study; this graphical structure allows domain experts to understand the underlying classification process without a deep knowledge of the theoretical issues involved. The various parameter probabilities estimated for the classifier from the data, moreover, often yield insight in the uncertainty of the studied problem. Various types of Bayesian network classifier have been developed, which constitute a hierarchy of classifiers of increasing complexity.

Learning a Bayesian network classifier involves searching the space of alternative graphical structures. This space in essence includes all possible structures over the variables involved. As we have argued in our introduction, however, not all feature variables are equally useful for the classification task at hand. To provide for focusing on the more useful variables, the search space also includes the possible structures over the various subsets of variables. Several different algorithms have been proposed to traverse the resulting space. With respect to feature selection, these algorithms basically take one of two approaches. Within the *filter approach*, the selection of relevant variables is based upon the characteristics of the data. For each feature variable, its ability to discriminate between the different classes is established. For this purpose, typically an information-theoretic measure such as conditional entropy or mutual information, is used. The selection of feature variables is performed in a pre-processing step to restrict the search space before the actual learning takes place with the selected subset of variables. Within the *wrapper approach*, on the other hand, feature subset selection is merged with the learning process: the selection of variables then takes the properties of the classifier to be learned into account. While with the filter approach the task of constructing the classifier is performed only once, it is performed iteratively with the wrapper approach where in each step a proposed selection of features is evaluated. The search of the space of alternative graphical structures aims at finding a structure that, when supplemented with estimates for its parameter probabilities, maximises the accuracy of the resulting classifier. With the filter approach the classification accuracy is maximised indirectly through the measure used and with the wrapper approach the accuracy is maximised directly through its use to guide the search.

In this paper, we consider different types of Bayesian network classifier. We construct the various classifiers from data using both the filter approach and the wrapper approach to feature selection. With the filter approach, we use the *mutual information* of a feature variable X_i and the class variable C, defined as

$$I(X_i, C) = \sum_{x_i, c} p(x_i, c) \log \frac{p(x_i, c)}{p(x_i)p(c)},$$

for the selection of variables to be included. Due to its tendency to favour densely connected structures, we use a cut-off value for the mutual information. To this end, we build upon the property that $2NI(X_i, C)$, where N is the number of instances, asymptotically follows a $\chi^2_{(r_i-1)(r_0-1)}$ distribution, where r_i is the number of values of X_i and r_0 is the number of class labels [7]. A feature variable X_i then is included in the classifier only if its value $2NI(X_i, C)$ serves to surpass a preset significance level α.

With the wrapper approach, we use a greedy hill-climbing algorithm for searching the space of alternative graphical structures. The algorithm uses the classification accuracy for its evaluation function.

We study three types of Bayesian network classifier; these are the (selective) Naive Bayes classifiers [8], the (selective) tree augmented Naive Bayes (TAN) classifiers [9], and the (selective) k-dependence Bayes classifiers [10].

Naive Bayes. The *Naive Bayes* classifier [8] assumes conditional independence of its feature variables given the class variable. The graphical structure of the Naive Bayes classifier over a given set of variables is fixed and does not include any arcs between the feature variables. Although the independence assumption is often violated in practice, good results are expected with Naive Bayes classifiers in many applications [11].

Selective Naive Bayes. A *selective Naive Bayes* classifier [12] has the same structure as a Naive Bayes classifier, yet includes just a subset of the feature variables. To learn a selective Naive Bayes classifier from data, we employ the filter approach as outlined above. For the wrapper approach, we start with an empty set of feature variables; in each step, a variable is added that serves to increase the accuracy the most, until no further improvement can be attained.

Tree Augmented Naive Bayes. While selective Naive Bayes inducers are able to detect and effectively remove irrelevant and redundant feature variables from their classifiers, they cannot discover or model dependences among these variables. There are some well-known datasets in fact for which Naive Bayes inducers yield classifiers with a very poor performance [13], perhaps because of this inability to identify and capture any relationships between the feature variables involved. A *tree augmented Naive Bayes* (TAN) classifier [9] now has for its graphical structure, a tree over the feature variables that is extended with the structure of a Naive Bayes classifier. For inducing a TAN classifier, the Chow-Liu algorithm [14] provides for constructing a maximum-likelihood tree over the feature variables. While the original TAN inducer enforces a connected tree over all feature variables, we allow for a forest of disjoint trees. To learn a selective TAN classifier, we build in essence upon the filter approach outlined before. A problem with applying the filter approach as suggested is that no statistic with a known distribution exists for establishing the significance of $2NI(X_i, X_j \mid C)$, where X_i and X_j are connected by an arc in the graphical structure. To circumvent this problem, we require $2N_cI(X_i, X_j \mid C = c)$, where N_c is the number of instances in which $C = c$, to surpass the $\chi^2_{(r_i-1)(r_j-1)}$ test, for at least one value c of the class variable. For the wrapper approach, we again start with the empty set of variables. After adding two variables in a greedy way, in each step either a new feature variable is added to the graphical structure or an arc is created between two feature variables that were added before.

***k*-Dependence Bayesian Classifier.** In the graphical structure of a TAN classifier, the number of parents allowed for a feature variable is limited: in addition to the class variable, a feature variable can have at most one other feature variable for its parent. This restriction on the number of parents strongly constrains the dependences that can be modelled between the various feature variables. A *k-dependence Bayes* (kDB) classifier [10] now relaxes the restriction by allowing a feature variable to have k parents in addition to the class variable. In practical applications, kDB inducers [10] require the number k to be fixed beforehand. For learning a selective kDB classifier, we use the filter approach as suggested above for TAN classifiers. Also the wrapper algorithm that we will use, is similar in essence to the one outlined for TAN inducers. The only addition to the algorithm is a test on the number of parents in each step in which the addition of an arc to the graphical structure is considered.

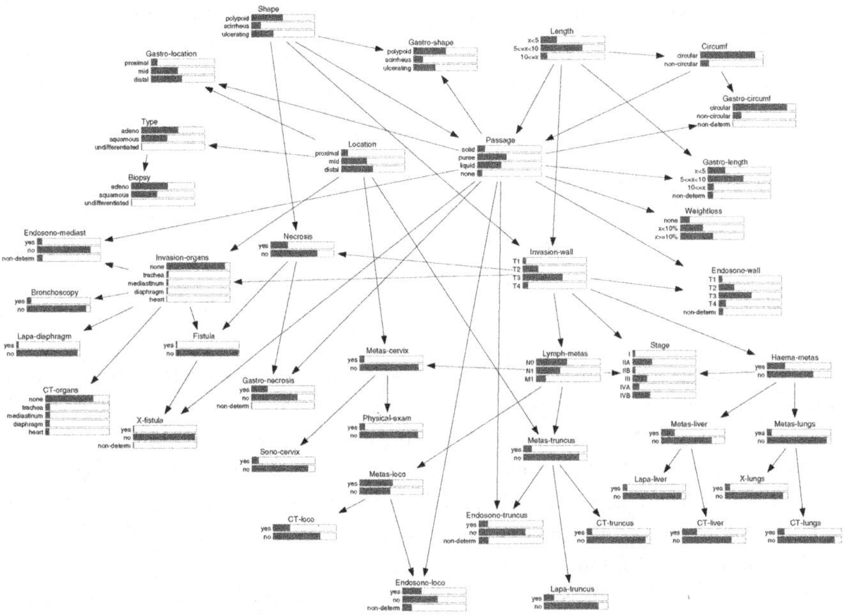

Fig. 1. The oesophageal cancer network.

3 The Domain of Oesophageal Cancer

In our study, we constructed various selective Bayesian network classifiers and compared their performance in terms of classification accuracy. For this purpose, we used a set of data from real patients suffering from cancer of the oesophagus. In this section, we provide some background knowledge of the disease and briefly describe the data that we had available for our study.

3.1 The Oesophageal Cancer Network

As a consequence of a chronic lesion of the oesophageal wall, for example as a result of frequent reflux or associated with smoking and drinking habits, a tumour may develop in a patient's oesophagus. The various presentation characteristics of the tumour, which include its location in the oesophagus and its macroscopic shape, influence its prospective growth. The tumour typically invades the oesophageal wall and upon further growth may invade such neighbouring structures as the trachea and bronchi or the diaphragm, dependent upon its location in the oesophagus. In time, the tumour may give rise to lymphatic metastases in distant lymph nodes and to haematogenous metastases in, for example, the lungs and the liver. The depth of invasion and extent of metastasis, summarised in the cancer's stage, largely influence a patient's life expectancy and are indicative of the effects and complications to be expected from the different available

Table 1. The confusion matrix established for the oesophageal cancer network with the available real patient data.

		network						
		I	IIA	IIB	III	IVA	IVB	*total*
	I	**2**	0	0	0	0	0	2
	IIA	0	**37**	0	1	0	0	38
data	IIB	0	2	**0**	2	0	0	4
	III	1	17	0	**28**	0	1	47
	IVA	1	1	0	9	**28**	0	39
	IVB	0	1	0	6	4	**15**	26
	total	4	58	0	46	32	16	156

treatment alternatives. To establish these factors in a patient, typically a number of diagnostic tests are performed, ranging from a gastroscopic examination of the oesophagus to a CT-scan of the patient's upper abdomen.

With the help of two experts in gastrointestinal oncology from the Netherlands Cancer Institute, Antoni van Leeuwenhoekhuis, we captured the state-of-the-art knowledge about oesophageal cancer in a Bayesian network. The network includes a graphical structure encoding the variables of importance and the probabilistic relationships between them. Each variable represents a diagnostic or prognostic factor that is relevant for establishing the stage of a patient's cancer. The probabilistic influences among the variables are represented by arcs; the strengths of these influences are indicated by conditional probabilities. The network currently includes 40 variables, 25 of which capture the results of diagnostic tests; the network further includes some 1 000 probabilities. For ease of reference, the network is reproduced in Figure 1.

3.2 The Patient Data

For studying the ability of the different classifiers to correctly predict the stage of a patient's cancer, the medical records of 156 patients diagnosed with oesophageal cancer are available from the Antoni van Leeuwenhoekhuis in the Netherlands. For each patient, various diagnostic symptoms and test results are recorded in the dataset. The number of data available per patient ranges between 6 and 21, with an average of 14.8. The data therefore are relatively sparse, including many missing values. For each patient, also the stage of his or her cancer, as established by the attending physician, is recorded. This stage can be either I, IIA, IIB, III, IVA, or IVB, in the order of advanced disease.

To establish a baseline accuracy to compare the accuracies of our classifiers against, we entered, for each patient from the data collection, all diagnostic symptoms and test results available into the oesophageal cancer network. We then computed the most likely stage of the patient's cancer and compared it against the stage recorded in the data. Table 1 shows the confusion matrix that we thus obtained. The table shows that the network predicted the correct stage for 110 of the 156 patients; the accuracy of the network established from the available patient data thus equals 71%.

4 Experimental Results

We describe the set-up of our experimental study. We further present the results that we obtained and discuss the conclusions to be drawn from them.

4.1 The Set-Up of the Experimental Study

For our study, we constructed a dataset of 2 000 artificial patient records by means of logic sampling from the oesophageal cancer network. Each such patient record includes values for all diagnostic variables as well as a value for the class variable modelling the cancer's stage. While in practice, it is very unlikely that all diagnostic tests available are performed with a patient, the constructed dataset nevertheless includes a value for each such test and therefore does not include any missing values. The constructed dataset can thus be considered the result of imputation given the probability distribution represented by the network.

Our study now is composed of two experiments. In the first experiment, we learn, from the generated artificial dataset, a full Naive Bayes, a full TAN classifier, and a full kDB classifier with $k = 3$, using 10-fold cross validation. Applying the same technique, we learn, for each type of classifier, five selective Bayesian network classifiers; the feature selection is performed by means of the wrapper approach and by the filter approach with $\alpha = 0.05$, $\alpha = 0.01$, $\alpha = 0.005$ and $\alpha = 0.001$, respectively. For each of these 18 classifiers, the parameter probabilities are estimated from the data by applying the Laplace correction to their maximum likelihood estimates. The experiment is repeated ten times. We record the classification accuracies of the various classifiers averaged over these ten runs. In the second experiment, we construct similar classifiers as in the first experiment, yet this time using the entire dataset of 2 000 artificial patient records. The accuracies of the resulting classifiers are established with the data of the 156 real patients.

4.2 The Results of the Experiments

The results of the two experiments as outlined in the previous section, are summarised in Table 2. The first column displays, for each type of classifier, the averaged accuracy over the ten runs of ten-fold cross-validation; the column also records the standard deviation of the averaged accuracy found. We applied the Mann-Whitney test to compare the differences in the accuracies of the various classifiers; in the table, the symbol † is used to denote a statistically significant difference at the 0.05 confidence level, with respect to the accuracy of the full Naive Bayes. The second column of the table reports, for each type of classifier, the classification accuracy found in the second experiment with the real patient data. The third column, to conclude, reports the numbers of feature variables selected for the classifiers resulting from the second experiment.

From the results of the first experiment, we observe that the classifiers that provide for modelling conditional dependence relationships among the various

Table 2. Averaged accuracy and standard deviation of ten-fold cross-validation (first column); accuracy and number of selected features upon training with the artificial dataset and testing with the real dataset (second and third columns).

		accuracy ten-fold cv	*accuracy real data*	*#selected features*
	Naive Bayes	70.95 ± 2.61	66.67	25
	TAN	72.15 ± 4.67	67.31	25
	kDB	70.10 ± 3.31	62.82	25
	Selective NB_{fs}	71.85 ± 2.89	66.67	17
$\alpha = 0.05$	Selective TAN_{fs}	73.85 ± 3.68	66.67	17
	Selective $k\text{DB}_{fs}$	$73.90 \pm 3.12^{\dagger}$	67.31	17
	Selective NB_{fs}	71.80 ± 2.15	67.31	16
$\alpha = 0.01$	Selective TAN_{fs}	73.80 ± 3.42	66.67	16
	Selective $k\text{DB}_{fs}$	$73.80 \pm 2.38^{\dagger}$	68.59	16
	Selective NB_{fs}	70.85 ± 3.14	67.31	15
$\alpha = 0.005$	Selective TAN_{fs}	$73.65 \pm 1.86^{\dagger}$	67.31	15
	Selective $k\text{DB}_{fs}$	73.30 ± 2.66	69.23	15
	Selective NB_{fs}	71.35 ± 2.64	67.31	15
$\alpha = 0.001$	Selective TAN_{fs}	74.00 ± 4.10	67.31	15
	Selective $k\text{DB}_{fs}$	73.65 ± 3.78	69.23	15
	Selective NB_{ws}	70.45 ± 3.34	50.64	10
	Selective TAN_{ws}	72.20 ± 2.97	52.56	7
	Selective $k\text{DB}_{ws}$	72.45 ± 3.58	54.56	7

features, have a higher accuracy on average than the corresponding full or selective Naive Bayes. For the selective k-dependence classifier $k\text{DB}_{fs}$ with $\alpha = 0.05$ and $\alpha = 0.01$, and for the TAN_{fs} classifier with $\alpha = 0.005$, more specifically, the averaged accuracy is significantly higher than that of the full Naive Bayes. The selective classifiers, moreover, show a slightly higher accuracy than their full counterparts. Despite the stronger reduction of dimensionality, however, the classifiers constructed with the wrapper approach do not exhibit significantly better performance than the classifiers constructed with the filter approaches.

The second experiment in essence reveals similar patterns of accuracy for the various classifiers as the first experiment. However, while in the first experiment the classifiers constructed with the wrapper approach perform comparably to the classifiers constructed with the filter approach, the wrapper-based classifiers exhibit a considerably worse accuracy with the real patient data.

4.3 Discussion

In our experimental study, we learned various Bayesian network classifiers from a complete dataset that was generated from the oesophageal cancer network and then simulated using the resulting classifiers in the original real-life setting where they are confronted with missing values. We observed that especially the classifiers that were constructed with the wrapper approach to feature subset selection, showed a poor accuracy with the real patient data.

To provide for explaining the relatively poor accuracy of the wrapper-based Bayesian network classifiers with the real patient data, we studied the associated confusion matrices for all constructed classifiers. As an example, we focus here

Table 3. The confusion matrix established from the real patient data for the selective Naive Bayes learned with the wrapper approach to feature selection; the classifier includes 10 features.

		selective Naive Bayes						
		I	IIA	IIB	III	IVA	IVB	*total*
	I	**1**	1	0	0	0	0	2
	IIA	0	**37**	0	0	0	1	38
data	IIB	0	2	**0**	2	0	0	4
	III	0	19	2	**23**	1	2	47
	IVA	0	11	0	23	**4**	1	39
	IVB	0	4	0	8	0	**14**	26
	total	1	74	2	56	5	18	156

Table 4. The confusion matrix established from the real patient data for the selective Naive Bayes learned with the filter approach to feature selection with $\alpha = 0.001$; the classifier includes 15 features.

		selective Naive Bayes						
		I	IIA	IIB	III	IVA	IVB	*total*
	I	**1**	1	0	0	0	0	2
	IIA	0	**38**	0	0	0	0	38
data	IIB	0	2	**0**	2	0	0	4
	III	0	19	2	**21**	3	2	47
	IVA	0	2	0	9	**27**	1	39
	IVB	0	0	0	4	4	**18**	26
	total	1	62	2	36	34	21	156

on the two matrices of Tables 3 and 4. Table 3 reports the confusion matrix for the Naive Bayes constructed with the wrapper approach; Table 4 reports the confusion matrix for the Naive Bayes constructed with the filter approach with $\alpha = 0.001$. Upon comparing the two confusion matrices, we observe that the poor accuracy of the wrapper-based classifier can be attributed almost entirely to its relative inability to identify patients with a stage IVA cancer.

To explain our finding, we consider the discriminating features of an oesophageal cancer of stage IVA. A stage IVA cancer can be distinguished from a cancer of stage IVB by the absence of secondary tumours in the lungs and the liver of the patient. The variables modelling the diagnostic tests that provide for establishing the presence of such secondary tumours have a high mutual information with the class variable and in fact are selected for each of the selective classifiers. An oesophageal cancer of stage IVA is distinguished from a stage III cancer, on the other hand, by the presence of secondary tumours in distant lymph nodes. To investigate whether or not the lymph nodes in the upper abdomen, that is, distant from the primary tumour, are affected by the cancer, three diagnostic tests are available: these are a CT-scan, an endosonographic examination and a laparoscopic examination of the upper abdomen. The laparoscopy is the most reliable among the three diagnostic tests, but as it involves a surgical procedure it is not performed with every patient. In fact, the procedure was performed in just 18 of the 156 patients from our dataset.

In the filter approach to feature selection, the importance of the three diagnostic tests for the identification of a stage IVA cancer is recognised. The three associated variables therefore are selected for inclusion in the selective Naive Bayes NB_{fs} with $\alpha = 0.001$. The resulting classifier as a consequence correctly identifies most patients with a stage IVA cancer. The wrapper approach to feature selection correctly identifies the relatively strong conditional dependence relationships between the three variables and selects just one of them. The selective classifier NB_{ws} includes just the variable capturing the result of the laparoscopic examination and does not include the variables modelling the CT-scan and the endosonographic examination. Since the laparoscopic procedure was performed only very infrequently, the classifier often is not able to identify a stage IVA cancer. The wrapper approach has in fact been too restrictive in its selection of features to be included in the classifier. We derived similar conclusions from the confusion matrices for the selective TAN and kDB classifiers.

5 Conclusions and Future Work

Real-life datasets often include missing values. To deal with these missing values, typically an imputation method is used to fill in the gaps in the data with plausible values. The thus completed dataset then is used for learning purposes. In this paper, we have studied the effect of learning selective classifiers from completed datasets, on their accuracy when confronted with real data that again includes missing values. For our study, we sampled a dataset of 2 000 artificial patient records from a Bayesian network in the field of oesophageal cancer. From this complete dataset, we constructed selective Bayesian network classifiers, using adapted filter and wrapper approaches to feature subset selection. We studied the accuracies of the resulting classifiers using the records of 156 real patients suffering from cancer of the oesophagus.

Our experimental results revealed that the wrapper approach can result in selective classifiers that show a relatively poor accuracy on real data with missing values. The poor behaviour of these classifiers can be attributed to the intrinsic characteristics of our data. As in many biomedical datasets, our data includes several feature variables that model the results of different tests that are performed to gain insight into the same underlying condition; these variables typically are mutually correlated. While the filter approach tends to select all of these correlated feature variables, the wrapper approach tends to select just one of them, since after inclusion of the first selected variable, the remaining variables do no longer contribute to the accuracy of the resulting classifier. The wrapper approach thus tends to remove any redundancy, based upon the data used for the learning process. The selection of feature variables that is induced from a completed dataset, however, may not be the best selection in view of real data with a large number of missing values. The wrapper approach can in fact be too restrictive in its selection of features.

Our experimental results suggest that when confronted with missing values in practice, a Bayesian network classifier should include some redundancy to arrive at a reasonable classification accuracy. We feel that knowledge of the occurrence of missing values should be taken into consideration when learning classifiers from data. The inclusion of such knowledge in the learning process is an interesting topic for further research.

Acknowledgments

The first, third and fourth authors are partially supported by the Ministry of Science and Technology, by the Fondo de Investigaciones Sanitarias, by the Basque Government and by the University of the Basque Country under grants TIC2001-2973-C05-03, PI021020, ETORTEK-GENMODIS project and 9/UPV 00140.226-15334/2003 respectively. The second author is partly supported by the Netherlands Organisation for Scientific Research (NWO).

References

1. Groves, R., Dillman, D., Eltinge, J., Little, R.: Survey Nonresponse. Wiley-Interscience (2002)
2. Kalton, G., Kasprzyk, D.: The treatment of missing survey data. Survey Methodology **12** (1986) 1–16
3. Kohavi, R., John, G.: Wrappers for feature subset selection. Artificial Intelligence **97** (1997) 273–324
4. Duda, R., Hart, P.: Pattern Classification and Scene Analysis. Wiley (1973)
5. Castillo, E., Gutiérrez, J., Hadi, A.: Expert Systems and Probabilistic Network Models. Springer-Verlag, New York (1997)
6. Jensen, F.: Bayesian Networks and Decision Graphs. Springer Verlag (2001)
7. Pardo, L.: Teoría de la Información Estadística. Hespérides (1997) In Spanish.
8. Minsky, M.: Steps toward artificial intelligence. Transactions on Institute of Radio Engineers **49** (1961) 8–30
9. Friedman, N., Geiger, D., Goldszmidt, M.: Bayesian network classifiers. Machine Learning **29** (1997) 131–164
10. Sahami, M.: Learning limited dependence Bayesian classifiers. In: Proceedings of the 2nd International Conference on Knowledge Discovery and Data Mining. (1996) 335–338
11. Hand, D., You, K.: Idiot's Bayes –not so stupid after all? International Statistical Review **69** (2001) 385–398
12. Langley, P., Sage, S.: Induction of selective Bayesian classifiers. In: Proceedings of the Tenth Conference on Uncertainty in Artificial Intelligence, Morgan Kaufmann (1994) 399–406
13. Pazzani, M.: Searching for dependencies in Bayesian classifiers. In: Artificial Intelligence and Statistics IV, Lecture Notes in Statistics, New York, Springer-Verlang (1997)
14. Chow, C., Liu, C.: Approximating discrete probability distributions with dependence trees. IEEE Transactions on Information Theory **14** (1968) 462–467

A Performance Comparative Analysis Between Rule-Induction Algorithms and Clustering-Based Constructive Rule-Induction Algorithms. Application to Rheumatoid Arthritis

J.A. Sanandrés-Ledesma[1], Victor Maojo[1], Jose Crespo[1], M. García-Remesal[1], and A. Gómez de la Cámara[2]

[1] Medical Informatics Group, AI Lab, School of Computer Science, Polytechnical University of Madrid, Spain
[2] Clinical Epidemiology Research Unit, Hospital 12 de Octubre, Madrid, Spain

Abstract. We present a performance comparative analysis between traditional rule-induction algorithms and clustering-based constructive rule-induction algorithms. The main idea behind these methods is to find dependency relations among primitive variables and use them to generate new features. These dependencies, corresponding to regions in the space, can be represented as clusters of examples. Unsupervised clustering methods are proposed for searching for these dependencies. As a benchmark, a database of rheumatoid arthritis (RA) patients has been used. A set of clinical prediction rules for prognosis in RA was obtained by applying the most successful methods, selected according to the study outcomes. We suggest that it is possible to relate predictive features and long-term outcomes in RA.

1 Introduction

Machine learning (ML) is an artificial intelligence research area that studies computational methods for mechanizing the process of knowledge acquisition from experience [1]. One of the main fields in ML is inductive learning (IL). IL is the process of acquiring knowledge by drawing inductive inferences from provided facts [2].

Statistical methods have been traditionally used in medical domains, but medical applications of ML have increased over the last few years [3–5]. These two approaches can be compared assessing issues such as comprehensibility and performance [5, 6] – e.g., classification and prediction accuracy, sensitivity, specificity, or learning speed.

Comprehensibility and accuracy are two of the most relevant parameters in medical applications of statistical methods and ML algorithms. Results presented in some comparative studies [7, 8] suggest that accuracy is similar for both families but comprehensibility is better for ML techniques, and more precisely, for the symbolic paradigm. Nevertheless, ML is not only based on a symbolic approach [1, 9, 10]. There are also other approaches such as the sub-symbolic

J.M. Barreiro et al. (Eds.): ISBMDA 2004, LNCS 3337, pp. 224–234, 2004.

– e.g. artificial neural networks [11] and Bayesian methods [12] – or those inspired from statistics – e.g. generalized linear models [13]. The most important drawback of statistical and ML approaches in medical studies is that they do not provide health professionals with an understandable explanation of the reasoning that was used. Furthermore, some of these methods behave like black boxes. This is a significant reason why physicians are sometimes reluctant to use these models in clinical practice. Conversely, models produced by symbolic ML approaches, such as rule-induction algorithms – or decision tree induction algorithms, since decision trees can be easily translated into rule sets – may be easier to be understood by health practicioners.

In this paper, two results are presented: i) an empirical performance comparative analysis – in the sense of prediction accuracy – between traditional rule-induction algorithms and clustering-based constructive rule-induction algorithms, and ii) a set of clinical prediction rules for prognosis in Rheumatoid Arthritis (RA). This set of clinical prediction rules was obtained by applying the best rule-induction algorithms – according to the results of the comparative analysis carried out in this work – to medical records from a local hospital in Madrid.

2 Methods

2.1 Description of the Study

As stated above, one of the main purposes of this study is to present an empirical performance comparative analysis between traditional rule-induction algorithms and clustering-based constructive rule-induction algorithms. The main idea behind the latter methods is to find dependency relations among primitive variables and use them to generate new features. These dependencies, corresponding to regions in the space, can be represented as clusters of examples. Unsupervised clustering methods [14] have been proposed for searching for these dependencies for two reasons: i) they are independent of expert knowledge, and ii) they only require the number of clusters that we are looking for as user parameters.

We applied some traditional unsupervised clustering algorithms to all pairs of numerical features. This decision was made to ensure that the dependencies generate a good graphical representation, that can be analyzed manually or with computers.

As stated above, the majority of clustering algorithms used in this study require the number of clusters that they must search for as input parameters. It is well-known that choosing the correct number of clusters is a key decision for any clustering algorithm. To determine the correct number of clusters for each pair of numerical features, the following procedure was used:

1. Cluster the pair of numeric predictive variables using the k-means algorithm (for efficiency reasons) with $k = 2, \ldots, 15$ (a number of clusters that we believe is enough). The k-means algorithm is executed multiple times for each k, and the best of these clusterings is selected based on sum of squared errors.

2. Apply a cluster validity index to each of the 15 clusterings obtained in step (1).
3. Select the best k for that pair of predictive variables according to the values of the indexes obtained in the previous step.

Two different clustering validity indexes were used in these experiments: i) Dunn's index [15], and ii) Davies-Bouldin's index [16]. When using Dunn's index, the value of k that maximizes the index must be selected. Conversely, when using Davies-Bouldin's index, one must choose the value of k that minimizes the index.

Once the correct number of clusters for each pair of numeric features was determined, several traditional clustering algorithms were applied. Concretely, the following algorithms were used: i) Single linkage method (Nearest neighbour), ii) Complete linkage method (Farthest neighbour), iii) Analysis of Cluster Centroids (Centroid), iv) Analysis of Cluster Medians (Median), v) Group Average Technique (Average), vi) Ward Technique (Ward), and vii) Minimum Spanning Tree Technique (MST). A detailed description of these clustering methods can be found in [14].

The application of one of these clustering algorithms to all pairs of numeric variables generates a new feature set, referred to as *set* from now onwards. This new *set* contains both the primitive and the new features – one new variable for each pair of numeric features clustered by using the current clustering algorithm. Taking only the new features and leaving out the primitive numerical and categoric features may lead to a dangerous loss of information.

One might wonder how these new features would look like. As an example, suppose that a pair of primitive features $[F_1, F_2]$ is clustered and three clusters have been found. Let us represent the new feature created from this clustering by NF_{F_1,F_2}. Thus, for a given example X, the new variable NF_{F_1,F_2} would take values on the set $\{1, 2, 3\}$ depending on the cluster to which the example X belongs.

We evaluated the performance of traditional rule-induction methods on each of the 8 different *sets* – the original set plus one new *set* for each of the seven abovementioned clustering algorithms. The original *set* includes the primitive 21 variables – 7 numeric and 14 categorical – while the others contain 42 features – the 21 primitive variables and the 21 new features (combinations of the seven numeric variables taken in pairs). We applied the following stateof-the-art rule-induction algorithms: i) C4.5 v8 (C4.5-25 and C4.5-80) [17], ii) FOIL [18], iii) InductH [19], and iv) T (T1 and T2) [20]. The labels beside some algorithm names are used to identify some variants. The labels C4.5-80 and C4.5-25 represent the algorithm C4.5 v8 applied with pruning factors 80 and 25 respectively. The latter generates more conservative trees, since it produces more pruning. Similarly, two variants of the T algorithm were used, producing one-level – label T1 – and two-level – label T2 – optimal trees respectively.

Each pair *[set, method]* was assessed by using 10-fold cross-validation [8]. The following parameters were used to evaluate the quality of each pair:

- **C**: Percentage of correctly classified examples.
- **I**: Percentage of incorrectly classified examples.

After analyzing and assessing the results from the validation process, we selected the pair *[set, method]* that performed best to generate a set of clinical prediction rules (CPR) for prognosis in Rheumatoid Arthritis.

2.2 Data

Data were obtained from a retrospective cohort epidemiological study, carried out at the 12 de Octubre Hospital in Madrid, Spain [21]. Two trained rheumatologists created a database from paper-based patient medical records. This database contains information about 434 patients diagnosed with RA from 1974 to 1995, with the following inclusion criteria: i) less than two years from the onset of symptoms to the first visit, and ii) no treatment with disease-modifying antirheumatic drugs (DMARDs) prior to the first visit. In all cases, diagnosis was made during the first visit to the hospital.

From these 434 patients, only 374 were selected for the study: i) those patients who died, and ii) those patients who answered – at least partially – the selfassessment questionnaires.

Medical experts in RA chose 21 predictive variables from an initial set of 40 features. A distinction between numerical and categorical predictive variables was made. If a value for a feature could not be extracted from the medical record, it was labeled as unknown. Summaries of categorical and numeric predictive variables are shown in tables 1 and 2 respectively. The values of 19 out of the 21 selected variables were measured just after the first year of follow-up. The two remaining variables (MESESFIR and ENFCRCON) were measured at the time of the study. Note that the variable MESESFIR – i.e., total number of months of use of DMARDs – ranges from 0 to 239 months.

A panel of rheumatologists selected the outcomes: death (categorical) and health status (numeric). From the 374 patients selected for the study, 41 were dead at the time of the study. The remaining patients filled in two self-assessment questionnaires to evaluate their health status: i) the general Medical Outcomes Study-Short Form (MOS-SF36) [22], and ii) the RA-specific Modified-Health Assessment Questionnaire (M-HAQ) [23]. The MOS-SF36 questionnaire includes 36 items grouped into 8 scales which measure different general health concepts: Role-Physical (RP), Physical Functioning (PF), Social Functioning (SF), Role-Emotional (RE), Bodily Pain (BP), Vitality (VT), General Health (GH), and Mental Health (MH). Scores for all scales range from 0 to 100, with higher scores indicating better health. On the other hand, the M-HAQ questionnaire is a measure of functional limitations in eight areas of life specifically created for scoring disability of patients with RA. The limitation in each area is scored from 0 to 3, from minimum to maximum disability. Scores are then averaged to produce an overall score which also ranges from 0 to 3.

All the rule-induction algorithms used in this study require the outcome variable to be dichotomous. For this reason, we dichotomized the HAQ and the MOS-SF36 scales, using median values as stratification points.

Table 1. Summary of categorical predictive variables.

Variable	*Description*	*Yes*	*No*	*Missing*
PRSEXO	Male gender.	108 (28.88%)	266 (71.12%)	0 (0.00%)
ARTIC	Both upper and lower joints involvement during the first year of follow-up.	303 (81.02%)	57 (15.24%)	14 (3.74%)
ART	Both small and large joints involvement during the first year of follow-up.	276 (73.80%)	84 (22.46%)	14 (3.74%)
PRAFSIME	Symmetric articular involvement during the first year of follow-up.	37 (9.90%)	335 (89.57%)	2 (0.53%)
PRAFMANO	Hands involvement during the first year of follow-up.	355 (94.91%)	18 (4.81%)	1 (0.28%)
EXPRNODU	Presence of rheumatoid subcutaneous nodules during the first year of follow-up.	42 (11.22%)	331 (88.50%)	1 (0.28%)
EXPRSICC	Presence of secondary sicca syndrome during the first year of follow-up confirmed by one of the following methods: Schirmer test, rose bengal staining, biopsy or parotic gammagraphic enlargement.	43 (11.50%)	309 (82.62%)	22 (5.88%)
EXPRIMER	Presence of extraarticular features during the first year of follow-up.	94 (25.14%)	260 (69.52%)	20 (5.34%)
PRCONTRO	The patient met at least one of the following control criteria during the first year of follow-up: i) morning stiffness of less than 15 minutes of duration, ii) no joint pain, iii) neither pain to pressure, nor to joint mobility, iv) there is no affection of soft parts neither in joints nor in tendinous insertions, and v) erythrocite sedimentation rate of less than 30 mm (20 mm) in women (men).	259 (69.25%)	80 (21.40%)	35 (9.35%)
PRCLFIV	Presence of III or IV Steinbrocker functional class during the first year of follow-up.	61 (16.31%)	297 (79.42%)	16 (4.27%)
PRFACREU	Rheumatoid factor positivity ($p \leq 0.05$ compared to general population by latex or nephelometry) during the first year of follow-up.	266 (71.13%)	108 (28.87%)	0 (0.00%)
USGFIR	Use of systemic glucocorticoids and DMARDs (gold salts, cloroquine, azathioprine, methotrexate, salazopyrine or D-penicilamine) for at least one month during the first year of follow-up.	322 (86.10%)	52 (13.90%)	0 (0.00%)
PREROSIO	Presence of erosions in antero-posterior view of hand radiographs blindly evaluated by a radiologist. These radiographs were done in the first visit.	150 (40.10%)	95 (25.40%)	129 (34.50%)
ENFCRCON	Presence of comorbid chronic diseases which required treatment. Unlike the other variables, this one was measured at the time of the study.	194 (51.88%)	178 (47.59%)	2 (0.53%)

3 Results

Regarding the optimum number of clusters according to Dunn's and Davies-Bouldin's criterias, both indexes agreed on the optimum number of clusters for 13 pairs of features. In the remaining cases, we followed the recommendations of Davies-Bouldin's index, since it is known that this index is more reliable than Dunn's criteria [24].

Table 2. Summary of numeric predictive variables.

Variable	*Description*	*Min/Max*	*Mean*	*StdDev*	*Missing*
EDAINPUT	Age at first visit.	18/83	52.30	14.08	0 (0.00%)
MSINTINP	Total number of months from onset of symptoms to the first visit.	0/23	8.31	6.95	2 (0.53%)
PRNOARTI	Total number of swollen joints during the first year of follow-up (28 joint count: 2 shoulders, 2 elbows, 2 wrists, 10 metacarpophalangical, 10 proximal interphalangical of hands and 2 knees).	0/28	15.73	9.31	20 (5.34%)
PRRIGIDE	Largest morning stiffness duration (in hours) during the first year of follow-up.	0/24	5.05	7.73	58 (15.50%)
PRNOCRIT	Total number of ACR 1987 RA diagnostic criteria fullfilled by the patient after the first year of follow-up.	0/7	4.69	1.34	157 (41.97%)
PRVSG	Highest erythrocite sedimentation rate value (in mm) during the first year of follow-up.	1/138	59.41	31.74	17 (4.54%)
MESESFIR	Total number of months of use of systemic glucocorticoids and DMARDs (gold salts, cloroquine, azathioprine, methotrexate, salazopyrine or D-penicilamine). Unlike the other variables, this one was measured at the time of the study.	0/239	56.45	47.34	29 (7.75%)

Table 3. Cross-validation results for best solutions for the original data set.

Outcome	*IL Algorithm*	*C*	*I*
DEATH	T1	88.85%	11.15%
SFUNCFIS	T1	51.67%	48.33%
SACTIVFI	C4.5-25	55.04%	44.96%
SDOLOR	T1	55.09%	44.91%
SSALUDG	C4.5-25	54.96%	45.04%
SVITALID	C4.5-25	58.47%	41.53%
SFUNCSOC	T1	58.26%	41.74%
SEMOCION	C4.5-25	55.34%	44.66%
SSALUDM	T1	63.93%	36.07%
HAQ	C4.5-25	53.14%	46.86%

Table 4. Cross-validation results for best solutions.

Outcome	*Clustering Algorithm*	*IL Algorithm*	*C*	*I*
DEATH	Ward	C4.5-25	89.11%	10.89%
SFUNCFIS	Mean	T2	60.02%	39.98%
SACTIVFI	Centroid	T2	61.50%	38.50%
SDOLOR	NONE	T1	55.09%	44.91%
SSALUDG	MST	C4.5-25	66.02%	33.98%
SVITALID	MST	T2	65.07%	34.93%
SFUNCSOC	Mean	C4.5-25	59.43%	41.57%
SEMOCION	Mean	T2	59.21%	40.79%
SSALUDM	NONE	T1	63.93%	36.07%
HAQ	MST	C4.5-80	55.39%	44.61%

Table 3 provides a summary including the cross-validation results for best solutions for the original data set – i.e. without clustering-based preprocessing. Similarly, table 4 provides the cross-validation results for best solutions.

3.1 Prognostic Rules and Their Utilization

In this section, an example of the prognostic rules developed for one of the outcomes considered in this study is presented. Our intention is to show the kind of rules that we have extracted, and what is more important, how to use them correctly. To show examples of the complexity of the rules, we selected the outcome DEATH. The model developed for this outcome is the simplest considering both the number of rules and the total number of selectors. For instance, a sample rule describing alive patients would be:

$$\begin{aligned} (DEATH == NO) \leftarrow \\ (EXPRNODU == YES) \wedge \\ (ENFCRCON == YES) \wedge \\ (PRRIGIDE - PRNOCRIT == 2) \wedge \\ (PRVSG \leq 68) \end{aligned} \tag{1}$$

As can be seen, some of the conditions involve features derived from clustering pairs of primitive variables. To evaluate these conditions it is necessary to plot the clustered examples corresponding to these pairs of primitive features. Any new example belong to the cluster of the nearest observation – according to the usual Euclidean distance – in the scatterplot . For example, suppose that there is a new observation, and we are interested in testing if this example would fire the rule (1). Thus, it will be needed to to determine if the new example meets the condition (PRRIGIDE-PRNOCRIT == 2). Figure 1 depicts this hypothetical situation. It is shown in this figure that the nearest example to the new observation belongs to cluster 2. The new observation will also belong to cluster 2, and therefore, it will satisfy the selector (PRRIGIDE-PRNOCRIT == 2).

4 Discussion

4.1 Technical Issues

For 8 of the 10 outcomes studied, the models developed by clustering-based rule-induction algorithms improved the performance of the models developed by applying only a ML rule-induction algorithm. They performed similarly in the other 2 outcomes, SDOLOR and SSALUDM. These results suggest that clustering-based data preprocessing may help to achieve more accurate and reliable results in ML tasks.

The use of Dunn's and Davies-Bouldin's clustering performance indexes was beneficial for the determination of the optimum number of clusters for each pair of numeric features. As shown in table 4, the clustering algorithms that performed better – i.e., they produced the data sets that achieved the best results – were MST, Mean, Ward and Centroid.

Several IL rule-induction algorithms were used. The algorithms that achieved the best results across all the outcomes were C4.5 v8 and T. The C4.5 v8 algorithm performed better with the 25% than with the 80% pruning confidence

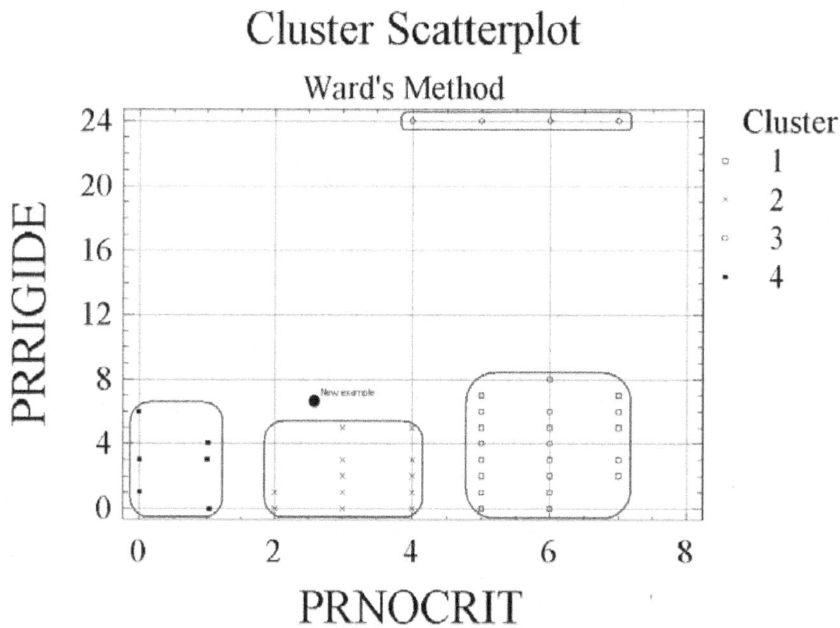

Fig. 1. Cluster scatterplot of PRNOCRIT vs PRRIGIDE.

level. The models developed by the other algorithms – and more concretely by FOIL – were complex, and presented strange feature matchings in the premises, such as comparing a cluster label with the value of a clinical variable.

The variables used in the study were selected by medical specialists from an initial set of more than 40 variables. However, there are other features in the database that may be useful in this prognosis task. A previous report [25], presents examples of cases in which some essential features were not considered due to experts prejudices, and this affected system performance. We believe that all the variables should be considered to develop more accurate prognostic models.

A limitation of the data set used in this study was the large number of features and the small number of patients [26]. The outcome DEATH is a good example, where there are only 33 patients in one of the classes. Another factor that heightened this shortage of examples was the high percentage of unknown values for some features. For instance, the variables PRNOCRIT and PREROSIO where the percentages of unknown values were 40.09% and 32.26% respectively. One could argue that if the percentage of unknown values for a given feature exceeds 25%, that variable should not be considered. However, that variable may have an excellent discriminant proficiency. Hence, it is preferable to let the IL algorithm decide how to use the available information.

There is a potentially interesting aspect which has not been considered in this study. Some variables such as PRCLFIV, PREROSIO, PRNOCRIT, and MESESFIR are time-dependent. We acknowledge that it would be interesting to give a solution to this difficulty. However, this line of research is outside the focus of this paper.

4.2 Clinical Issues

Rheumatoid arthritis is a disease with different outcomes. The models that we have developed indicate that the clinico-epidemiological features evaluated in the first year of evolution of the disease can explain most of these outcomes. In the case of the outcome DEATH, the variables EXPRNODU (subcutaneous nodules), ENFCRCON (chronic comorbid diseases), and PRVSG (highest erythrocite sedimentation rate) are the most useful for prognosis. The most significant features of the developed model for the outcome HAQ are: PRNOARTI (number of swollen joints), MESESFIR (months of DMARDs use), PRVSG, PRNOCRIT (number of ACR 1987 RA diagnostic criteria fullfilled by the patient), and EDAINPUT (age at the first visit). Considering the set of solutions for all the MOS SF-36 questionnaire sections, the most influential features are: EDAINPUT, MESESFIR, PRSEXO (male gender), PRNOARTI (number of swollen joints), PRVSG, and MSINTP (number of months from onset of symptoms to the first visit).

The simplest model was the developed for the outcome DEATH, with 16 rules. Each rule had three conditions in the premise on average. Conversely, the most complex models were those developed for the outcomes HAQ and SSALUDG – General health (GH SF-36) – with 160 and 103 rules respectively. Both outcomes measure the general health status. Perhaps these models are more complex because the associated outcomes reflect the influence of many subjective patient features, and this influence may result in noisy data.

5 Conclusions and Future Work

In this paper, a performance comparative analysis between traditional ruleinduction algorithms and clustering-based rule-induction algorithms is presented. The most successful methods according to this study were used to build a set of clinical prediction rules for prognosis in RA. Unsupervised clustering algorithms were used to find relationships between each pair of numeric predictive features. The number of clusters was chosen using Dunn's and Davies-Bouldin's clustering performance indexes.

We found that clustering-based data preprocessing improved the performance of traditional rule-induction algorithms for 8 of the 10 outcomes considered in this study. 10-fold cross-validation was used for evaluation purposes. The models that we have developed indicate that the clinical features evaluated in the first year of follow-up may be helpful in prognosis.

Regarding future work, we believe that another study with more patients may help to improve the results presented in this paper.

References

1. Langley, P., Simon, H.: *Applications of machine learning and rule induction.* Communications of the ACM 38 (11) (1995) 55–64.
2. Michalski, R.S.: *A theory and methodology of inductive learning.* Artificial Intelligence 20 (1983) 111–161.
3. Kononenko, I., Bratko, I., Kukar, M.: *Application of machine learning to medical diagnosis.* In: Michalski, R.S., Bratko, I., Kubat, M. (Eds.). Machine learning and data mining: Methods and applications. John Wiley & Sons Ltd., 1997.
4. Grošelj, C., Kukar, M., Fettich, J., Kononenko, I.: *Machine learning improves the accuracy of coronary artery disease diagnostic methods.* In: Proc. Computers in Cardiology 24 (1997) 57–60.
5. Lavrač, N., Keravnou, E., Zupan, B.: *Intelligent data analysis in medicine and pharmacology: An overview.* In: Lavrač, N., Keravnou, E., Zupan, B. (Eds.). Intelligent data analysis in medicine and pharmacology. Kluwer, 1997.
6. Long, W., Griffith, H., Selker, H., D'Agostino, R.: *A comparison of logistic regression to decision-tree induction in a medical domain.* Computers and Biomedical Research 26 (1993) 74–97.
7. Michie, D., Spiegelhalter, D.: *Machine learning, neural and statistical classification.* Ellis Horwood, 1994.
8. Weiss, S., Kapouleas, I.: *An empirical comparison of pattern recognition, neural nets, and machine learning classification methods.* In: Proceedings of the Eleventh International Joint Conference on Artificial Intelligence (1989) 806–812.
9. Duda, R.O, Hart, P.E., Stork, D.G.: *Pattern classification.* Wiley & Sons, 2000.
10. Mitchell, T.M.: *Machine learning.* McGraw-Hill, 1997.
11. Príncipe, J.C., Euliano, N.R., Lefevre, W.C.: *Neural and adaptive systems.* Wiley & Sons, 2000.
12. Cowell, R.G., Dawid, A.P, Lauritzen, S.L., Spiegelhalter, D.J.: *Probabilistic networks and expert systems.* Springer Verlag, 1999.
13. Fahrmeir, L., Tutz, G.: *Multivariate statistical modeling based on generalized linear models.* Springer Verlag, 2001.
14. Everitt, B.: *Cluster Analysis*, Edward Arnold, London, 1993.
15. Dunn, J.C.: *Well separated clusters and optimal fuzzy partitions.* Journal of Cybernetics 4 (1974) 95–104.
16. Davies, D.L., Bouldin, D.W.: *A cluster separation measure.* IEEE Transactions on Pattern Analysis and Machine Intelligence 1 (4) (1979) 224–227.
17. Quinlan, J.C.: *C4.5: Programs for Machine Learning*, Morgan Kauffman, San Mateo, CA, 1992.
18. Quinlan, J.C.: *Induction of logic programs: FOIL and related systems.* New Generation Computing 13 (1995) 287–312.
19. Gaines, B.R.: *An ounce of knowledge is worth a ton of data: quantitative studies of the trade-off between expertise and data based on statistically well-founded empirical induction*, in: Proceedings of the 6th InternationalWorkshop on Machine Learning, Morgan Kauffman, 1989, pp. 156–159.
20. Auer, P., Holte, R.C., Maas, W.: *Theory and applications of agnostic pac-learning with small decision trees*, Tech. Rep. NC-TR-96-034, NeuroCOLT (1996).
21. Gómez de la Cámara, A., Ciruelo Monge, E., de la Cruz Bértolo, J., Serrano Díaz, J.M., Pato Cour, E., Gómez-Reino Carnota, J.J.: *Pérdida de fiabilidad en la extracción de datos de las historias clínicas: origen de los defectos y utilidad del adiestramiento.* Medicina Clínica 10 (108) (1997) 377–381.

22. Ware, J.E., Sherbourne, C.D.: *The MOS 36-item short-form health survey.* Medical Care 30 (6) (1992) 473–83.
23. Estelle-Vives, J., Batlle-Gualda, E., Reig, A.: *Spanish version of the Health Assessment Questionnaire: reliability, validity, and transcultural equivalency.* Journal of Rheumatology 20 (12) (1993) 2116–2122.
24. Theodoridis, S., Koutroumbas, K.: *Pattern Recognition.* Academic Press, 1999.
25. Glymour, C., Madigan, D., Pregibon, D., Smyth, P.: *Statistical themes and lessons for data mining,* Data Mining and knowledge discovery 1 (1997) 11–28.
26. Wasson, J., Sox, H., Neff, R., Goldman, L.: *Clinical prediction rules: applications and methodological standards,* The New England Journal of Medicine 313 (13) (1985) 793–799.
27. Sanandrś-Ledesma, J.A., Maojo, V., Crespo, J., Gómez de la Cámara, A.: *A clustering-based constructive induction method and its application to rheumatoid arthritis.* in: Quaglini, S., Barahona, P., Andreassen, S. (Eds), Artificial intelligence in medicine, Vol. 2101 of Lecture Notes in Artificial Intelligence, Springer Verlag, 2001, pp. 59–62.
28. Maojo, V., Crespo, J., Sanandrés-Ledesma, J.A., Billhardt, H.: *Computational intelligence techniques in medical diagnosis and prognosis: the data mining perspective.* in: L. Jain (Ed.), Computational Intelligence Techniques in Medicine, Springer Verlag (in press).
29. Maojo, V., Sanandrés-Ledesma, J.A.: *A survey of data mining techniques.* in: R. Brause, E. Hanisch (Eds.), Medical Data Analysis, Vol. 1933 of Lecture Notes in Computer Science, Springer Verlag, 2000 pp. 17–22.

Domain-Specific Particularities of Data Mining: Lessons Learned

Victor Maojo

Biomedical Informatics Group, Artificial Intelligence Laboratory,
Universidad Politecnica de Madrid, Spain
vmaojo@fi.upm.es

Abstract. Numerous data mining methods and tools have been developed and applied during the last two decades. Researchers have usually focused on extracting new knowledge from raw data, using a large number of methods and algorithms. In areas such as medicine, few of these DM systems have been widely accepted and adopted. In contrast, DM has obtained a considerable success in recent genomic research, contributing to the huge tasks of data analysis linked to the human genome project and related research. This paper presents a study of relevant past research in biomedical DM. It is proposed that traditional approaches used in medical DM should apply some of the lessons learned in decades of research in disciplines such as epidemiology and medical statistics. In this context, novel methodologies will be needed for data analysis in the areas related to genomic medicine, where genomic and clinical data will be tightly collected and studied. Some ideas are proposed for new research design, considering those lessons learned during the last decades.

Keywords: Medical data mining. Medical data analysis. Knowledge discovery in databases. Epidemiology. Medical statistics. Genomics. Genomic medicine medicine.

1 Introduction

During the last two decades the field of Knowledge Discovery in Databases (KDD) has attracted considerable interest for extracting knowledge from biomedical databases. According to classical KDD methodologies [1], Data Mining (DM) is a step in the KDD process, carried out using large amounts of data, usually from a single organization [2]. Within health environments, DM can be used to extract knowledge from institutional data warehouses –e.g.,for financial purposes–, or in CPRs or clinical databases –e.g., to identify clinical prediction rules, or in diagnostic or prognostic tasks.

In this paper, we analyse the particularities of a specific area, in this case biomedicine, by using two different approaches: (1) Medical DM may have suffered some drawbacks because of the lack of standard methodologies, adapted to the special characteristics of the area. Some suggestions will be presented. (2) A comparison of DM in the areas of medical informatics (MI) and bioinformatics (BI) gives important clues, by showing the different underlying theoretical background and special characteristics of applications of DM in both fields.

This paper does not present a thorough review of the field, already available elsewhere with numerous and different perspectives [3–11]. It addresses significant past projects and extract some useful lessons from these experiences. In the next section an analysis of previous DM research projects in medicine is carried out. This kind of

J.M. Barreiro et al. (Eds.): ISBMDA 2004, LNCS 3337, pp. 235–242, 2004.

analysis should provide clues to improve certain aspects of future directions of medical research and practice, particularly interesting for future genomic medicine, where the analysis of combined clinical and genomic databases will be fundamental.

2 Past Research in DM in Medicine

Taking a retrospective view of KDD or DM –from now, both terms are similarly considered, although there are differences between them, as stated above– in medicine, it can be seen an antecedent of these areas in the work carried out during the 70 and 80s to analyse large clinical databases. Various research projects [12][13] attempted to demonstrate the feasibility of analysing large clinical databases, using statistical and other techniques [14]. A significant example if the project carried out at the Brighman and Women's hospital, in Boston, USA, to create decision trees using recursive partioning methods in myocardial infarction. They generated algorithms and clinical procedures that were routinely used in clinical care [15]. Other scholars developed formal methodologies to develop clinical prediction rules, with relative success [16].

Since the 1970s, Artificial Intelligence (AI) researchers met the "bottleneck" of knowledge acquisition from medical specialists. Developers of pioneering expert systems like CASNET, MYCIN, INTERNIST, or PIP [17], recognized the difficulties of acquiring knowledge from medical experts. Since the time of the investigations carried out by researchers in cognitive science [18], it was clear that it would be difficult to capture the knowledge and problem solving methods in a specific domain. Given this scenario, researchers realized that automated methods such as machine learning techniques could provide new approaches to extract useful knowledge from data sets, with or without human supervision.

An example of pioneering work in machine learning for knowledge acquisition in medical expert systems was the KARDIO system [19]. This program, for cardiological diagnosis and treatment, used an inductive algorithm to extract rules from large clinical databases. It aimed to eliminate subjective biases in the knowledge base contents. Since that time, clinical databases have been mined with AI techniques for purposes such as diagnosis, screening, prognosis, monitoring, therapy support or overall patient management [4][9]. In many cases, data sets were in the public domain and sample sizes were not longer than a few hundreds of cases. Since this kind of demonstration systems served only for academic purposes, not clinically relevant, developers suggested that larger samples may improve outcomes and be used in clinical routine.

In this regard, some significant examples, using large data samples – over 5000 patients – can be cited. For instance, studies carried out in Pittsburgh [20] for extracting clinical predictors in pneumonia mortality and in Boston [21] for patient classification in cardiac ischemia. In the Pittsburgh study, researchers used a number of different techniques, including decision trees, Bayesian networks, logistic regression, rule-based approaches, neural networks and k-nearest neighbours. Outcomes of statistical and machine learning techniques were quite similar. In the Boston study outcomes – using logistic regression and the C4.5 algorithm– were slightly worse than those obtained by physicians. In both cases researchers envisioned the use of the combination of some of these techniques, i.e. hybrid methods, to improve their performance.

Neural neworks have been also applied to large patient data sets. A comprehensive review has been reported [11]. Some of these applications have been successfully applied to different medical issues, particularly for image – e.g., in SPECT or mammograms – and signal analysis – e.g., for EEG or ECG [22]. In oncology, various applications have been introduced into clinical routine, for issues such as cervical cytologic studies. Nevertheless, it seems that only a small part of applications reach commercial and clinical use, arising doubts about their real impact on clinical practice. For instance, in another project performed in various US hospitals to study mortality after coronary artery bypass surgery [23], researchers could not obtain significant improvements over logistic regression. In their conclusions, these researchers doubted of the reliability of previous studies reporting that neural networks performed better than traditional statistical methods. They claimed that researchers conducting these previous experiments may have failed to detect some errors.

Other studies have reported research carried out with clinical databases that included more than 40000 patient records [24][25]. In these studies, larger sample sizes did not significantly improve the final outcomes. In general, it seems that using larger sizes or different algorithms do not provide an improvement in DM. This issue will be discussed in the next section.

3 The Reduced Impact of Medical DM

Since MYCIN, research reports have claimed that AI systems outperform physicians in diagnostic accuracy [26]. Machine learning reports have frequently shown a similar trend regarding medical applications, stating that physicians routinely accept DM systems and outcomes [4][8][9][27]. Nevertheless, these optimistic estimations have been seriously disputed [28]. According to these views, it seems that some requirements and biases may have not been accurately considered in many experiments [11][23][28]. In fact, most medical DM systems are still not routinely used in clinical practice, with few exceptions. A surprising similarity may be established between medical expert systems and DM: in many occasions, health professionals highly considered their performance and outcomes, but not enough to use them in their routines.

Various researchers have stated [27] that some machine learning techniques outperform others – e.g., that belief networks outperform decision trees. According to this view, the type of DM technique that is adopted for each case is fundamental to obtain a satisfactory response from physicians. Other reviews [28] and our own experience do not seem to support this assertion. Although quite different statements can be found in the scientific literature, it seems that most machine learning systems can generate quite similar outcomes and users' responses.

In a project carried out at the Universidad Politecnica of Madrid, Spain, over the last years, clinical prediction rules were extracted for prognosis of patients with rheumatoid arthritis. It has been reported elsewhere [29]. Although results were promising from a medical DM point of view, outcomes have not been introduced yet in clinical routine. Working in this DM project, the author and his colleagues realized about some of the limitations of current approaches in medical DM. Departing from these own research results and experience, it can be suggested that there are many issues that are not properly considered when applying computing methods to medical data analysis.

One might wonder if DM is providing the kind of information and knowledge that medical practitioners expect in order to advance science and practice. These professionals base their arguments in much more things than just a collection of external signs and symptoms. The thorough evaluation of patient appearance, personal circumstances, accounts or psychological traits are rarely included in databases or medical records. They are a fundamental basis for medical diagnosis and patient management in clinical routine. Furthermore, physicians collect data with subjective thoughts about the patient and using different theories, evidence-based models, knowledge representations and problem solving strategies to base their judgments. This information is rarely registered.

It has been previously proposed [30] that KDD researchers should consider studies from cognitive psychology in order to adapt KDD methodologies to specific application domains. In the case of medical applications it should also include considerations about medical reasoning and the kind of heuristics and biases that are frequently used by physicians in their routine. This approach might result that in a better acceptance of DM by medical practitioners.

In many medical DM papers, researchers have used a wide range of medical datasets in the public domain for their concrete DM methods and algorithms. In medicine, researchers have scarcely searched for the best solutions for specific scientific problems, that may advance the scientific foundations of medicine. This kind of statement could be also valid, in general, for MI, where an application-driven purpose has dominated the discipline during the last four decades [31][32].

Less efforts have been dedicated in medical DM to purely scientific research that may have led to improvements in medical physiology and pathology, not directly useful for clinical practice, but paying off in the long run. A comparison with DM in genomics could provide interesting insights.

4 A Comparison Between DM in Medicine and Biology

An interesting example from the history of AI is DENDRAL, the first expert system. Some of their developers later created MYCIN, one of the first medical expert systems. The objectives of both projects were quite different [33]. Whereas DENDRAL aimed to contribute to model the process of scientific creation and discovery, MYCIN was built as a decision aid for clinical practice. It did not intend to advance medical knowledge in its application domain, but rather to develop an innovative methodological approach to clinical diagnosis and practice. It is interesting to see how early, research in MI and BI – or computational biology – was separated in terms of their primary goals – scientific in biology, practical or clinical in medicine. We have extended this view elsewhere [31][32].

One of the overall objectives of DM in genetics is to reduce complexity and extract information from large datasets as. In general, DM in genomics aims to generate descriptive and predictive models to understand patterns or relationships in the data, that can lead to achievements in genomic research.

Practically all machine learning methods and algorithms have been applied to different biological topics [33]. The complexity and volume of genomic and proteomic information has implied that researchers have tested many different techniques for information management and analysis. For instance, neural networks were used in areas such as prediction of protein structures and signal peptides, sequence encoding and output interpretation; various probabilistic techniques were used for creating phylogenetic trees; hidden markov models are useful for multiple alignments, classification of sequences or structural analysis; genetic algorithms for classifying protein segments, and so on [33].

While the techniques and goals may be considered similar to those of data mining in medicine, there are some clear differences between both fields. In medical DM there has been a predominant trial and error approach, usually aiming to develop clinical applications for decision support. The scientific foundations of the biology, stronger than in medicine, have given different perspectives and goals to the area. In biology, DM researchers have focused their efforts in advancing knowledge and science in the genomic area [31].

Genetic data are collected considering different assumptions, based on more clear scientific theories and models, but also including uncertainty, which must be managed in probabilistic terms. Research on phylogenetic structures and systems biology demonstrate the influence of various kinds of interactions among genes and proteins. These interactions make difficult to model these processes. While projects are based on more theoretical assumptions and models, compared to medical applications, research in biology also implies trial and error approaches and uncertainty management.

For instance, past research in biology labs using PCR has implied the use of numerous heuristics. Thus, it is not surprising that BI and researchers in DM in biology are demanding more theories to support their efforts [33]. Given these differences, the integration of clinical and genomic data poses various challenges for research and development, including the design of specific, genomic-based clinical trials. Various examples of linking genomic and clinical information can be given, such as the recollection of data carried out in the Iceland population [34].

In biology, it has been reported [36] that comparing data from different databases without realizing their underlying differences may damage the future development of fields such as microarrays. To avoid this problem, there is a need to standardize comparable experimental designs and database systems [36]. In this regard, there is a significant challenge in the area concerning the creation of the infrastructures and methods needed to integrate databases to connect information, from genetic and medical sources. Applications may include, for instance, drug development by pharmaceutical companies, multicentric clinical trials or functional genomics projects.

5 Establishing Methodological Variations for Medical DM

There are already research efforts on the road to integrate clinical and genomic data in expanded databases that could be analysed to extract biomedical knowledge. Using the lessons learned in twenty years of research in medical DM – and a few less years in BI – investigators may introduce novel approaches for DM in future integrated genomic and clinical databases. This research direction introduces significant and difficult challenges –e.g., data integrity, standards, concept mapping, etc. The use of new approaches to data pooling and the development of integrated medical/genomic ontologies might help in data integration tasks.

From a pure medical perspective, there are lessons learned in years of previous experiences that should be considered. Correcting these issues in medical DM may improve system performance and users' acceptance. Below, a few examples of tips and considerations are proposed. They should be taken into account when designing and carrying out medical DM projects:

- Elaborate or control a correct study design, from a epidemiological perspective. In order to ensure clinicians' acceptance, DM study designs should be made, as long as possible, according to classical clinical and epidemiological research. This approach includes randomised clinical trials – although they may not be affordable for most DM projects – or adapt, as much as possible, the classical DM methodology, to include epidemiological principles and methodologies.
- Control patient eligibility for inclusion in a clinical data set to be mined
- Evaluate sample sizes by statistical methods. DM studies need an adequate sample, in terms of data quality and quantity, for performing correct analyses.
- Avoid biases in variable and predictor selection. DM developers may introduce their own biased models of the domain and cognitive and problem solving methods when they select variables and the kind of outcomes they are looking for.
- Include comments in data sets about changes in clinical aproaches to specific diseases, including variations in measurements, diagnostic tests and therapeutic procedures over the years, socioeconomic characteristics, if data come from state-of-the-art academic hospitals, level of technological resources and so on.
- A formal validation should be made, considering both clinical and software results.

A comparison with medical statistics and epidemiological research may give interesting insighths to medical DM, creating a synergy between both perspectives, by exchanging methods, tools and best practices.

6 Conclusions

From a pure medical perspective, there are lessons learned in years of previous experiences that should be considered. Correcting these issues DM may improve system performance and users' acceptance. Meanwhile, significant results in biological studies including DM, that have contributed to advance science and accelerate studies such as the Human Genome Project.

To improve the quality of DM in medicine – and genomic medicine, of course – new methodologies must be developed. In this regard, greater emphasis should be dedicated to study designs. As stated above, many medical DM have not paid attention to this issue, forgetting the importance of variability in clinical practice. Randomized clinical trials are an example of the kind of medical studies that have been succesfully carried out for decades. The lessons learned in this methodological approach should be considered.

The recent success of DM applications in genomics suggests that shifting objectives towards long-term scientific goals – e.g., relating genomic research to phenotypic and clinical characteristics and diseases –, should improve scientific results and recognition. In this regard, recent issues of scientific journals emphasize the need for integrated biomedical approaches, leading to genomic medicine [37].

Acknowledgments

Dr. Maojo's research is supported by the INFOBIOMED European Network of Excellence in Biomedical Informatics (IST directorate, European Commission).

Bibliography

1. Fayyad, U., Piatetsky-Shapiro, G., and Smyth P. (1996), "From Data Mining to Knowledge Discovery: An Overview", In: Fayyad, U., Piatetsky-Shapiro, G., Smyth, P., and Uthurusamy, R. (eds.), *Advances in Knowledge Discovery and Data Mining*, pp. 1-34. AAAI Press/The MIT Press, Menlo Park, California.
2. Han, J. and Kamber, M. Data Mining: Concepts and Techniques, Morgan Kaufmann Publishers. 2000.
3. Cios, K. and Kacprzyk, J. (Eds.) (2001), *Medical Data Mining and Knowledge Discovery*, Springer Verlag, New York, USA.
4. Lavrac, N., Keravnou, E., and Zupan, B. (1997), "Intelligent data analysis in medicine and pharmacology: An overview", In: *Intelligent Data Analysis in Medicine and Pharmacology*, pp. 1-13, Kluwer.
5. Maojo, V. (2000), "A Survey of Data Mining in Medicine. Methods and Limitations", Keynote speech at ISMDA 2000, Frankfurt.
6. Maojo, V.; Sanandres, J.; Billhardt, H.; Crespo, J.. Computational Intelligence Techniques: The Data Mining Perspective. In Jain. L (Ed.): Computational Intelligence Techniques in Medical Diagnosis and Prognosis. Springer Verlag. 2001
7. Cios, Krzysztof J., ed. *Medical Data Mining and Knowledge Discovery.* New York: Physica-Verlag, 2001.
8. Kononenko, I.: Machine learning for medical diagnosis: history, state of the art and perspective. Artif Intell Med 2001 Aug;23(1):89-109.
9. Lavrac N.: Selected techniques for data mining in medicine. Artif Intell Med. 1999 May;16(1):3-23.
10. Zupan B, Lavrac N, Keravnou E. Data mining techniques and applications in medicine.Artif Intell Med. 1999 May;16(1):1-2
11. Lisboa, PJG.: A review of evidence of health benefit from Artificial Neural Networks in medical intervention.. Neural Networks 2002, 15,11-39.
12. Rosati RA, Wallace GG, Stead EA: The way of the future. Arch Intern Med 1973; 131:285-288.
13. Fries J: Time oriented patient records and a computer data bank. JAMA 1972; 222:1436-1542.
14. Breiman, L., Friedman, J., Olshen, R., and Stone, C. (1984), *Classification and Regression Trees*, Wadsworth International Group.
15. Goldman L, Cook EF, Brand DA, Lee TH, Rouan GW, Weisberg MC, Acampora D, Stasiulewicz C, Walshon J, Terranova G, et al. (1988), A Computer Protocol to Predict Myocardial Infarction in Emergency Department Patients with Chest Pain, The New England Journal of Medicine, Vol.318, 13, 797-803.
16. Wasson, J.H., Sox, H.C., Goldman. L., and Neff, R.K. (1985), Clinical Prediction Rules; Applications and Methodologic Standards, New England Journal of Medicine, 313:793-9.
17. Clancey, W. and E.H. Shortliffe (Eds).: Readings in Medical Artificial Intelligence: The First Decade. Reading: Addison Wesley. 1984
18. Anderson J. Cognitive Psychology and Its Implications (5th Ed). Worth Publishing. 1999.
19. Bratko, I., Mozetic, I., and Lavrac, N. (1989), KARDIO: A Study in Deep and Qualitative Knowledge for Expert Systems, The MIT Press, Boston, MA.

20. Cooper GF, Aliferis CF, Ambrosino R, Aronis J, Buchanan BG, Caruana R, Fine MJ, Glymour C, Gordon G, Hanusa BH, Janosky JE, Meek C, Mitchell T, Richardson T, Spirtes P. (1997): An Evaluation of Machine–Learning Methods for Predicting Pneumonia Mortality, Artificial Intelligence in Medicine, 9, 107-138.
21. Long, W.J., Griffith, J.L., Selker, H.P., and D'Agostino R.B.: A comparison of logistic regression to decision-tree induction in a medical domain, Computers and Biomedical Research 1993, 26:74-97.
22. Sacha JP, Goodenday LS, Cios KJ.: Bayesian learning for cardiac SPECT image interpretation. Artif Intell Med 2002 Sep-Oct;26(1-2):109-143.
23. Tu JV, Weinstein MC, McNeil BJ, Naylor et al. CD (1998), Predicting Mortality after Coronary Artery Bypass Surgery, Medical Decision Making, 18, 229-235.
24. Prather JC, Lobach DF, Goodwin LK, Hales JW, Hage ML, Hammond WE.: Medical data mining: knowledge discovery in a clinical data warehouse. Proc AMIA Annu Fall Symp. 1997;:101-5.
25. Ennis M, Hinton G, Naylor D, Revow M, Tibshirani R.: A comparison of statistical learning methods on the Gusto database.Stat Med. 1998 Nov 15; 17(21):2501-8.
26. Teach, R.L. and Shortliffe, E.H. (1981), An Analysis of Physician Attitudes regarding Computer-Based Clinical Computation Systems, Computers and Biomedical Research, 14 (6):542-558.
27. Keravnou E., Lavrac, N.: AIM portraits: tracing the evolution of artificial intelligence in medicine and predicting its future in the new millennium. Artif Intell Med. 2001 Aug;23(1):1-4.
28. Schwarzer G, Vach W, Schumacher M:. On the misuses of artificial neural networks for prognostic and diagnostic classification in oncology. Stat Med. 2000 Feb 29;19(4):541-61.
29. Sanandrés, J., Maojo, V., Crespo, J., and Gomez, A.: A Clustering-Based Constructive Induction Method and its Application to Rheumatoid Arthritis. In S. Quaglini, P. Barahona and S. Andreassen (Eds). Proc. of Artificial Intelligence in Medicine 2001
30. Pazzani, M. Knowledge discovery from data? IEEE Intelligent Systems 15(2): 10-13 (2000)
31. Maojo, V. and Kulikowski, C.: Medical Informatics and Bioinformatics: On the Road to Genomic Medicine. Journal of the American Medical Informatics Association. 2003.
32. Maojo, V., Iakovidis, I., Martín F., Crespo, J. and Kulikowski, C.: Medical informatics and bioinformatics: European efforts to facilitate synergy. J Biomed Inform 2001, 34(6):423-7.
33. Newell, A. Foreword. In Buchanan, B. and E.H. Shortliffe.: Rule-Based Expert Systems: The Mycin Experiments of the Stanford Heuristic Programming Project. New York: Addison-Wesley. 1984.
34. Baldi, P. and Brunal, S.: 2001. Bioinformatics: The Machine Learning Approach, Second Edition (Adaptive Computation and Machine Learning). The MIT Press.
35. Annas GJ.: Rules for research on human genetic variation--lessons from Iceland. N Engl J Med 2000 Jun 15;342(24):1830-3.
36. Bertone P, and Gerstein M.: Integrative data mining: the new direction in bioinformatics. IEEE Eng Med Biol Mag. 2001 Jul-Aug;20(4):33-40.
37. Maojo, V., and Crespo, J.: Challenges for future intelligent systems in biomedicine. Journal of Intelligent and Fuzzy Systems 12 (1): 1-3 (2002).

A Structural Hierarchical Approach to Longitudinal Modeling of Effects of Air Pollution on Health Outcomes

Michael Friger[1], Arkady Bolotin[1], and Ulrich Ranft[2]

[1] Epidemiology Department, Ben-Gurion University of the Negev, Beersheba, Israel
[2] Department of Environmental Epidemiology and Biomonitoring
Medical Institute of Environmental Hygiene, Heinrich Heine University, Duesseldorf, Germany

Abstract. In the paper we present the methodology of construction and interpretation of models for the study of air pollution effects on health outcomes and their applications. According to the main assumption of the model, every health outcome is an element of the multivariate hierarchical system and depends on the system meteorology, pollution, geophysical, socio-cultural and other factors. The given model is built on system approach using GEE-technique and time-series analysis. The model is tested by the data collected from lung function measurements of the group of 48 adults with vulnerable respiratory system in Leipzig, Germany, over the period from October 1990 till April 1991 (the total of 10,080 individual daily records). The meteorological variables comprise temperature and humidity, while the pollution variables are made of the Total Suspended Particulate Matter and Sulfur Dioxide airborne concentration. Results of the models, constructed separately for morning, noon, and evening, demonstrate direct and indirect influence of air pollution on the lung function under the certain meteorological, individual factors and seasonal changes.

1 Introduction

Influence of the environment on human health is a problem of fundamental magnitude deeply concerning all mankind. Year by year, this problem only becomes more acute one, painful and financially consuming. As a matter of fact, at stake is survival of human race. Majority of the studies on in this problem were concentrated on efforts to expose adverse effects of urban air pollution on health outcomes [6, 1, 8, and many others]. The adverse affects included enlarged mortality and morbidity rates, pulmonary function decrements, visits to emergency departments and hospital admissions, and increased medication use. The association between air pollution and the adverse effects revealed in these studies is mostly consistent, despite differences in definitions of exposure and outcome measurements and the statistical methods used to model the relationship between air pollution and health outcomes.

It is obvious nowadays that to analyze the above link one has to include multiple aspects into a statistical model, such as geophysical factors (periodical change in the seasons, geomagnetic field magnitude, sun radiation level, ...), meteorological factors (humidity, temperature, wind strength and direction, ...), socio-cultural factors (all-national cycles in life stile, for example: sequences of working days and weekends, holydays and regular days, ...), individual factors (genetic background, body mass index, smoking, physical fitness, ...), and others. But the question of principle is how to do it?

However, to construct more adequate model it is necessary to not just consider all the model factors mentioned above but also their hierarchical and other relationships

J.M. Barreiro et al. (Eds.): ISBMDA 2004, LNCS 3337, pp. 243–250, 2004.

obtained from a-priori knowledge about the model. Such approach (based on structural hierarchical models and partially described in [3] and [2]) is certainly more adequate reflection of reality than previous one.

In this paper, basing on the techniques of generalized linear models (GLM), generalized estimation equations (GEE) [7, 4, 9], and time-series technique we build a longitudinal model of the structural hierarchical kind mentioned above.

A model of that kind does not have one but several complicatedly related functional patterns of independent variables. Therefore, any conventional epidemiologically sound interpretation of the model results becomes impossible. Explaining the model in epidemiologically meaningful terms we propose the interpretation we call "multi-layer" one. In the paper we develop the strategy and methodology of this interpretation.

To computerize employing of the structural hierarchical approach to longitudinal modeling we constructed and published the program module `quickmodel_interact` implemented as an ado-file of Stata statistical software (version 8.2, Stata Corp, 2003).

We applied the model on the data collected from lung function measurements of the group of 48 adults with vulnerable respiratory system in Leipzig, Germany, over the period from October 1990 till April 1991 (the total of 10,080 individual daily records).

2 Constructing the Model

2.1 Structural Hierarchical Model

Let us consider term "health" as an outcome of our major interest.

We assume that "health" is a factor of a multi-factor hierarchical system, which also includes meteorology, pollution and other factors (Figure 1).

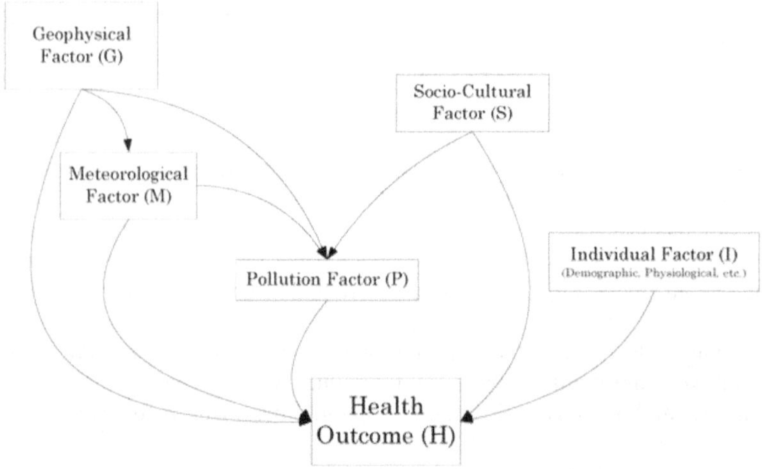

Fig. 1. Hierarchical Structural Model of Relation between Health Outcome and Geophysical, Meteorological, Socio-Cultural, Pollution factors

Such a hierarchical system can be considered as a *hierarchical structural model* describing relations between the factors.

The model is resulted from basic system analysis based upon a-priori knowledge of the considered system [3].

For example, geophysical factor G can directly affect health H: G→H; besides, factor G can indirectly affect H through meteorology M and pollution P as well: G→M→P→H.

At this stage we will only consider periodical components of factor G (i.e. seasonal changes) and similar component of factor S (i.e. week day's variation).

Obviously, formalization of the structural hierarchical model can be achieved by many ways. One of them is using one of the axiomatic rules of path analysis [5], namely: parallelism of paths (fragments) interpreted as the paths' sum.

Doing so we get the following formalization of our structural hierarchical model:

$$\begin{aligned} H_t = {} & F_1^{GH}(\mathbf{G_t},t)+F_2^{SH}(\mathbf{S_t},t)+F_3^{MH}(\mathbf{M_t},t)+ \\ & +F_4^{GM}(\mathbf{G_t},t)\circ F_4^{MH}(\mathbf{M_t},t)+ \\ & +F_5^{GM}(\mathbf{G_t},t)\circ F_5^{MP}(\mathbf{M_t},t)\circ F_5^{PH}(\mathbf{P_t},t)+ \\ & +F_6^{SP}(\mathbf{S_t},t)\circ F_6^{PH}(\mathbf{P_t},t)+F_7^{PH}(\mathbf{P_t},t)+F_8^{IH}(\mathbf{I_t},t) \end{aligned} \quad (2.1.1)$$

where:

t is the time variable; Gt, St, Mt, Pt, It are the vectors of geophysical, socio-cultural, meteorological, pollution and individual variables, respectively; Ht is the "health" outcome (dependent variable); the terms F_1^{GH}, F_2^{SH}, F_3^{MH}, F_7^{PH}, F_8^{IH} are the functions expressing the "direct" effects of geophysical G, socio-cultural S, meteorological M, pollution P and individual I components on "health" H. The terms describing "indirect effects" are: F_4^{GM} - geophysical component G effect on meteorology M; F_4^{MH} - meteorological component M effect on "health" H (after removing influence of geophysical component G on meteorology M); F_5^{GM} - geophysical component G effect on meteorology M; F_5^{MP} - meteorological component M effect on pollution P and after removing influence of geophysical component G on meteorology M; F_5^{PH} - pollution P effect on "health" H (after removing influence of geophysical component G and meteorological component M on pollution P); F_6^{SP} - socio-cultural component S effect on pollution P; F_6^{PH} - pollution P effects on "health" H (after removing influence of socio-cultural component S on pollution P).

Sign "$\circ$" depicts a hierarchical consequential link between factors. Such a link can be formalized by using another axiomatic rule of path analysis: consequential relation between terms interpreted as the terms' product (we will call this formalization *multiplicative-additive* one) or as a superposition of functions (in this case we will call the formalization *functional-additive* one). In this paper we will use the first type of the formalization; implementation and description of the second type may be found in [2].

The next step in model building is determining the type of all functions F_i^{****} of the model.

Let's consider the functions which relate to component G.

We hypothesize that the periodic seasonal changes (caused by geophysical processes) have an effect on the weather, pollution P and "health" H. Weather, in its turn, also influences pollution P and health outcome H. So, the relationship between P and H has both direct and indirect links.

Hence follows that all the functions of G can be presented by pairs of sinusoidal and co-sinusoidal functions with various periods. We pick out just 4 periods built on the annual cycle.

Periodical changes in socio-cultural component S are described by pairs of sine and cosine functions with seven-day period. Furthermore, periodic changes in S can be described by a set of 6 dummy variables representing each day of the week. Other model functions can be constructed using a spline approach or, in the particular case, polynomial and/or logarithmic functions.

Bellow we apply the described general approach to our particular case.

Let $M=(M_1,M_2,\ldots,M_{r_m})$, $P=(P_1,P_2,\ldots,P_{r_p})$ and $I=(I_1,I_2,\ldots,I_{r_i})$ be variables representing meteorological M, pollution P and individual I components, respectively. Then we get the following formalization of (2.1.1)

$$\begin{aligned} H_t &= q_0+\sum_{j=1}^{r_m} q_j M_j+\sum_{k=1}^{r_p} q_k P_k+\sum_{l=1}^{r_i} q_l I_l+\sum_{i=1}^{g}\left(a_i\cos(\omega_i t)+b_i\sin(\omega_i t)\right)+ \\ &+\sum_{j=1}^{r_p}\left(c_j P_j\cos(\omega_7 t)+d_j P_j\sin(\omega_7 t)\right)+\sum_{j=1}^{r_m}\sum_{i=1}^{g}\left(a_{ij} M_j\cos(\mathrm{T}_i\cdot\omega t)+b_{ij} M_j\sin(\omega_i t)\right)+ \\ &+\sum_{j=1}^{r_p}\sum_{i=1}^{g}\left(c_{ij} P_j\cos(\omega_i t)+d_{ij} P_j\sin(\omega_i t)\right)+\sum_{k=1}^{r_p}\sum_{j=1}^{r_m}\sum_{i=1}^{g}\left(a_{ij}^k M_j P_k\cos(\omega_i t)+b_{ij}^k M_j P_k\sin(\omega_i t)\right) \end{aligned} \quad (2.1.2)$$

where: t is the time variable; ω_i denotes frequency of the periodic oscillation with period T_i: $\omega_i=2\pi/T_i$ $(i=1,2,3,4)$, here T_i is the time period built on the fundamental annual cycle. In our case, T_1 is the year period, T_2 is the half-year period, T_3 is the period of season, T_4 is the month period; that is $T_1\approx 365.4, T_2=T_1/2, T_3=T_1/4, T_4=T_1/12$; ω_7 represents weekly cycling of socio-cultural component S; $q_i, a_i, b_i, c_j, d_j, a_{ij}, b_{ij}, c_{ij}, d_{ij}, a_{ij}^k, b_{ij}^k$ are the constants obtained from an appropriate multiple regression.

2.2 Modeling Strategy

We realized time-series approach by using repeated-measures regression models. Specifically, we applied generalized estimating equations (GEE) models with an exchangeable working correlation matrix to estimate the population-averaged effect of air pollution on the health outcome. The resulting GEE models could take into account seasonal changes and meteorological variables.

Since dependent variable PEF has a normal distribution, we use the Gaussian family of GEE models.

2.3 Interpretation of the Model

The model we have built is not easy for interpretation, especially when it sets against standard linear models

The model (2.1.2), which is an application of the structural hierarchical model (2.1.1), does not have one but several complicatedly related functional patterns of independent variables. Hence follows, that interpretation of the model should use some sort of "multi-layer" interpretation.

Let us explain such strategy and methodology of interpretation.

We will start reminding that in our case we use GEE-approach to the generalized linear model

$$E(y_{it}) = \mathbf{b} \cdot f_{it}(\mathbf{x}) \tag{2.3.1}$$

of y_{it} with covariates $f_{it}(\mathbf{x})$, where vector $\mathbf{b} = (b_1, b_2, \ldots, b_N)$ with coefficients b_i connected with the certain normal distribution model ($\mathbf{x}$ is the vector of all independent variables).

To realize the approach, we split the whole set of the model independent variables into two sub-sets of "main factors" and "cofactors" (covariates) in accordance with a particular problem of the general study.

For example, assume that we want to evaluate the influence of pollution factor P on health outcome H. Then, we define pollutant variables $P_1, P_1, \ldots P_k$ as "main factors" and consider the rest of independent variables as "co-factors".

Because of multiplicative-additive structure of the GEE model we got, we can transform Equation (2.1.2) into the following form:

$$Y_t = F_0(\mathbf{X}_t, t) + F_1(\mathbf{X}_t, t) \cdot P_1 + F_2(\mathbf{X}_t, t) \cdot P_2 + \ldots + F_k(\mathbf{X}_t, t) \cdot P_k \quad , \tag{2.3.2}$$

where $\mathbf{X}_t$ is the vector of "cofactors" variables.

Let us replace all the coefficients b_i of (2.3.3) included in the functional patterns $F_i(\mathbf{X}_t, t)$ $(i = 0, 1, \ldots, N)$ by their standardized regression coefficients $\beta_i = b_i (\sigma_{x_i} / \sigma_Y)$, and then redefine "new" $F_i(\mathbf{X}_t, t)$ as functions $\phi_i(t)$ (we will call the function $\phi_i(t)$ "profile" of "main factor" P_i).

Now we are ready to introduce the new function $\Phi_{P_i}(t)$ called "cumulative profile" of "main factor" P_i:

$$\Phi_{P_i}(t) = \int_{t_0}^{t} \phi_i(\tau) d\tau \quad . \tag{2.3.3}$$

where t_0 is the start time of the observation period, t is the current time. This function tells us about an overall effect of the particular "main factor" P_i over the period of time $[t_0, t]$. Using the standard calculus of functional analysis for studying minimums and maximums of function $\Phi_{P_i}(t)$, its intervals of increasing and decreasing and so on, we can get the value of contribution of each "main factor" as well as its behavior in the course of observation time.

3 Results

We implemented the described approach for group of 48 adult residents of Leipzig, Germany with vulnerable respiratory system. There were 10,080 individual daily records collected over seven months between October 1990 and April 1991.

The dataset comprised the following types of variables.

Health outcome individual parameters:

- Peak expiration flow (PEF in l/min) measured 3 times a day (in the morning, noon and evening);
- Number of cigarettes smoked daily;
- Hours spent outdoor daily;

(Individual records might start at different times and last for different periods of time.)

Air pollution and meteorological data:

- Daily averaged concentration of sulfur dioxide SO_2 (in mg/m^3)
- Daily averaged concentration of air pollution particle matter (PM) (in mg/m^3);
- Daily maximum, minimum, and mean local temperatures (in centigrade);
- Daily averaged local humidity (in %).

At the first stage of our study, we analyzed temporal behavior of the dependent variable (PEF). Harmonic analysis performed for each of 48 individuals observed in the study and for the whole group has shown up apparent periodic changes in PEF.

To analyze variations between pollution effects at the different time of the day, we modeled the values measured in the morning, noon and evening separately. Results of modeling show, that in the morning both SO2 and PM have significant effects on PEF, while in the afternoon and evening hours only PM pollution has statistically significant effect on PEF; due to the lack of space we present the model results for the morning only (Table 1). The Stata program module `quickmodel_interact` we developed allows automatic optimization of the original model (2.1.2) in accordance with interactions and a given level of significance.

As one can see from Tables 1 some model terms (representing pollutants) have positive coefficients. It would seem confusing and even absurd (pollutants positively affect lungs performance!) if we interpreted the results in the standard way. However, calculating the "cumulative profile" $\Phi_{P_i}(t)$ for pollutants SO2 and PM by taking the integrals of their profiles

$$\Phi_{SO_2}(t)\Big|_{\text{morning}} = \int_{t_0}^{t} \left(0.042 - 0.001 \cdot \text{hmdt}(\tau)\right) d\tau \ , \tag{4.1}$$

$$\Phi_{PM}(t)\Big|_{\text{morning}} = \int_{0}^{t} \Big(0.051 - 0.021 \cdot \sin(\omega_3 \tau) - 0.034 \cdot \cos(\omega_2 \tau) - \\ - 0.042 \cdot \sin(\omega_2 \tau) - 0.093 \cdot \sin(\omega_1 \tau)\Big) d\tau \ , \tag{4.2}$$

we get a meaningful interpretation of the modeling results. In Figures 2-3 we present pictures of the "cumulative profiles" for SO2 and PM in the morning.

Since all the curves of the "cumulative profiles" never leave the negative semi-plane, all the cumulative effects of pollution are negative. Besides, we see that in Figures 2 the curves monotonically descend, while in Figure 3 the curve rises at the end of the observation period. The falling curve apparently represents worsening of adverse effects of the pollutants, meanwhile the growing curve mirrors lessening of those effects.

Table 1. GEE population-averaged model for association between PEF and air pollutants in the mornings (reduced model: terms with $p > 0.1$ removed)

PEF (morning)	Coef.	p-Value	C.I. Min	C.I. Max
outdoor	1.60	0.00	1.16	2.04
So2	17.65	0.15	-6.40	41.69
Pm	49.12	0.04	2.10	96.15
hmdt	0.13	0.02	0.02	0.24
Tmpr	-3.14	0.00	-4.66	-1.62
$sin(\omega_7 t)$	-1.13	0.62	-5.61	3.34
$cos(\omega_3 t)$	1.94	0.03	0.18	3.69
$sin(\omega_3 t)$	5.87	0.00	3.30	8.44
$cos(\omega_2 t)$	4.43	0.09	-0.76	9.61
$sin(\omega_2 t)$	-4.25	0.37	-13.46	4.96
$cos(\omega_1 t)$	7.94	0.22	-4.77	20.66
$sin(\omega_1 t)$	-1.05	0.91	-19.19	17.10
$so2 \times cos(\omega_2 t)$	5.87	0.23	-3.70	15.44
$so2 \times sin(\omega_2 t)$	8.93	0.24	-5.90	23.76
$so2 \times cos(\omega_1 t)$	-3.28	0.78	-26.46	19.91
$so2 \times sin(\omega_1 t)$	8.21	0.61	-23.22	39.63
$pm \times sin(\omega_3 t)$	-19.90	0.00	-31.96	-7.84
$pm \times sin(\omega_2 t)$	-32.54	0.01	-55.99	-9.10
$pm \times cos(\omega_1 t)$	-40.73	0.02	-73.46	-7.99
$pm \times sin(\omega_1 t)$	37.57	0.11	-8.08	83.22
$pm \times sin(\omega_2 t)$	-90.28	0.01	-157.64	-22.92
$hmdt \times sin(\omega_7 t)$	0.04	0.25	-0.03	0.11
$tmpr' cos(\omega 3t)$	-0.61	0.00	-0.94	-0.27
$tmpr' sin(\omega 3t)$	0.57	0.00	0.28	0.86
$tmpr' cos(\omega 2t)$	1.36	0.00	0.64	2.08
$tmpr' sin(\omega 2t)$	2.01	0.00	0.99	3.03
$tmpr' cos(\omega 1t)$	-2.16	0.00	-3.48	-0.84
$tmpr' sin(\omega 1t)$	4.19	0.00	2.12	6.25
$so2' hmdt$	-0.30	0.01	-0.52	-0.09

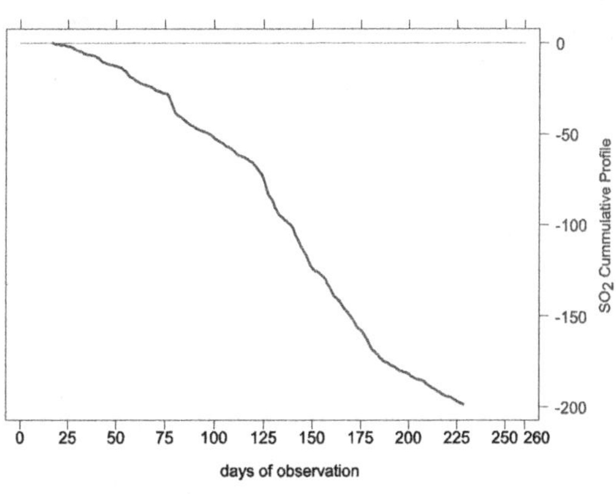

Fig. 2. Cumulative Profile for SO2 in the morning

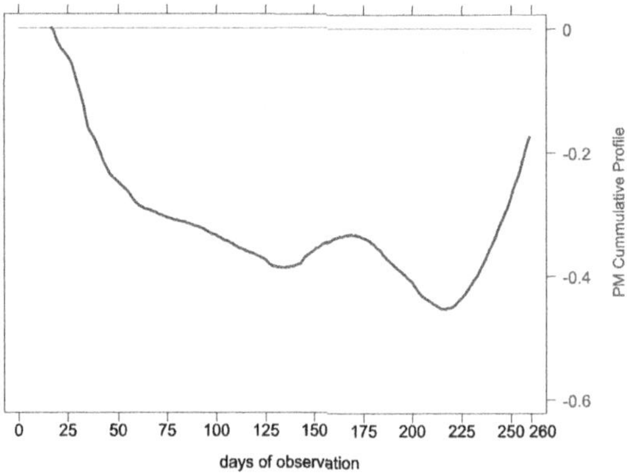

Fig. 3. Cumulative Profile for PM in the morning

References

1. DOMINICI, F., ZEGER, S., SAMET J.(2000) A measurement error model for time-series studies of air pollution and mortality. *Biostatistics*, **1** (2), 157-175.
2. FRIGER, M., NOVACK, Y. & RANFT, U. (2001) Quasi-Fourier Modeling for Individual and Count Outcomes. *Medical Data Analysis,* LNS 2199, 95-10.
3. GOLDSMITH, J., FRIGER, M., ABRAMSON, M.(1996) Associations between Health and Air Pollution a Time-Series Analyses. *Arch Environ Health*, **51**, 358-367.
4. GRAUBIL, F. (1976) *Theory and Application of Linear Models*. New-York: Duxbury Press.
5. LI, C. C. (1975) *Path analysis: A Primer*. Pacific Grove, CA: Boxwood Press.
6. POPE III, C., SCHWARTZ, J.(1996) Time series for the analysis of pulmonary health data. *Am J_Respir Crit Care Med*. **154**, S229-S233.
7. WEDDERBURN, R. (1974) Quasi-likelihood functions, generalized linear models, and the Gauss-Newton method. *Biometrika*, **61**, 439-447.
8. ZEGER S.L., DOMINICI F., MCDERMOTT A., SAMET J.M. (2002) Modeling the Health Effects of Environmental Exposures: Particulate Air Pollution and Mortality in Urban America *in Monitoring the Health of Populations: Statistical Methods for Public Health Surveillance, (Edited by Brookmeyer R. and Stroup D.)*, Oxford University Press, 1-18
9. ZEGER, S., LIANG, K., ALBERT, P. (1988) Models for longitudinal data: a generalized estimating equation approach. *Biometrics*, **44,** 1049-1060.

Replacing Indicator Variables by Fuzzy Membership Functions in Statistical Regression Models: Examples of Epidemiological Studies

Arkady Bolotin

Ben-Gurion University of the Negev, Beersheba, Israel
arkadyv@bgumail.bgu.ac.il

Abstract. The aim of this paper is to demonstrate the possibility of substitution of indicator variables in statistical regression models used in epidemiology for corresponding membership functions. Both methodological and practical aspects of such substitution are considered in this paper through three examples. The first example considers the connection between women's quality of life and categories of Body Mass Index. In the second example we examine death incidence among Bedouin children of different age categories. The third example considers the factors that can affect on high hemoglobin HbA(1c) in diabetic patients.

Nowadays there are many applications of fuzzy sets and systems in many fields such as artificial intelligence, automatic control, pattern recognition, etc. But if there is one domain where fuzzy sets are rather seldom used, that must be statistical analysis. The literature shows that main efforts to bring fuzzy sets into statistical methods are concentrating in two different directions. The first direction (which can be called theoretical one as it is devoted to generalizations of statistical hypotheses to vague hypotheses) investigates attempts to replace the set defining the null hypothesis by a fuzzy set [1-3]. The second direction studies the problem of the data characterization [4, 5]. Despite the importance of both directions, they are quite far from everyday needs of statistical analysis. In our work we want to do with fuzzy sets something more practical. The main purpose of this paper is to consider the possibility to replace indicator variables in statistical regression models by corresponding membership functions. Categorical and indicator variables occur so often in medical data that perhaps they make up the main feature of medical information. A continuous variable measures something, for instance a person's age, height; a city's population or land area. A categorical variable identifies a group to which the thing belongs. For example, one can categorize persons according to their race or ethnicity. An indicator variable denotes whether something is true. For example, is a person's blood pressure high? Indicator variables allow controlling for the effect of a variable in a regression model. For instance, instead of the linear regression

$$y = \alpha + \beta[x]\cdot \mathbf{X} + \beta[z]\cdot z + \varepsilon \qquad (1)$$

where $\mathbf{X}$, z are some variables; y is the outcome (dependent variable); $\beta[x]$, $\beta[z]$ are the regression coefficients; α is the constant (intercept); and ε is the residual; we can control for z in the following regression

J.M. Barreiro et al. (Eds.): ISBMDA 2004, LNCS 3337, pp. 251–258, 2004.

$$y = \alpha + \boldsymbol{\beta}[x]\cdot \mathbf{X} + \beta[z\,1,]\cdot \delta[z\,1,] + \beta[z\,2,]\cdot \delta[z\,2,] + \ldots + \beta[n\,z-1]\cdot \delta[n\,z-1] + \varepsilon \;, \qquad (2)$$

where $\delta[z,j]$ is 1 if z is in category j and 0 otherwise. However, the lack of medical information, and its imprecise, and sometimes contradictory can make the process of converting continuous to indicator variables very difficult one. For example, systolic blood pressure above 150 mmHg generally considered high. Does it mean that a person's blood pressure equal to, say, 149.999 mmHg would be normal? At the same time, fuzzy sets are known for their ability to introduce notions of continuity into deductive thinking. In fuzzy logic, the truth of any statement becomes a matter of degree. In other words, fuzzy sets allow the use of conventional symbolic systems in continuous form. Practically, this means that we can try to replace the crisp set of categories of a variable in a regression model by the corresponding fuzzy set. For example, we can replace the equation (2) by the following one

$$y = \alpha + \boldsymbol{\beta}[x]\cdot \mathbf{X} + \beta[z\,1,]\cdot \mu[z\,1,] + \beta[z\,2,]\cdot \mu\,[z\,2,] + \ldots + \beta[n\,z-1]\cdot \mu\,[n\,z-1] + \varepsilon, \qquad (3)$$

where $\mu[z,j] \in [0,1]$ determines the degree to what z is in category j. It is necessary to emphasize that statistical regression model (3) has nothing to do with fuzzy linear regression (FLR) models. Even though we replace indicator variables in (2) by the membership functions, model (3) is still a traditional regression model with all the strict assumptions of the statistical model. On the other hand, FLR, which was first introduced by Tanaka et al. [6], relaxes some of the statistical model assumptions. The basic FLR model supposes a fuzzy linear function as

$$\tilde{Y} = \tilde{\beta}\,[0]\cdot X\,[0] + \tilde{\beta}\,[1]\cdot X\,[1] + \ldots + \tilde{\beta}\,[N]\cdot X\,[N] = \tilde{\beta}\cdot \mathrm{X}\,, \qquad (4)$$

where $\mathbf{X}$ is a vector of independent variables; $\tilde{\beta}$ is a vector of fuzzy coefficients presented in the form of symmetric triangular fuzzy numbers denoted by the form

$$\tilde{\beta}\,[i] = \{\, b[i],\, c[i]\} = \{\, \tilde{\beta}\,[i]\colon b\,[i] - c[i] \le \tilde{\beta}\,[i] \le\; b[i] + c[i]\,\}\,, \qquad (5)$$

where $b\,[i]$ is the center and $c\,[i]$ is the half-width of $\tilde{\beta}[i]$. One of the explanations of the width c is that $c = 0$ means that X directly influences $\tilde{Y}$, and $c \neq 0$ means X indirectly influences $\tilde{Y}$. In other words, the relationship between X and $\tilde{Y}$ cannot be expressed as a simple linear function because many other factors may be included in the relation. Since the FLR analysis can be applied to many real-life problems in which the strict assumptions of classical regression analysis cannot be satisfied, there are many researchers devoted to the field of FLR. However, there are critiques regarding FLR models such as: no proper interpretation about the fuzzy regression interval [7]; issue of forecasting has yet been addressed [8]. In this paper we will concentrate on the proposed fuzzy approach to traditional statistical modeling, and through three examples we will show how it works in practice.

Example 1. Connection Between Quality of Life and Body Mass Index

In the first example we use records collected with the help of the World Health Organization (WHO) Quality of Life Short Version Questionnaire QOL in the group of 104 women (aged in the interval from 17 to 62 years old) with school or university background (the study was a part of the Longitudinal Investigation of Depression Outcome conducted by Prof. Lily Neumann at the Ben-Gurion University of the

Negev [9]). We have data on women's quality of life value (`qol`) and Body Mass Index (`bmi`).

Experts of WHO generally consider a BMI bellow 20 to be underweight and a BMI of 20 to 25 to be healthy. BMIs of 25 to 30 are generally considered overweight as a BMI over 30 is generally considered very overweight (obese). Assume we wish to predict a woman's quality of life on the basis of which one of the following four categories her BMI belongs to: (1) underweight BMI, (2) healthy BMI, (3) overweight BMI, or (4) obese BMI. We can do it by estimating the following four linear regression models:

$$\mathtt{qol}[j] = \alpha[j] + \beta[j] \cdot \mathtt{bmi}[j] + \varepsilon[j], \quad \text{(E1.1)}$$

where $j = 1, 2, 3, 4$; $\alpha[j]$ are the constants (or intercepts), $\beta[j]$ are the regression coefficients, and $\varepsilon[j]$ are the residuals. Within the frame of classical (crisp) approach, `bmi`$[j]$ are indicator (dummy) variables specifying whether is true (`bmi`$[j] = 1$) that a woman's BMI is in category j or otherwise (`bmi`$[j] = 0$), while in accordance with fuzzy approach, `bmi`$[j]$ are membership functions (MFs) specifying the degree ($0 \leq$ `bmi`$[j] \leq 1$) a woman's BMI belongs to category j.

For fuzzification, we use the simplest straight line MFs: triangular and trapezoidal ones; they are shown in Figure 1.

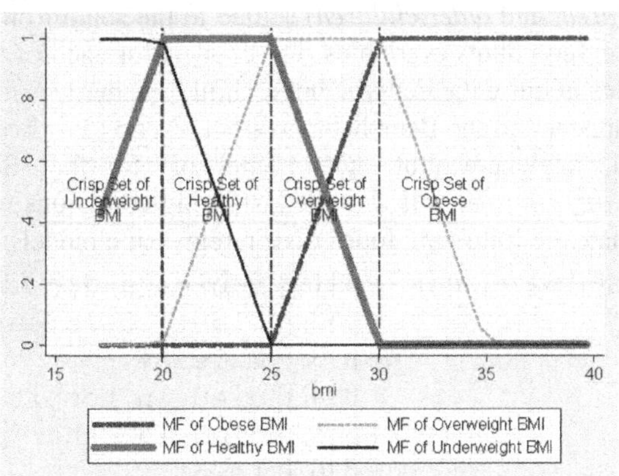

Fig. 1. Crisp and fuzzy sets of BMI categories

The results of the linear regression models on indicator variables or MF are given away in Table 1.

As one can see from the table, the regression models of `qol` on indicator variables `bmi`$[j]$ failed to estimate the coefficients for underweight and overweight BMIs (with the significance less than 0.05), but the regression models on MFs did not. According to the late ones, women with definitely underweight BMIs have the highest linear prediction of quality of life: 29.07 + 61.73 = 90.8.

Example 2. Analysis of Death Incidence Among Bedouin Children

In the second example, we want to analyze the number of deaths of: (1) home injures, (2) sudden deaths, (3) deaths of road injures, and (4) deaths of other causes among

Table 1. Table of the estimated regression coefficients (β), standard errors (Δβ) and two-sided significance level (p-value) for the quality of life value on different categories of BMI

Variables in equation	Crisp Set of **BMI** categories		Fuzzy Set of **BMI** categories	
	$\beta \pm \Delta\beta$	p-value	$\beta \pm \Delta\beta$	p-value
			Model 1	
Underweight BMI	13.26 ± 12.78	0.302	29.07 ± 5.12	0.000
constant	69.02 ± 2.17	0.000	61.73 ± 2.31	0.000
			Model 2	
Healthy BMI	24.15 ± 3.65	0.000	24.52 ± 3.68	0.000
constant	59.41 ± 2.35	0.000	57.72 ± 2.51	0.000
			Model 3	
Overweight BMI	-7.29 ± 8.55	0.396	16.54 ± 5.56	0.004
constant	69.89 ± 2.22	0.000	64.56 ± 2.63	0.000
			Model 4	
Obese BMI	-23.09 ± 3.64	0.000	-24.43 ± 3.61	0.000
constant	80.72 ± 2.55	0.000	81.92 ± 2.57	0.000

Bedouin children of different age categories (such as *babies and toddlers*, *early school years children*, and *older children*) settled to the south from Beersheba, Israel. We have the observed counts (variables `deaths[j]`) for each of these four events *j*, and other variables in our data are: whether a child's gender was masculine (`males`), whether death happened in the Beersheba hospital (`died_in_hospital`), whether death happened anywhere but not home or in the Beersheba hospital (`died_in_other_place`), whether the last living conditions were urban (`town`). We wish to estimate the following four Poisson regression models:

$$\begin{aligned}\texttt{deaths}[j] = \exp\{\, \alpha[j] \; & + \beta[1,j]\cdot \texttt{babies\_and\_toddlers} + \\ & + \beta[2,j]\cdot \texttt{older\_children} + \\ & + \beta[3,j]\cdot \texttt{males} + \\ & + \beta[4,j]\cdot \texttt{died\_in\_hospital} + \\ & + \beta[5,j]\cdot \texttt{died\_in\_other\_place} + \\ & + \beta[6,j]\cdot \texttt{town}\} \end{aligned} \tag{E2.1}$$

(j = 1, 2, 3, 4). Variables `babies_and_toddlers` and `older_children` are either indicator ones (specifying whether is true that an individual was in the respective age category), or MFs (specifying the degree an individual belonged to the respective age category). In the study, which was carried out at the Ben-Gurion University of the Negev [10], the following indicator variables denoting the age categories were made:

$$\begin{aligned} \texttt{babies\_and\_toddlers} &= \begin{cases} 1, & 0 \le \texttt{age} \le 4 \\ 0, & \texttt{otherwise} \end{cases} \\ \texttt{early\_school\_years\_children} &= \begin{cases} 1, & 4 \le \texttt{age} \le 9 \\ 0, & \texttt{otherwise} \end{cases} \\ \texttt{older\_children} &= \begin{cases} 1, & \texttt{age} \le 9 \\ 0, & \texttt{otherwise} \end{cases} \end{aligned} \tag{E2.2}$$

where age is given in years. The fuzzy sets of the age categories are determined by the following MFs:

$$\texttt{babies\_and\_toddlers} = \exp(-\texttt{age})$$

$$\texttt{early\_school\_years\_children} = \exp\left(\frac{(7-\texttt{age})^2}{4}\right)$$

$$\texttt{older\_children} = \begin{cases} 0, & \texttt{age} < 7 \\ \frac{\texttt{age}-7}{7}, & 7 \le \texttt{age} \le 14 \\ 1, & \texttt{age} > 14 \end{cases} \qquad \text{(E2.3)}$$

The results of the Poisson maximum-likelihood regression of `deaths`[*j*] on indicator variables (E2.2) or MFs (E2.3) are presented in Table 2.

We can see from this table that the models on the fuzzy sets of the age categories are better in a sense than those build on indicator variables (E2.2). Indeed, as it follows from Table 2, only with the fuzzy sets we can predict the rate at which deaths of home injures among Bedouin babies and toddlers occur home (i.e when a child was pronounced dead at the scene and not later in the hospital or on the way to the hospital): *rate* = *exp*(-0.96-1.94) = 0.055. Also, models on the indicator variables failed to estimate the incidence rate ratio for sudden deaths, deaths of road injures and other causes among Bedouin babies and toddlers. For instance, with the help of fuzzy approach we estimate that the rate of sudden death is *exp*(1.79) = 5.99 times larger for babies and toddlers than for early school years children.

Example 3. Study on High Hemoglobin HbA(1c) in Diabetic Patients

In the previous examples we discussed regression models on (independent) indicator variables which were being replaced by fuzzy membership functions (MFs). Now we will consider the possibility to replace a dependent indicator variable of a regression model by a corresponding MF. We will use the data obtained from the panel study of hemoglobin HbA(1c) levels in diabetic patients done by Prof. S. Weitzman of the Ben-Gurion University of the Negev and his colleagues [11]. These data were collected in the calendar period January 1997 through November 2003. Participants were adult patients with diabetes mellitus living in Israel. Each patient completed two interviews and several tests in different time before and after the interviews. The independent variables in the data are: the current age of a patient in years (`age`), elapsing years of diabetes (`years_of_diabetes`), whether a patient was treated with insulin (`insulin_treatment`), whether the tests were done after the second interview (`second_interview`), whether the tests and interviews were carried out in one of the clinics situated in the South of Israel (`south`). We want to know if any of the above mentioned independent variables has influence on the high level of hemoglobin HbA(1c) (`high_hba1c`). We wish to estimate the following random-effects linear models:

Table 2. Table of the estimated Poisson regression coefficients (β), standard errors (Δβ) and two-sided significance level (p-value) for death incidence on different age categories

Variables in equation	Crisp set of **age** categories		Fuzzy set of **age** categories	
	$\beta \pm \Delta\beta$	p-value	$\beta \pm \Delta\beta$	p-value
	(1) Deaths of home Injures			
Babies and toddlers	-1.10 ± 0.48	0.023	-1.94 ± 0.55	0.000
Older children	0.35 ± 0.61	0.560	0.31 ± 0.65	0.640
Males	-0.30 ± 0.35	0.385	-0.37 ± 0.34	0.284
Died in hospital	-1.52 ± 0.39	0.000	-1.15 ± 0.38	0.003
Died in other place	-1.76 ± 1.00	0.079	-1.83 ± 0.99	0.065
Town	-0.47 ± 0.39	0.903	-0.01 ± 0.38	0.984
constant	-0.72 ± 0.40	0.058	-0.96 ± 0.31	0.002
	(2) Sudden Deaths			
Babies and toddlers	0.97 ± 0.95	0.310	1.79 ± 0.51	0.000
Older children	-13.84 ± 1.01	0.000	-59.62 ± 7.67	0.000
Males	0.15 ± 0.37	0.692	0.23 ± 0.35	0.512
Died in hospital	-3.89 ± 0.73	0.000	-4.35 ± 0.75	0.000
Died in other place	-18.44 ± 0.28	0.000	-21.73 ± 0.27	0.000
Town	0.01 ± 0.38	0.988	-0.12 ± 0.34	0.715
constant	-2.28 ± 1.00	0.023	-2.67 ± 0.77	0.000
	(3) Deaths of Road Injures			
Babies and toddlers	-2.22 ± 0.67	0.001	-3.10 ± 0.99	0.002
Older children	-1.11 ± 0.63	0.078	-0.45 ± 0.55	0.413
Males	0.18 ± 0.50	0.713	0.29 ± 0.43	0.497
Died in hospital	15.02 ± 0.27	0.000	15.62 ± 0.80	0.000
Died in other place	(not estimated)		18.05 ± 0.73	0.000
Town	0.61 ± 0.34	0.076	-0.06 ± 0.33	0.844
constant	-17.41 ± 0.28	0.000	-18.19 ± 0.79	0.000
	(4) Deaths of Other causes			
Babies and toddlers	0.43 ± 0.23	0.057	0.14 ± 0.07	0.028
Older children	0.34 ± 0.24	0.158	-0.16 ± 0.22	0.485
Males	-0.00 ± 0.03	0.899	-0.01 ± 0.03	0.855
Died in hospital	0.50 ± 0.10	0.000	0.48 ± 0.10	0.000
Died in other place	-0.03 ± 0.18	0.849	-0.02 ± 0.18	0.907
Town	-0.01 ± 0.03	0.731	**-0.01 ± 0.03**	**0.759**
constant	-0.97 ± 0.24	0.000	-0.63 ± 0.11	0.000

$$\begin{aligned}\texttt{high\_hba1c}[t\,i] = \alpha &+ \beta[1]\cdot\texttt{age}[t\,i] + \\ &+\beta[2]\cdot\texttt{years\_of\_diabetes}\ [t\,i] + , \\ &+\beta[3]\cdot\texttt{insulin\_treatment}[t\,i] + \\ &+\beta[4]\cdot\texttt{second\_interview}\ [t\,i] +, \\ &+\beta[5]\cdot\texttt{south}[t\,i] + , \\ &+\nu[i\,] + \varepsilon[t\,i\,]\end{aligned} \tag{E3.1}$$

where index i specifies the unique patient number; index t specifies time of observation; $\nu[i\,]$ is the random effect; and $\varepsilon[i,t\,]$ is the residual. Outcome high_hba1c$[i,t\,]$ is either the indicator variable specifying whether a patient's hemoglobin is high, or the MF specifying to what extent a patient's hemoglobin is high. Medical experts on diabetes generally consider the hemoglobin HbA(1c) level above 9.5 high. So, the definition of outcome `high_hba1c`$[i,t]$ as an indicator variable could be as follows

$$\texttt{high\_hba1c}[i,t] = \begin{cases} 1, & \texttt{hba1c}[i,t] \geq 9.5 \\ 0, & \text{otherwise,} \end{cases} \tag{E3.2}$$

and the definition of outcome `high_hba1c`$[i,t]$ as a membership function could be as follows

$$\texttt{high\_hba1c}[i,t] = 1 - \exp\left[-\left[\frac{\texttt{hba1c}[i,t]}{9.5}\right]^8 \right] \tag{E3.3}$$

Calculating the regression model of indicator variable (E3.2) and the regression model of MF (E3.3) we get the result presented in Table 3.

Table 3. Table of the longitudinal regression coefficients (β), standard errors (Δβ) and two-sided significance level (p-value) for high hemoglobin HbA(1c)

Variables in equation	Crisp set of **high HbA(1c)** (Model of (E3.2))		Fuzzy set of **high HbA(1c)** (Model of (E3.3))	
	$\beta \pm \Delta\beta$	p-value	$\beta \pm \Delta\beta$	p-value
Age (in years)	-0.004 ± 0.002	0.012	-0.004 ± 0.002	0.007
Years of diabetes	0.003 ± 0.002	0.139	0.004 ± 0.001	0.026
Insulin treatment	0.113 ± 0.058	0.051	0.130 ± 0.051	0.012
Second interview	-0.060 ± 0.028	0.028	-0.040 ± 0.019	0.039
South	-0.068 ± 0.033	0.044	-0.075 ± 0.030	0.012
constant	0.481 ± 0.111	0.000	0.578 ± 0.104	0.000

Unlike of the model of indicator variable (E3.2), the model of MF (E3.3) reveals that all of the independent variables in the study have an effect on high hemoglobin HbA(1c). For instance, this model estimates that the advance in years of diabetes increases the degree a patient's hemoglobin is high at the rate 0.004 per year; that insulin treatment lifts up this degree by, all things held constant, approximately 13%.

Assessing goodness of fit we calculated the linear prediction including random effect (fitted values) for each model, the results of this calculation is graphically presented in Figure 2.

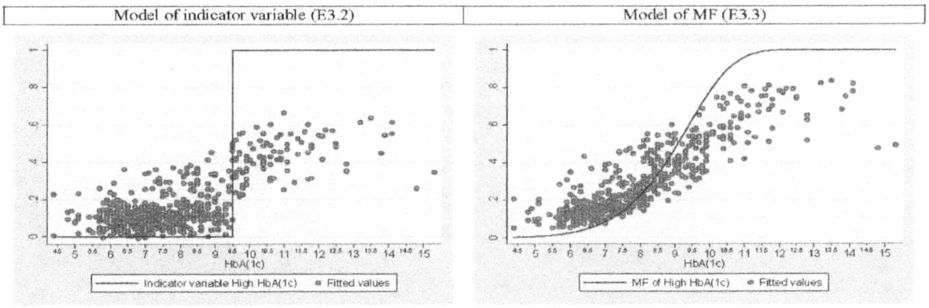

Fig. 2. Outcome `high_hba1c` vs. fitted values

As we can see, the model based on fuzzy approach is also better in terms of goodness of fit.

References

1. Arnold B.F.: Statistical tests optimally meeting certain fuzzy requirements on the power function and on the sample size. Fuzzy Sets and Systems 75 (1995) 365–372
2. Slowinski R. (ed.): The Handbooks of Fuzzy Sets Series. Fuzzy Sets in Decision Analysis, Operations Re- search and Statistics. Kluwer Academic Publishers, Boston London Dordrecht (2001)
3. Holena M.: Fuzzy hypotheses testing in the framework of fuzzy logic. Fuzzy Sets and Systems 145 (2004) 229–252
4. Manton K., Woodbury M., Tolley H.: Statistical applications using fuzzy sets. Wiley, New York, (1994)
5. Loslever P, Popieul J.C., Simon P.: From classic statistical characterization to fuzzy windowing based char- acterization for the exploratory analysis of miscellaneous time variables: example in the field of car driving studies. Fuzzy Sets and Systems 137 (2003) 271–296
6. Tanaka H., Ishibuchi H.: Possibilistic regression analysis based on linear programming, in: Fuzzy Regres- sion Analysis. Omnitech Press, Warsaw and Physica-Verlag, Heidelberg (1992) 47-60
7. Wang H.-F., Tsaur R.-C.: Insight of a fuzzy regression model. Fuzzy Sets and Systems 112 (2000) 355-369
8. Pedrycz W., Savic D.A.: Evaluation of fuzzy regression models. Fuzzy Sets and Systems 39 (1991) 51-63
9. Neumann L., Sukenik S., Bolotin A., Abu-Shakra M., Amir M., Flusser D., Buskila D.: The effect of bal- neotherapy at the Dead Sea on quality of life of patients with fibromialgia syndrome. Clinical Rheumatology 20 (2001) 15-16
10. Broides A; Assaf M.: Home accidents in Arab Bedouin children in southern Israel. J Child Health Care 7(3) (2003) 207-214
11. Bilenko N., Shahar D., Shai I., Weitzman S., Fraser D.: Prevalence and characteristics of myocardial infarc- tion, diabetes and hypertension in the adult Jewish population: results from the Negev Nutritional Study. Harefuah 142(1) (2003) 17-21

PCA Representation of ECG Signal as a Useful Tool for Detection of Premature Ventricular Beats in 3-Channel Holter Recording by Neural Network and Support Vector Machine Classifier

Stanisław Jankowski[1], Jacek J. Dusza[1], Mariusz Wierzbowski[1], and Artur Oręziak[2]

[1] Warsaw University of Technology, Institute of Electronic Systems,
ul. Nowowiejska 15/19, 00-665 Warszawa, Poland
{sjank,jdusza}@ise.pw.edu.pl, mwierzbo@elka.pw.edu.pl
[2] 1st Department of Cardiology, Medical University of Warsaw,
ul. Banacha 1 A, 02-097 Warszawa, Poland
artur.oreziak@amwaw.edu.pl

Abstract. In the paper classification method of compressed ECG signal was presented. Classification of single heartbeats was performed by neural networks and support vector machine. Parameterization of ECG signal was realized by principal component analysis (PCA). For every heartbeat only two descriptors have been used. The results of real Holter signal were presented in tables and as plots in planespherical coordinates. The efficiency of classification is near to 99%.

1 Introduction

The shape analysis of ECG signal is one of basic non-invasive diagnostic method [9]. It allows making an assessment of myocardium state. The examination of arrhythmia and sporadically episode detection requires the analysis of long sequences of heartbeats. It corresponds to the number of ECG cycles up to more than 100 000. Review of such long records is rather hard task. Therefore, automatic morphological analysis of Holter ECG recordings can be considered as a useful diagnostic tool.

In this work automatic classifiers based on neural multi-layer perceptron (MLP) and support vector machine (SVM) are presented. The Classifier Efficiency defined as a quotient of correctly classified patterns to total number of testing patterns in both cases reaches 99%.

The computation speed of classification and its effectiveness is obtained due to signal compression and particular parameterization method. For each heartbeat description only two parameters were used. Such a small number of descriptors allow us to apply a training set containing not too many patterns. For parameterization of 3-channel ECG Holter recording, Principal Component Analysis (PCA) method was applied [1, 4, 7].

In section 2 the dataset considered in this paper is taken from 3-channel Holter monitor that registers three quasi-orthogonal components of electric potential from the heart action. We attempt to reconstruct the trajectory of heart potential in three dimensional phase space by using signals from each channel as ($x(t)$, $y(t)$, $z(t)$) components. In sections 3 and 4 we present preprocessing (filtration and segmentation) and parameterization of single heartbeats by covariance matrix calculation and its

J.M. Barreiro et al. (Eds.): ISBMDA 2004, LNCS 3337, pp. 259–268, 2004.

eigenvalues and eigenvectors. The results of classification for MLP and SVM with linear separating function are presented in section 5.

2 ECG Signal Recording

A pair of electrodes placed on the patient body can record potential of the connecting point caused by electric charge stored in myocardium, which is variable in the time. It is a basis of operation of Holter monitor, which serves us to 24-hours monitoring of heart action. Usually Holter monitor has 3 pairs of electrodes performing quasi-orthogonal system of coordinates. An example of 3-channel ECG Holter recording containing 19 heartbeats is presented in Fig. 1.

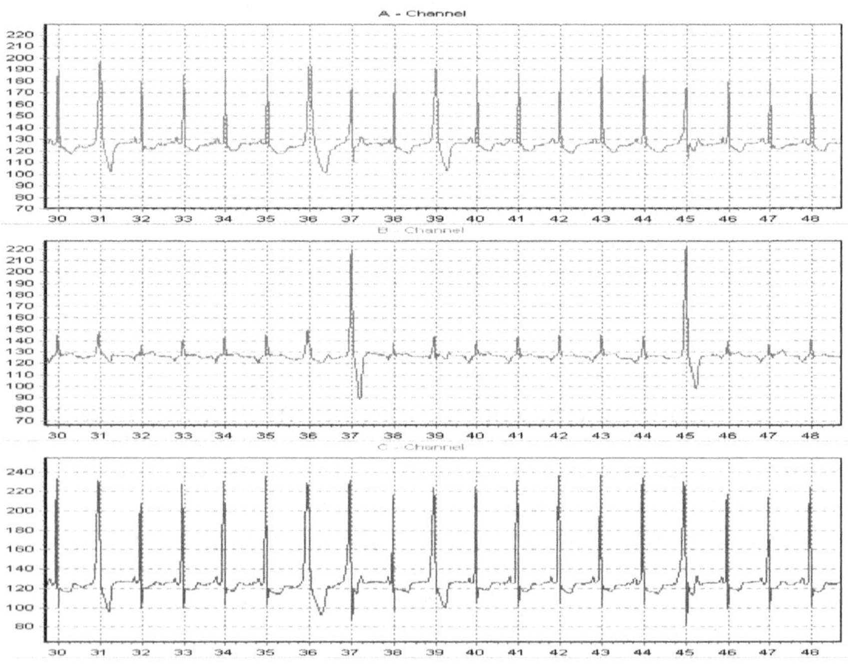

Fig. 1. Example of 3-channel Holter recording

Suppose that each signal is a parametric function of the time x(t), y(t) and z(t). At any moment t_0 three coordinates of the points in 3-dimmensional space can be calculated. In this way we can reconstruct the trace of the electric vector in 3-dimmensional space as a trajectory, which is shown in Fig 2. The time is a parameter. For any single normal heartbeat the trajectory consist of 3 loops. The greatest one corresponds on QRS wave and two small loops represent P and T waves respectively. Single trajectory as a 3- dimensional object can be places into rectangular prism. The lengths of the edges are proportional to eigenvalues and orientation of rectangular prism depends on eigenvectors of covariance matrix. The trajectory is not regular or symmetrical object but we can indicate the direction of its greatest changes. It is the same as a direction of one from 4 diagonals of the rectangular prism.

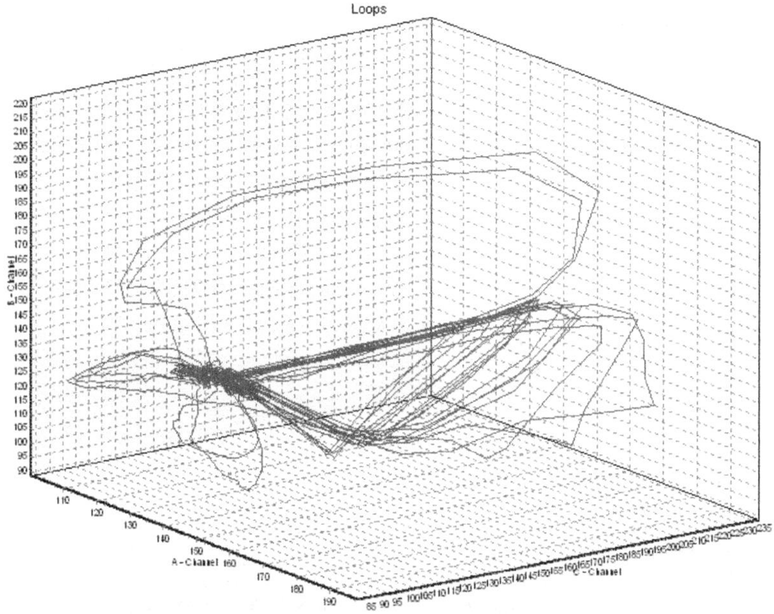

Fig. 2. Vectocardiograms of 19 ECG cycles presented as a time series in Fig. 1. The greatest loops correspond to QRS waves of two types of heartbeats, two small loops represents T waves. The third loop (P wave) is almost invisible

This direction can be determined, when calculation of eigenvectors of covariance matrix of phase space trajectory are provided. It depends on the shape of trajectory. Therefore is related to the morphology of Holter signals.

3 Principal Component Analysis for Parameterization of ECG Cycles

We take into account that:

The direction of the electric vector field of the heart averaged over duration time of separated beat depends on the propagation of excitation signal in the conduction system of myocardium.

The ECG Holter recording is subjected to segmentation into intervals corresponding to single heartbeats. Every cycle is related to R wave of ECG and contains 30% of $R_{n-1}R_n$ interval and 70% of R_nR_{n+1} interval. For each heartbeat the Holter signal can be presented as a signal matrix $S^k = [s_{ij}]^k$, where:

k - number of heartbeat,

i – number of channel,

j – number of samples in single beat recording.

Now if covariance matrix is calculated as follows:

$$\mathbf{C}^k = \frac{1}{N}\mathbf{S}^k \cdot \left(\mathbf{S}^k\right)^T, \tag{1}$$

where N – number of samples, we obtain compressed signal, but information about its energy (the elements on diagonal are proportional to the square of RMS values of each channel) and correlation between the pairs of signal (the rest of elements of matrix C are dot product of every two signals) is not lost. The elements of covariance matrix not depend on the time and can be considered as an integral of time measures or average of sample values.

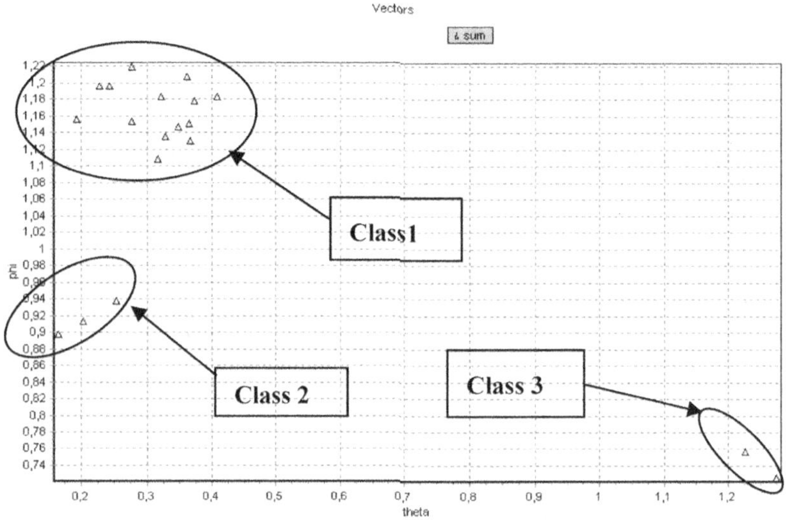

Fig. 3. Directions of resultant vectors in planespherical coordinates

After calculation of eigenvalues λ_i and unit eigenvectors $\mathbf{v}_i$ (i = 1, 2, 3) of covariance matrix **C** one can obtain the resultant vector of electric field of charge distribution in myocardium and averaged over time, as bellow

$$\mathbf{W} = \lambda_1\mathbf{v}_1 + \lambda_2\mathbf{v}_2 + \lambda_3\mathbf{v}_3 \tag{2}$$

For the signal shown in previous figures, vectors **W** were calculated and presented in Fig. 3. Planespherical coordinates show us two angles (*theta* and *phi*) which are identical to those of spatial polar coordinates, but the absolute value of vector is not indicated.

This initial analysis indicates a very strong relation of the direction of the resultant vector of electric field to the shape of ECG signal recorded by the Holter monitor.

4 Data Preparation

The patient P101 suffered from arrhythmia was observed in Department of Cardiology, Medical University of Warsaw. 24-hour ambulatory ECG monitoring was performed using a 3-channel Oxford Medilog FD3 recorder and was evaluated by an Oxford Medilog Excel 2 analysis system [8]. Approximately 120000 heartbeats were registered; the average heart rate was 83 bpm (range 56-92 bpm). The sinus rhythm, ventricular premature beats from 3 foci and couplet episodes were observed in the analysis of ECG. Therefore at least 2 types of pathological beats were recorded.

Especially for this publication from whole Holter recording a part containing 1000 consecutive heartbeat, where all 3 types of shapes appear, was chosen. There are 3 digital signals corresponding to 3 channels. Data sets are written as integer numbers from 0 to 255 in `txt` format. The sampling frequency was 128 Hz. All signals was filtered in order to eliminate high-frequency disturbance (noise, crashes and electromagnetic interference) and low-frequency disturbance (respiration and patient motion components). Also isoelectic line (zero level) has been specified. The separation into single heartbeats is performed by determination of R waves.

For each heartbeat the covariance matrix, eigenvalues and unit eigenvectors were calculated. The obtained resultant vectors (3) were transformed into spatial polar coordinates (□, □, □). Hence, each heartbeat can be represented as a pair of descriptors (□, □). This form is useful to present on the plane or as a three-dimensional vector. On the basis of initial result presented in part 2 we made an assumption that two-parameter representation (defining only the direction of resultant vector) of single heartbeat is sufficient for automatic classification of ECG cycles shape.

5 Results of Classification

Automatic classification of heartbeat shape was performed using two methods: MLP [1] and SVM [6, 10]. In both cases the simplest separating function was chosen, e.i. linear function. The set of 1000 examples (two-dimensional vectors) was separated in two subsets. The training set consisted of 100 initial heartbeats. Cardiologist distinguished three classes of heartbeat shapes: Ist – normal (70 examples); IInd – ventricular beats from 1st focus (VPB_1) (9 examples); IIIrd – ventricular beats from 2nd focus (VPB_2) (21 examples). Their distribution in planespherical coordinates is shown in Fig. 4.

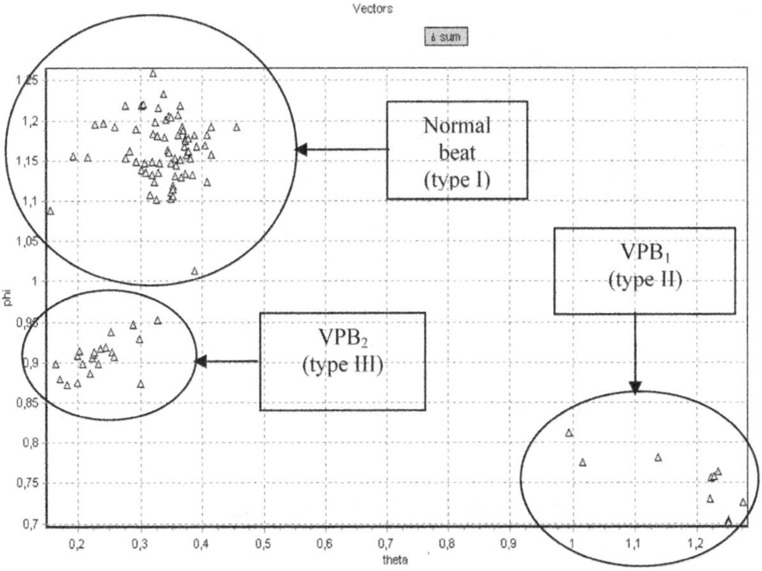

Fig. 4. Distribution of training examples in (phi-theta)-plane (ECG cycles from 1 to 100)

The shapes of Holter recording in 3 channels and corresponding phase trajectories for 3 classes defined earlier were shown in Fig. 5.

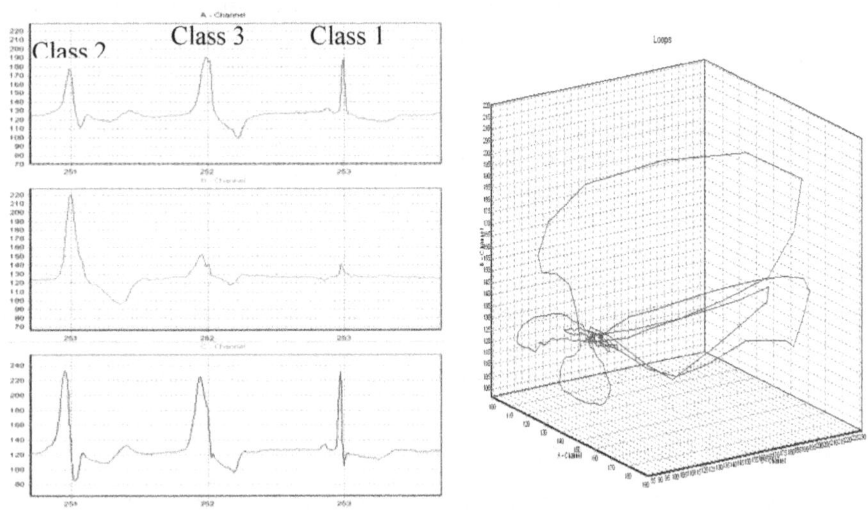

Fig. 5. 3-channel Holter recording and phase space trajectory for individual classes

5.1 Result of Neural Network Classification

The first type o f classifier was a neural multilayer perceptron composed of 2 inputs, 2 hidden neurons and 3 output neurons, as shown in Fig. 6.

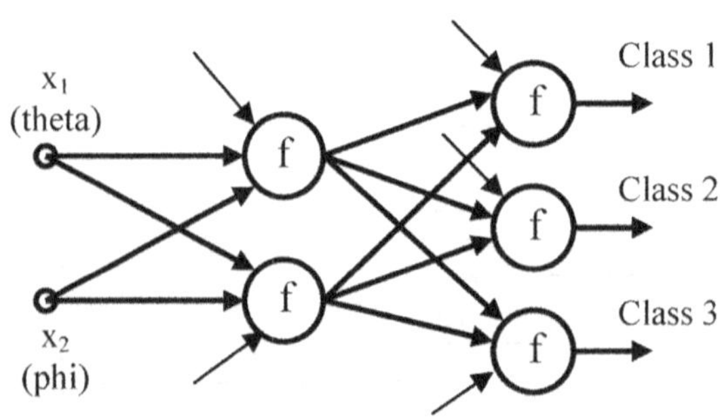

$$f(x) = \frac{2}{1+e^{-2x}} - 1$$

$$x_j = \sum_i w_{ij} x_i$$

Fig. 6. Neural network diagram and its activation function, biases are shown by thin arrows

The result of classification of the test set containing 900 heartbeat examples (from 101 to 1000) is presented in Fig.7 and in tables I. The classification quality defined as a quotient of well-classified patterns to all patterns was calculated for each class separately and totally.

5.2 Result of Support Vector Machine Classification

The next tested classifier was SVM with linear kernel. This type of kernel we chose because of small dimension of the parameter space and result of previous observation

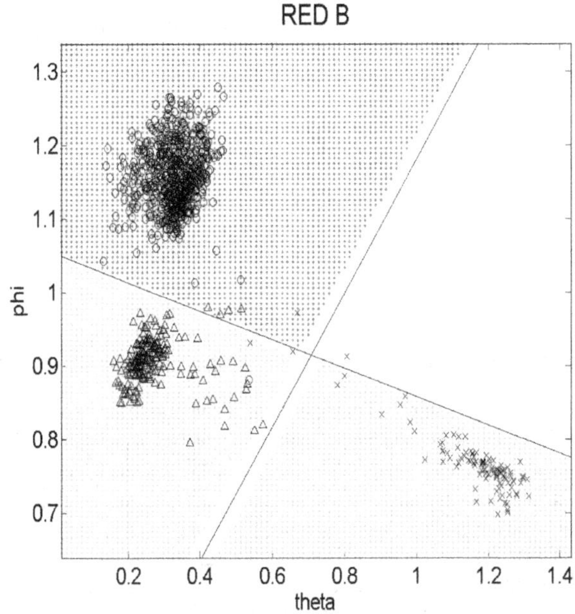

Fig. 7. Result of neural classifier for the test set of 900 examples

Table 1. Testing and verification of MLP B

	Class 1	Class 2	Class 3	TOTAL
Number of examples	619	96	185	900
Good classification	618	92	180	890
Wrong classification	1	2	4	7
Not classified	0	2	1	3
Score [%]	99,8	95,8	97,3	98,9

of eigenvectors directions. The classification type "one class against the others" was performed 3 times. The training set was the same like in the case of MLP classifiers. The following figures present separating lines between particular classes and positions of the support vectors. It can be seen that in every case the separating line and margins are defined by 3 support vectors.

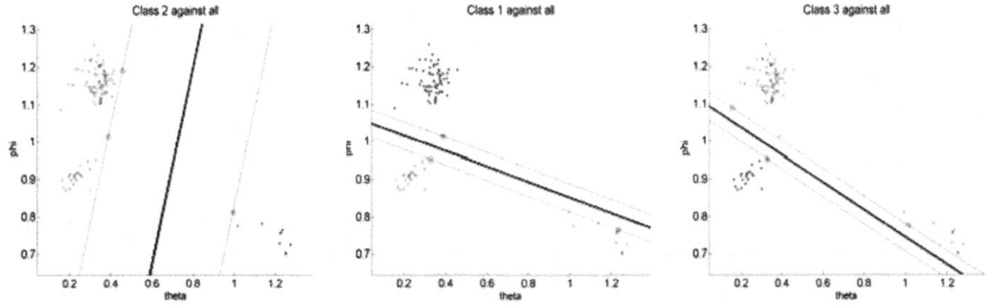

Fig. 8. Results of SVM training

The results of SVM classification for testing set are shown in Fig. 9 and in table II.

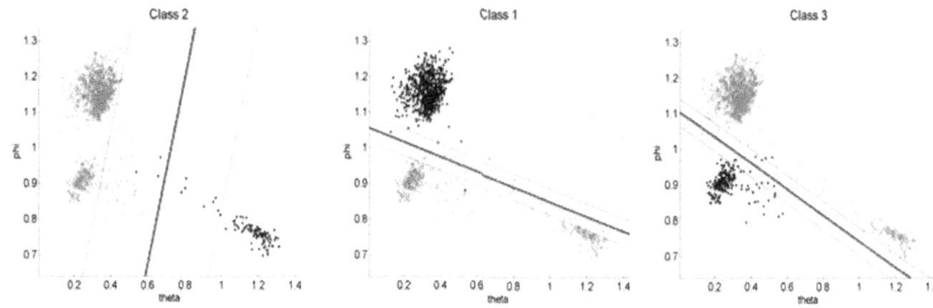

Fig. 9. Result of SVM classification for the test set of 900 examples

Table 2. Test results of SVM classifier

	Class 1	Class 2	Class 3	TOTAL
Number of examples	619	96	185	900
Support vectors	3	3	3	
Correct classification	618	94	181	893
Incorrect classification	1	0	4	5
Not classified	0	2	0	2
Score [%]	99,8	97,9	97,8	99,2

In order to explain the reason of wrong classification cases we compared Holter recording of 3 successive cycles, where the central one was classified incorrectly to similar sequence well classified. Both plots are presented in Fig. 10.

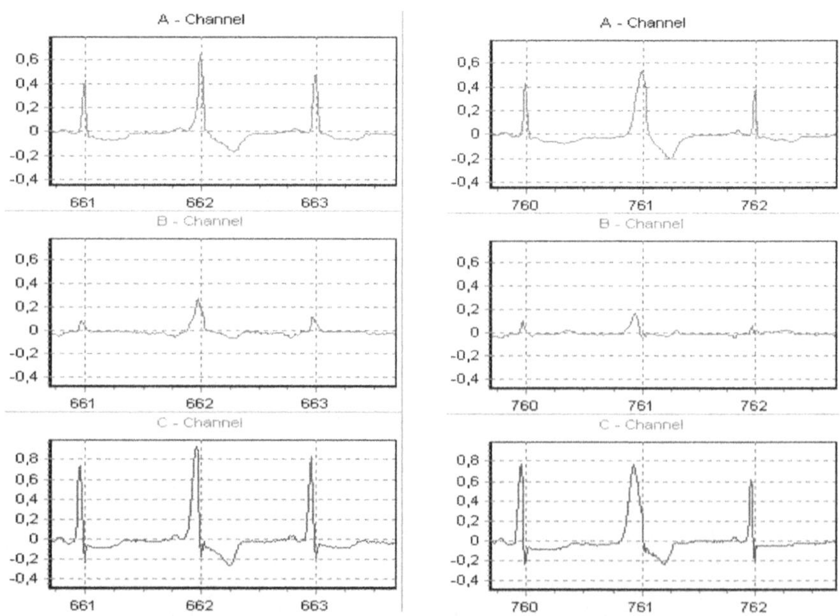

Fig. 10. Incorrect (on the left) and correct (on the right) classification of sequence 1, 3, 1. The central heartbeat on the left chart was classified as class 1 (normal)

We can notice that the central beat in both plots have different shapes. It is very subjective question to decide if the central cycle on the left plot is more similar to normal heartbeat or to the central cycle on the right plot, which is assigned to pathology 3. This is the case of an intermediate signal shape.

6 Discussion and Conclusions

The main result of presented research is that PCA representation of single heartbeats obtained from 3-channel Holter monitoring enables very efficient automatic classification of normal and pathological cases.

Application of principal component analysis to data parameterization allowed us to design simply and effective classifier based on neural network or support vector machine. The efficiencies for both types of classifiers are similar and reach 99% of patterns classified correctly.

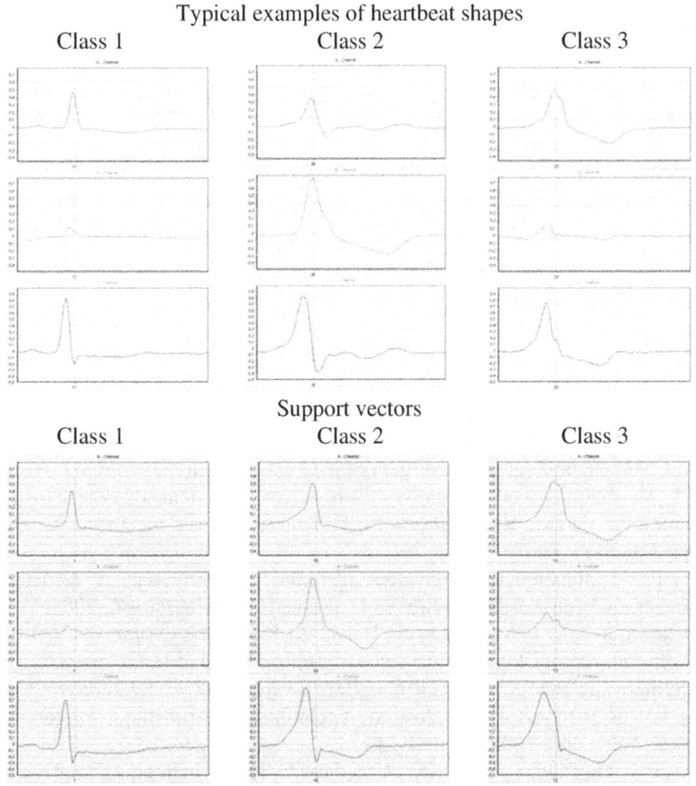

Fig. 11. Examples of heartbeat shape and corresponding support vectors

Number of parameter reduction is very important for classification or detection of unique cases. There are some diseases when one pathological cycle appears among dozens of normal heartbeats. As the number of such cycles in the entire Holter recording is small, we reduced the space dimension in order to guarantee proper number of training examples according to the Cover theorem [3].

The methodology of investigation consisting in treating some number of initial successive heartbeats as training set can be important in perpetual patient monitoring. A classifier can be design quickly in the first minutes of the patient observation and then we can use it for the same patient for automatic recognition of pathological beats, during long time monitoring.

We noticed that some cycles have the features specific for two different classes. In our tests that case occurs very seldom (less than 3% tested patterns). It is possible to eliminated or reduce this effect by increasing the training set. In our case, as said, the first 100 cycles of complete recording was chosen. The intermediate shapes occurrence is a main reason of classification errors.

The prototypes of considered classes of ECG signal shapes and selected support vectors are shown in Fig. 11. The visual inspection does not significant differences in signal shapes. Hence, it can be concluded that the PCA application for morphological classification can enhance significant features of studied cases.

Due to high information compression the feature space is reduced to a plane. The main result of our approach is that in all considered cases the optimal classifiers are linear. The results of neural classification coincides with SVM one that is evident from Figs. 7 and 9. Also, the number of support vectors is minimal. This fact is encouraging for further studies.

Acknowledgments. The authors acknowledge Prof. Dr. Med. Grzegorz Opolski, Medical University of Warsaw and Dr. Brigitte Quenet and Dr. Rémi Dubois, Ecole Supérieure de Physique et Chimie Industrielles de la ville de Paris, for discussions and useful suggestion concerning this paper.

References

1. Bausá Lamazares, D.: Morphological Classification of ECG Holter Recording by Principal Component Analysis (PCA) and Support Vector Machine (SVM), Final Project (SOCRATES/ERASMUS), Warsaw Institute of Technology, 2003
2. Bishop, C. M.: Neural networks for pattern recognition, Clarendon Press, Oxford
3. Cover T. M.: Geometrical and Statistical Properties of Systems of Linear Inequalities with Application in Pattern Recognition, IEEE Transaction on Electronic Computers, June 1965, pp.326-334
4. Dubois, R.: Application des nouvelles méthodes d'apprentissage à la détectionprécoce d'anomalies en électrocardiographie, Ph.D. thesis, Université Paris 6, 2003
5. Jankowski, S. Tijink, J., Vumbaca, G., Balsi, M., Karpiński, G.: Morphological analysis of ECG Holter recordings by support vector machines, Medical Data Analysis, Third International Symposium ISMDA 2002, Rome, Italy, October 2002, "Lecture Notes in Computer Science LNCS 2526" (eds. A. Colosimo, A. Giuliani, P. Sirabella) Springer-Verlag, Berlin Heidelberg New York 2002, pp. 134-143
6. Jankowski, S., Oręziak, A., Skorupski, A., Kowalski, H., Szymański, Z., Piątkowska-Janko, E.: Computer-aided Morphological Analysis of Holter ECG Recordings Based on Support Vector Learning System, Proc. IEEE International Conference Computers in Cardiology 2003, Tessaloniki, pp. 597-600
7. Jaworski, R.: Factoring of ECG Cycles by Computing Eigenvectors and Eigenvalues of Covariance Matrixes (in Polish), M. Sc. Thesis, Warsaw Institute of Technology, 2004
8. Medilog Oxford Management Systems - http://www.scanmed.co.uk/oxford.htm
9. Wagner, G. S.: Marriot's Practical Electrocardiography, Williams & Wilkins, 1994
10. Vapnik, N. V.: Statistical Learning Theory, John Wiley & Sons Inc., New York, 1998

Finding Relations in Medical Diagnoses and Procedures

David Riaño and Ioannis Aslanidis

Department of Computer Sciences and Mathematics
Universitat Rovira i Virgili
Tarragona, Spain

Abstract. A graph-based probability model has been defined that represents the relations between primary and secondary diagnoses and procedures in a file of episodes. This model has been used as a basis of an application that permits the graphical visualization of the relations between diagnoses and procedures. The application can be used by physicians to detect diagnosis or procedure structures that are hidden in the data of assisted patients in a health care center and to perform probability data analysis. The application has been tested with the data of the Hospital Joan XIII in Tarragona (Spain).

1 Introduction

When people arrive to a hospital due to some medical reason, the physician analyzes the signs and the symptoms and proposes a diagnostic which is the most feasible cause of the disease. At this particular moment if some medical or surgical treatment is needed or recommended, the visiting person becomes a patient who is optionally admitted to the hospital depending of whether the diagnostic is referred to a complex disease or not. The diagnostic with which a patient is admitted to the hospital is known as the *primary diagnostic*. During the evolution of the patient's disease in the treatment, some other diseases may appear or find out which affect the treatment but which are not the ones that define the primary actions over the patient. These diagnoses that appear as a result of the evolution of a patient are called *secondary diagnostics*. Therefore, a diagnostic is secondary to another when it appears after the patient is diagnosed or if it is detected at the beginning but it is not the one that must direct the main medical or surgical actions. Although secondary diagnoses do not direct the main medical actions on the patient, they are taken into account in order to adjust the main treatment to the patient particularities.

When analyzing the relations among medical diagnoses, it is difficult to know whether these relations are usual or casual, at a first glance. On the one hand, the relation between two diagnoses is *usual* when it is observed in the evolution of many patients. That is to say, many patients with the same primary diagnosis end up with the same or similar secondary diagnoses. On the other hand, the relation between two diagnoses is *casual* when there are few occurrences of a secondary diagnosis among the patients with the same primary diagnosis.

J.M. Barreiro et al. (Eds.): ISBMDA 2004, LNCS 3337, pp. 269–280, 2004.

For medical purposes and foreseing, it is interesting to find out which are the most common relations among primary and secondary diagnoses in order to anticipate which would be the most probable evolution of a patient which is admitted with a particular disease.

Once a patient is diagnosed, a treatment or therapy is scheduled in order to cure or to improve the health of that patient. A treatment is described as a sequence of drug prescriptions and medical or surgical procedures. A *medical procedure* is an action taken by a physician to achieve as result the improvement or resolution of the diagnosis given to a patient. A *surgical procedure* is a type of medical procedure which involves the use of instruments to incise a patient and it is performed to repair damage or arrest disease to the patient. The treatment of a patient is directed by a single procedure which is called the *primary procedure*. Often, this main procedure comes together with other *secondary procedures* that can change according to the patient evolution along the complete treatment. On the contrary, the main procedure remains the same during the whole treatment.

For quality assessment and cost analysis, it is interesting to study the relations between primary and secondary procedures (and their related costs) in the treatment of a disease. Since procedures are part of the treatment, this study is also interesting for anticipating medical actions for new admitted patients.

Medical diagnoses and procedures follow a classification that is worldwide recognized. In the studies about mortality data, the *ICD* (International Classification of Diseases) codification is used. However, in the studies about morbidity data, the *ICD-CM* (ICD with a Clinical Modification) codification, which is based on the ICD, is used. Nowadays, two main versions of the ICD-CM coexist: the ICD-9-CM (ninth revision) and the ICD-10-CM (tenth revision).

Historically, the ICD was formalized in 1893 as the Bertillon Classification or International List of Causes of Death and it has been continuously updated by the World Health Organization (WHO) approximately every ten years, adding new morbidity causes. The ICD-9-CM was published in 1977 by NHS in the USA with guidelines set by the American Hospital Association (AHA) and maintained compatible with the international system of ICD-9 established by WHO. The ICD-9-CM was developed to provide a way for indexing of medical records, medical case reviews, and ambulatory and other medical care programmes, as well as for basic health statistics. Since then, it has been revised and updated annually. In 2003, a draft version of the ICD-10-CM appeared with main changes in the amount and the names of the ICD-9-CM categories.

In a Hospital, all the information about the treatments of the admitted patients is stored in complex databases. For this work, the most important file in these databases is the one that stores the medical and surgical episodes. An *episode* is formally defined as a happening that is distinctive in a series of related medical events. Usually, the concept of episode is combined with the one of *minimum basic data set* which proposes fifteen data in order to describe a patient medical situation: hospital id, patient id, birth date, sex, residence, way of financing, admission date, admission circumstances, *primary and secondary diagnoses*, *primary and secondary procedures*, discharge date and reason, and id of the physician that discharged the patient. Therefore, the file of episodes contains the primary and secondary diagnoses and procedures of the treatments of all the patients admitted to the hospital in an period of time.

The file of episodes can be used to analyze the relations between primary and secondary diagnoses and procedures in order to find out hidden dependencies that could help physicians to asses the quality of the treatments, to detect feasible improvements, and also to make decisions about future patient therapies.

In this framework, evidence-based medicine is described as the conscientious, explicit, and judicious use of current best evidence in *making decisions* about the care of individual patients [8]. The health-care community has developed some methodologies which are mainly based on clinical trials [5] to conclude about *evident* cause-effect relations between diagnoses (i.e. disease, ailment, etc.) and procedures (i.e. drug, treatment, etc.) [2]. The high cost of clinical trials makes them impractical in the sort of analysis that this paper proposes.

Simultaneously, the AI community has developed well known statistical models as belief networks [4] or influence diagrams [1] to solve the same sort of problems. Unfortunately, the relations between primary and secondary diagnoses and procedures are not of the type cause-effect and the above models are not appropriate to face the problem. Other flowchart models [6, 7] are neither applicable.

Here, a new probabilistic model is introduced that permits the analysis a file of episodes in order to obtain the relations between medical diagnoses and between medical procedures, to detect the cross-relations between diagnoses and procedures, to find out chains of closely related diseases (or medical procedures), to study the *usualness* and *casuality* of those relations, to detect *nosocomial* diseases, to identify clusters of diseases or procedures, and to check the correct use of the ICD-CM classification, among other possible uses.

The model is based on two internal probability directed graphs which are generated from the file of episodes. One graph describes the relations between all the diagnoses, and the other one those relations between medical procedures. These internal structures are used by a computer-based data analysis system to study and to conclude about all the items mentioned in the above paragraph.

In section 2 the formal aspects of the graph structure from both the graph theory and the probability theory are introduced and related to the direct medical implications. Section 3 is devoted to the description of the system functionality. Some remarks about the best exploitation of the system analysis capabilities are also provided. Section 4 contains the results obtained for the analysis of the data of a real hospital. The paper finishes with some conclusions in section 5.

2 Formal Descriptions

The relations between diagnoses and procedures in health-care are well studied by *evidence-based medicine* formal methodologies as randomized, cross-over or double-blinded clinical trials [2, 5]. However, this sort of tests is inadvisable to study cause-effect relations as belief networks [4] and other models do. Unfortunately, the relation between primary and secondary diagnoses (or procedures) is not causal and a new probabilistic model is required.

A complete formalization of this model must contain a description of the sort of input data used to generate the model (i.e. episodes), the structure that supports the model (i.e. probability graph), and the feasible analysis that are possible with the model (i.e. functionality). As far as the last ones are concerned, two levels must be discussed: the structural and the probabilistic.

2.1 The Input Data

One of the interesting features of the medical data analysis system proposed is that the data it uses to find relations in medical diagnoses and procedures comes directly from the databases of health-care centers without any complex pretreatment. This means that on one side, the analysis process can be performed simultaneously to the daily activities of the hospital and on the other side, the results of the analysis can easily be maintained actual.

A *clinical episode* contains all the relevant information about the treatment of a patient between the admission and the discharge times. An episode is structured as a sequence of one or more *episode steps*. The length of this sequence is an indicator of the episode complexity. Each episode step describes the medical actions taken during each phase of the treatment (e.g. stage in a hospital service, gravity, etc.). In 1973, the *minimum basic data set* (MBDS) was introduced by the National Committee on Vital and Health Statistics (USA) to describe a medical situation by means of fifteen variables: hospital id, patient id, birth date, sex, residence, way of financing, admission date, admission circumstances, primary and secondary diagnoses, primary and secondary procedures, discharge date, discharge reason, and id of the physician discharging the patient. Among these variables there are four which remain the same for all the MBDS versions developed since then: primary diagnosis, secondary diagnoses, primary procedure, and secondary procedures.

Here, these four variables are defined to be part of the episode steps. Therefore, a file of episodes E is a sequence of episodes e_1, e_2, ..., e_k; e_i being a tuple (pd_i, pp_i, S_i) with pd_i a primary diagnosis, pp_i a primary medical procedure, and S_i a sequence of episode steps s_{i1}, s_{i2}, ..., s_{ik_i} where s_{ij} is a tuple (sd_{ij}, sp_{ij}); sd_{ij} being a set of secondary diagnoses, and sp_{ij} a set of secondary procedures.

Then, for any episode e_i in the file of episodes E, equations in 1 stand for the primary and secondary diagnoses and procedures of e_i, respectively.

$$pd(e_i) = pd_i, \quad sd(e_i) = \bigcup_{s_j \in S_i} sd_{ij}, \quad pp(e_i) = pp_i, \quad \text{and } sp(e_i) = \bigcup_{s_j \in S_i} sp_{ij} \qquad (1)$$

In the context of diagnoses (or procedures), let (a, b) represent the relation '*a is primary of the secondary b*', $n_e(a, b)$ the number of times that this relation is observed in the steps of the episode e (i.e. $n_e(a, b) = 0, 1, 2, ...$), $d_e(a, b)$ the discriminant value that is 1 if $n_e(a, b) > 0$ and 0 otherwise, $n(a, b) = \sum_e n_e(a, b)$ the number of times that (a, b) is observed in E, and $d(a, b) = \sum_e d_e(a, b)$ the number of episodes in which (a, b) is observed. Notice that $n(a, b) \neq d(a, b)$ if there are several secondary b's in an episode with a as primary.

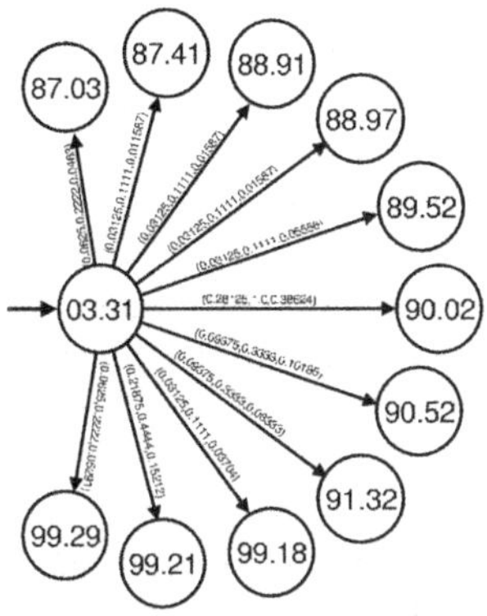

Fig. 1. Graph representation.

2.2 Structural Analysis

Given an input data file with episodes E as the one described in the previous section, the set $\{(a,b) : a \text{ primary of } b \text{ in } E\}$ can represent the edges of a directed graph with diagnoses (or procedures) as vertices. See, for instance, in figure 1 the graph of procedures obtained for the file of single step episodes in table 1.

There, 03.31 stands for the ICD-9-CM code of the procedure *spinal tap, lumbar puncture for removal of dye* (ST) that acts as primary of the secondaries 90.02 (*microscopic examination-1 of nervous system medullar culture*, μEMC), 99.21 (*antibiotic injection*), etc. So, the edge (03.31, 90.02) represents the relation ST is primary of the secondary procedure μEMC, and (03.31, 99.21) the fact that ST is primary procedure of the secondary procedure *antibiotic injection*. This last fact is observed in the first, third, forth, and eighth episodes.

Observe that under the above assumptions, the graphs obtained for either diagnostics and procedures are directed, but not necessarily acyclic or connected. Nevertheless, the graph theory [3] can be used to find some other interesting features as starting nodes, terminal nodes, isolated graphs, and one-separable graphs, among some others which are not described here.

In a (a,b) relation the vertex a is called *primary* (diagnosis or procedure) and the vertex b, *secondary*. A vertex which is never primary or secondary is respectively called *terminal* or *starting* diagnosis or procedure. Determining starting and terminal vertices allows physicians to detect three levels of relevance of diagnoses and procedures. Those which are starting have a high relevance, those which are terminal have a low relevance, and the rest have a medium relevance.

The one-connectivity set of a vertex a is defined as the set of edges that contain a as primary or secondary, i.e. $C_a = \{(x,y) : x = a \text{ or } y = a\}$. The transitive closure of the one-connectivity set in equation 2 defines the connectivity set of a. Isolated graphs are connected subgraphs whose vertices are not related to vertices out of the subgraph. Formally, there is a partition $\{V_i\}_{i=1,\ldots,k}$ of the set of edges $V = \{(a,b) : a \text{ primary of } b \text{ in } E\}$ such that $V_i = C^*_{a_k}$, for some a_k.

$$C^*_a = C_a \cup \bigcup_{b \in C_a} C_b \tag{2}$$

This means that there are clusters of diagnoses or procedures that can be studied independently of the rest of diagnoses or procedures because they are never related. In other words, this means that the file of episodes can be divided into subfiles of mutually independent sorts of patient (i.e. diseases) and sorts of treatment (i.e. procedures).

Finally, the concept of one-separability refers to connected graphs which are close to be the union of two isolated graphs, but there is a relation that prevents this to happen. Formally speaking, a connected graph with a set of edges V is one-separable if it contains (a, b) such that $C_a^* \cup C_b^* = \emptyset$ when the relation is removed. The one-separability feature permits the physicians to detect outliers, i.e. patients with diagnosis or procedure relations that are not observed in any other patient in the file of episodes.

2.3 Probabilistic Analysis

As figure 1 shows, the edges of the graph can be labeled with a value $P(a, b)$, representing the probability of (a, b) in the file of episodes. Let $p(a)$ stand for the number of times that a is primary in the file of episodes. Then, $P(a, b)$ can have three interpretations:

a) the proportion of times that b appears as secondary of the primary a.

$$P(a,b) = \frac{n(a,b)}{\sum_i n(a,i)} \tag{3}$$

b) the proportion of episodes in which b is secondary of the primary a.

$$P(a,b) = \frac{d(a,b)}{p(a)} \tag{4}$$

c) the proportion of secondariness that b has with respect to the primary a.

$$P(a,b) = \frac{\sum_e \frac{n_e(a,b)}{\sum_j n_e(a,j)}}{p(a)} \tag{5}$$

d) the proportion that b is secondary and a is primary in the file of episodes.

$$P(a,b) = \frac{n(a,b)}{\sum_i \sum_j n(i,j)} \tag{6}$$

For example, table 1 shows the nine cases of *lymphocytic choriomeningitis* registered at the Hospital Joan XXIII (Spain) in 2002. Observe that some data as the patient id, the residence, and others have been removed for space reasons and also because it is not relevant to this explanation. The hospital id has been changed by the service id; *p.d.*, *s.d.*, *p.p.* and *s.p.* stand for the primary and secondary diagnoses and procedures, respectively, and phys. contains the id of the physician that discharged the patient.

Table 1. Episodes of *lymphocytic choriomeningitis* in 2002.

e	service	age	sex	days	*p.d.*	*s.d.*	*p.p.*	*s.p.*	phys.
1.	1010	33	W	6	049.0	305.1	03.31	90.02 90.52 91.32 87.03 99.21 99.21	1113
2.	1010	24	M	4	049.0	-	03.31	90.02 90.52	1113
3.	1050	0	M	3	049.0	-	03.31	90.02 90.52 91.32 99.21	4007
4.	1010	19	M	8	049.0	305.1	03.31	90.02 87.03 99.21 99.21	1113
5.	1010	28	W	6	049.0	-	03.31	90.02 91.32 99.18	3831
6.	1050	4	W	2	049.0	-	03.31	90.02 99.18 99.29	4007
7.	1010	25	M	5	049.0	998.89 724.2	03.31	90.02 89.52	579
8.	1010	21	W	17	049.0	013.20 276.8	03.31	90.02 88.91 87.41 88.97 99.29 99.21 99.21	1113
9.	1010	34	M	3	049.0	-	03.31	90.02	886

Therefore, $n(03.31, 99.21) = n_1(03.31, 99.21) + n_3(03.31, 99.21) + n_4(03.31, 99.21) + n_8(03.31, 99.21) = 7$, and $d(03.31, 99.21) = d_1(03.31, 99.21) + d_3(03.31, 99.21) + d_4(03.31, 99.21) + d_8(03.31, 99.21) = 4$. Likely, $n(03.31, 90.02) = d(03.31, 90.02) = 9$. Finally, $P(03.31, 99.21)$ is $7/32$, $4/9$, $115/756$, and $7/32$ according to equations 3, 4, 5, and 6. The first value is obtained dividing the number of appearances of the relation (03.31,99.21) by the total number of secondary procedures of the primary 03.31. The second value divides the number of episodes that contain (03.31,99.21) by the total number of episodes that contain 03.31 as primary. The third value adds the proportion of 99.21 procedures in each episode and divides the obtained number by the total number of episodes that contain 03.31 as primary. The last value is the proportion of times that (03.31,99.21) appears in the file of episodes. Likely, the values for $P(03.31, 90.02)$ are $9/32$, 1, $73/189$, and $9/32$, respectively.

For all the interpretations, $P(a, b)$ is null only if the relation (a, b) is not observed in the file of episodes. That is to say, a is never primary of the secondary b. On the contrary, the reasons for the probability $P(a, b)$ to be one are different depending on the interpretation: for equations 3, 5 and 6 it means that (1) a is not primary of any secondary out of b and (2) a has always b as secondary, one or more times. For equation 4 it means only (2). The difference between the first two ones is that in equation 3 all the secondary diagnoses and procedures contribute equally to the global probability whereas in equation 5 this contribution must be divided by the number of secondary diagnoses or procedures in the episode.

$P(a, b)$, $P(b, c)$ and $P(a, c)$ are independent probabilities since the variable b means a different concept whether it is in the left side (primary diagnosis or procedure) or in the right side (secondary diagnosis or procedure). Therefore, $P(a, b)$ cannot be operated as a conditional probability $P(b|a)$, and the graph is not a Bayesian network.

Concerning all the outgoing edges of a vertex, $\sum_i P(a, b_i)$ is one only for the first interpretation, is greater than or equal to one for the second and third interpretations, and is equal to the probability of a to be primary, for the last interpretation. For incoming edges, $\sum_i P(b_i, a)$ represents the probability of a being secondary only for the last interpretation. The meaning of these additions are depicted in figures 2(a) and 2(b).

As we have shown, equation 6 defines a probability function of (a, b) that has several advantages with respect to the other ones. For the rest of the paper, this will be the interpretation to be used in the analysis of medical episodes.

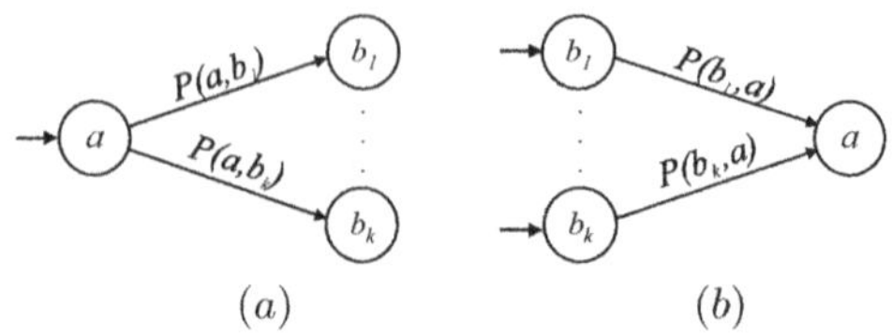

Fig. 2. Meaning of outgoing and incoming edges.

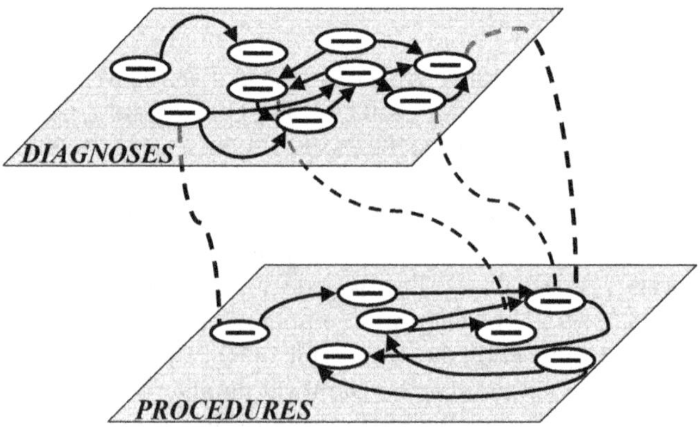

Fig. 3. Join analysis of diagnoses and procedures.

2.4 Diagnosis, Procedure and Join Analysis

The structure of the representation model described in the above subsections permits the physician to mine the data about medical episodes at three levels: diagnosis, procedures, and join analysis.

When the vertices of the graph represent diagnoses, the relations (a, b) are about the influences of one primary diagnosis on the secondary diagnoses. Some of these influences may be casual, and some other usual. Unexpected usual influences are those ones more valuable to detect by physicians. The structural and probabilistic interpretation of the graph can serve to calculate to what extent a primary diagnosis influences in the happening of a secondary disease.

If the graph is about the medical and surgical procedures, the relations (a, b) being a a fixed procedure represent the complexity of a treatment. Once again, the detection of usual relations among one primary procedure and several secondary procedures can drive the user to realize about complex treatments.

There is a third approach represented by figure 3 that permits the join analysis of diagnoses and procedures. Although this alternative is not considered in detail in this paper, it is worthwhile mentioning that the possibilities of a combined analysis of diagnoses (i.e. diseases) and procedures (i.e. treatments) represents a more powerful potential source of information than the marginal studies of diagnoses and procedures separately.

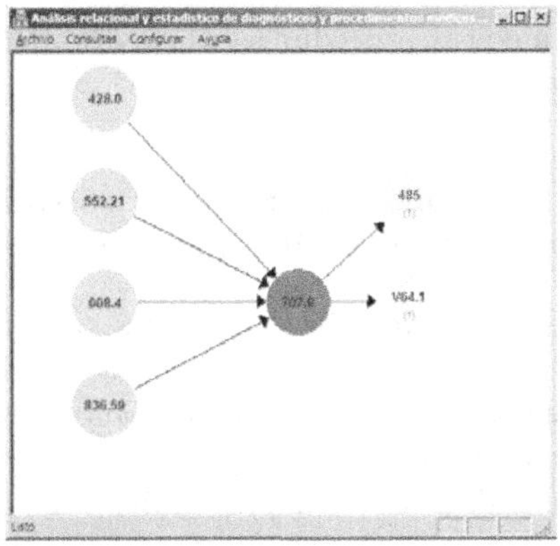

Fig. 4. Main screen of the implemented visual application.

3 The Implemented System

The representation model described in the section 2 has been used as a basis for the construction of a decision support system that helps physicians to analyze the clinical episodes in health-care centers in order to take evidence-based decisions. This analysis can be carried out through the use of some functions that are integrated in an application whose main appearance is shown in figure 4. The graph shows the disease *Chronic ulcer of unspecified site* with ICD-9-CM code 707.9 together with the primary diagnoses for which that is a secondary diagnoses (nodes in the left hand side), and also the secondary diagnoses for which that disease is primary (nodes in the right hand side).

The physician can move though the graph by clicking on the disease he is willing to focus on, and apply any of the functions explained below. Some other functions as detection of one-separated groups or detection of weak diagnoses have been implemented, but they are not considered in this paper.

3.1 Detection of Starting and Terminal Diagnoses and Procedures

Starting and terminal diagnoses were described in subsection 2.2 as graph vertices that are never primary or secondary, respectively.

The system is capable of detecting the starting and terminal medical diagnoses and procedures from the file of episodes.

3.2 Detection of Isolated Groups of Diagnoses and Procedures

Another interesting function that the system provides is to find isolated groups of diagnoses and procedures. With this function we can detect medical diagnoses (or procedures) that are interconnected among them, but not with the rest of the graph. When we analyze the graph of medical diagnoses, isolated groups represent diseases that on the one hand use to occur simultaneously, and on the other hand they never coexist with other diseases out of the group. A similar result can be observed for medical procedures, where the detected groups represent potential models of medical treatments.

3.3 Detection of Relations with Strong Probability Between Non-compatible Diagnoses or Procedures

Some relations can exist between two diagnoses (or procedures) with distant ICD-9-CM codifications and still with a very high probability that a patient with one of those diagnoses might end having the other one. Finding such relations helps the physician to detect that there is a potential relation among two apparently independent diagnoses (or procedures). The system can be used to analyze whether that fact is by chance or if there is some reason that justifies it.

3.4 Detection of Sequential Chains of Strongly Related Diagnoses

The relations among diagnoses can be chained in a sequence $(a_1, a_2) \to (a_2, a_3) \to \dots \to (a_i, a_{i+1})$. If all the single relations in the chain have a high probability, the sequence shows a justified indirect relation between the diagnoses a_1 and a_{i+1} that can be compared with the direct relation (a_1, a_{i+1}).

From the structural viewpoint, detecting all the chains between two diagnoses informs about all the ways a disease can become secondary of a primary one. That is to say, all the routes of developing a disease given another one or, in other words, all the possible evolutions of one disease towards another one.

From the probability viewpoint, a measure of how probable a route between two diseases is can be calculated.

4 Tests and Results

The above functions have been tested on the file of episodes of the Hospital Joan XXIII in Tarragona (Spain) in the years 2001, 2002, and 2003. These files contained 19020, 19307, and 20295 episodes, respectively.

The analysis of starting and terminal diagnoses and procedures produced the results indicated in table 2 where the last three columns contain the number of cases that are observed in all three years, two years or one year. For example, 38 procedures are starting procedures all three years, and 116 are only starting procedures two years out of the three analyzed.

Table 2. Coincidences of starting and terminal diagnoses and procedures.

	3 years	2 years	1 year
starting diagnoses	57	209	1048
terminal diagnoses	397	698	1641
starting procedures	38	116	436
terminal procedures	56	206	591

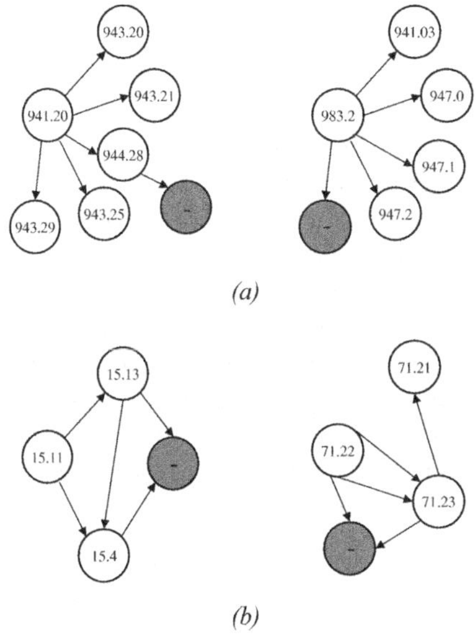

Fig. 5. Isolated groups of (a) diagnoses and (b) procedures.

As it was expected, the importance of those diagnoses that only appear as primary with respect to those which are only secondary is evident. In the first group there are diseases as *malignant neoplasms of colon* (151-153) or *bone* (171-174), and *noninfectious esterilitis and colitis* (555-556). In the second group diseases as *bacterial infection* (041) or *nondependent abuse of drugs* (305). A similar result is obtained with the procedures.

As far as the isolated groups is concerned, the system was able to separate the diagnoses related to burns from the rest in the years 2001 and 2003, but not in 2002. Nevertheless, the two isolated groups presented several differences as the graphs in figure 5(a) show. For the procedures the system isolated the *operations on extraocular muscles* (15) and the *operations on vulva and perineum* (71) in the graphs displayed in figure 5(b).

Many strong relations between diseases that are codified in different classes in ICD-9-CM are found. For example, *tuberculosis of lung* (011) is highly connected to the secondary *acute and chronic respiratory failure* (518), or *Boutonneuse fever* (082) to *tobacco use disorder* (305). Among the connections found, the physicians identified some that are evident and therefore not interesting. However, there were also other strange and still frequent that they found very interesting and whose reasons are currently being under study.

The last sort of tests performed were on the detection of sequential chains of strongly related diseases. Here, some of the most interesting ones according to the physicians' criterion are reported. For example, in the *disorders of the globe* (360) the sequence *purulent endophthalmitis* $\rightarrow$ *retinal detachment* $\rightarrow$ *senile cataract*, and in the *benign neoplasm of connective tissue* (215) the sequence *other specified sites* $\rightarrow$ *pain in thoracic spine* $\rightarrow$ *cyst of kidney acquired*.

5 Conclusions

A graphical probabilistic model to represent relations between primary and secondary diagnoses and procedures has been proposed for the analysis of hospital data coming from the files of clinical episodes. Several functions on the model have been implemented and integrated into an graphical application to ease the analysis. The application has been used with real data about the patients assisted at the Hospital Joan XXIII (Spain) in three consecutive years.

Although according to the physicians at the hospital we have obtained interesting results, the work presented must be considered as part of a work in progress that still has not exploited all the potential of the model presented. Also, there are still several complex conclusions that have to be studied and validated before they can be taken for sure by physicians.

The authors want to thank Dr. X. Allué his work in the analysis of the results. The work was funded by the projects TIC2001-0633-C03 and TIC2003-07936.

References

1. A. P. Dawid, Influence diagrams for causal modelling and inference. *International Statistical Review* 70: 161–189, 2002.
2. A. L. Cochrane, Effectiveness and efficiency (Spanish version), Salvat (Ed.), 1985.
3. J. L. Gross, J. Yellen, Handbook of Graph Theory, CRC Press, 2003.
4. J. Pearl, Causality: Models, Reasoning, and Inference, Cambridge University Press, NY, 2000.
5. S. Piantadosi, Clinical Trials: A Methodologic Perspective, John Wiley & Sons, 1997.
6. D. Riaño, S. Prado, The Analysis of Hospital Episodes, ISMDA, LNCS 2199, 2001.
7. D. Riaño, S. Prado, Improving HISYS-1 with a DSS, AIME, LNAI 2101, 2001.
8. D.L. Sackett, et al., Evidence based medicine: what it is and what it isn't. BMJ 312 (7023): 71–72, 1996.

An Automatic Filtering Procedure for Processing Biomechanical Kinematic Signals

Francisco Javier Alonso[1], José María Del Castillo[1], and Publio Pintado[2]

[1] University of Extremadura, Escuela de Ingenierías Industriales, Avda de Elvas s/n 06071, Badajoz, Spain
fjas@unex.es
[2] University of Castilla La Mancha, Escuela Técnica Superior de Ingenieros Industriales, Ciudad Real, 13071, Spain

Abstract. In biomechanics studies it is necessary to obtain acceleration of certain parts of the body in order to perform dynamical analysis. The motion capture systems introduce systematic measurement errors that appear in the form of high-frequency noise in recorded displacement signals. The noise is dramatically amplified when differentiating displacements to obtain velocities and accelerations. To avoid this phenomenon it is necessary to smooth the displacement signal prior to differentiation. The use of Singular Spectrum Analysis (SSA) is presented in this paper as an alternative to traditional digital filtering methods. SSA decomposes original time series into a number of additive time series each of which can be easily identified as being part of the modulated signal, or as being part of the random noise. An automatic filtering procedure based in SSA is presented in this work. The procedure is applied to two signals to demonstrate its performance.

1 Introduction

The systems for motion capture used in biomechanical analysis introduce measurement errors that appear in the form of high-frequency noise in the recorded displacement signals. The noise is dramatically amplified when differentiating the displacements to obtain velocities and accelerations [1]. This fact could cause unacceptable errors in the Inverse Dynamic Analysis of biomechanical systems [2, 3]. It is necessary to filter the displacement signal prior to differentiation to avoid this phenomenon.

The filtering of displacement signals to obtain noiseless velocities and accelerations has been extensively treated in the literature. Traditional filtering techniques include Digital Butterworth filters, splines, and filters based on spectral analysis [4-9]. Nonetheless, traditional filtering methods are not well-suited for smoothing non-stationary biomechanical signals such as the the impact–like floor reaction forces [10-12].

In order to filter non–stationary signals, advanced filtering techniques like Discrete Wavelet Transforms [13], the Wigner Function [11] and Singular Spectrum Analysis [14] have been used. These methods produce better results than

J.M. Barreiro et al. (Eds.): ISBMDA 2004, LNCS 3337, pp. 281–291, 2004.

conventional techniques. Nevertheless, its application is more complex and a number of additional parameters must be chosen. In fact, a mother wavelet function must be selected when using Discrete Wavelet Transforms, and the filtering function parameters must be chosen when using the Wigner Function. Singular Spectrum Analysis requires the appropriate selection of window length and grouping strategy. One of the main drawbacks of advanced filtering techniques is the difficulty to automate its application.

The goal of this paper is to demonstrate the advantages of smoothing methods based on Singular Spectrum Analysis (SSA) techniques and to provide an automatic and systematic filtering procedure procedure based in such techniques. The filtering procedure will be applied to two different signals: one of them taken from the literature, and the other acquired with our own motion capture system.

2 Methods

2.1 Background: Singular Spectrum Analysis

Singular Spectrum Analysis (SSA) is a novel non–parametric time series analysis technique based on principles of multivariate statistics. Its has been successfully used in the processing of climatic, meteorological and geophysical time series [15]. SSA was first applied to extract tendencies and harmonic components in meteorological and geophysical time series [16, 17], as well as to identify periodic motion in complex dynamic systems [18]. A concise description of the method will be given in this section. In their book, Golyandina et al. [15] have presented a complete derivation.

The method starts by producing a Hankel matrix from the time series itself by sliding a window that is shorter in length than the original series. This step is referred to as "embedding". The columns of the matrix correspond to the terms inside the window for each position of the window. This matrix is then decomposed into a number of elementary matrices of decreasing norm. This step is called Singular Value Decomposition (SVD). Truncating the summation of elementary matrices yields an approximation of the original matrix. The approximation eliminates those elementary matrices that hardly contribute to the norm of the original matrix. This step is called "grouping". Thus, the result is no longer a Hankel matrix, but an approximated time series may be recovered by taking the average of the diagonals. This new signal is the smoothed approximation of the original. This step is the "reconstruction"or the "diagonal averaging".

The above description may be stated in formal terms as follows:

Step 1. Embedding
Let $\mathbf{F} = (f_0, f_1, \ldots, f_{N-1})$ be the length N time series representing the noisy signal. Let L be the window length, with $1 < L < N$ and L an integer. Each column $\mathbf{X_j}$ of the Hankel matrix corresponds to the "snapshot" taken by the sliding window: $\mathbf{X_j} = (f_{j-1}, f_j, \ldots, f_{j+L-2})^T, j = 1, 2, \ldots, K$, where $K = N - L + 1$ is the number of columns, that is the number of different possible positions

of said window. The matrix $\mathbf{X} = [\mathbf{X_1}, \mathbf{X_2}, \ldots, \mathbf{X_K}]$ is a Hankel matrix since all elements in diagonal $i+j = constant$ are equal. This matrix is sometimes referred to as the trajectory matrix.

Step 2. Singular Value Decomposition (SVD) of the trajectory matrix.
It can be proven that the trajectory matrix (or any matrix, for that matter) may be expressed as the summation of d rank one elementary matrices $\mathbf{X} = \mathbf{E_1} + \ldots + \mathbf{E_d}$, where d is the number of non-zero eigenvalues of the $L \times L$ matrix $\mathbf{S} = \mathbf{X} \cdot \mathbf{X^T}$. The elementary matrices are given by $\mathbf{E_i} = \sqrt{\lambda_i}\mathbf{U_i}\mathbf{V_i^T}$, $(i = 1, \ldots, d)$, where $\lambda_1, \ldots, \lambda_d$ are the non-zero eigenvalues of $\mathbf{S}$, in decreasing order, $\mathbf{U_1}, \ldots, \mathbf{U_d}$ are the corresponding eigenvectors, and vectors $\mathbf{V_i}$ are obtained from $\mathbf{V_i} = \mathbf{X^T} \cdot \mathbf{U_i}/\sqrt{\lambda_i}$, $i = 1, \ldots, d$

The norm of elementary matrix $\mathbf{E_i}$ equals $\sqrt{\lambda_i}$. Therefore, the contribution of the first matrices to the norm of $\mathbf{X}$ is much higher than the contribution of the last matrices, and it is likely that these last matrices represent noise in the signal. The plot of the eigenvalues in decreasing order is called the singular spectrum and is essential in deciding the index from where to truncate the summation. For further explanations, see [14].

Step 3. Grouping
This step is very simple when the method is used for smoothing a time series. It consists of approximating matrix $\mathbf{X}$ by the summation of the first r elementary matrices. More complex types of grouping may be necessary when one intends to extract tendencies from the time series behavior. In our case, matrix $\mathbf{X}$ is approximated by $\mathbf{X} \approx \mathbf{E_1} + \mathbf{E_2} + \ldots + \mathbf{E_r}$.

Step 4. Reconstruction (Diagonal Averaging)
The approximated matrix described above is no longer a Hankel matrix, but an approximated time series may be recovered by taking the average of the diagonals. Nevertheless, it may be more practical to carry out this averaging for each elementary matrix independently in order to obtain time series that represent the different components of the behaviour of the original time series. These "elementary"time series are referred to as "principal components".

Let $\mathbf{Y}$ be any of the elementary matrices $\mathbf{E_i}$, the elements of which are y_{ij}, $1 \leq i \leq L$, $1 \leq j \leq K$. The time series $g_0, \ldots, g_{N-1}$ (principal component) corresponding to this elementary matrix is given by:

$$g_k = \begin{cases} \dfrac{1}{k+1} \displaystyle\sum_{m=1}^{k+1} y_{m,k-m+2} & \text{for } 0 \leq k < L^* - 1 \\ \dfrac{1}{L^*} \displaystyle\sum_{m=1}^{L^*} y_{m,k-m+2} & \text{for } L^* - 1 \leq k < K^* \\ \dfrac{1}{N-k} \displaystyle\sum_{m=k-K^*+2}^{N-K^*+1} y_{m,k-m+2} & \text{for } K^* \leq k < N. \end{cases} \tag{1}$$

where $L^* = min(L, K)$, and $K^* = max(L, K)$. The smoothed time series is obtained by adding the first r principal components.

It is worth pointing out that the application of the basic SSA algorithm requires selecting the values of just two parameters: the window length L, and the number r of principal components to be retained in the reconstruction.

2.2 Filtering Automation

As it has been pointed out [14, 15], one of the drawbacks of SSA application is the lack of general rules for selecting the values of the parameters L and r that arise in the SSA algorithm. Their values depend on the type of signal to be analyzed, and on the type of information to be extracted from the signal: tendencies, harmonics, noise. Golyandina et al. [15], again, have presented a complete description of parameter selection. An automatic filtering procedure is presented in this paper to make the choice of L and r automatic.

The procedure is based on the fact that raw-displacement acquired signals present a very large signal-to-noise ratio. In this situation, the contribution of the first matrices to the norm of $\mathbf{X}$ is much higher than the contribution of the last matrices, that represent noise. To eliminate the noise present in the displacement signal it is sufficient to choose the leading eigenvalues that represent a large percentage of the entire singular spectrum. In fact, for an arbitrary window length L, the grouping strategy r will retain a large percentage of the sum of eigenvalues. Thus, the automatic procedure starts by choosing an arbitrary window length L. The grouping strategy r was fixed in order to account for the 99.999% of the sum of the eigenvalues.

As has been pointed out [14, 15], in some cases, a choice of a large window length L produces a poor separation between signal trend and noise. In other words, trend components would be mixed with noise components in the reconstruction of the signal. For small L, we would extract the trend but obtain mixing of the other series components which are to be extracted [15]. A way to to overcome the uncertainty in the choose of L is to apply sequential SSA. This means that we extract some components of the initial series by the standard SSA and then extract the components of interest applying SSA smoothing to an already smoothed record. A recursive SSA application produces a gradual elimination of the noise present in the signal.

Sequential SSA was applied, using the same window lengths and grouping strategies in each decomposition. The stop criterion is imposed over the obtained acceleration signals. In fact, when the difference between RMS values of accelerations signals in two iterations is sufficiently small, the SSA sequential application is stopped. Such a procedure produces a gradual elimination of the noise in each iteration independently of window length. The stop criterion prevents an excessive smoothing of the acceleration signal.

The automatic filtering procedure is summarized in the following way:

- Choose an arbitrary window length L.
- Apply sequential SSA (Grouping strategy r is fixed to account for the 99.999% of the sum of the eigenvalues in each iteration).
- Calculate the acceleration signal numerically in each iteration.

– Stop the procedure when the difference between RMS values of accelerations signals in two iterations is sufficiently small, namely smaller than 1%.

2.3 Test Data

Two different signals will be smoothed using the procedure described in the previous section. A double differentiation is performed on the signals in order to quantify the effect of smoothing. First order finite differences are used to calculate the higher derivatives [19]. In order to study the performance of the filtering procedure two reference acceleration signals were used. The aim is to compare the acceleration obtained from filtered signals with reference acceleration. Nevertheless the reference acceleration signal is usually not available in practical situations. The observed signals and reference accelerations are briefly described in the following.

Signal 1: Stationary sinusoidal signal

A reflective marker was attached to a uniformly rotating crank. The marker motion was captured for 8 seconds at a frequency of 100 Hz using three infrared cameras (Qualisys Medical AB). The vertical component of this motion is a raw sinusoid (Fig. 1a). The reference acceleration signal is a pure sinusoid of the same frequency.

Signal 2: Signal with impact ([11, 20])

This second signal has been taken from the literature. The signal is a measure of the angular coordinate of a pendulum impacting against a compliant wall [11, 20]. The angular acceleration obtained from the motion capture system is compared to that obtained directly (after dividing by pendulum length) from accelerometers. Three accelerometers were used in order to average their measurements to reduce noise. The average signal, logged at a sampling rate of 512 Hz is used as the acceleration reference signal.

3 Results

3.1 Signal 1: Stationary Sinusoidal Signal

The first time series has a total of 800 elements. The signal-to-noise ratio is very large in this example, see figure 1a. Nonetheless, this small noise heavily contaminates the numerically obtained acceleration signal, and it is here, in the acceleration, where the efficiency of the method can be tested. The acceleration obtained using the original raw signal is plotted in Figure 1b. It is clear that smoothing or filtering is absolutely mandatory in order to obtain meaningful acceleration signals.

Figure 2 shows the evolution of singular spectrum using the automatic filtering procedure and the calculated acceleration after the smoothing for four different initial window lengths. The grouping strategy was fixed in order to account for the 99.999% of the sum of the eigenvalues. The algorithm stops when the difference between the current and previous values of the RMS acceleration

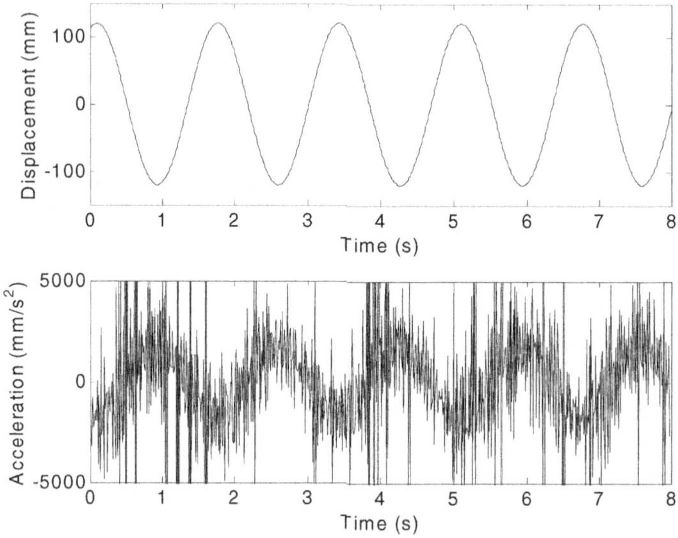

Fig. 1. (Top) Noisy displacement signal 1. (Bottom) Acceleration calculated from noisy displacement signal 1.

is sufficiently small, namely 1% . It has been mentioned that the norm of the elementary matrices into which matrix **X** may be decomposed equals the square root of the eigenvalues of **S**. The singular spectrums in Figure 2 are plotted in logarithmic scale. The contribution of the first few eigenvalues to the norm of **X** is much higher than the contribution of the rest. This fact justifies the automatic filtering procedure. By choosing the most significant eigenvalues , we are eliminating the noise of the signal. The bulk of the contribution to the noise arises from the lower slightly changing set of eigenvalues [15]. This fact can be appreciated in Figure 2, where this set is continuously diminished in each iteration.

Four initial window lengths were chosen, $L = 10$, $L = 50$, $L = 100$ and $L = 200$. The obtained RMS errors respect to reference acceleration signal are respectively $55.43mm/s^2$, $31.65mm/s^2$, $28.41mm/s^2$ and $28.51mm/s^2$. The automatic filtering procedure yields similar results for different chosen window lengths. Moreover, SSA calculated accelerations do not present the so-called end-point errors. Methods based on signal extension have been proposed to reduce end-point error [11]. No extension is necessary in the case of SSA smoothing. Errors due to this phenomenon are negligible (Fig. 2).

3.2 Signal 2: Signal with Impact ([11, 20])

The record of 600 elements from motion capture was processed using the automatic algorithm. Grouping strategy was fixed in order to account for the 99.999% of the sum of eigenvalues. The algorithm stops when the difference between the

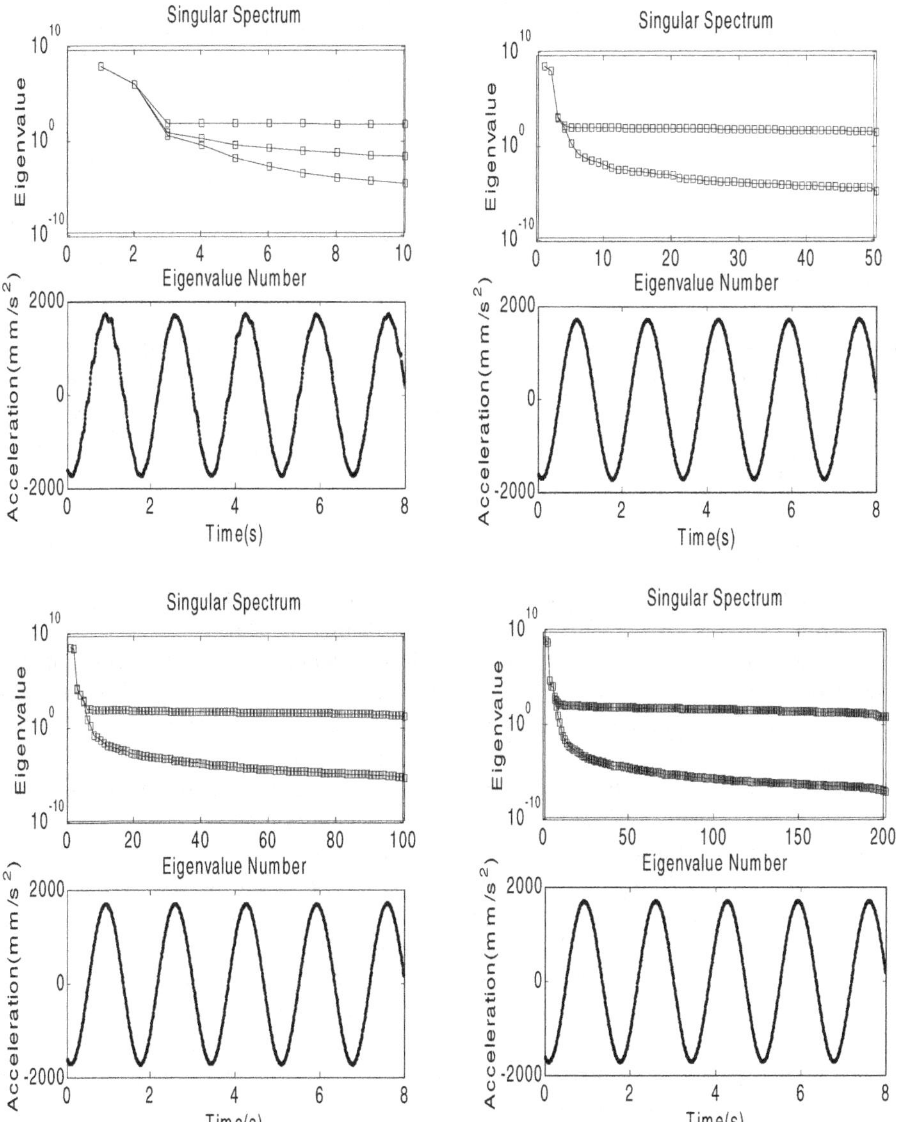

Fig. 2. In the upper part of each of the four graphics are represented singular spectrum evolution of signal 1 using window lengths $L = 10$, $L = 50$, $L = 100$ and $L = 200$. Each branch of singular spectrum correspond to an iteration of sequential SSA procedure. In the lower part of each graphic it is represented accelerations obtained from reference acceleration signal 1 (continuous line) and acceleration calculated from raw displacement data applying SSA based filtering procedure (dotted line).

current and previous values of the RMS acceleration is smaller than 1% in order to prevent excessive smoothing.

Four initial window lengths were chosen, $L = 10$, $L = 20$, $L = 50$ and $L = 100$. The obtained RMS errors respect to reference acceleration signal are respectively $25.03 rad/s^2$, $26.20 rad/s^2$, $31.37 rad/s^2$ and $24.52 rad/s^2$ (see Fig. 3). The automatic filtering procedure obtain similar results for different chosen window lengths. The result is similar to the value $RMSE = 23.60 rad/s^2$ obtained by Giakas et al. [11] with the help of the Wigner distribution. Our reconstruction right at the instant of impact is a little worse, but our signal in the vicinity of this time instant is more accurate. The slight loss of accuracy in the SSA method is compensated by the ease with which the method is applied: no need to select parameters, and no need to extend the ends of the record in order to eliminate end–point errors. Moreover, we do not use any information of the reference acceleration signal, such as the impact instant, to apply the filtering procedure.

4 Discussion

The results of our study show the superiority of the SSA based smoothing algorithm over automatic filtering techniques found in the literature. The SSA algorithm decomposes the original signal into independent additive components of decreasing weight. This fact allows the method to successfully extract the latent trend in the signal from the random noise inherent to the motion capture system.

One of the main advantages to the method is the fact that the algorithm requires the selection of just two parameters. Namely, the window length and the number of components to use for reconstruction. The method is also very intuitive in the sense that the appearance of the corresponding singular spectrum is a very good indicator for distinguishing signal from noise. It has also been shown that the method works properly on both stationary and non–stationary signals. Moreover, the method can be very easily programmed as a stand–alone automatic algorithm. The sequential process can also be made automatic with little effort. Convergence is measured by means of the difference between the current and previous values of the acceleration RMS. The algorithm stops when this difference is sufficiently small. Moreover, this method doesn't use any of the reference acceleration signal to perform the smoothing.

As drawbacks one may mention the fact that there are no fixed, objective rules for selecting the window length, grouping strategy and stop criterion. Nevertheless, it has been shown in the examples that the results are not very sensitive to the initial window length. Future studies will focus on developing rules to chose the optimum window length, the grouping strategy, and the stop criterion in each iteration of sequential procedure for a given signal.

In conclusion, we believe that the biomechanics community will benefit from this new automatic smoothing technique that has proven its effectiveness with complex signals. Future studies will need to focus on the possibilities of embedding the procedure in commercial biomechanical analysis packages.

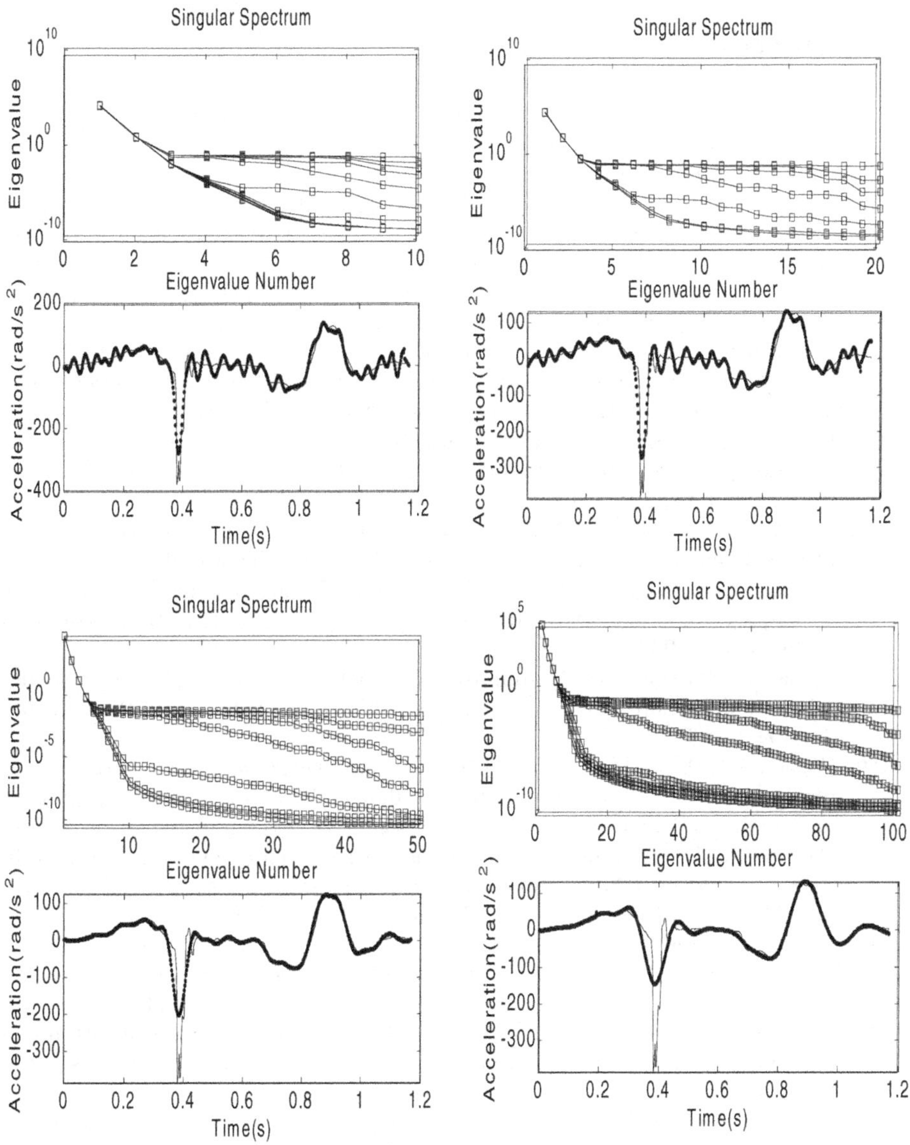

Fig. 3. In the upper part of each of the four graphics are represented singular spectrum evolution of signal 2 using window lengths $L = 10$, $L = 20$, $L = 50$ and $L = 100$. Each branch of singular spectrum correspond to an iteration of sequential SSA procedure. In the lower part of each graphic it is represented accelerations obtained from reference acceleration signal 1 (continuous line) and acceleration calculated from raw displacement data applying SSA based filtering procedure (dotted line).

References

1. Vaughan, C.L.: Smoothing and differentiation of displacement-time data: an application of splines and digital filtering. International Journal of Bio-Medical Computing **13** (1982) 375–386
2. Bogert, A.J. van den, de Koning J.J.: On optimal filtering for inverse dynamics analysis. Proceedings of the 9th Canadian Society of Biomechanics Congress. Burnaby, B.C., (1996) 214–215
3. Hatze, H.: The fundamental problem of myoskeletal inverse dynamics and its implications. Journal of Biomechanics **35** (2002) 109–115
4. D'Amico, M., Ferrigno, G.: Tecnique for the evaluation of derivatives from noisy biomechanical displacement data using a model-based bandwith-selection procedure. Med. and Biol. Eng. and Comp. **28** (1990) 407–415
5. D'Amico, M., Ferrigno, G.: Comparison between the more recent techniques for smoothing and derivative assesment in biomechanics. Med. and Biol. Eng. and Comp. **30** (1992) 193–204
6. Giakas, G., Baltzopoulos, V.: A comparison of automatic filtering techniques applied to biomechanical walking data. Journal of Biomechanics **30** (1997) 847–850
7. Giakas, G., Baltzopoulos, V.: Optimal digital filtering requires a different cut-off frequency strategy for the determination of the higher derivatives. Journal of Biomechanics **30** (1997) 851–855
8. Giakas, G., Baltzopoulos, V.: Improved extrapolation techniques in recursive digital filtering: a comparison of least squares and prediction. Journal of Biomechanics **31** (1998) 87–91
9. Walker, J.A.: Estimating velocities and accelerations of animal locomotion: a simulation experiment comparing numerical differentiation algorithms. The Journal of Experimental Biology **201** (1998) 981–995
10. Woltring, H.J.: Smoothing and differentiation techniques applied to 3-D data. In: Allard, P., Stokes, I.A.F., Blanchi, J.P. (eds.): Three Dimensional Analysis of Human Movement. Human Kinetics, Champaign, IL (1995) 79–99
11. Giakas, G., Stergioulas, L.K., Vourdas, A.: Time-frequency analysis and filtering of kinematic signals with impacts using the Wigner function: accurate estimation of the second derivative. Journal of Biomechanics **33** 2000 567–574
12. Georgiakis, A., Stergioulas, L.K., Giakas, G.: Wigner filtering with smooth roll-off boundary for differentiation of noisy non-stationary signals. Signal Processing **82** 2002 1411–1415
13. Adham, R.I., Shihab, S.A.: Discrete wavelet transform: a tool in smoothing kinematic data. Journal of Biomechanics **32** (1999) 317–321
14. Alonso, F.J., Del Castillo, J.M., Pintado, P.: Application of singular spectrum analysis to the smoothing of raw kinematic signals. Journal of Biomechanics In Press, Corrected Proof, Available online 15 July 2004
15. Golyandina, N., Nekrutkin, V., Zhigljavsky, A.: Analisys of Time Series Structure - SSA and Related Techniques. Chapman & Hall/CRC, Boca Raton, Florida (2001) 13–78
16. Vautard, R., Ghil, M.: Singular spectrum analysis in nonlinear dynamics, with applications to paleoclimatic time series. Physica D: Nonlinear Phenomena **35** (1989) 395–424
17. Vautard, R., Yiou, P., Ghil, M.: Singular-spectrum analysis: A toolkit for short, noisy chaotic signals. Physica D: Nonlinear Phenomena **58** (1992) 95–126

18. Pasmanter, R.A.: Variational search of periodic motions in complex dynamical systems. Chaos, Solitons and Fractals **6** (1995) 447–454
19. Burden, R.L., Faires, J.D., Reynolds, A.C.: Numerical Analysis. PWS Publishers, Boston (1981)
20. Dowling, J.: A modelling strategy for the smoothing of biomechanical data. In: Johnsson, B. (ed.): Biomechanics, Vol. XB. Human Kinetics, Champaign, IL, (1985) 1163–1167

Analysis of Cornea Transplant Tissue Rejection Delay in Mice Subjects

Zdenek Valenta[1,*], P. Svozilkova[2,3,**], M. Filipec[2], J. Zvarova[1,***], and H. Farghali[3]

[1] European Center for Medical Informatics, Statistics and Epidemiology, Prague, Czech Republic
[2] Department of Ophthalmology, 1st Faculty of Medicine, Charles University, Prague, Czech Republic
[3] Institute of Pharmacology, 1st Faculty of Medicine, Charles University, Prague, Czech Republic

Abstract. In this paper we present statistical analysis of cornea transplant tissue rejection delay in mice subjects resulting from using one of five types of immunosuppressive agents or placebo. The therapy included FK506 (tacrolimus), MMF (mycophenolate mofetil), AMG (aminoguanidine) and combinations FK506+AMG and FK506+MMF. Subjects were randomized to receiving one of the post-transplant regimens and were followed for up to two months until either rejection of the transplant tissue or censoring occurred. Due to complexity and personnel limitations the trial was performed in four stages using groups of either high risk or regular subjects. We used covariate-adjusted Gray's time-varying coefficients model for analyzing the time to transplant tissue rejection. At several occasions the type of the outcome (failure or censoring) could not be unambiguously determined. Analyses resulting from the two extreme interpretations of the data are therefore presented, leading to consistent conclusions regarding the treatments efficacy.

1 Introduction

Due to both trial complexity and personnel limitations the study was conducted during four separate calendar periods of 2003 extending for up to two months each. The four periods began in January, March, May and November of 2003, respectively. During the first two periods regular mice subjects were used, while the latter two involved subjects classified as high risk. Efficiency of three alternative therapies, FK506, AMG and MMF, was compared with that of placebo

* Correspondence to: Zdenek Valenta. EuroMISE Center, Institute of Computer Science, Academy of Sciences of the Czech Republic, Pod Vodarenskou vezi 2, Prague, Czech Republic. E-mail: valenta@euromise.cz, Phone: 420,266053099, Fax: 420,286581453.

** Contract/grant sponsor: GA CR, contract/grant number: 305/03/D130. Contract/grant sponsor: IGA MZ, contract/grant number: NI 7531-3.

*** Contract/grant sponsor: Ministry of Education of the CR, contract/grant number: LN00B107.

J.M. Barreiro et al. (Eds.): ISBMDA 2004, LNCS 3337, pp. 292–298, 2004.

(saline solution). The dosage used with the FK506 therapy was 0.2 mg/kg per day, MMF used 30 mg/kg per day and AMG 100 mg/kg per day. The multiple additive therapies FK506+AMG and FK506+MMF combined the corresponding monotherapy dosages. They were added at stages three and four of the trial, respectively, which might have resulted in lower power in assessing efficacy of these additive treatments.

Both stratified and covariate-adjusted models for time to rejection have indicated departure from the proportional hazards assumption. Gray's time-varying coefficients (TVC) model [1] was therefore employed for analyzing time to transplant tissue rejection. Here we present results from fitting the covariate adjusted Gray's TVC survival model which appeared to yield more power and flexibility than the model stratified for the four seasonal periods. In a small number of instances (12 out of 154) it could not be unambiguously determined whether the failure or censoring occurred. The two extreme alternatives have led to two alternative ways of analyzing the data which provided consistent results regarding the treatments efficacy.

2 Methods

As mentioned earlier, the complexity of the clinical trial resulted in seasonal stratification, which had to be accounted for at the analysis stage. Furthermore, during the first two stages of the trial regular subjects were used, while the latter two saw subjects classified as being at high risk.

One obvious way of accounting for both of these effects simultaneously would be by fitting a stratified survival model with four strata corresponding to seasonal periods. Note that in our case the full seasonal stratification would account for the type of subject as well. Using this approach, both seasonal effects and differences resulting from using the two types of subjects would be modelled by the baseline hazard in each of the four strata. Consequently, they would not be directly estimated by the model.

Alternatively, we could model the seasonal differences as well as the effect of using different types of subjects as covariate effects. In this paper we will discuss the results we obtained by adopting this alternative modelling approach. In this case one common baseline hazard function will be modelled for all data.

The advantage of this approach would potentially be twofold. First, the seasonal effects as well as the differences between the two types of subjects will actually be estimated. Second, because the seasonal effects will be estimated, only those showing significant departure from the baseline (say, November 2003 strata) will need to be modelled.

Incorporating both types of subjects (i.e. *regular* and *high risk*) in the study is in our situation equivalent to assuming that the relative effect of each treatment will remain the same independently of which type of subject is being used. Although this would appear to be a reasonable assumption, its validity could not actually be tested in our data, because the two multiple therapies were used only with the high risk subjects.

Several covariates have shown significant departure from the assumption of proportionality of the hazard functions over time. We therefore used an extension of the Cox proportional hazards model [2] proposed by R. J. Gray which allows for modelling time-varying covariate effects. Gray's time-varying coefficients model has the following form:

$$\lambda(t|z) = \lambda_0(t) \exp\{\beta(t)'z\}, \tag{1}$$

where $\lambda(t|z)$ represents the conditional hazard function given the covariate vector with values in z and $\lambda_0(t)$ denotes the baseline hazard function. Time-varying regression coefficients are denoted by $\beta(t)$.

We used a piecewise-constant implementation of Gray's time-varying coefficients model where the covariate effects are assumed to remain constant between each two consecutive knots. The knots are selected from among the observed failure times so that the number of failures occurring between each pair of consecutive knots is approximately the same.

Under the piecewise-constant implementation of model (1) we have $\beta(t) = \beta(\tau_j)$ for $t \in [\tau_j; \tau_{j+1})$, $j = 0, \ldots, q$, where $\tau_j, j = 1, \ldots, q$, denote the internal knots, $\tau_0 = 0$, and $\tau_{q+1} = T$ denotes the maximum observed (survival or censoring) time. Parameter estimates $\beta(\tau_j)$ are obtained via maximizing the penalized partial likelihood. Gray's time-varying coefficients model with 4 knots and 2 degrees of freedom for fitting piecewise-constant penalized splines was used throughout the paper.

3 Results

In comparison with the survival model fully stratified according to individual seasonal periods the covariate adjustment method of modelling the cornea transplant tissue rejection delay in mice subjects proved slightly more efficient, as well as more informative.

One disadvantage of the stratified approach lies in inseparability of the seasonal and subject-type related effects, which are not directly estimated by the model, since they are absorbed into the baseline hazard. Furthermore, the covariate adjustment method revealed virtually no seasonal differences between the response of subjects used in January and March of 2003, respectively, so the treatment effects could actually be pooled across the two strata.

As mentioned earlier, in twelve out of one hundred fifty four cases the outcome could not be unambiguously determined as either rejection or censoring. This led to two extreme interpretations of the data. Results from the two corresponding analyses are summarized in Tables 1 and 2. The two columns of Table 1 labelled "Overall" show the overall significance level of the corresponding effect from Gray's TVC model. The columns labelled "Non-prop." report the significance level of a formal test of non-proportionality of the hazard functions over time. Time-varying estimates of the hazard ratio are shown in Table 2, where statistical significance of the estimate at the $\alpha = 0.05$ level is denoted by "*".

Table 1. Modelling Results from Gray's Time-Varying Coefficients Model.

Model Significance (p-value)	**Ambiguous Observations Coded As:** Events		Censored Observations	
Treatment	Overall	Non-prop.	Overall	Non-prop.
AMG	0.868	0.639	0.789	0.666
MMF	0.034	0.025	0.009	0.021
FK506	0.009	0.147	0.001	0.578
FK506+AMG	0.362	0.377	0.227	0.537
FK506+MMF	0.017	0.093	0.010	0.078
Risk Group	0.000	0.912	0.000	0.855
November 2003	0.008	0.046	0.005	0.019

Table 2. Time-Varying Estimates of the Hazard Ratio of Cornea Transplant Tissue Rejection.

Hazard Ratio * $p < 0.05$	**Coding A.O.**	**Time Frame in Days** 1-14	15-21	22-28	29-34	35-60
AMG		0.944	0.983	0.876	0.899	1.182
MMF		0.340*	0.346*	0.559	0.842	0.628
FK506		0.182*	0.207*	0.344*	0.393*	0.544
FK506+AMG	**Events**	0.462	0.732	1.031	1.031	1.031
FK506+MMF		0.383	0.308	0.087*	0.051*	0.046*
Risk Group		14.79*	16.39*	16.38*	10.87*	10.02*
November 2003		3.306*	3.199*	0.982	0.684	0.636
AMG		0.868	0.835	0.759	0.776	1.044
MMF		0.208*	0.233*	0.467	0.621	0.508
FK506		0.111*	0.124*	0.202*	0.213*	0.240*
FK506+AMG	**Censored**	0.405	0.612	0.745	0.745	0.745
FK506+MMF		0.336	0.278*	0.077*	0.038*	0.035*
Risk Group		50.20*	35.80*	26.44*	25.10*	23.39*
November 2003		3.686*	3.064*	0.811	0.499	0.470

The results shown in Tables 1 and 2 indicate that, after adjusting for seasonal and subject-type effects, the use of FK506 therapy brought about a most significant departure from the placebo effect. Over the two-months follow-up period adopted in our study the benefit of the FK506 therapy appeared to be relatively stable. In contrast, the other two outstanding therapies, namely MMF and FK506+MMF, have both indicated that their effect possibly changed over time.

Estimates of temporal trends in the hazard associated with each therapy and other model covariates are plotted separately for both ways of coding ambiguous observations, as shown in Figures 1 and 2, respectively. The log-hazard ratio plots suggest that a major improvement over the placebo was achieved using the FK506 therapy. Note that the upper limit of the log-hazard ratio appears to have remained below zero for most of the time. We further observe that an initial preventive effect of the MMF therapy is eventually somewhat reduced over time.

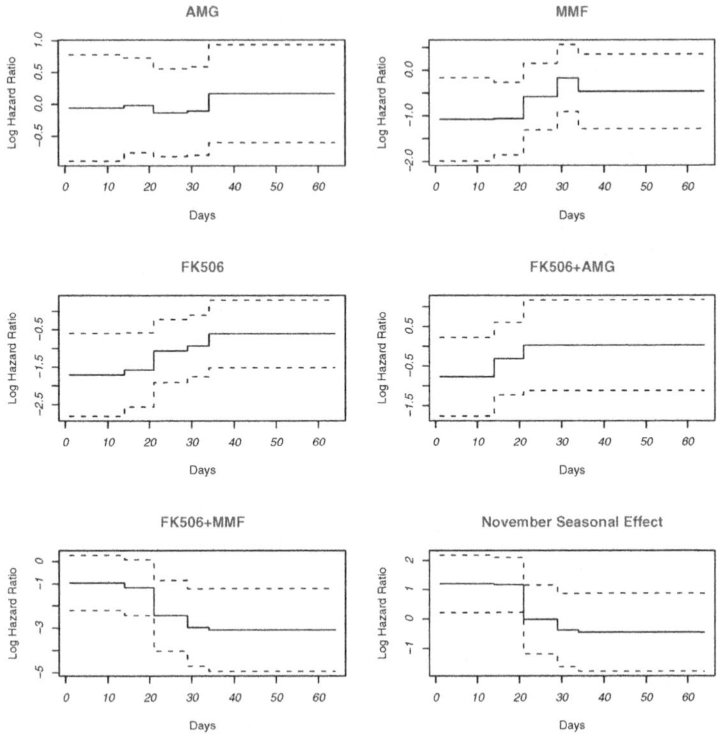

Fig. 1. Log-hazard ratios for model covariates with ambiguous observations coded as failures.

In contrast, the plots showing the estimated change in the log-hazard ratio over time indicate that the initial hazard reduction associated with the use of combined therapy FK506+MMF further increased after about three weeks of follow up. This finding should, however, be weighted very carefully.

First of all, we have to bear in mind that this combination therapy was applied only once at the November stage of the trial. Probably for this reason the seasonal effect of the November follow-up period could not be well separated from that of utilizing the FK506+MMF therapy itself. At least partially this is demonstrated when comparing the temporal trend in the log-hazard ratio associated with the FK506+MMF therapy with that associated with the November period. Both temporal trends seem to reflect a very similar underlying shape.

As mentioned earlier, the fact that the two combination therapies FK506+MMF and FK506+AMG were added during the later stages of the trial not only reduced power to detect the existing treatment differences, but in this case also undermined our capability of testing whether the treatment effect was possibly modified by using the different types of subjects or by conducting the trial during different seasonal periods.

Finally, we observe that both the monotherapy AMG as well as its combination with FK506, that is FK506+AMG, indicated no improvement over the placebo treatment.

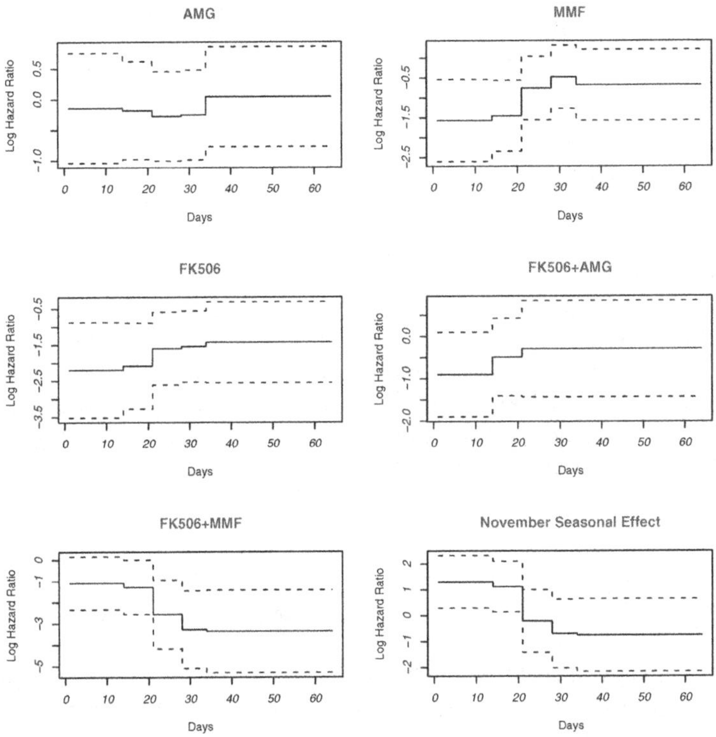

Fig. 2. Log-hazard ratios for model covariates with ambiguous observations coded as censored.

4 Discussion

Because the assumption of the Cox proportional hazards model appeared to be violated for several of our model covariates, we employed Gray's time-varying coefficients model for analyzing the survival data from our clinical trial. The trial used two types of subjects (regular and high risk) and due to both its complexity and personnel limitation data was collected over the four seasonal periods of 2003. Covariate adjustment method was used for both the type of subject and seasonal effects. Several outcome readings of cornea transplant tissue rejection status could not be unambiguously resolved which lead to two alternative codings of the survival status variable, thus prompting two alternative statistical analyses of the data.

Both ways of coding the ambiguous readings of the survival status variable lead at the analysis stage to a consistent finding, by which FK506 emerged as the most effective therapy in terms of preventing or rather delaying the autoimmune reaction of rejecting the cornea transplant tissue in mice subjects. Furthermore, the MMF therapy as well as multiple therapy combining the individual dosages of FK506 and MMF have both shown some improvement over the placebo effect. However, because the FK506+MMF therapy was only utilized during the

November stage of the trial, a follow-up study would seem to be necessary in order to properly assess its effectiveness relative to other treatments used in the clinical trial.

Acknowledgments

Tacrolimus (FK506) was kindly supplied by Fujisawa GmbH, Munich, Germany and Mycophenolate Mofetil (MMF) by Roche s.r.o., Prague, Czech Republic. We would also like to thank Dr. Robert J. Gray from Harvard University and Dana Farber Institute for making his own implementation of the modelling routine for Gray's time-varying coefficients model available to us. All computations were performed using R for Windows [3], rel. 1.9.0. This work was supported by the Internal Grant Agency of the Ministry of Health of the Czech Republic, grant No. 7531-3, and Grant Agency of the Czech Republic, grant No. 305/03/D130 and by the grant No. LN00B107 from the Ministry of Education of the Czech Republic.

References

1. Robert J. Gray. Flexible methods for analyzing survival data using splines, with applications to breast cancer prognosis. *Journal of the American Statistical Association*, 87:942–951, 1992.
2. D. R. Cox. Regression models and life tables (with discussion). *Journal of the Royal Statistical Society, Ser. B*, 34:187–220, 1972.
3. Ross Ihaka and Robert Gentleman. R: A language for data analysis and graphics. *Journal of Computational and Graphical Statistics*, 5(3):299–314, 1996.

Toward a Model of Clinical Trials

Laura Collada Ali[1], Paola Fazi[1], Daniela Luzi[2], Fabrizio L. Ricci [2], Luca Dan Serbanati[3], and Marco Vignetti[1]

[1] Centro Dati Gruppo Italiano Malattie Ematologiche dell'Adulto – GIMEMA ONLUS, Dip. di Biotecnologie Cellulari ed Ematologia, Università Roma – La Sapienza, Via Benevento, 6, 00161 Rome, Italy
{collada_ali,fazi,vignetti}@bce.uniroma1.it
[2] IRPPS-CNR, Via Nizza, 128, 00198 Rome, Italy
{d.luzi,f.ricci}@irpps.cnr.it
[3] "Politehnica" University, Spl. Independentei,313, 060032 Bucharest, Romania
l.serbanati@flashnet.it

Abstract. In the paper some results of the modelling of the clinical trial (CT) process are presented. CT research is a complex process which includes the protocol editing, its use and implementation in the CT experimentation, and the evaluation of the results. To improve the medical research, it is necessary to consider the CT research process as a whole. We structured the CT research process in three subprocesses: a) clinical trial management; b) management of statistical units; and c) patient health care delivery process. Each process has different objectives and is enacted in different environments, carried out by its own agents and resources, and influenced by specific rules characterising each process. The model is supported by three perspectives on the CT process: functional, structural, and behavioural views.

1 Introduction

Research and innovation in the pharmaceutical drug and new treatment/diagnostic strategies development involve three distinct worlds: the industry, the health care delivery system, and patients. These stakeholders consider innovation from different points of view: the industry is concerned with the identification of new market segments, the health care delivery system puts particular attention on the effectiveness of treatments and finally general public looks for new liable health care treatment. Medical research carried out through clinical trials (CT) has to agree upon these three points of view: the new drug has to be innovative, but also not dangerous and effective. Moreover, for its correct use it is necessary to identify new guidelines, considering applications and costs. CTs are carried out in four phases of study, each one is devoted to verify a specific aspect of the drug development, for instance its toxicity, effectiveness, and dosage. CTs may last from 1 to 13 years, they cost between \$600 and \$800 million and only one molecule among 4000 becomes a marketable product. Thus, all stakeholders are concerned to achieve reliable results as soon as possible (in case of both unsuccessful and successful results), and to avoid repetitions in experimentation. A computer-supported and standard based management of the process connected to the CTs (protocol definition, diffusion, execution, result evaluation as well as the related professional training of health care operators) becomes fundamental for shortening periods of regular drug introduction, diffusing a punctual knowl-

J.M. Barreiro et al. (Eds.): ISBMDA 2004, LNCS 3337, pp. 299–312, 2004.

edge on new clinical trials, avoiding duplications, comparing the various aspects of the results (biological, medical, ethical, economical, etc.), and developing the guidelines necessary to diffuse the best practice linked to the innovation. Such approach enables to facilitate the interaction between the different centres participating to CT.

There is an increasing number of research on CTs, which demonstrates the converging interest and need in achieving a standardised model and a common terminology [13, 12]. Due to the complexity of CT research, these studies generally address single, specific issues in order to improve locally the process linked with some of the major steps of the protocol design and management. For instance there are studies and applications focused on the protocol's eligibility criteria [1, 9], drug treatments [8], task scheduling [16]. Other authors have addressed the problem of helping medical investigators to authoring protocols [3, 6], or to improve the communication between the participating and the co-ordinator centres [14]. However, there is a strong demand on integrating research and systems in a unique approach, able to support the whole process of the CT research. In order to achieve this objective a comprehensive model of the CT process is needed.

The aim of this paper is to present our first results on the modelling of the CT process as a whole. The model has been elaborated using the standard UML (Unified Modelling Language) version 2.0 [7].

2 Rationale

The starting point of our research project has been the analysis of CT protocols in the field of oncology and haematology [2]. The role of the protocol cannot be underestimated in CT research. As known, the CT represents an assessment process of a previously obtained product (drug or treatment strategies). This process is carried out according to criteria of evaluation derived from both well-defined objectives and existing standards [5]. Like any assessment process, a CT has to be described in a detailed, coherent and consistent way. The description has to contain all the information necessary to carry out the assessment process. This information is embedded in the protocol. This is why the elaboration of a protocol is one of the most important tasks of CTs. In order to have the approval of the experimentation by the scientific and ethic committees and the starting of the medical research a coherent and correct protocol is needed. Such a protocol is also an essential requirement for a uniform multicentre CT execution as well as to obtain a correct evaluation of the test results. Moreover, the protocol and all the documents annexed to it (we called them *CT Master file*) reflect different perspectives based on managerial and/or scientific concerns of stakeholders as well as on the various collaborations and expertise needed to organise and carry out a CT research. For instance the Case Report Form (CRF) templates are produced to match the views of the data centre and single investigators, while toxicity criteria derive from the physicians' view in the CT process. The protocol in particular is a complex, multifaceted document where concerns of various stakeholders converge.

One of the results of our research was the understanding that the analysis and design of a IT system, which helps the collaborative writing of a protocol in a coherent and consistent way, cannot disregard a detailed analysis of the whole CT research process [4]. This analysis constitutes the baseline to model the tightly coupling of the protocol, as a planning document, and its implementation within CT research. For this reason we decided to model the entire process of the CT research as a business process.

As known, a business process is defined as a collection of related structural activities that produce a specific outcome for a particular customer. A business process can be part of a larger, encompassing process and can include other business subprocesses that are specified in its method [10]. In business modelling, models provide ways of expressing business processes or strategies in terms of business activities and collaborative behaviour, so that we can better understand the CT process, and the agents participating in the process. This technique has helped us to understand the business processes of the CT organisations supporting the process by: a) identifying the business or domain objects involved in the CT, b) establishing the competencies required in each process of the workers: investigators, physicians, writing committee, statisticians, etc. and their responsibilities, and c) the activities the agents perform in the encompassing process.

CT modelling has several advantages. On the one hand, models are helpful for documenting, comprehending and communicating complexity. By documenting business processes from various perspectives, business models help stakeholders to better specify their views on the CT domain and managers to understand their environment. On the other hand, we know that every time a new protocol is experimented, some changes related to the patient treatment are introduced in the participating centres. These changes often imply a redefinition of the health care delivery process. For this reason business modelling would enable to introduce a higher level of flexibility in the centres participating to the CTs.

Our model is described using UML, which is the standard language for system modelling. It is a visual modelling language, which enables system developers to specify, visualize, document, and exchange models in a manner that supports scalability, security, and robust execution. UML provides a set of diagrams and features which have all proven valuable in real-world modelling. Our business modelling is supported by three types of models: functional, structural and behavioural descriptions, which are the three complementary views adopted by UML for system modelling.

3 Clinical Trial as a Business Process

3.1 Overview

As already mentioned, to improve the quality of CTs, it is necessary to consider the CT research process as a whole. However, CT research is a complex process, which includes other processes and activities, like the protocol development, the protocol use and implementation in the CT experimentation, and the evaluation of the CT results. Each process/activity has different objectives and is enacted in different environments, carried out by its own agents and resources, and governed by specific rules. Figure 1 introduces three process types we identified in the CT research:

- Management of clinical trial (CTMP), which carries out activities related to the set up, co-ordination and monitoring of the CT participating centres, and the final evaluation of CT results. This process is carried out within the Coordinator Centre (CC) environment.

- Management of statistical units (SUMP) includes the activities of managing the CT in the participating centre. Each instance of the process is carried out in a peripheral, participating centre (PhC). Its main functions are: patient enrolment and filling in the CRF extracted from the patient's healthcare record (HCR).
- Patient health care delivery process (PM) is related to the diagnostic and therapeutic activities necessary to treat an enrolled patient, following the instructions defined in the protocol. It is carried out within the clinical ward (CW).

Figure 1 describes the relationship between instances of these process types. As soon as the clinical protocol is developed by the writing committee and approved by the scientific and ethical committees, the CC allows the PhCs to start the activities connected with the official opening of the clinical trial. As the figure shows, the CTMP triggers the SUMP for each PhCs.

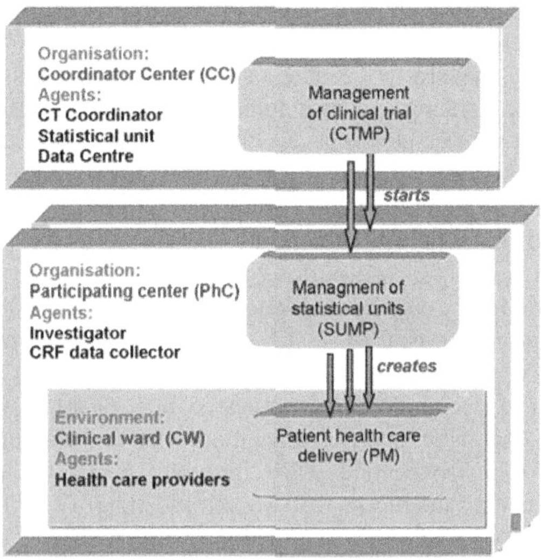

Fig. 1. Process types in the clinical trial process

In each PhC environment, a MPTP process instance is created for each enrolled patient. This means that at a certain point in the SUMP process we have as many MPTP instances as the number of the enrolled patients in treatment. For the SUMP process these instances correspond to anonymous statistical units, which will be evaluated during the analysis of the Clinical trial results.

Each process type has its own agents, which collaborate with each other in order to carry out the process. In Figure 1 the agents are associated to the process they carry out. The majority of these processes are concurrent and their interaction is based on the achievement of specific clauses/conditions, the production of certain information/documents or the occurrence of specific events. Figure 2 shows the information flow between the instances of the CT process and specifies the different types of information exchanged between processes: data, resources, commands/directives, workflows/process specifications. In the figure, the following shared documents and highly structured data are emphasised: a) the CT master file containing the approved protocol, the associated CRF templates as well as auxiliary documents, for instance: informed consent, PhCs list, clinical trial design, etc.; b) the CRF database, which gathers the CRF from all PhCs, and c) the patient's HCR.

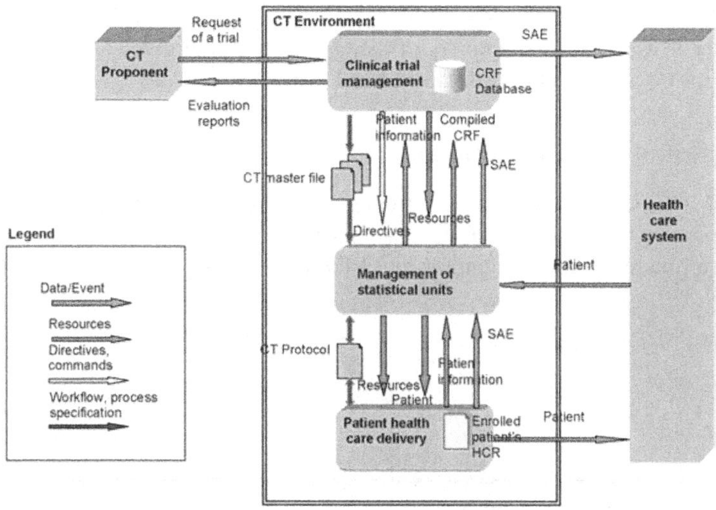

Fig. 2. Data flow of the clinical trial

3.2 Clinical Trial Management

The whole process starts with a request for a clinical trial execution and terminates when the CT results have been published. Figure 3 introduces the main subprocesses of the CTMP process: 1. the protocol development process, 2. the co-ordination and control process, the monitoring process for data exchange with PhC and 4. the evaluation process of CT results.

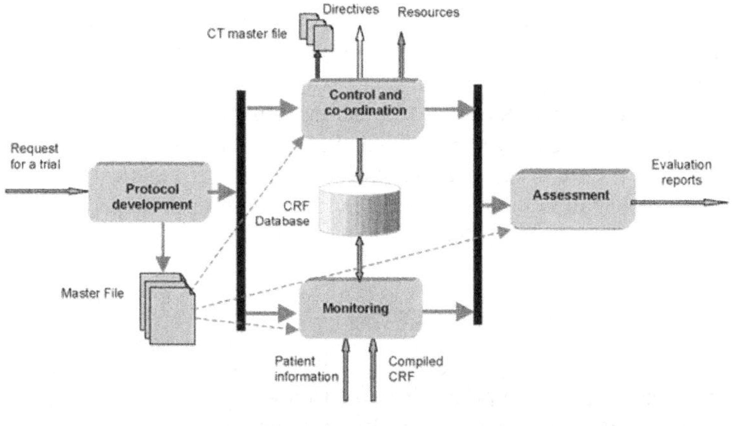

Fig. 3. Clinical Trial Management Process

The coordination and control process and the monitoring process are concurrent and they communicate indirectly through the CRF database.

The first activity to be implemented is the protocol development, which produces the CT master file. All other activities of the CT process will be driven by the documents contained in the CT master file. Among these documents the most important one is the CT protocol. In order to model the whole process of the CT, we modelled the protocol itself. The complexity of using such a model gives an idea of the difficulty in the development of clinical protocols.

3.3 Statistical Units Management

The SUMP process represents all activities carried out in a PhC. Figure 4 introduces the subprocesses of the SUMP process: 1 process starting up procedures, 2 patient enrolment management, 3. monitoring of the patient treatment and 4. closing of the CT.

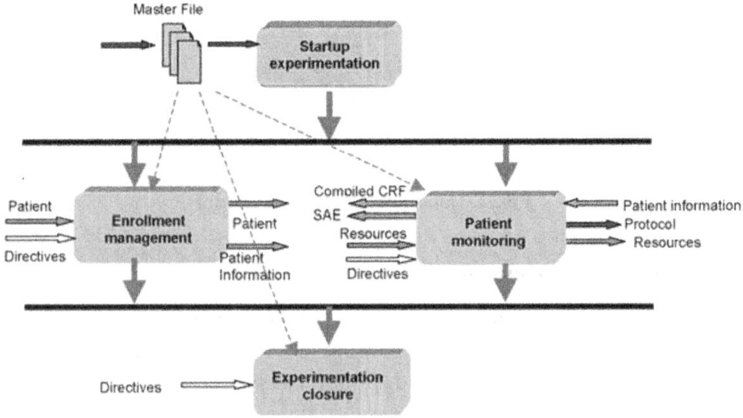

Fig. 4. Management of statistical units process

As already mentioned all the activities are driven by documents included in the CT master file. As the figure shows patient enrolment management and patient monitoring are parallel activities, even if for a single patient the enrolment precedes the monitoring of her/his disease progression. Patient enrolment selects patients applying the selection criteria included in the protocol and gives the patient a *sequential identification code* (SIC). As a consequence the patient becomes a statistical unit for CT. Patient monitoring has the function of verifying that the information contained in a patient's HCR has been correctly reported in the CRF.

3.4 Patient Health Care Delivery Process

Figure 5 shows the main subprocesses of the PM process: the start-up of treatment process, the patient treatment process and the follow-up process.

An instance of this process is created for each patient: The physician treats the patient according to the treatment plan described in the protocol. The physician is constrained to guarantee the patient's life safety and to notify SAE as soon as they occur. The clinical data related to the patient are stored in her/his HCR.

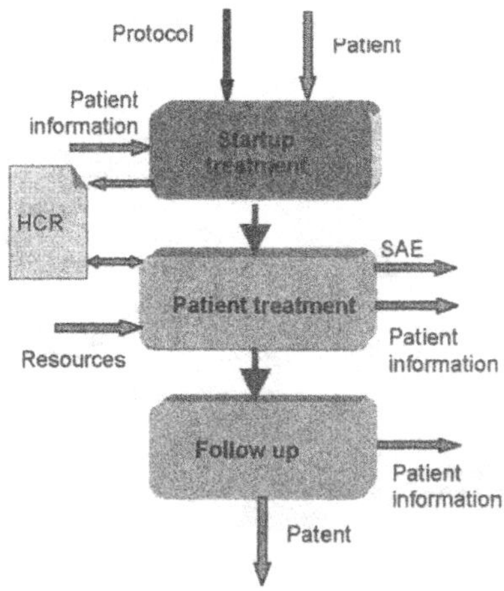

Fig. 5. Patient health care delivery process

4 Modelling Clinical Trials

In this section we present the main UML diagrams used in our model of the CT process. Due to editorial space limits we present our model at a high level of abstraction. A more detailed description of the model can be found in [11]. Our CT model considers the process under at least three views: the functional, the structural, and the behavioural ones. The views may be external (*black box view*) or internal (*white box views*). In order to model various stakeholders' concerns, other views have been added. A multifaceted model [10] closely related to reality has resulted [11]. To describe these different perspectives we use the following diagrams: a) use case and activity diagrams for the functional CT description; b) class diagram for the CT structural description, and c) interaction overview and sequence diagrams for the behavioural CT description.

4.1 The CT User's Functional View

Functional views specify the logic of a system; its main functions can be identified by the perspective of either a user, who interacts with the system (user's or black box view), or a system's designer, i.e. the stakeholder, who decides how the system is built (designer's or white box view).

The use case diagram is used to model how actors (people and other systems) interact with the system. A use case denotes a set of scenarios where the user interacts with the system. A UML use case diagram shows the relationships among actors/agents and use cases within a system. One or more actors can participate to a use case, but only one is the user case trigger, who makes the user case start. Use cases provide the functional requirements of the system/organisation [15].

Figure 6 shows the main scenario of the CT research process from the perspectives of actors/agents involved in the process. The main actors/agents of a CT process are: the writing committee, the data centre, the CT coordinator, the statistical unit and the participating centres.

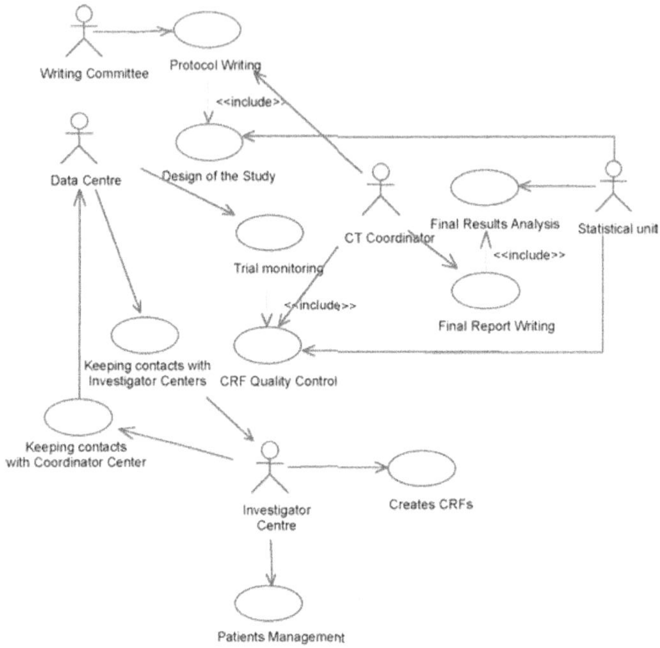

Fig. 6. The Use case diagram of the CT process

The analysis of this diagram highlights the fundamental role played by the CC, which collaborates with other actors to perform the protocol definition, the control of the CT execution, and the evaluation of results. In the diagram, the patient treatment activities and the CRF creation are loosely coupled, they are carried out independently.

4.2 The CT Structural View

The class diagram stands at the centre of the object-modelling process. It is the diagram used for: a) capturing all the relationships between objects in the system and rules that govern the use of these objects [15],b) explore domain concepts in the form of a domain model,c) analyse requirements in the form of a conceptual model, and d) depict the detailed design of business objects.

It is well known that objects are abstractions of real world entities. Our objects may be: laboratory tests, drugs, adverse events, etc. Figure 7 describes one of these objects: the CT master file. As the figure shows, in the protocol we distinguish between information related to scientific aspects from those connected with the administrative-organisational ones. This information is mandatory for CT approval by the scientific and ethical committees according to international standardised rules [5]. Giving some examples, scientific information are particularly useful for the investigator to enrol the patient (the protocol section "Patient selection criteria"), for the elaboration of statistical analysis (the section "statistical consideration"), for physicians to perform the therapeutic plan (the sections "therapeutic regiments" and "clinical evaluation"), etc. Administrative and organisational information can be more easily standardised and consequently CT writing authoring tools can support its reuse. A more detailed structure of the CT master file can be found in [11].

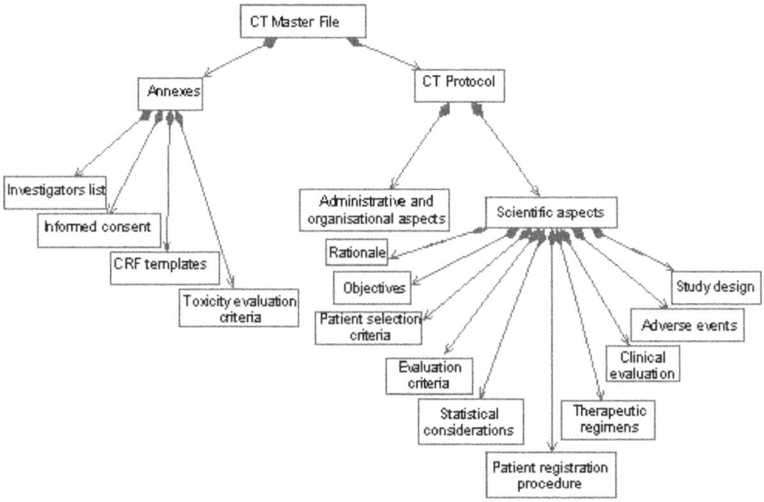

Fig. 7. The Class diagram of the CT process

Our analysis of the protocol has resulted in the development of a collaborative Writer System of CT (WITH) [3]. This analysis was based on the identification of the semantic relationships between CT sections [4]:

4.3 The CT Designer's Functional View

The activity diagram is often seen as part of the functional view of a system because it describes logical processes, or functions. UML activity diagrams are the object-oriented equivalent of flow charts and data-flow diagrams from structured development [15]. In our model the activity diagrams are used to describe the process and objects flows in a CT research. An example of the use of this UML activity diagram is presented in Figure 8, which describes the whole CT process at a high level of abstraction emphasising the communication between the CC and the PhCs.

The first activity in the process flow is related to the feasibility of a CT research and produces a list of potential PhCs as well as an approved outline. This gives the start of a protocol writing activity, which finishes when the protocol and its annexes (CT master file) are evaluated and approved. Now parallel activities are performed: database creation, writing of standard operating procedures manual, stipulations of contracts with investigators and with pharmaceutical industry for drug supply. Each one produces a specific object/document (for example the standard operating procedures manual). From the CRF templates contained in the annexes of the master file, a database is developed to store CT patient data (CRF). When all these activities are finished, the experimentation can start. An event launched by the Coordinator Centre triggers the start-up activity in all PhCs. Once a PhCs are activated, the enrolment procedures can be performed sending the registration CRF for the first enrolled patient. The patient enrolment continues until the coordinator centre sends a message to

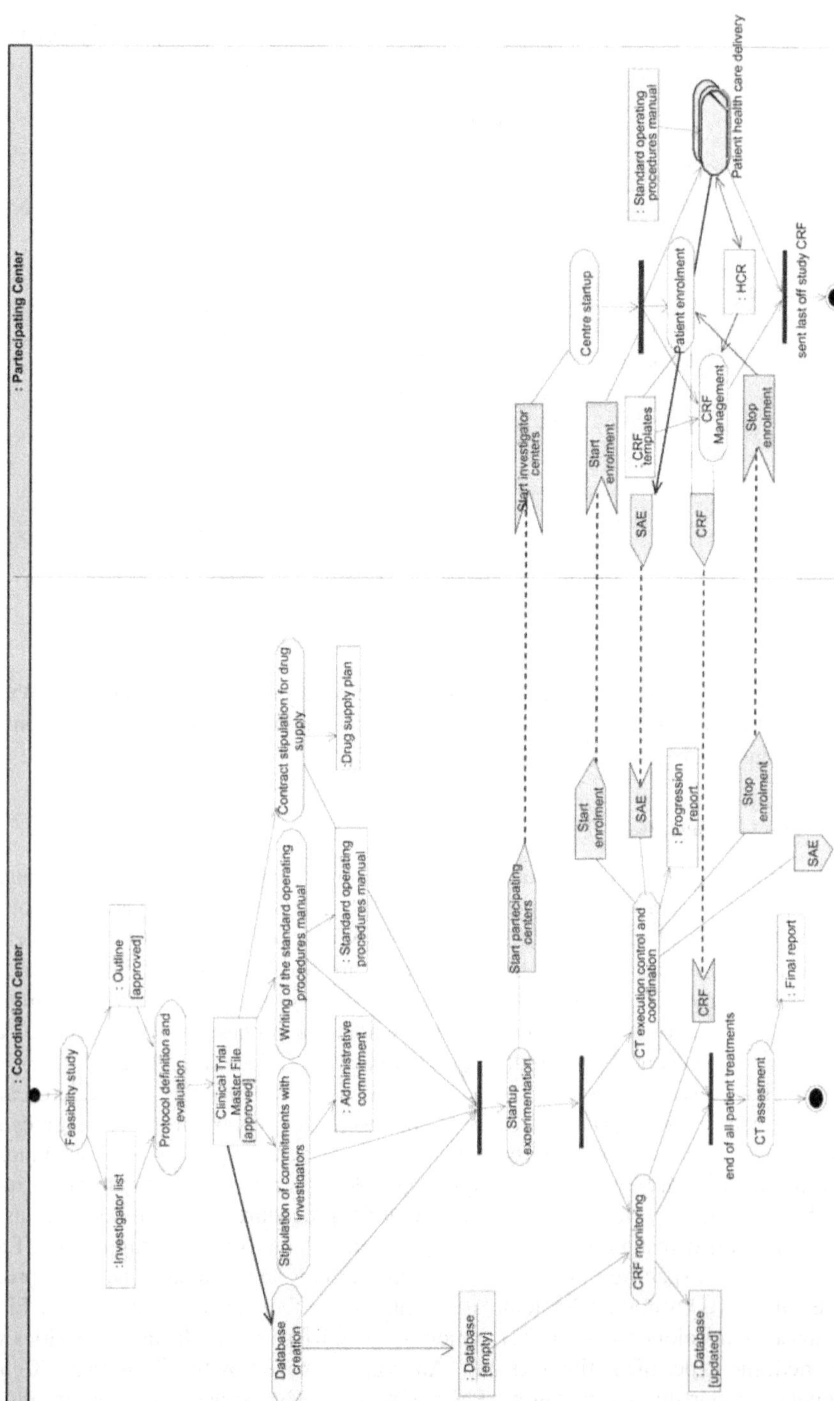

Fig. 8. The Activity diagram of the CT process

stop enrolment, because the number of patients foreseen in the statistical analysis has been reached. The instances of the business process "Patient health care delivery" are seen as a *black box*. The results of the activities carried out in this black box are stored in the HCR of the single patient. The investigator operating in each PhC fills in CRF with data extracted from HCRs. The activities of CRF management and patient treatment are performed in parallel and are concluded when the last CRF of the enrolled patients is sent. While the PhCs are performing their activities, the Coordinator Centre executes two parallel activities: CRF monitoring and CT execution control and coordination. The CRF monitoring is performed evaluating the quality of the CRF received, the number of forms associated to each patient, and the form associated to his/her treatment step. The control of CT implies the assignment of a code to each enrolled patient, the evaluation of the adverse events (sent to the Health Care Ministry in case of serious adverse events (SAE)), and the elaboration of the progress reports. When the last *off study form* is sent to the CC, the sequence of activities necessary to elaborate the final reports and the publication of results are performed.

The analysis of this diagram emphasises the separation between the activities carried out during the patient treatment and those connected with the protocol execution. The link between these activities is represented by the use of HCR. Clinical data are input during the patient treatment, while the investigators fills in the CRFs afterwards. The quality of data depends from this link, generally the trial coordinator(s) and the data centre are not in contact with the patient, but they can ask the physicians for explications.

A special case of communication between processes involved in the CT is represented by the occurrence of a SAE during the patient health care delivery. The consequences of this event can be modelled in UML as an *exception handling mechanism*. The event occurs in an instance of the patient health care delivery process and is immediately sent to the corresponding PhC, which on its turn redirects it to the CC. Finally the CC notifies the SAE to the Health Care Ministry.

4.4 Behavioural View

Behavioural models specify a time-oriented view of the interaction between components of a system. A UML sequence diagram is used to model system behaviour. An interaction may be modelled at any level of abstraction within the system design, from subsystem interactions to instance-level interaction for a single operation or activity. Sequence diagrams are typically used to validate the logic and completeness of a usage scenario, or to detect bottlenecks within an object-oriented design [15].

UML 2.0 introduces a valuable conceptual tool: the interaction overview diagram, which combines sets of interactions represented by sequence diagrams in one or more control flows, in same way the activity diagrams do [15].

Figure 8 shows an interaction overview diagram, which specifies interactions between the CC and the PhCs: These interactions are based on exchange of synchronous and asynchronous messages: CRF, information requests, notifications, etc. They are connected in control flows by different control operators: sequence (strict), iteration (loop), weak sequencing (seq), not mandatory activities (opt) etc.

The events "start participating centres" and "sent last off study CRF" are examples of asynchronous communication between centres.

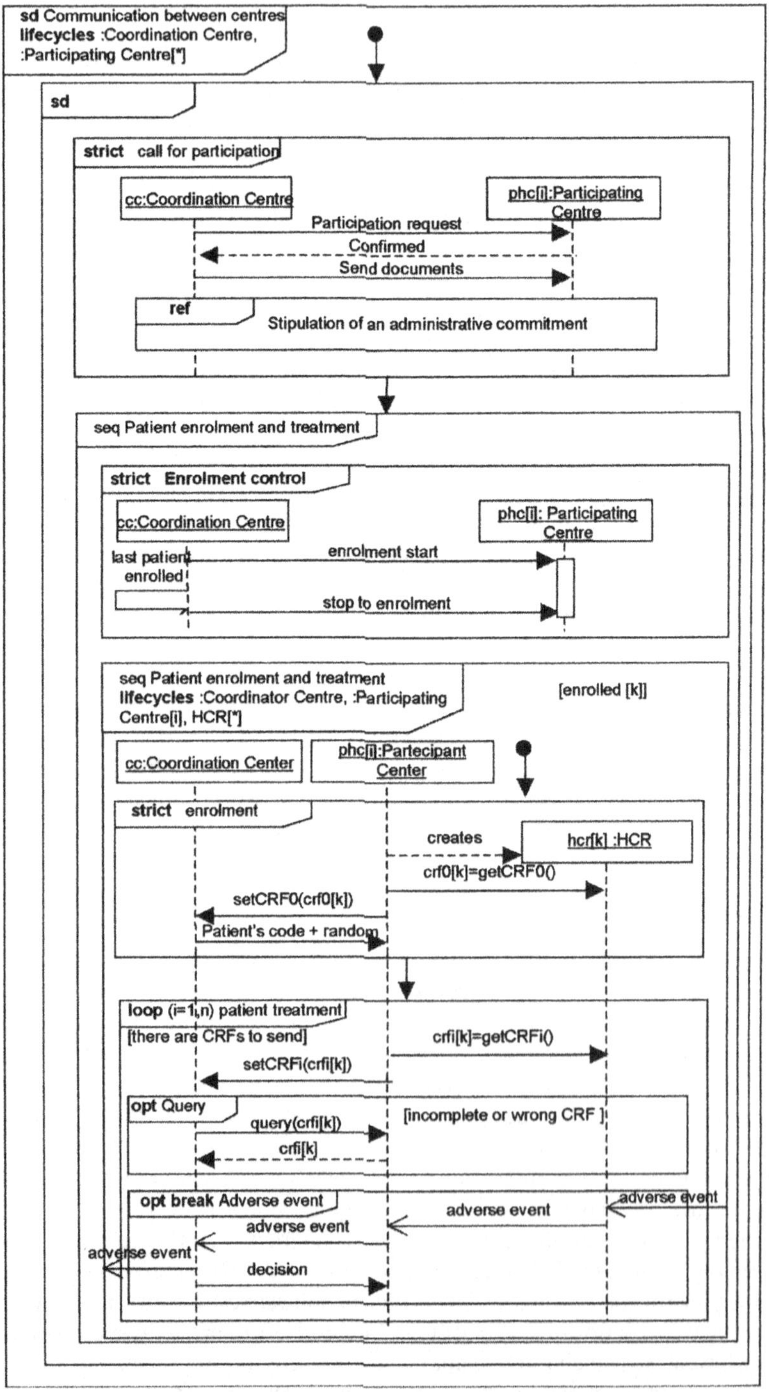

Fig. 9. The Sequence diagram of the CT process

The analysis of this diagram identifies the collection of CRF as a bottleneck of a CT research. In fact, there are two nested interactions of "weak sequencing" type. This operator indicates that several interactions may evolve in parallel without any mutual synchronisation. The interactions "PhC enrolment" and "Patient enrolment and treatment" show that there are no constraints on the order of collecting the forms of a single patient. The asynchronous communication between the CC and the PhCs should require special control mechanism provided by communication management. To overcome this difficulty we are testing a solution based on a dynamic model of CRF objects. Each CRF is viewed as an entity with its own lifecycle represented by a UML state diagram.

5 Conclusions

CT research is a complex process which includes definition, writing, evaluation, and approval of the CT protocol, its use for CT execution, and analysis of results. In order to enhance the clinical research, it is compulsory to consider it as a whole. This approach allows us to define a complete, coherente protocol model at an accurate level of abstraction as well as to identify new requirements for enhancing the WITH system.

The use of UML as a modelling language for the CT process allows us to develop a description able to be understood by all stakeholders. We claim that this research can be a stimulus for approaching the problem of the exchange of models which permits the interoperability between systems supporting activities of CT research.

The model creates a CT standard description which offers a framework to be customised for various experimentation environments (hemathology, oncology, cardiology, etc.). This model can also offer a base for applications which support CT single subprocesses or activities, for instance applications for communications between and inside centres, tools for supporting collaborative protocol writing, tools for CRF and SAE management, tools for CT execution monitoring.

References

1. Breitfeld P.P., Weisburd M., Overhage M.M., Sledge G., Tierney W.M.: Pilot Study of a Point-of-use Decision Support Tool for cancer Clinical Trial Eligibility. JAMIA, 6(6) (1999).
2. Fazi P., Luzi D., Ricci F.L., Vignetti M.: Supporting Writing and Diffusion of Clinical Trials. Proc. Information and Communication Technology Conf. 2001, (2001).
3. Fazi P., Luzi D., Manco M., Ricci F.L., Toffoli G., Vignetti M.: WITH: a System to Write Clinical Trials using XML and RDBMS.. Proc. AMIA Symp. 2002 (2002) 240-244.
4. Fazi P., Luzi D., Ricci F.L., Vignetti M.: The conceptual Basis of WITH, a Collaborative Writer System of Clinical Trials. Proc. ISMDA Symp. 2002. In: Colosimo A., Giuliani A. Sirella P. (eds.) Medical Data Analysis. Lecture Notes in Computer Science, Vol. 2526. Springer-Verlag, Berlin Heidelberg New York (2002) 86–97.
5. Guideline for good clinical practice. Available at http://www.eortc.be/documents (2000).
6. Modgil S., Hammond P., Wyatt J.C., Potts H.: Developing a Knowledge-based Tool for Authoring Clinical Trial Protocols. Proc. EWGLP, 2000 (2000).
7. Pender T.: UML Bible. John Wiley (2003).
8. Rubin D.L., Gennari J.H., Musen M.A.,: Knowledge Representation and Tool Support for Critiquing Clinical Trial Protocols. In Proceedings of the AMIA Symp. 2000, (2000).

9. Rubin D.L., Gennari J.H., Srinivas S., Yuen A., Kaizer H., Musen M.A., Silva J.S.: Tool Support for Authoring Eligibility Criteria for Cancer Trials. Proc. AMIA Symp. 1999 (1999) 369-373.
10. Serbanati L.D.: Integrating Tools for Software Development. Yourdon Press Computing Series, Prentice Hall, Englewood Cliffs, New Jersey (1992).
11. Serbanati L.D., Ricci F.L., Luzi D.: A New Approach for Modelling Clinical Trial Research. Working Paper WP IRPPS-CRR 3/2004, June (2004).
12. Silva, J. Wittes, R. Role of Clinical Trials Informatics in the NCI's Cancer Informatics Infrastructure. Proc. AMIA Symp. 1999 (1999) 950-954.
13. Standardizing Information Flow in Clinical Trial Protocols. Panel organizer: John Gennari, Available at http://www.amia.org/pubs/syposia/D200544.pdf (2000).
14. Unutzer J., Choi Y., Cook I.A., Oishi S.: Clinical Computing: a Web-based Data Management System to Improve Care for Depression in a Mulicenter Clinical Trial. Psychiatric Services, June (2002).
15. UML Superstructure version 2.0. Available at http://www.omg.org/docs/ptc/03-08-02.pdf (2003).
16. Weng C., Kahn M., Gennari J.H.: Temporal Knowledge Representation for Scheduling Tasks in Clinical Trial Protocols. Proc. AMIA Symp. 2002 (2002) 879-883.

Predicting Missing Parts in Time Series Using Uncertainty Theory

Sokratis Konias[1], Nicos Maglaveras[1], and Ioannis Vlahavas[2]

[1] Laboratory of Medical Informatics, Medical School, Aristotle University of Thessaloniki, POB 323, 54124 Thessaloniki, Greece
{sokratis,nicmag}@med.auth.gr
[2] Department of Informatics, Aristotle University of Thessaloniki, 54124 Thessaloniki, Greece
vlahavas@csd.auth.gr

Abstract. As extremely large time series data sets grow more prevalent in a wide variety of applications, including biomedical data analysis, diagnosis and monitoring systems and exploratory data analysis in scientific and business time series, the need of developing efficient analysis methods is high. However, essential preprocessing algorithms are required in order to obtain positive results. The goal of this paper is to propose a novel algorithm that is appropriate for filling missing parts of time series. This algorithm, named FiTS (Filling Time Series), was evaluated over 11 congestive heart failure patients' ECGs (Electrocardiogram). Those patients using electronic microdevices with which were recording their ECGs and sending them via telephone to a home care monitoring system, over a period of 8 to 16 months. Randomly missing parts in each ECG were introduced in the initial ECG. As a result, FiTS had 100% of successfully completion with high reconstructed signal accuracy.

1 Introduction

Time series can be defined as sequences of recorded values, which are usually real numbers recorded at regular intervals, such as weekly, daily, hourly and so on. Massive time series data are commonplace in a variety of monitoring application in medicine, finance, engineering, meteorology and other. Hence, there are several examples of the above applications generating this type of data like the mission operations for NASA's Space Shuttle, where approximately 20,000 sensors are telemetered once per second to mission control at Johnson space center, Houston [1] and the AT&T long distance data stream which consists of approximately 300 million records per day from 100 million customers [2].

Currently, there are a large number of different techniques for efficient subsequence matching. In [3] the problem of sequence similarity for applications involving one dimensional time series data, is addressed. An intuitive notion of sequence similarity is introduced, which allows non matching gaps, amplitude scaling and offset translation. The [1] illustrates a probabilistic approach for pattern matching in time series databases, which is a search algorithm using a distance measure to find matches for a variety of patterns on a number of data sets. In [4] several algorithms for efficient mining of partial periodic patterns in time series database needing only two scans over the data are proposed.

In a broad diversity of fields like medicine, financial, meteorology and so on, massive time series data sets are collected, as it has already mentioned. Missing parts are

J.M. Barreiro et al. (Eds.): ISBMDA 2004, LNCS 3337, pp. 313–321, 2004.

frequently appeared in this type of data. For instance, in a home care monitoring system, where heart failure patients send their ECGs (Electrocardiogram) via telephone. In such applications, missing values are due mainly to technical problems or improper use of the various interfaces and are considered random. The paper sets off by illustrating a novel algorithm for filling missing parts in time series. The new algorithm, called FiTS (Filling Time Series), was evaluated over several congestive heart failure patients' ECGs since they can be considered as time series.

The remaining part of the paper is organized as follows. In Section 2 the problem of missing values is presented. Section 3 presents measurements of time series similarity. In Section 4 the new algorithm for filling ECGs' missing parts, is illustrated. In Section 5 the results of an experimental evaluation of FiTS algorithm on an ECG home care database are described. Finally, in Section 6 we conclude the possibility of using our algorithm in the cleaning step of the KDD (Knowledge Discovering in Database) process appropriate for multimedia data as time series are.

2 Dealing with Missing Values

As it has already mentioned the problem of the missing values in databases of many fields is frequent. There are various reasons why missing values exist [5]. In some cases, values recorded are missing because they were too small or too large to be measured. In other cases, it is common for recorded values to be randomly missed because they have been forgotten or they have been lost. Furthermore, in applications where no human activity is taking part in the procedure of collecting data, random missing values result from the existence of technical problems or inappropriate use of the various interfaces.

There are two key ways to deal with missing values, internally or externally of a data mining technique. At present, treatments are often specific and internal to the algorithms which limits their flexibility. In [6] [7] [8] new algorithms handling missing demographic (i.e. age, pressure, weight etc) data, are proposed. The [7] presents an uncertainty rule algorithm in which the main idea upon tackling the problem of missing values was to ignore records containing them for each corresponding itemset separately, in order to avoid missing important information. For that scope new metrics were introduced correspondingly to the well known notion of support and confidence [9]. In [8] an improvement of the aforementioned algorithm is illustrated. The originality of that algorithm lies in its new adaptive threshold that is used in order to mine the most efficient rules amongst the data. Finally, in [10] nine different popular approaches coping internally with missing values are compared.

On the contrary, in [11][12] several universal approaches are described to replace missing values prior (external) to the data mining step. In [11] a method, namely MVC (Missing Values Completion), based on extracted association rules for filling demographic missing values are described. The core of MVC is an algorithm of association rules enabling it to be used for the data cleaning step of the KDD process. Furthermore, in [12] numerous general well known approaches are illustrated to replace the missing values prior the mining phase:

- Estimate values using simple measures derived from means and standard deviations or regression

- Augment each feature with a special value or flag that can be used in the solution as a condition for prediction

All previous algorithms for dealing with missing values (internally or externally) were appropriate for demographic data. In this paper, we focus on the missing values problem suitable for time series data proposing FiTS, a novel external data mining algorithm based on uncertainty theory. In other words, FiTS is an algorithm for the data cleaning step of the KDD process in time series data, like an ECG. Its important advantage is the additional capability to deal with the missing parts by an internal way. The reason is that it is common for the initial data to have multiple missing parts, i.e. more than one missing part in an ECG time series. FiTS involves two main phases, during the first the time series is converted into an alphabet, while during the second, association rules are extracted.

3 Measurements for Time Series Similarity

To cluster a given time series into similar subsequence (i.e. into alphabet), distance notions are needed. For that principle the given sequence $s=(x_1, x_2, \ldots, x_n)$ is separated into equal in number subsequences $s_i=(x_i, x_{i+1}, \ldots, x_{i+w-1})$ using a window of width w. All subsequences obtained by s are denoted as $W(s)=\{s_i / i= 1, 2, \ldots, n-w+1\}$. In this section some possible distance measures for clustering W(s) are described.

The simplest possibility is to treat the subsequences of length w as elements of R^w and use the Euclidean distance (i.e. the L_2 metric). Let $\overline{x}=(x_1,\ldots,x_w)$ and $\overline{y}=(y_1,\ldots,y_w)$ then $L_2(\overline{x},\overline{y})=\sqrt{\sum_i (x_i - y_i)^2}$ is defined as the Euclidean distance. Although L_2 is used most often for time series [13], other alternative distance measures between time series can provide interesting results too. For instance, the general L_p metrics defined by $L_p(\overline{x},\overline{y})=(\sum_i (x_i - y_i)^2)^{1/p}$ for $p \geq 1$ and $L_\infty = \max_i |x_i - y_i|$.

Nevertheless, the shape of time series is the first thing someone can observe from a time series plot. It is regular for many applications similarity search for time series data. In [14] some of those applications are indicated:

- In finance, where a trader is interested in finding all socks whose price movements follow the pattern of a particular stock in the same trading day.
- In music, where a vender wants to decide whether a new musical score is similar to any copyrighted score to detect the existence of plagiarism.
- In business management, where spotting products with similar selling patterns can result in more efficient product management.
- In environment science, for example comparing the pollutant level in different sections of a river, scientists can have a better understanding of the environmental changes.

Concerning with the shape, for humans it is easy to see the similarity among time series by just looking at their plots. Such knowledge must be encoded in the computer, if we desire to automate the detection of similarity among time series. The aforementioned distance measures are not adequate as a flexible similarity measure among time series since two time series can be very similar even though they have different base lines or amplitude scales. One way of achieving this is by normalizing the subsequences and then using the L_p metrics on the normalizing subsequences.

A simple and well known way to normalize a sequence is by shifting the time series by its mean and then scaling by its standard deviation.

$$\hat{x} = \frac{\overline{x} - avg(\overline{x})}{std(\overline{x})} \quad (1)$$

where $avg(\overline{x})$ is the average of $\overline{x}$ and $std(\overline{x})$ is the standard deviation for $\overline{x}$.

An alternative way of accomplishing the problem of the different base lines or amplitude scales between the time series is the Pearson Correlation Coefficient similarity measure. This measure is widely used in statistical analysis, pattern recognition and image processing [15].

$$corr(\overline{x}, \overline{y}) = \frac{avg(\overline{x} * \overline{y}) - avg(\overline{x})avg(\overline{y})}{std(\overline{x})std(\overline{y})} \quad (2)$$

where $\overline{x} * \overline{y}$ is the inner product between $\overline{x}$ and $\overline{y}$.

The Pearson Correlation Coefficient ranges from –1 to 1. A negative coefficient indicates a negative relation, while a positive coefficient identifies a positive relation. Lastly, a coefficient equal to zero indicates that the compared time series do not have any relation. In this paper the Pearson Correlation Coefficient is chosen in order to find similar parts among an ECG. The final purpose is to fill missing parts among an ECG due the rest of the signal.

4 The FiTS Algorithm

The primary step of FiTS algorithm is to define three parameters. The first parameter is a percentage of extension for the missing part from both sides. For example if 100 values are missing and 100% extension has been selected, then the compared subsequences will have 300 values length (i.e. 100 values from both sides additionally to the missing part). Continuously, the parameter of moving window k has to be defined. The reason is to scan and find similar parts among the sequence and the specified missing part. Thus, if k is equal to 10 then the first subsequence that will be compared with the missing part, will be $s_1=(x_1, x_2, \ldots, x_{300})$ while the second one will be the $s_{10}=(x_{10}, x_{11}, \ldots, x_{310})$. Finally, a threshold for the correlation criterion is needed, which means that two subsequences will be considered as correlated if their Pearson Correlation Coefficient is higher than the specified threshold.

Latter than defining the required parameters, the missing parts of the initial sequence are located. For each missing part the extended subsequence is compared based on the correlation between the extended part and the corresponding part, with each subsequence W(s) of the initial sequence. At the previous example, the moving window parameter was defined as 10, thus the first compared subsequence would be s_1, the second s_{10} and so on. The subsequences with correlation higher than the specified threshold for the extended parts (i.e. the first 100 values and the last 100 values of the subsequences) are added to a list with the candidate similarly subsequences.

In the next step the similar candidate subsequences are scanned in order to be categorized according to the correlation among their correspondingly missing part. In other words, for each created category all contained subsequences have higher correlation in pairs than the specified threshold. For instance, if the list with the similar candidate subsequences consists of (x_{10} , x_{11} ,..., x_{310}), (x_{40} , x_{41} ,..., x_{340}) and (x_{80} , x_{81} ,..., x_{380}) then their categorization is based on the middle 100 values which are the corresponded values with the initial missing part.

Afterwards, the categorized similar candidate subsequences, among their correlation that have been computed in the previous step, are combined using the uncertainty theory to find the most similar subsequence category [16][17] for the missing part. As the certainty factor in this study can be interpreted the Pearson Correlation Coefficient (see equation 2). For each similar candidate subsequences the part of the middle values (correspondingly to the missing part) is considered as the hypothesis Y while the rest of the subsequence is considered as evidence X. So, each subsequence can be assumed as a rule "IF X THEN Y WITH CF(X,Y)", where CF(X,Y) its certainty factor. When X is also predicted based on other evidence Z then the following function can be used to calculate the certainty factor.

$$CF(Z,Y) = CF(X,Y) \times \max\{0, CF(Z,X)\} \tag{3}$$

Where CF(Z,Y) represents the certainty factor of predicting Y based on known evidence Z, similarly for CF(X,Y) and CF(Z,X).

In case where there are two or more matching rules for a missing part (hypothesis Y) of the sequence the combination function below is required:

$$CF(XcoZ,Y) = \begin{cases} CF(X,Y) + CF(Z,Y)(1 - CF(X,Y)), CF(X,Y), CF(Z,Y) > 0 \\ \\ \dfrac{CF(X,Y) + CF(Z,Y)}{1 - \min\{|CF(Z,Y)|.|CF(X,Y)|\}}, -1 < CF(X,Y) \cdot CF(Z,Y) \le 0 \\ \\ CF(X,Y) + CF(Z,Y)(1 + CF(X,Y)), CF(X,Y), CF(Z,Y) < 0 \end{cases} \tag{4}$$

This combination function is commutative and associative in its first argument, so the order in which production rules are applied has no effect on the final result.

After finding the category based on the uncertainty theory the average subsequence of all subsequences including in this category, is calculated. The task following is to compute the variation between the extended subsequence and the corresponding part of the average subsequence in order to fill the missing part based on this variation. The main idea of the FiST algorithm is shown in the following pseudo code.

The main scheme for the FiTS algorithm is demonstrated in the following C line notation of pseudo code.

```
void FiST(float threshold, int movingWindow, float
precedence)
{
  int i;
  float corr;
  for(i=0; i<wholeNumber; i=i+movingWindow)
  {
    corr=correlation(s_i, extending_missing_subsequence)
    if(corr>=threshold)
      add to similar candidate subsequences
```

```
    }
    for each cand_s_i similar candidate subsequence
    {
      if(i==1)
      {
        define the first category
      }
      else
      {
        for all already defined cand_s_j
        {
          corr=correlation(cand_s_i, cand_s_j);
          if(corr>=threshold)
           define it into the correspondingly category j;
        }
        if(no already defined category match)
          define a new category;
      }
    }
    for each category defined above
    {
      compute the certainty factor;
    }
    find the most similar category msc using the
    Uncertainty Theory;
    compute avg_s=average(cand_s_msc);
    for(i=0; i<length_of_missing_part; i++)
      predicted_s_i = predicted_s_i-1 + avg_s_i - avg_s_i-1;
  }//end function
```

5 Experimental Results

In order to evaluate our algorithm we used the ECGs' database, created at the laboratory of medical informatics in the Aristotle University of Thessaloniki, Greece. It consists of records of patients who participated in the Citizen Health System (CHS) project between September 2001 and January 2003 [18]. CHS is a home care system constructed around an automated contact center functioning as a server. Patients can communicate with it via a variety of interfaces, like public telephone, internet or a mobile device (through WAP). In this project, patients record the values of their vital parameters (continuous variables) and their ECGs with the help of electronic micro-devices and transmit them to the contact center along with some yes/no answers to simple questions regarding mostly the occurrence of certain symptoms (dichotomous variables).

As coherence in this database, missing values are due mainly to technical problems or improper use of the various interfaces and are considered random. During the period of this study, 11 congestive heart failure patients were monitored for a period of 8-13 months and they were sending their ECG once a week while their values of the parameters three times a week. Table 1 describes the previous parameters. The chief function was to monitor the condition of the patients and help them to avoid hospital readmissions.

Table 1. Data transmitted to the Contact Center by congestive heart failure patients

Vital parameters (continuous)
Systolic blood pressure
Diastolic blood pressure
Pulse
Weight
Temperature
Questions asked (dichotomous)
Did you feel breathless during the night?
Are your feet swollen?
Do you feel more tired today?
Do you have dyspnoea today?
Did you take your heart failure medication?
ECG signals

We ran the FiTS algorithm for each ECG separately. The used dataset consisted of 160 ECGs. We used different values for the required parameters. The moving window parameter was selected to be one, so that we could obtain higher accuracy. The values between 0.75 and 0.95 in proportion with the quality of the corresponding ECG, were used for the threshold correlation parameter. As better quality a specific ECG had as higher threshold correlation was selected. Finally, the percentage of extension parameter was selected between 100% and 200%. For each ECG, randomly missing parts were introduced between 50%-100% of the ECG's device sample rate. The results show that we obtained 100% of successfully completion with most of the times small variation hard to be recognized even by a quick look at their plots (in most cases less than 2% variation). Figure 1 shows three examples of ECG's predictions from three different patients.

6 Conclusion

In this paper the FiTS algorithm was presented, which is an algorithm for filling missing parts of a time series according to the rest dataset. This algorithm was tested over 11 congestive heart failure patients' ECGs. As we can observe, the mainly reasons of randomly missing values in some important fields, like in telemedicine where the medical data are transferred all the time through the health centers, are caused usually by technical problems. So in these cases, algorithms for improving the quality of medical data like ECGs are required in order to assist doctors' work.

Experimental results illustrated in previous section show that the proposed algorithm has high effectiveness in filling missing parts in ECGs. The major idea that proposed in this paper was to implement an algorithm for time series datasets appropriate for the cleaning step of the KDD process. Hence, an improved for FiTS could be developed in the future, which will not need to predefine any thresholds by the users and the most suitable thresholds would be defined automatically.

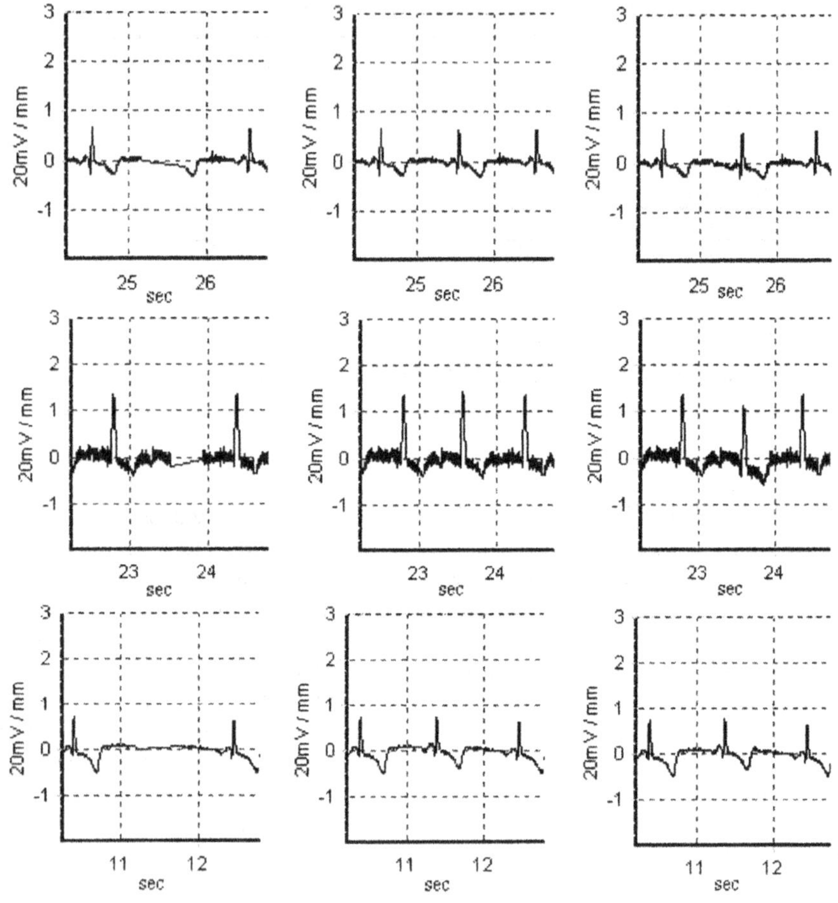

Fig. 1. On the left side the ECGs with about one second introduced missing values for each case are shown. In the middle part the initial ECGs are shown while on the right side the predicted ECG are shown. The reconstructed signal variation correspondingly in each case is 0.57%, 1.32% and 0.20%

Acknowledgments

This work was supported in part by the EC projects IST-1999-13352-CHS, IST-2001-33369-PANACEIA-ITV, as well as, by PROMESIP and IRAKLITOS both funded by the Greek Ministry of Education (EPEAEK I & II).

References

1. Keogh, E., Smyth, P.: A probabilistic Approach to Fast Pattern Matching in Time Series Databases. In Proc. of 3rd Int. Conference on Knowledge Discovery and Data Mining (1997) 24-30

2. Cortes, C., Fisher, K., Pregibon, D., Rogers, A.: Hancock: a language for extracting signatures from data streams. In ACM SIGKDD Int. Proc. of Conference on Knowledge Discovery and Data Mining (2000) 9-17
3. Agrawal, R., Lin, K., Sawhney, H.S., Shim, K.: Fast Similarity Search in the Presence of Noise, Scaling, and Translation in Time Series Databases. In Proc. of 21st Int. Conference on Very Large Databases (1995) 490-501
4. Han, J., Dong, G., Yin, Y.: Efficient Mining of Partial Periodic Patterns in Time Series Database. In 15th Int Conference on Data Engineering, Sydney (1999) 106-115
5. Konias, S., Bamidis, P.D., Maglaveras, N., Chouvarda, I.: Treatment of Missing Values Using Uncertainty in Medical Data. Eur J Med Res 7 (Suppl I), Regensburg Germany, (2002) 39-40
6. Konias, S., Bamidis, P.D., Maglaveras, N.: An Uncertainty Rule Generation Algorithm for Dynamic Medical Data. In Proc. of 11th World Congress on Medical Informatics (medinfo), San Francisco USA (CD), (2004) 1690
7. Konias, S., Giaglis, G.D., Gogou, G., Bamidis, P.D., Maglaveras, N.: Uncertainty Rule Generation on a Home Care Database of Heart Failure Patients. In Proc. of Computers in Cardiology, IEEE Comp. Soc. Press, (2003), 30, 765-768
8. Konias, S., Bamidis, P.D., Maglaveras, N.: Efficient Mining of Uncertainty Rules using Adaptive Thresholds in Medical Data. In Proc. of 3rd Hellenic Conference on Artificial Intelligence (2004) 32-41
9. Agrwal, R., Swami, A.: Fast Algorithm for Mining Association Rules. In Proc. of 20th Int. Conference on Very Large Data Bases. (1994) 487-499
10. Grzymala-Busse, J.W., Hu, M.: A Comparison of Several Approaches to Missing Values in Data Mining. RSCTC 2000, LNAI 2005, (2001) 378-385
11. Ragal, A., Cremilleux, B.:MVC- apreprocessing method to deal with missing values. Knowledge-Based Systems (1999),12; 378-385
12. Pyle, D.: Data Preperation for Data Mining. Morgan Kaufmann, San Francisco (1999)
13. Das, G., Lin, K., Mannila, H., Renganathan, G., Smyth, P.: Rule Discovery from Time Series. In Proc. of Int Conference on Knowledge Discovery and Data Mining (1998) 16-22
14. Agrawal, R., Faloutsos, C., Swami, A.N.: Efficient Similarity Search in Sequence Databases. In Proc. of 4th Int Conference of Foundations of Data Organization and Algorithms, Chicago (1993) 69-84
15. Rodgers, J.L., Nicewander, J.L, Nicewander, W.A.: Thirteen Ways to Look at the Correlation Coefficient. American Statistician 42, (1995) 59-66
16. Cohen, E., Datar, M., Fujiwara, S., Gionis, A., Indyk, P., Motwani, R., Ullman, J.D, Yang, C.: Finding Interesting Association without Support Pruning, ICDE (2000) 489-499
17. Das, G., Gunopulos, D., Mannila, H.: Finding Similar Time Series. In Proc. of Practice of Knowledge in Databases PKDD (1997) 88-100
18. Maglaveras, N., Koutkias, V., Chouvarda, I., Goulis, D.G., Avramides, A., Adamidis, D., Louridas, G., Balas, E.A.: Home Care Delivery through the Mobile Telecommunications Platform: The Citizen Health System (CHS) Perspective, International Journal of Medical Informatics 68, (2002) 99-111

Classification of Long-Term EEG Recordings

Karel Kosar[1], Lenka Lhotska[1], and Vladimir Krajca[2]

[1] Gerstner Laboratory, Czech Technical University in Prague
Technicka 2, 166 27 Prague 6, Czech Republic
lhotska@fel.cvut.cz
[2] University Hospital Bulovka, Budínova 2, 18081 Prague 8, Czech Republic
krajca@fnb.cz
http://cyber.felk.cvut.cz

Abstract. Computer assisted processing of long-term EEG recordings is gaining a growing importance. To simplify the work of a physician, that must visually evaluate long recordings, we present a method for automatic processing of EEG based on learning classifier. This method supports the automatic search of long-term EEG recording and detection of graphoelements – signal parts with characteristic shape and defined diagnostic value. Traditional methods of detection show great percent of error caused by the great variety of non-stationary EEG. The idea of this method is to break down the signal into stationary sections called segments using adaptive segmentation and create a set of normalized discriminative features representing segments. The groups of similar patterns of graphoelements form classes used for the learning of a classifier. Weighted features are used for classification performed by modified learning classifier fuzzy k-Nearest Neighbours. Results of classification describe classes of unknown segments. The implementation of this method was experimentally verified on a real EEG with the diagnosis of epilepsy.

1 Introduction

Computer assisted processing of long-term EEG recording is gaining a growing importance. The aim is to simplify the work of a physician that must visually evaluate many-hour EEG recordings. At present, EEG is recorded at patients 24 or 48 hours. The automatic systems cannot fully replace a physician but they are to make his/her work more efficient. They identify segments of the signal where there are deviations from standard brain activity and in this way they shorten the time required for visual inspection of the whole recording.

We illustrate our approach on classification of EEG signal of epileptic patients. The analysis and evaluation of long-term EEG recordings have recently gained increasing importance. One of the problems that are connected with the evaluation of EEG signals is that it necessitates visual checking of such a recording performed by a physician. In case the physician has to check and evaluate long-term EEG recordings computer-aided data analysis might be of great help. Our case study work deals with the issue of application of artificial intelligence methods to the analysis of EEG signals. The work describes the design and implementation of a system, which performs an automatic analysis of EEG signals.

Several attempts to detect epileptic seizures have already been made. They use formalisms such as conventional temporal and frequency analyses [1], [2], [3], quanti-

J.M. Barreiro et al. (Eds.): ISBMDA 2004, LNCS 3337, pp. 322–332, 2004.

tative characterization of underlying non-linear dynamical systems [4], local texture features in conjunction with wavelet transform [5], neural networks [6].

In the next sections we describe used theoretical methods, proposed approach that combines the methods, and give some details about the implemented system. Finally we present experiments and obtained results.

2 Problem Domain – Long-Term EEG Recordings of Epileptic Patients

The electroencephalogram (EEG) is a recording of spontaneous brain electrical activity by means of electrodes located on the scalp. The location of electrodes origins from natural physical limits -size of electrodes, which limits the maximum number of electrodes. Another limitation is mutual influence of electrodes located close to each other. Standardized placement of basic number of electrodes is based on scheme designed by Dr. Jaspes and nowadays it is called International 10-20 system.

In frequency domain we can distinguish four basic frequency bands on an EEG signal, namely delta, theta, alpha, and beta activities.

Delta band - corresponds to the slowest waves in the range of 0-4 Hz. Its appearance is always pathological at an adult in the waking state. Pathological significance increases with increasing amplitude and localization. Existence of delta wave is normal at children up to three years of age, in deep sleep and hypnosis. During sleep the waves can have amplitude higher than 100μV.

Theta band - corresponds to waves in the range of 4-8 Hz. Their existence is considered as pathological if their amplitude is at least twice as high as alpha activity or higher than 30 μV if the alpha activity is absent. The presence of theta wave is normal if its amplitude is up to 15 μV and the waves appear symmetrically. At healthy persons they appear in central, temporal and parietal parts. This activity is characteristic for certain periods of sleep.

Alpha band - corresponds to waves in the range of 8-13 Hz. In waking state at mental and physical rest the maximum appears in the occipital part of the brain. Its presence is highly influenced by open or closed eyes. The amplitude is in the range of 20-100 μV, most frequently around 50 μV.

Beta band - corresponds to the fastest waves in the range of 13-20 Hz. Maximum of the activity is mostly localized in the frontal part and it decreased in backward direction. The rhythm is mostly symmetrical or nearly symmetrical in central part. The amplitude is up to 30 μV. The activity is characteristic for concentration, logical reasoning and feelings of anger and anxiety.

The term epilepsy refers to a group of neurologic disorders characterized by the recurrence of sudden reactions of brain function caused by abnormalities in its electrical activity, which is clinically manifested as epileptic seizures. Manifestations of epileptic seizures vary greatly, ranging from a brief lapse of attention to a prolonged loss of consciousness; this loss is accompanied by abnormal motor activity affecting the entire body or one or more extremities. The basic classification of epilepsy and epileptic seizures into partial and generalized ones is widely accepted [7]. Among generalized epilepsy, grand mal and petit mal seizures are the most prevalent.

The ictal EEG features of the grand mal attack are characterized by a fall of amplitude of the signal, followed by a rhythmical activity at about 10 Hz in all leads, with rapidly increasing amplitude. Then, slower frequencies, in the delta range (0-4 Hz), as an expression of the postseizure stupor, precede normalization of the EEG, which coincides with return to the waking state. In the petit mal or absence seizure, the EEG is pathognomic, showing brief 3 Hz spike-and-wave discharges, which appear synchronously throughout all the leads (see Figure 1). Interictal EEG background activity is frequently normal in grand mal and petit mal epilepsy.

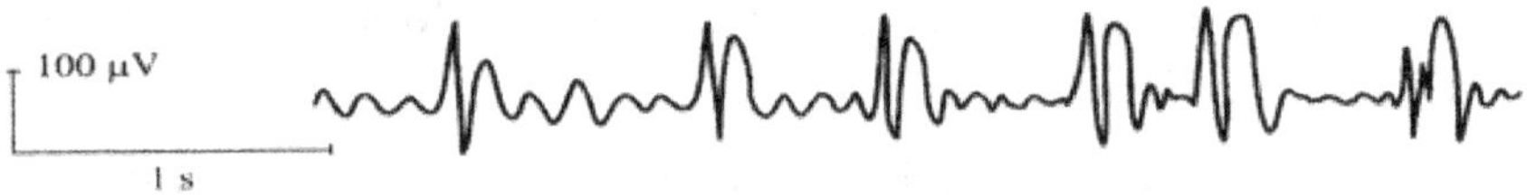

Fig. 1. Example of the spike-and-wave graphoelement

3 Phases of EEG Signal Processing

EEG signal processing represents a complex process consisting of several subsequent steps, namely data acquisition and storing, pre-processing, visualization, segmentation, extraction of descriptive features, and classification. We will briefly describe individual steps and in next sections we will focus on segmentation and classification as the most important steps that are decisive for the success of the whole process.

Data acquisition. EEG signal is recorded digitally and saved in defined format in files on a PC.

The aim of **pre-processing** is to remove noise and thus prepare the signal for further processing. The operations include, for example removal of DC part of the signal, signal filtration, removal of certain artefacts [8].

Segmentation. If we use signal divided to intervals of constant length for acquisition of informative attributes, non-stationariness of the signal may cause distortion of characteristics estimation. Segments defined in this way may contain mixture of waves of different frequencies and shapes. It is preferable to divide signal to segments of different interval length that are stationary. There exist several approaches to adaptive segmentation [9], [10] which divide signals to stationary segments.

Extraction of descriptive features is closely linked with segmentation. In automatic signal analysis, extraction of informative features with the greatest possible discriminative ability belongs to important tasks. Ordered set of features constitutes the feature vector. Values of individual features may differ in several orders and therefore feature normalization is performed. Output of this step is a vector of normalized features for each segment.

Classification means to assign class to unknown objects. A class is a group of objects with certain specific properties. In our case the objects are segments described by vectors of normalized features and classes correspond to different groups of graphoelements. Result of classification is signal divided into segments where each segment is assigned to a certain class.

4 Segmentation

EEG signal belongs to stochastic signals. Stochastic signals can be divided into two basic groups, namely stationary and non-stationary signals. Stationary stochastic signals do not change their statistic characteristics in time. Non-stationary signals may have variable quantities in time, for example mean value, dispersion, or frequency spectrum. EEG signal is non-stationary as most of real signals. Therefore such signals are considered stationary whose statistic parameters remain constant over sufficiently long time. This is the main idea of signal segmentation. In principle, there exist two basic approaches, namely constant segmentation and adaptive segmentation.

Constant segmentation divides signal into segments of constant length. In genereal, this type of segmentation is the simplest one. However, its disadvantage is that the resulting segments are not necessarily stationary. Our modification suggests to use overlapping of individual segments. Using small shift and suitable length of segments, we can reach very good results for correct division directly into individual graphoelements.

Constant segmentation performs division of signal x[n], where n = 0, 1,..., N-1, into segments $s_i[m]$, where m = 0, 1,..., N_i-1. Length of segment $s_i[m]$ is then N_i. Assume constant P be value of shift during segmentation and constant step M. If we allow M < P we reach segment overlapping. For length of segments N_i and total number of segments S it holds

$$\forall i : N_i = D, \quad i = 0, 1, ..., S - 1, D \in N.$$

Constant segmentation is based on division of signal into segments of length D at successive shift of starting point in each step by the value M. For exact classification, it would be advantageous to acquire segments that contain a single graphoelement each. In such a way we would reach the most precise results in automatic detection of graphoelements. Therefore we have to set small values of the step M and mean value D. Constant value of D is not optimal and therefore it is impossible to reach exactb results. Moreover, an excessive number of segments is generated which results in increased demands on computation. Consequently, adaptive segmentation is used preferably.

Adaptive segmentation is based on the principle of division of the signal into quasi-stationary segments. These segments are relatively stationary and in general they have different length N_i for each segment in dependence on presence of individual stationary parts in the signal. The method utilizes the principle of sliding two joint windows [10] where both windows have the same fixed length D. It is based on calculation of differences of defined signal parameters of two windows. Following procedure enables to indicate segment borders: Two joint windows slide along the signal. For each window the same signal characteristics are calculated. Measure of difference is determined from the differences of signal characteristics in both windows. This measure corresponds to difference of signals in both windows. If the measure of difference exceeds defined threshold, the point is marked as segment border. The difference is frequently calculated from spectra of both windows, using FFT. The method is very slow because the difference is calculated using FFT for each window shift.

For our implementation two modifications have been proposed. Method 1 is based on [11] modified in [12]. It uses two characteristics for computation of measure of difference of both windows. Principle of the method is illustrated in Figure 2. Both characteristics reflect certain properties of the signal both in time and frequency domains.

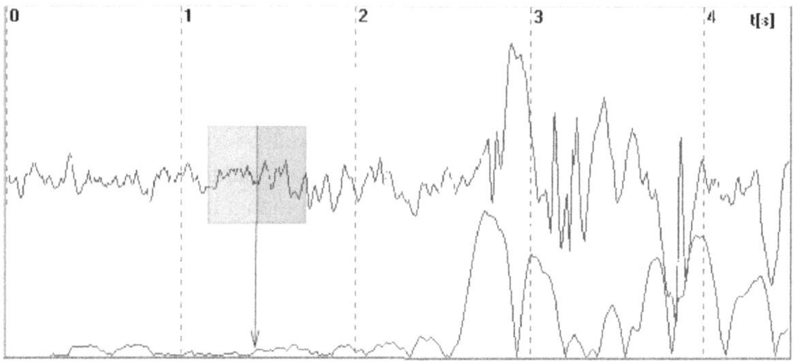

Fig. 2. Illustration of joint sliding windows and measure of difference

The first characteristic is based on estimation of average frequency in the segment

$$A_s = \sum_{j=0}^{N_i-1} | s_i[j] |$$

The second characteristic is the value of mean amplitude in the window

$$f_s = \sum_{j=0}^{N_i-1} | s_i[j] - s_i[j-1] |$$

The measure of difference is then computed as

$$G(n) = k_A \, |A1_s(n) - A2_s(n)| + k_F \, |f1_s(n) - f2_s(n)|$$

The coefficients k_A and k_F influence impact of individual characteristics, or partially compensate different scales of characteristics. Direct detection of local maxima of these characteristics leads to generation of relatively lower number of segments. For speeding up the computation of segments it is possible to shift both windows by step having value of several samples. Further it is possible to define a condition for minimum length of the segment. If the segment does not satisfy this condition it is attached to one of the neighbouring segments.

Method 2 is modification of method 1 proposed in [13]. Basic principle of segmentation remains, only the way of computing the measure of difference, applied characteristics and finding the segment borders is different. A single characteristic, nonlinear energy operator [14], is used for computation of difference. This quantity is more robust with respect to noise.

5 Set of Features for EEG Classification

After segmentation, attributes that will be used for classification are selected. There are considered characteristics in both time and frequency domains and basic properties of EEG. The following attributes describing signal can be used: average AC amplitude in the segment, variance of AC amplitude in the segment, maximum positive and minimum negative values of amplitude in the segment, maximum value of the first derivation of the signal in the segment, maximum value of the second derivation of the signal in the segment, average value of frequency in the segment, amplitude values in defined frequency bands (e.g. for EEG in alpha, beta, theta, and delta bands), frequency-weighted energy (it is based on nonlinear energy operator; the resulting value is proportional to amplitude and frequency). All attribute values are normalized because values of different attributes may vary in several orders and thus they are incomparable. Normalized attributes are dimensionless quantities with normal distribution N(0,1).

6 Classification

In our study we have decided to use for classification two methods, namely k-NN (nearest neighbour) [15] and fuzzy k-NN [16]. k-NN method is a relatively simple and frequently used method. However, it has several disadvantages. It is slow because the algorithm has to search the whole training set when classifying an unknown vector; it has high memory demands because the whole training set is stored in the memory. On the other hand, the classification error is in most cases comparable to classification error of neural networks. Fuzzy k-NN is similar to k-NN but it differs in the output information. It does not return number of class but class membership values. The class membership value can be determined in several ways. We have used two ways, namely plain determination of class membership and determination of class membership by nearest neighbours.

Plain determination of class membership values is based on the assumption that the vectors in the training set are characteristic vectors of the given class and thus they do not belong to the other classes. Plain learning keeps exactly information about the class. The vector has unambiguous membership to the given class and null to all other classes.

Determination of class membership by nearest neighbours is based on the assumption that the given value of class in the training set need not characterise exactly corresponding vector. Therefore the algorithm tries to find class membership according to distribution of neighbouring vectors in the feature space using k-NN algorithm. It tries to keep classes defined in the training set but at the same time it respects surrounding k nearest neighbours of the given vector in the feature space. In case of a representative vector of the given class (in its neighbourhood there are only vectors of the same class) the method corresponds to plain determination of the class membership.

7 Experimental Data and Results

The efficiency of developed algorithms has been tested using a training set created from 931 classified signals that contain 177 segments with epileptic graphoelements and 734 non-epileptic graphoelements. Epileptic graphoelements are of the type spike-and-wave. Class 0 denominates non-epileptic graphoelements and class 1 epileptic graphoelements. As a testing set we have used a signal containing 12610 EEG samples in 20 channels recorded with sampling frequency of 128 Hz. The signal contains two epileptic seizures having different length. Beginning of the seizure 1 is in 3rd second and beginning of seizure 2 is in 72nd second of the recording. The main aim of the experimental part has been verification of the influence of parameters of individual parts of processing to classification error. Different setups of segmentation, types of classifiers and feature weights have been tested.

Table 1. Classification error for different setting of classifier using weighted parameters

Classifier	Classification error (%)	Difference P (%)
1-NN	39.95	-
3-NN	17.45	-
fuzzy 3-NN (plain)	15.06	36.51
fuzzy 3-NN (3-NN)	18.36	69.26
fuzzy 3-NN (5-NN)	15.92	76.77
5-NN	6.33	-
fuzzy 5-NN (plain)	6.33	45.55
fuzzy 5-NN (3-NN)	12.24	78.65
fuzzy 5-NN (5-NN)	8.41	86.59
fuzzy 5-NN (7-NN)	6.05	84.54
7-NN	5.49	-
fuzzy 7-NN (plain)	5.42	48.33
fuzzy 7-NN (5-NN)	5.77	84.98
fuzzy 7-NN (7-NN)	5.22	85.88
fuzzy 7-NN (9-NN)	4.59	86.86
9-NN	5.59	-
fuzzy 9-NN (plain)	5.15	49.37
fuzzy 9-NN (7-NN)	5.08	87.07
fuzzy 9-NN (9-NN)	5.42	88.11
fuzzy 9-NN (11-NN)	5.49	89.92
11-NN	5.70	-
fuzzy 11-NN (plain)	5.70	59.76
fuzzy 11-NN (9-NN)	6.05	89.50
fuzzy 11-NN (11-NN)	5.84	90.82

7.1 Testing Classifier Parameters

In the first step we determine the impact of k value on classification error. With respect to the training set containing two classes it is suitable to choose k odd because then we will not face the problem of indecision. Let us start with k=3. Signal has been segmented using adaptive segmentation (method 1). Length of the window is 32, minimum length of segments is 30 samples, filtration is not applied. Threshold setting is adaptive, for features FFT=128 samples and Hanning window are used. For computation of difference, sum of mean amplitude with coefficient $k_A=1$ and mean frequency $k_f=20$ is applied. Classification results of 1438 segments are presented in Tables 1 and 2. Table 2 shows results reached using standard weight and Table 1 shows results reached using following values of weights:

1. Maximum amplitude value = 0.0
2. Minimum amplitude value = 0.0
3. Mean frequency = 0.9
4. Mean amplitude = 1.1
5. Amplitude variance = 0.5
6. First derivation = 1.5
7. Second derivation = 1.2
8. Alpha activity = 1.0
9. Beta activity = 1.5

10. Delta activity = 1.3
11. Theta activity = 1.0
12. Frequency-weighted energy = 0.8

These values have been set up experimentally by minimization of cross-validation error of classification for different values of weights. For verification of classification error, a reference table containing information about correct classification has been created for the given segments. The value of class membership has been set to 100%. Symbol P in tables represents number of segments where the computed value of class membership does not agree with the real value. This quantity is meaningful only in fuzzy k-NN classifiers.

The disadvantage of k-NN classifier is that it is not able to determine validity of results in percentage. Application of fuzzy k-NN classifier has been very advantageous and has allowed acquire certain idea about real results. Plain learning has mostly reached comparable results to k-NN learning. Moreover k-NN learning has frequently created higher uncertainty of resulting class and manifested higher time demands.

Table 2. Classification error for different setting of classifier using standard parameters

Classifier	Classification error (%)	Difference P (%)
1-NN	16.13	-
3-NN	7.51	-
fuzzy 3-NN (plain)	7.58	18.43
fuzzy 3-NN (3-NN)	7.30	49.44
fuzzy 3-NN (5-NN)	6.88	53.20
5-NN	6.61	-
fuzzy 5-NN (plain)	6.40	21.84
fuzzy 5-NN (3-NN)	6.40	56.19
fuzzy 5-NN (5-NN)	6.05	60.08
fuzzy 5-NN (7-NN)	5.91	60.92
7-NN	6.12	-
fuzzy 7-NN (plain)	5.96	23.64
fuzzy 7-NN (5-NN)	6.26	63.35
fuzzy 7-NN (7-NN)	6.26	64.19
fuzzy 7-NN (9-NN)	6.12	70.17
9-NN	6.26	-
fuzzy 9-NN (plain)	6.33	25.66
fuzzy 9-NN (7-NN)	6.40	67.52
fuzzy 9-NN (9-NN)	6.40	72.11
fuzzy 9-NN (11-NN)	5.91	73.37
11-NN	6.26	-
fuzzy 11-NN (plain)	6.33	26.84
fuzzy 11-NN (9-NN)	6.26	73.37
fuzzy 11-NN (11-NN)	6.40	74.83

7.2 Testing Segmentation Algorithms

Considering the results of previous testing, we have selected values of k=5, 7, 9 for testing of segmentation algorithms. Parameters not mentioned in this section have been set up to values according to section 7.1.

First test has been performed with adaptive segmentation using method 1. Length of window is 32, minimum length of one segment is 30 samples, filtration of length 5 is used, user defined threshold (=25). For computation of attributes, FFT length of 128 samples and Hanning window have been used. For computation of difference, sum of mean amplitude with coefficient k_A=1 and mean frequency k_f=20 is applied. The best results (lowest value of classification error) have been reached for 5-NN with weighted parameters (error = 7.17%) and fuzzy 5-NN (plain) with standard parameters (error = 11.53%).

Second test has been performed with adaptive segmentation using method 2. Length of window is 32, minimum length of one segment is 30 samples, difference filtration of length 7 is used, adaptive setting of threshold using 16 samples. For computation of attributes, FFT length of 128 samples and Hanning window have been used. 1216 segments have been found. The best results (lowest value of classification error) have been reached for 7-NN with weighted parameters (error = 3.85%) and 9-NN with standard parameters (error = 6.17%).

Third test has been performed with adaptive segmentation using method 2 with different settings. Length of window is 32, minimum length of one segment is 30 samples, difference filtration of length 7 and signal filtration of length 5 are used, user defined threshold (=10). For computation of attributes, FFT length of 128 samples and Hanning window have been used. 779 segments have been found. The best results (lowest value of classification error) have been reached for fuzzy 7-NN with weighted parameters (error = 7.71%) and 9-NN with standard parameters (error = 10.15%).

Finally, the constant segmentation has been tested. The value of shift has been set to 50 samples; length of segment has been set to 80 samples to reach overlapping. The reason for the particular value of shift is to reach reasonable number of segments. Length of segment corresponds roughly to the length of some epileptic graphoelements. In this way, the algorithm has found 5020 segments. The best results (lowest value of classification error) have been reached for fuzzy 9-NN (7-NN) with weighted parameters (error = 3.04%) and fuzzy 9-NN (7-NN) with standard parameters (error = 4.15%). Comparison of results is summarized in Table 3.

Table 3. Overview of results for different settings of segmentation

Segmentation	Mean error (%)
Adaptive, method 1, adapt. threshold, 1438 seg.	6,55
Adaptive, method 1, threshold 20, filtr.=5, 892 seg.	8,60
Adaptive, method 2, adapt. threshold, 1216 seg.	4,42
Adaptive, method 2, threshold 10, filtr.=5, 779 seg.	8,42
Constant, segment length 80, shift 50, 5020 seg.	3,94

The best results have been reached by constant segmentation. It is understandable because the classified segments have similar length and parameters as the segments used for learning. However, great disadvantage of constant segmentation is necessity to classify several times higher number of segments than when using the adaptive segmentation. Adaptive segmentation has reached comparable results with both methods (1, 2) for computation of difference. Both methods have worked better with adaptive setting of the threshold.

Misclassification has appeared at extremely long segments containing several thousands of samples. It is probable that the characteristics are not similar to learned patterns that have length of several tens or hundreds of samples. Further, misclassification has occurred in presence of artefacts if they have been similar to studied graphoelements.

8 Conclusion

One of the aims of signal classification system development is to ease work (in the described application work of medical doctors). These systems are to help the doctor interpret long-term EEG records correctly and successively to propose the most appropriate treatment. Further applications of these systems can be in education of new doctors.

The developed system has been tested using a real EEG signal containing epileptic graphoelements. Classification into two classes has been used. Based on individual experiments we can compare properties of applied methods for EEG processing. First test has been aimed on evaluation of impact of the value of constant k in k-NN algorithm and K in fuzzy k-NN with K-NN learning. The classifier reaches better results with higher value of k. However, if k exceeds a certain limit the classification error increases again. From the tests it has followed that the most suitable values of k are 5, 7 or 9. These values have been used for further tests when segmentation methods have been evaluated.

Methods of adaptive segmentation have generated similar numbers of segments that have been several times lower than the number of segments generated by constant segmentation. Constant segmentation has reached the lowest classification error at the expense of high number of insignificant segments. The error has been mainly influenced by the length of segments in the training set. Adaptive segmentation has mostly divided signal into more segments in parts with epileptic activity and less segments in areas of normal EEG activity. Misclassification has appeared for long segments or segments with present artefacts with similar shape as graphoelements. In most cases it has been advantageous to apply non-standard weights. The error has decreased by several per cents.

The system has reached very good results in detection of graphoelements. The whole processing has reached mean testing error of 6%. More exact results have been reached by mutually advantageous combination of setups of individual parts of the system.

Future work can be divided into following main directions:

- improved generation and representation of segments;
- utilisation of decision trees for classification;
- application of data mining and knowledge discovery methods in order to find possibly new relations among signal features;
- more efficient implementation of applied algorithms for increasing performance of the system.

Acknowledgments

The research of K. Kosar and L. Lhotska was supported by the research program No. MSM 210000012 "Transdisciplinary Research in the Area of Biomedical Engineering" of the CTU in Prague, sponsored by the Ministry of Education, Youth and Sports of the Czech Republic. The research of V. Krajca was supported by grants No. 7511 and 7586 IGA CR.

References

1. Davey B.L.K. et al., 1989, "Expert system approach to detection of epileptiform activity in the EEG", Med. Biol. Eng. Comput. 27(4), pp. 365-370
2. Gotman J., 1982, "Automatic recognition of epileptic seizure in the EEG", Electroencephalogr. Clin. Neurophysiol. 83, pp. 271-280
3. Qu H.; Gotman J., 1993, "Improvement in seizure detection performance by automatic adaptation to the EEG of each patient", Electroencephalogr. Clin. Neurophysiol. 86, pp. 79-87
4. Mayer-Kress G., 1994, "Localized measures for nonstationary time-series of physiological data", Integrative Physiological Behav. Sci. 29 (3), pp. 205-210
5. Petrosian A.; Homan R.W.; Pemmaraju S.; Mitra S., 1995, "Wavet-based texture analysis of EEG signal for prediction of epileptic seizure", SPIE Proceedings on Wavelet Applications in Signal and Image Processing, Vol. 2569, San Diego, CA, pp. 189-194
6. Weng W.; Khorasani K., 1996, "An adaptive structure neural networks with application to EEG automatic seizure detection", Neural Networks 9(7), pp. 1223-1240
7. Hornero R., Espino P., Alonso A., Lopez M.: Estimating Complexity from EEG Background Activity of Epileptic Patients. IEEE Engineering in Medicine and Biology, Nov./Dec. 1999, pp. 73-79
8. Smith S.W., 1997, "Digital Signal Processing", California Technical Publishing, San Diego, CA, USA
9. Bodenstein G.; Praetorius H.M., 1977, "Feature extraction from the electroencephalogram by adaptive segmentation", Proc. IEEE, 65, pp. 642-652
10. Krajca V.; Petranek S.; Ondruska V.; Doruzkova J.; Pecharova D., 1992, "Multichannel adaptive segmentation – basis for EEG record pre-processing", Lekar a technika, 2, 23, pp. 28-34 (in Czech)
11. Varri A. Digital Processing of the EEG in Epilepsy. Tampere University of Technology, 1988.
12. Krajca V., Petranek S., Patakova I., Varri A. Automatic identification of significant graphoelements in multichannel EEG recordings by adaptive segmentation and fuzzy clustering. Int. Journal Biomed. Comput., 1991, 28, pp. 71-89.
13. Agarwal R., Gotman J., Flanagan D., Rosenblan B. Automatic EEG analysis during long-term monitoring in the ICU. Electroencephalography and Clinical Neurophysiology. 1998, Vol. 107, Issue 1, pp. 44-58.
14. Plotkin E.I., Swamy M.N.S. Nonlinear signal processing based on parameter invariant moving average modeling. In Proceedings CCECE '21. September 1992, Toronto, Canada, pp. TM3.11.1-TM3.11.4.
15. Cover T.M., Hart P.E. Nearest neighbour pattern classification. IEEE Transaction Inform. Theory. January 1967, vol. IT-13, pp. 21-27.
16. Keller J. M., Gray M. R., Givens J. A. A Fuzzy K-Nearest Neighbor Algorithm. IEEE Transactions on systems, man. and cybernetics. July/August 1985, vol. SMC-15, no. 4, pp. 580-585.

Application of Quantitative Methods of Signal Processing to Automatic Classification of Long-Term EEG Records

Josef Rieger[1], Lenka Lhotska[1], Vladimir Krajca[2], and Milos Matousek[3]

[1] Gerstner Laboratory, Czech Technical University in Prague
Technicka 2, 166 27 Prague 6, Czech Republic
lhotska@fel.cvut.cz
[2] University Hospital Bulovka, Budínova 2, 18081 Prague 8, Czech Republic
[3] Psychiatric Center Prague, Ustavni 98, Prague 8, Czech Republic
krajca@fnb.cz
http://cyber.felk.cvut.cz

Abstract. The aim of the work described in the paper has been to develop a system for processing long-term EEG recordings, especially of comatose state EEG. However with respect to the signal character, the developed approach is suitable for analysis of sleep and newborn EEG too. EEG signal can be analysed both in time and frequency domains. In time domain the basic descriptive quantities are general and central moments of lower orders, in frequency domain the most frequently used method is Fourier transform. For segmentation, combination of non-adaptive and adaptive segmentation has been used. The approach has been tested on real sleep EEG recording for which the classification has been known. The core of the developed system is the training set on which practically depends the quality of classification. The training set containing 319 segments classified into 10 classes has been used for classification of the 2hour sleep EEG recording. For classification, algorithm of nearest neighbour has been used. In the paper, the issues of development of the training set and experimental results are discussed.

1 Introduction

The aim of the work described in the paper was to develop a system for processing long-term EEG recordings, especially of comatose state EEG. However with respect to the signal character, the developed approach is suitable for analysis of sleep and newborn EEG too.

Classical "paper" electroencephalography consumes a large amount of paper for recording. Using standard speed of shift of 3 cm/s, 20 minute recording represents length of 36 meters of paper. However, during such a short time there need not manifestate, for example, epileptic activity. When studying sleep disorders, length of recording may reach several hundreds meters of paper. During long-term (e.g. 24 hour) monitoring the data load is even much higher.

It is logical and natural that development of information and computer technology has contributed to EEG signal processing in recent years. Capacity of hard disks, DVDs and optical disks, etc., enables incomparably more efficient storing of EEG recordings.

Digital signal form enables computational signal processing that was in paper form unrealizable. We can find examples, such as simple statistical methods, filtering,

J.M. Barreiro et al. (Eds.): ISBMDA 2004, LNCS 3337, pp. 333–343, 2004.

segmentation, automatic classification, computation of coherence between individual electrodes; advanced methods such as EEG signal mapping to 3D head (brain mapping). All these applications are being developed for enhancing efficiency of medical doctors' work when analyzing EEG recordings.

This paper is organised as follows. Section 2 presents a brief description of the medical problem domain – coma. Section 3 describes used methods for data preprocessing and processing. Section 4 describes unconventional procedure of preparation of the training set. Section 5 describes the experiments and analyses the results obtained. Finally, section 6 summarises the conclusions.

2 The Problem Domain – Coma

Coma is a state of brain function. It can be very roughly compared to sleep. However, an individual cannot awaken purposefully from coma, using either internal, or external stimulus. Comatose state may have a number of causes, starting from head injury at a serious accident, over cerebral vascular diseases, infectious diseases, brain tumours, metabolic disorders (failure of liver or kidney), hypoglycemia, to drug overdosing, degenerative diseases, and many more. A patient in coma does not manifest any notion of higher consciousness, does not communicate and frequently functions of his/her inner organs are supported by devices. There has been great effort devoted to scaling comatose states into different levels according to seriousness, depth, and to prediction of probable development of patient state. In practice, there have been usually used relative terms as mild, moderate and severe coma that cannot serve to more extended research because of non-existence of exact definition and are source of misunderstandings. First trial to unify coma classification was the Glasgow classification of unconsciousness (Glasgow Coma Scale - GCS) described in 1974 [1]. GCS has become widely used and reliable scale for classification of coma depth. It is highly reproducible and fast and it is a suitable tool for long-term monitoring of patient coma. During next decades, further systems of coma classification have been developed, for example Rancho Los Amigos Scale, Reaction Level Scale RLS85 [21] both classifying into 8 levels, Innsbruck Coma Scale, Japan Coma Scale, etc. Individual systems of coma classification differ in number of levels, way of examination, precision, etc.

In addition to different scales for classification of coma depth, a number of scales for classification of health state of the patient that aroused from coma have been developed. They are used for long-term research of patient state changes, for state prediction, etc. Glasgow Outcome Scale (GOS), Rappaport's Disability Rating Scale [3] are examples of them.

Glasgow Coma Scale was the first trial to unify classification of coma depth. The authors developed a simple and fast procedure of examination that did not require additional demanding training of hospital staff. The examination consists of three steps (tests):

- Motor response - usually examined on upper limbs since they manifest richer spectrum of responses than the lower limbs. The doctor must consider the patient state, e.g. injured spinal cord after an accident, fracture; differentiate volitional reaction from pure spinal reflex; select suitable intensity and location for a painful stimulus, etc.

- Eye opening response - similarly to motor response it requires from the expert evaluation of secondary influences. The doctor has to evaluate reactions of face muscles and eye-ball when a painful stimulus is applied.
- Verbal response - probably the most frequent manifestation of the end of a comatose state is the ability of the patient to communicate reasonably because it shows correct integration of higher parts of the neural system.

Each of the described three steps is rated by a certain number of points (see Table 1) and the resulting level of coma is determined as a sum of these numbers, practically it is a value in the interval 3 to 15, from a deep coma without any observable reaction (level 3) to mild coma (level 15) more or less characterised by confusion of the individual. If the sum is less then 8 points the state is identified as severe traumatic brain injury.

Table 1. Glasgow Coma Scale

step of examination	description	rate
motor response	obeys commands for movement	6
	purposeful movement to painful stimulus	5
	withdraws from pain	4
	abnormal (spastic) flexion, decorticate posture	3
	extensor (rigid) response, decerebrate posture	2
	none	1
eye opening response	spontaneous--open with blinking at baseline	4
	opens to verbal command, speech, or shout	3
	opens to pain, not applied to face	2
	none	1
verbal response	oriented	5
	confused conversation, but able to answer questions	4
	inappropriate responses, words discernible	3
	incomprehensible speech	2
	none	1

The resulting coma level is usually presented in a graph in dependence on time, together with additional information about the patient state, as temperature, pulse rate, blood pressure, breathing rate, diameter of eye pupils, etc. Evaluation of individual patient reactions is in Table 1 simplified; in practice higher level of expert evaluation is required (presence of fracture, injury of spinal cord, tracheotomy, injury of trigeminus, etc.). The presented procedure of coma depth evaluation has been proved by practice and till now it is used for its simplicity and speed.

2.1 Conventional EEG During Comatose State

EEG record represents record of brain cell activity and thus it is theoretically applicable to evaluation and prediction of course of coma. We use the term "theoretically" because views of the possibility to use EEG differ significantly among authors. There have appeared many studies supporting use of EEG, on the other side there exist studies that reject the former ones. However in general they agree on the opinion that EEG record is suitable and may be used for estimation of coma depth level but it cannot be used for detailed prediction of its long-term development.

When using conventional EEG [4], there have been described several distinguishable courses in comatose EEG: alpha pattern coma, theta pattern coma, sleep-like coma, spindle coma, burst suppression coma etc. [5]. According to presence of these courses it is possible (in some cases) to roughly estimate further development of the patient health state, as recovery or death (e.g. burst suppression pattern has in general negative prognosis, alpha and theta pattern comas are transient states and they do not supply applicable information about long-term development [6]). Examination using evoked potentials [7] is relatively frequent as well.

In general, conventional EEG is applicable to rough estimation of patient state, however considering the paper form it is limited to qualitative estimation. It depends on subjective experience of the doctor and in addition it is not suitable for long-term monitoring of patients at ICU.

2.2 Quantitative EEG in Comatose State

Due to expansion of computer technology in electroencephalography, it is possible to perform quantitative processing of comatose EEG nowadays, especially in frequency domain (computation of power spectrum in basic EEG bands, mutual coherence of electrodes, using results in the form of compressed frequency fields, etc.) that as a consequence remove subjective influence of evaluating experts.

A number of studies have been performed. Individual authors have approached the problem differently and with different results. Some have tried to estimate coma depth only using quantitative EEG [8], [9], others have predicted its long-term development [10]. However from many evaluating studies [4], [11] it follows that it is not very suitable to use only EEG for this purpose. EEG differs at different individuals and depends significantly on physiological changes as swelling, bleeding into brain, skull fracture and other damages of nervous tissue. On the other hand, EEG examination is relatively simple and cheap, it reflect state of brain functionality, therefore it is worth continuing the research in this field. Some of the recent studies use combination of functional brain examination using EEG and examination of the state of its structure using CT or MRI [12], [13].

2.3 Burst Suppression Pattern

State of deep coma (the highest level of unconsciousness) appears in patient EEG as specific rhythms called "burst suppression pattern" when periods of suppressed brain activity (interburst) with periods of sudden increase of brain activity (burst) alternate periodically (see Figure 1). This activity is usually relatively synchronised in the whole brain, similarly to epileptic seizures.

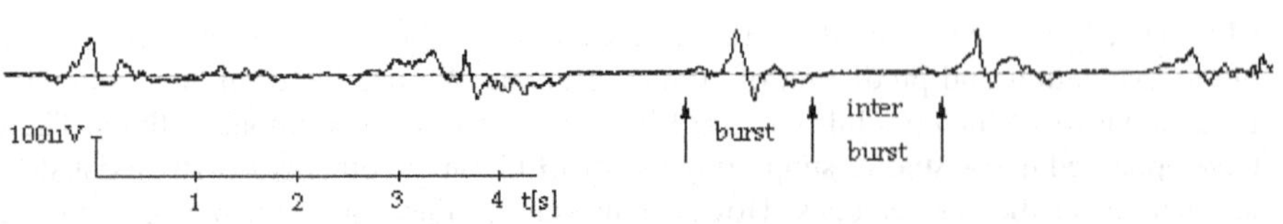

Fig. 1. Example of the course of burst suppression pattern

3 Methods of EEG Signal Processing and Analysis

EEG signal can be analysed both in time and frequency domains. In time domain the basic descriptive quantities are general and central moments of lower orders, in frequency domain the most frequently used method is Fourier transform.

Adaptive segmentation. Application of all methods of pattern recognition is based on correct extraction of discriminative features describing characteristics of classified objects. Each method of automatic classification is as good as used features are. It is well-known that EEG signal has non-stationary character. Its both frequency and amplitude characteristics change with time. In the signal, there may appear artefacts, non-stationarities (transients), as epileptic graphoelements, etc. If we divide the long-term EEG records for the purpose of feature extraction into periods of constant length, the borders of these periods have no relation to the signal character. There may appear hybrid segments containing, for example, a mixture of waves of different shapes and frequencies. Therefore it is more suitable to divide the signal into partially stationary periods of variable length in dependence on occurrence of non-stationarities in the signal. Solution of this problem brings adaptive signal segmentation, designed for the first time by Bodenstein and Praetorius [14]. A modification of the original algorithm is adaptive segmentation based on two joint windows sliding along the signal [15].

To reduce the dimensionality of the signal, the multiple channels were projected to the first principal component (PC). The adaptive segmentation was performed on this PC curve and the segment boundaries were projected back to all original EEG channels (Fig 2).

Principal Component Analysis (PCA) [16] is a statistical method that tries to discover dependencies in the structure of high-dimensional stochastic observations and to acquire more compact description of this structure. It is applicable to compression, dimension reduction and data filtering.

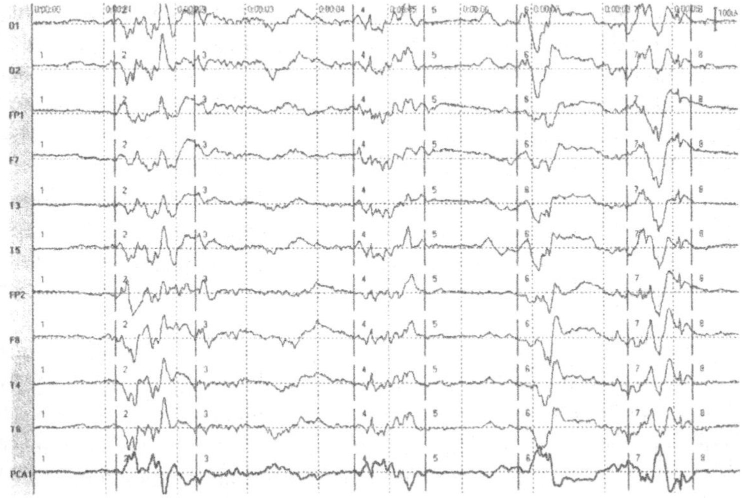

Fig. 2. Adaptive segmentation of PCA curve (bottom line). The segment boundaries are projected to the original EEG traces

Classification of EEG signal. Segmented EEG signal is successively classified using feature-based pattern recognition methods. Features describing the object can be arranged into a n-dimensional vector that is called feature vector. Objects are then represented by points in n-dimensional space. The classifier maps the object feature space into a set of class indicators. In our study, k-NN classifier and RBF neural network have been used for classification. It is well known that quality of classification of a supervised learning method highly depends on the training set. Therefore we have focused in the study on the preparation of the training set. It has been developed in a non-traditional way using expert background knowledge.

4 Preparation of the Training Set

The core of the developed system is the training set on which practically depends the quality of classification. In the implementation we have developed the user can create the training set during the program execution. However in the case of classification of comatose EEG we have decided to create the training set in a different way. Individual fragments have been acquired from sleep EEG that is comparable to comatose EEG. The basic steps can be described as following:

1. We have saved in total 453 eight-second periods of 18-electrode sleep EEG where the classification into levels 1 thru 10 (provided by professor Milos Matousek, MD) has been known.
2. Since the created training set has shown inacceptable cross-validation error it has been necessary to edit the training set to become acceptable.
3. The segments unsuitable for further processing, for example those containing artefacts, have been excluded from the training set. The number of segments has decreased to 436.
4. The core of the training set has been generated by cluster analysis - only such segments have been included for that the classification by cluster analysis has agreed with original classification of professor Milos Matousek. At repeated clustering, it has been searched for such a metrics of the feature space that results in correspondence in classification at the highest number of segments. The core of the training set generated in this way contains 184 segments.
5. Using auxiliary scripts in Matlab realizing classification by nearest neighbour and parallel visual control of results some of the segments excluded in the previous step have been added to the training set, however frequently their classification has been changed by 1 to 2 levels. The resulting training set has had 349 segments.
6. Using RBF implementation of a neural network [17] the cross-validation error has been computed. Data has been randomly divided in 1:1 ratio into training and testing sets. RBF network has been learned on the training set and the error has been computed using the testing data. This procedure has been repeated many times (in the order of hundreds) for different random distributions training/testing set. The resulting error has been computed as an average error of these distributions. Repeatedly incorrectly classified segments in the second phase of computation have been excluded from the resulting training set.

7. The resulting training set created in previous steps contains 319 segments classified into levels 1 thru 10 of coma. Average cross-validation error computed using RBF neural network does not exceed the value of 3 percent.

The training sets generated in individual steps have been saved in the format compatible with the format of the training set of resulting application and thus they are applicable to classification of comatose EEG and accessible in the application itself. For illustration, segments of several classes of the resulting training set are shown in Figure 3.

5 Experiments

The approach has been tested on real sleep EEG recording for which the classification has been known. It is necessary to stress that the comatose EEG is similar to sleep EEG. For segmentation, combination of non-adaptive and adaptive segmentation has

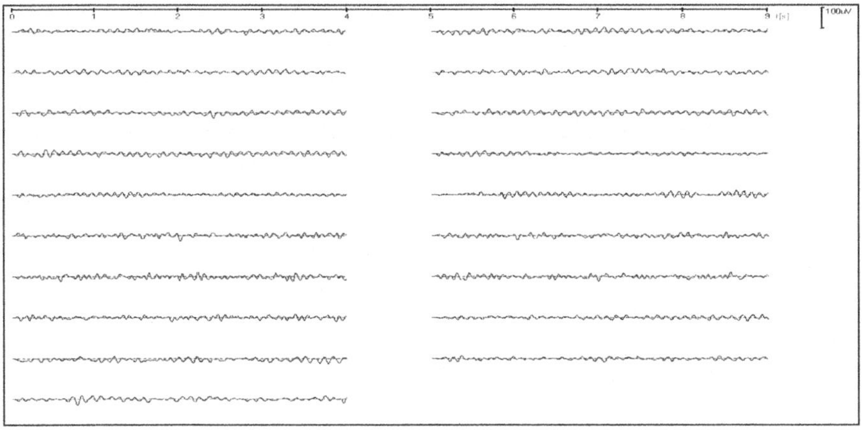

Class 1

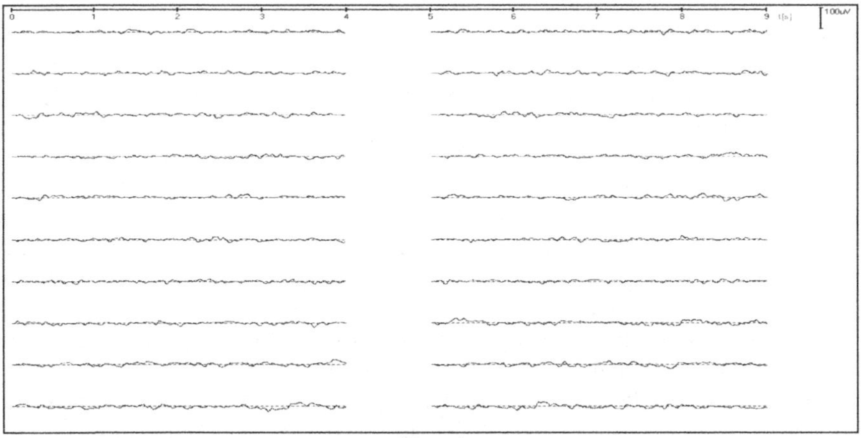

Class 4

Fig. 3. Segments of the classes 1, 4, 7, and 10 of the resulting training set

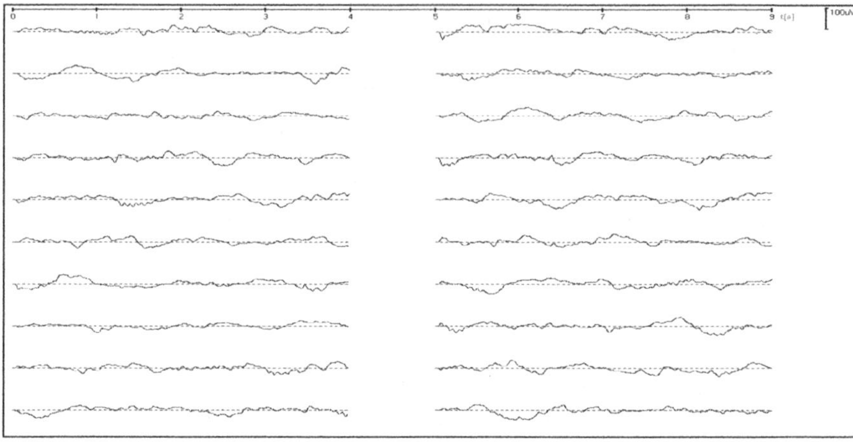

Class 7

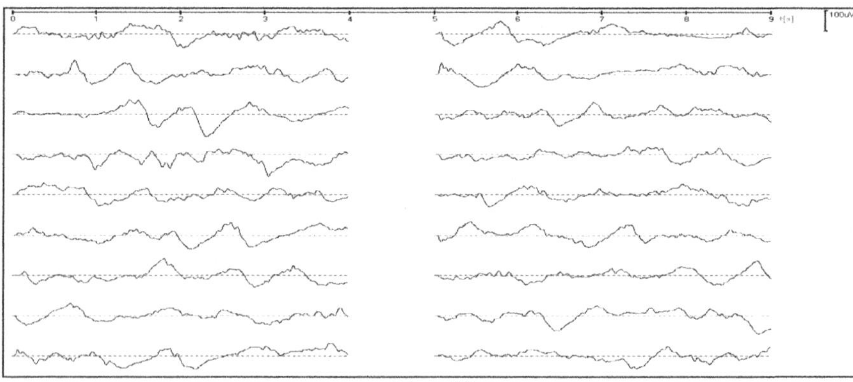

Class 10

Fig. 3. (Continued)

been used. Length of segments for non-adaptive segmentation has been set up to 32 seconds (at sampling rate of 256 Hz 8192 samples correspond to 32 seconds, this value has been selected with respect to successive computation of FFT). Intervals containing artefacts have been determined by adaptive segmentation.

The training set developed according to procedure described in Section 4 and containing 319 segments classified into 10 classes has been used for classification of the 2hour sleep EEG recording. For classification, algorithm of nearest neighbour has been used. The whole classification has lasted 2 minutes. In Table 2 the success rate of the classification is presented. The classified signal has contained levels 1 thru 7. P1 is a number of segments classified by professor Matousek to the level, P2 is a number of successfully classified segments with no error, U1 represents success rate in per cents (P2/P1), P3 contains number of successfully classified segments with tolerance of one level, and U2 represents success rate in per cents (P3/P1).

The presented results can be summarized as follows. With respect to the character of the application we cannot expect 100% success rate. When requiring exact classification we reach success rate of approximately 80%. When allowing tolerance of one level of coma the success rate increases to 90%. More exact evaluation of the error has no practical sense because the manual estimation of classification done by professor Matousek is burdened by a non-zero error according to his view. In literature we can find similar rough estimations ([5], [9], [11], summary in [4]) when long-term trends are more important than exact results.

Table 2. Success rate of the classification

level	P1	P2	U1	P3	U2
1	36	27	75%	33	92%
2	24	19	79%	21	88%
3	15	14	93%	15	100%
4	43	36	84%	40	93%
5	18	12	66%	15	83%
6	45	41	91%	42	93%
7	23	14	61%	20	87%

6 Conclusions

One of the aims when developing an EEG classification system is to ease the work of medical doctors. These systems are to help the doctor interpret EEG records correctly, and then to propose the most appropriate treatment. Further applications of these systems can be in educating new doctors, in evaluating long-term EEG records, at intensive care units, or neurological clinics. There are a number of algorithms that may be employed to classify unknown EEG signals. Basically, they can be divided into two groups.

The first group is based on rules defined by human experts. Since there is no exact algorithm or gold standard specifying EEG signals of healthy persons and patients with different diagnoses, the rules are biased towards human expertise. The same situation arises when a single EEG recording is evaluated by several human experts. EEG is not periodic and is non-stationary. Its shape depends on many factors such as mental or motoric activities (even blinking eyes cause artefacts in EEG), pathologies (e.g. epilepsy), awakeness, or sleep, etc. Therefore more steps in pre-processing are required before we get description in the form of attribute values.

The second group utilises various forms of learning, thus avoiding human biasing. Both groups of algorithms have their advantages and drawbacks. Attempts have been made to combine rules defined by human experts with rules generated by the See5 program [38]. The experiments showed that a knowledge base originally created from expert rules refined with generated rules gives better results than the original knowledge base and decision tree as separate systems.

Proper selection of attributes plays a very important role in classification systems. It may significantly influence the success rate of classification. Use of irrelevant and weakly relevant attributes can decrease the accuracy. The attributes can be selected either automatically or manually. Automatic selection can be viewed as a state space search where each state represents a single combination of attributes. The goal of the search is to find the state with the highest value of the evaluation function that characterises the success rate of classification with the corresponding attributes. It is obvious that such an evaluation function is only an estimation of the success rate of the classification, because the training set is limited. The transition operator is attribute adding or deleting. The average accuracy of cross-validation is usually used as an evaluation function. Manual selection, on the other hand, is a more or less intuitive process based on experience.

One of the most important aspects of the EEG classification systems is reliable analysis of EEG records, which enables significant values to be identified on the measured signal. This analysis is a necessary condition for correct classification.

It is necessary to stress that not only the selection of a pre-processing method is a very important step in data mining process, especially when working with continuous signals, but also careful generation of the training set. In such complex tasks as classification of EEG records, experience of a human expert that can modify, for example, a training set generated by cluster analysis may contribute to more successful classification.

Acknowledgement

The research of J. Rieger and L. Lhotska paper was supported by the research program No. MSM 210000012 "Transdisciplinary Research in the Area of Biomedical Engineering" of the CTU in Prague, sponsored by the Ministry of Education, Youth and Sports of the Czech Republic. The research of V. Krajca and M. Matousek was supported by grants No. 7511 and 7586 IGA CR.

References

1. TEASDALE, G., JENNET, B. Assessment of coma and impaired consciousness. A practical scale. *The Lancet*, July 1974, ii, pp 81-84.
2. STARMARK, J. E., STÅLHAMMAR, D., HOLMGREN, E. The Reaction Level Scale (RLS85). Manual and Guidelines. *Acta Neurochirurgica*, January 1998, vol. 91, no. 1, pp 12-20.
3. *Traumatic Brain Injury Resource Guide: Assesment Scales* [online]. [cit. 2004-4-12].
4. WALLACE, E. B., et al. A history and review of quantitative electroencephalography in traumatic brain injury. *The Journal of Head Trauma Rehabilitation*, April 2001, vol. 16, no. 2, pp 165-191.
5. YOUNG, G. B., ROPPER, A. H., BOLTON, CH. F. *Coma and impaired consciousness: a clinical perspective*. New York: McGraw-Hill. Health Professions Division, 1998. 665 p. ISBN 0-07-072371-0.
6. YOUNG, G. B., et al. Alpha, theta and alpha-theta coma: a clinical outcome study utilizing serial recordings. *Electroencephalography and clinical Neurophysiology*, August 1994, vol. 91, no. 2, pp 93-99.
7. CHIAPPA, K. H, HILL, R. A. Evaluation and prognostication in coma. *Electroencephalography and clinical Neurophysiolology*, February 1998, vol. 106, no. 2, pp 149-155.
8. THATCHER, R. W., et al. EEG discriminant analyses of mild head trauma. *Electroencephalography and clinical Neurophysiolology*, August 1989, vol. 73, no. 2, pp 94-106.
9. MATOUSEK, M., et al. Quantitative EEG analysis as a suplement to the clinical coma scale RLS85. *Acta Anaesthesiologica Scandinavica*, 1996, vol. 40, pp 825-831.
10. KANE, N. W., et al. Quantitative electroencephalographic evaluation of non-fatal and fatal traumatic coma. *Electroencephalography and clinical Neurophysiolology*, March 1998, vol. 106, no. 3, pp 244-250.

11. THATCHER, R. W. QEEG and Traumatic Brain Injury: Present and Future. *Brain Injury Source*, Fall 1999, vol. 4, no. 3, s. 20-23.
12. THATCHER, R. W., et al. Biophysical Linkage between MRI and EEG Amplitude in Closed Head Injury. *Neuroimage*, May 1998, vol. 7, no. 4, pp 352-367.
13. THATCHER, R. W., et al. Biophysical Linkage between MRI and EEG Coherence in Closed Head Injury. *Neuroimage*, November 1998, vol. 8, no. 4, pp 307-326.
14. BODENSTEIN, G., PRAETORIUS, H. M. *Feature extraction from the electroencephalogram by adaptive segmentation*. Proceedings of IEEE, May 1977, vol. 65, no. 5. pp 642-652.
15. Krajča V., Petránek S., Patáková I., Värri A., (1991): 'Automatic identification of significant graphoelements in multi-channel EEG recordings by adaptive segmentation and fuzzy clustering', Int. J. Biomed. Comput., 28, pp71-89
16. Jolliffe I.T.: *Principal Component Analysis*. 2nd edition. Springer-Verlag 2002. 502 p., ISBN 0-38-795442-2
17. Haykin S.: *Neural Networks: A Comprehensive Foundation*. Prentice Hall 1999. 842 p., ISBN 0-13-273350-1

Semantic Reference Model in Medical Time Series

Fernando Alonso, Loïc Martínez, César Montes, Aurora Pérez, Agustín Santamaría, and Juan Pedro Valente

Facultad de Informática. Universidad Politécnica de Madrid. Campus de Montegancedo, 28660 Boadilla del Monte. Madrid. Spain
{falonso,loic,cmontes,aurora,jpvalente}@fi.upm.es
Agustin.Santamaria@sun.com

Abstract. The analysis of time series databases is very important in the area of medicine. Most of the approaches that address this problem are based on numerical algorithms that calculate distances, clusters, index trees, etc. However, a domain-dependent analysis sometimes needs to be conducted to search for the symbolic rather than numerical characteristics of the time series. This paper focuses on our work on the discovery of reference models in time series of isokinetics data and a technique that transforms the numerical time series into symbolic series. We briefly describe the algorithm used to create reference models for population groups and its application in the real world. Then, we describe a method based on extracting semantic information from a numerical series. This symbolic information helps users to efficiently analyze and compare time series in the same or similar way as a domain expert would.

Domain: Time series analysis
Keywords: Time series characterization, semantic reference model, isokinetics

1 Introduction

There are many databases that store temporal information as sequences of data in time, also called temporal sequences. They are to be found in different domains like the stock market, business, medicine, etc. An important domain for the application of data mining (DM) in the medical field is physiotherapy and, more specifically, muscle function assessment based on isokinetics data.

Isokinetics data is retrieved by an isokinetics machine (Fig. 1), on which patients perform strength exercises. The machine has the peculiarity of limiting the range of movement and the intensity of effort at constant speed. We decided to focus on knee exercises (extensions and flexions) since most of the data and knowledge gathered by sport physicians is related to this joint. The data takes the form of a strength curve with additional information on the angle of the knee (Fig. 1b). The positive values of the curve represent extensions (knee angle from 90º to 0º) and the negative values represent flexions (knee angle from 0º to 90º).

This work is part of the I4 Project (Intelligent Interpretation of Isokinetics Information) [1], which provides sport physicians with a set of tools to visually analyze patient strength data output by an isokinetics machine. The I4 system cleans and preprocesses the data and provides a set of DM tools for analyzing isokinetics exercises in order to discover new and useful information for monitoring injuries, detecting potential injuries early, discovering fraudulent sickness leaves, etc.

However, a lot of expertise in the isokinetics domain is needed to be able to correctly interpret the I4 output. After observing experts at work, we found that they

J.M. Barreiro et al. (Eds.): ISBMDA 2004, LNCS 3337, pp. 344–355, 2004.

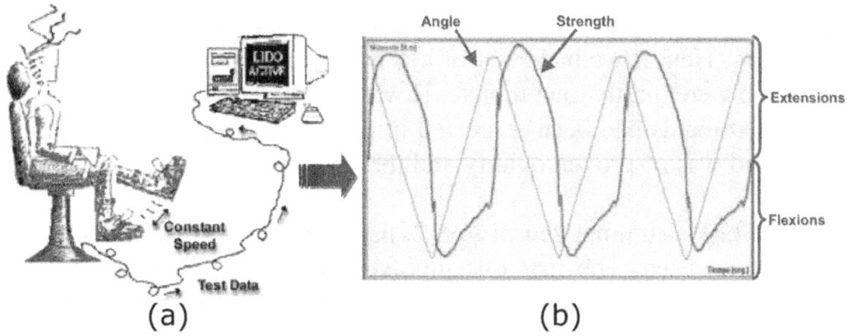

Fig. 1. Isokinetics machine (a) and collected data (b)

apply their knowledge and expertise to focus on certain sections of the series and ignore others. Therefore, we looked for a way of bringing this output closer to the information sport physicians deal with in their routine work, since they demand a representation related to their own way of thinking and operating. Hence, symbolic series have been researched as an alternative that more closely resembles expert conceptual mechanisms.

This paper focuses on our work on the discovery of reference models in time series and the development of a technique that transforms the numerical time series into symbolic series. The paper is arranged as follows. Section 2 describes the process to create reference models for population groups. Section 3 introduces the importance of domain-dependent analysis and symbolic time series and describes the Symbols Extraction Method (SEM). Section 4 shows the results and evaluation of the Semantic Reference Model and, finally, section 5 presents some conclusions and mentions future lines of research.

2 Creating Reference Models for Population Groups

One of the most common tasks involved in the assessment of isokinetic exercises is to compare a patient's test against a reference model created beforehand. These models represent the average profile of a group of patients sharing common characteristics. Representative models can be created, for example, of different sports, by age groups, sex, or even grouping patients that have suffered the same injury. When we have a model that represents a particular group, it can be used for comparison against individual exercises to ascertain whether an athlete fits a profile for a given sport, whether the complaints of an athlete may be due a specific injury, etc.

Model creation is a three-stage process: initial data preparation, model creation and, finally, transformation of the model into a symbolic representation as an aid for later comparisons.

2.1 Initial Data Preparation

A good preparation of the initial data is crucial for achieving useful results in any DM or discovery task. But no universally valid standard procedure can be designed for this stage, so solutions vary substantially from one problem to another.

Data preparation in I4 is as follows. The available isokinetics test data sets have been used to assess the physical capacity and injuries of top competition athletes since the early 90s. An extensive collection of tests has been gathered since then, albeit immethodically. Hence, we had a set of heterodox, unclassified data files in different formats, which were, partly, incomplete. However, the quality of the data was unquestionable: the protocols had been respected in the huge majority of cases, the isokinetics system used was of proven quality and the operating personnel had been properly trained.

A series of tasks, summarized in Fig. 2, had to be carried out before the available data set could be used. The first one involved decoding, as the input came from a commercial application (the isokinetics system) that has its own internal data format. Then, the curves had to be evaluated to identify any that were invalid and to remove any irregularities entered by mechanical factors of the isokinetics system. Two data cleaning tasks were performed using expert knowledge: removal of incorrect tests (the ones that did not follow the test protocol) and elimination of incorrect extensions and flexions (because of lack of concentration by the patient). Having validated all the exercises as a whole and each exercise individually, they have to be filtered to remove noise introduced by the machine itself. Again expert knowledge had to be used to automatically identify and eliminate flexion peaks, that is, maximum peaks produced by machine inertia. This process outputs a database in which tests are homogeneous, consistent and noise free.

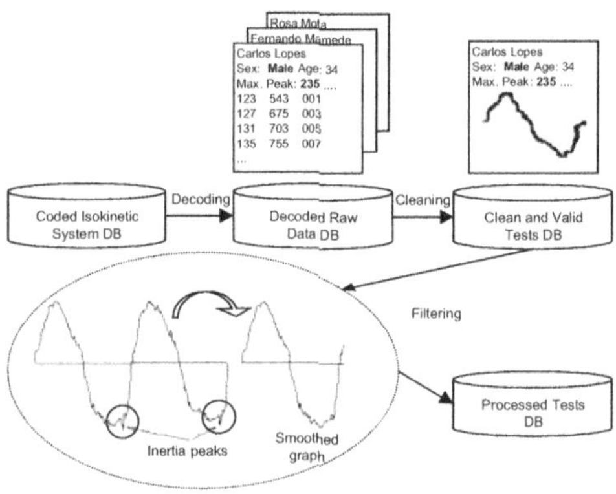

Fig. 2. Data pre-processing tasks

2.2 Creating the Model

All the exercises done by individuals with the desired characteristics of weight, height, sport, sex, etc., must be selected to create a reference model for a particular population. There may be some heterogeneity even among patients of the same group. Some will have a series of particularities that make them significantly different from the others (in American football, for instance, players have very different physical characteristics). Therefore, exercises have to be discriminated and the reference model has to be created using exercises among which there is some uniformity.

An expert in isokinetics was responsible for selecting the exercises that were to be part of the model. It is not easy to manually discard exercises that differ considerably from others and so this was mostly not done. The idea we aim to implement is to automatically discard the exercises that are different before creating the model.

The problem of comparing exercises can be simplified using the discrete Fourier transform to transfer the exercises from the time domain to the frequency domain. The fact that most of the information is concentrated in the first components of the discrete Fourier transform will be used to discard the remainder and simplify the problem. The advantage of the discrete Fourier transform is that there is an algorithm, known as the fast Fourier transform, that can calculate the required coefficients in a time of the order of O(n log n) when the number of data is a "power of 2". In our case, we restricted the strength values of the series to 256 values, which is roughly two leg flexions and extensions and, therefore, sufficient to characterize each exercise.

The time it takes to make the comparisons is drastically reduced using this technique, a very important factor in this case, since there are a lot of exercises for comparison in the database and comparison efficiency is important.

Once the user has selected all the tests of the patient population to be modeled, the process for creating a reference model is as follows (Fig. 3):

1. All the series are pruned to 256 values (approximately 3 full repetitions for a speed of 60°/s) to be able to apply the fast Fourier transform.
2. The Fourier transform is applied for each of the series, and the first four coefficients of each one are selected (these are representative enough).
3. A divisive k-means clustering algorithm (whose essential parameters have been established a priori after running numerous tests) is applied to this data set, which outputs a set of classes grouping patients depending on their muscle strength. The majority classes define the standard profile or profiles of each sport, whereas the minority classes represent athletes that are atypical within their sport. The former are used to create a reference model, unifying all the common characteristics.
4. The next step is normalization of the exercises. This step levels out the size (in time) of the different isokinetics curves and adjusts the times when patients exert zero strength (switches from flexion to extension and vice versa), as these are singular points that should coincide in time. This would not be necessary if the exercises were strictly isokinetic. However, slight variations do unfortunately occur.
5. The last step is the calculation of the mean value of the curves point to point.

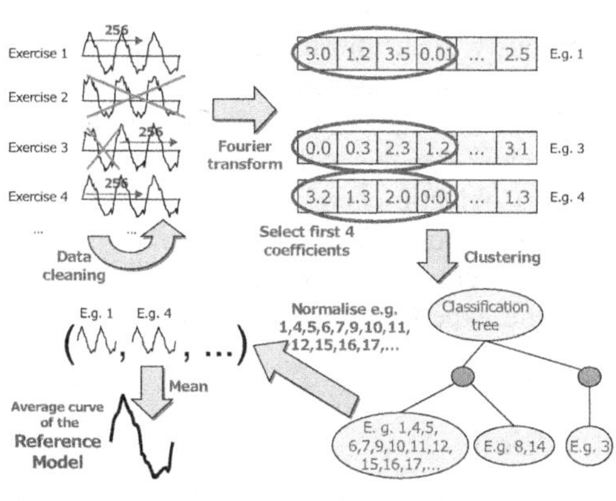

Fig. 3. Process for creating reference models

2.3 Transforming the Model

Having completed the first two stages, we have a numerical model that is representative of the group of patients in question. In earlier versions of this project, this system was basically used to run numerical comparisons between a model and individual exercises. Fig. 4 shows an example comparing a model (left) and a patient exercise (right). The system provides different kinds of comparison: total or partial (comparing flexions, extensions or curve portions). Similar regions are highlighted for ease of visualization.

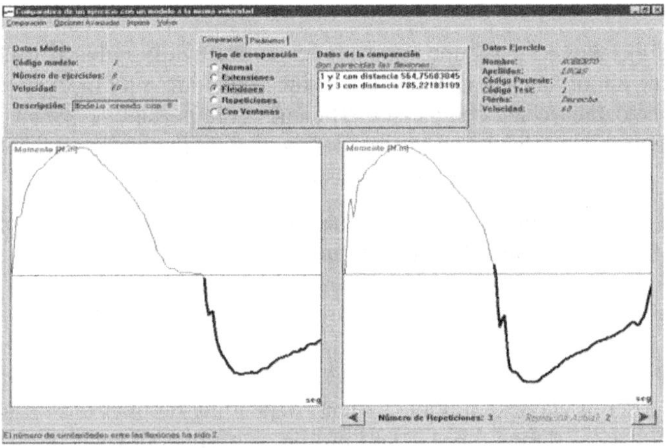

Fig. 4. Comparison of a numerical model (left) with a patient (right)

This kind of comparison is very helpful for isokinetics experts as it enables them to determine what group patients belong or should belong to and identify what sport they should go in for, what their weaknesses are with a view to improvement or how they are likely to progress in the future. However, this kind of comparison, based exclusively on numerical methods, could overlook some curve features that are numerically inconsequential, but very significant for experts, for example, small peaks in the intermediate region of the curve, a steeper upward slope than normal, etc. These features needed to be finer tuned in the numerical comparison algorithm parameters to be properly weighted. Obviously, such adjustments inflated the more regular cases.

To overcome this problem, we designed a method whose goal was to take into account all the relevant features of the curve, irrespective of whether or not they had a high absolute strength value. For this purpose, we designed a semantic method of extracting features from isokinetic curves, a method that transforms the numerical series (whether this is a model or an individual exercise) into a symbolic series containing the features of each curve that are most significant from the medical viewpoint. This means that the expert can interpret and compare the curve more effectively.

3 Semantic Extraction

In this section we describe the method that transforms the numerical time series (a reference model or isokinetic exercise) into a symbolic time series.

3.1 Time Series Comparison Issues

The problem we face then is to compare time series. There has been a lot of research in this area, introducing concepts like distance (needed to establish whether two series are similar), transformations (designed to convert one time series into another to ease analysis), and patterns (independently meaningful sections of a time series that explain a behavior or characterize a time series). Many papers have been published analyzing which are the best techniques for calculating distances [2,3], what transformations have to be used to match series [4] and what techniques should be used to find patterns [5].

The comparisons of these methods are based on point values of each series, not only the overall appearance of these series. Fig. 5 shows an example in which a traditional method is likely to indicate that series b1 and b2 resemble each other more closely than a1 and a2.

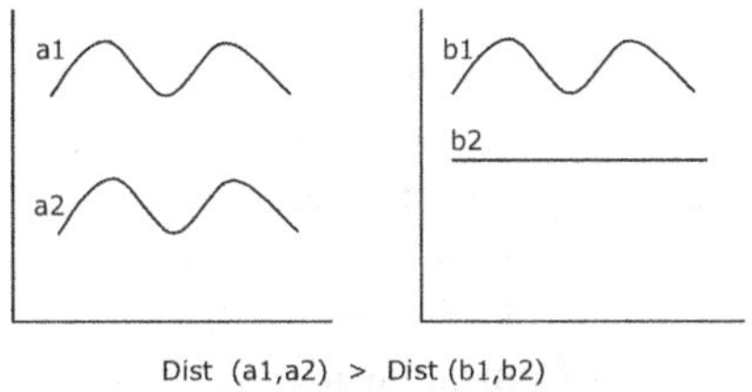

Fig. 5. Example in which traditional similarity methods would not be suitable

This would clearly not be the case in the isokinetics domain, where we are interested in the morphology of the curves rather than the strength value exercised at any given point in time. It could be argued that a simple time translation would solve the problem for the example in Fig. 5. However, this translation would overlook the patients' strength value (which is not unimportant) and would not be a valid solution in all cases or for all parts of the sequence.

Work by Agrawal, Faloutsos and Swami [2] takes a different approach to this issue. They present a shape definition language, called SDL, for retrieving objects based on shapes contained in the histories associated with these objects. This language is domain independent, which is one of the main differences from the work that we present in this paper.

In our case, an important point is that time series should, in most cases, be analyzed by an expert in the isokinetics domain. The expert will have the expertise to interpret the different features of the time series. When analyzing a sequence, most experts instinctively split the temporal sequence into parts that are clearly significant to their analysis and may ignore other parts of the sequence that provide no information. So, the expert identifies a set of concepts based on the features present in each part of the time series that are relevant for explaining its behavior.

After observing isokinetics domain experts at work, we found that they focus on sections like "ascent, curvature, peaks..." These are the sections that contain the concepts that must be extracted from the data. To achieve this, we developed SEM (Symbol Extraction Method), whose goal is to translate the numerical time series into a symbolic series incorporating expert knowledge.

3.2 Symbols Extraction Method

We will first describe the Isokinetics Symbols Alphabet (ISA), which includes the symbols used to build the symbolic sequences. Then, we will describe the method used for symbol extraction.

3.2.1 Isokinetics Symbols Alphabet (ISA)

It does not make much sense to start to study data depicted in time, if there is no knowledge of the domain that is to be analyzed. Some interviews with the isokinetics expert, who is specialized in analyzing isokinetics temporal sequences of some joints like the knee or the shoulder, had to be planned to elicit expert knowledge as the research advanced.

After the first few interviews, the expert stated that there were two visually distinguishable regions in every exercise: knee extension and flexion. Both had a similar morphology (the shape shown in Fig. 6), from which we were able to identify the following symbols:

- *Ascent*: part where the patient gradually increases the strength applied.
- *Descent*: part where the patient gradually decreases the strength applied.
- *Peak.* A prominent part in any part of the sequence.
- *Trough.* A depression in any part of the sequence.
- *Curvature.* The upper section of a region.
- *Transition.* The changeover from extension to flexion (or vice versa).

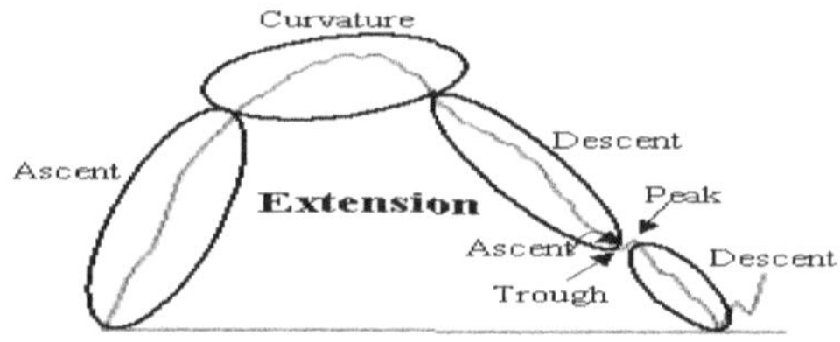

Fig. 6. Symbols of an isokinetics curve

After identifying the symbols used by the expert, the symbols needed to be typed. The symbol types have to be taken into account when translating a numerical temporal sequence into a symbolic series. The types were elicited directly from the expert as he analyzed a set of supplied sequences that constituted a significant sample of the whole database. As the expert separated an extension from a flexion, each symbol had to be labeled with its type and also with the keyword "Ext" or "Flex". The set of symbols, types and regions form an alphabet called ISA (Isokinetics Symbols Alphabet), shown in Table 1.

Table 1. Isokinetics Symbols Alphabet

Zone	Symbol	Types		
EXT	*Ascent*	Sharp		Gentle
	Descent	Sharp		Gentle
	Trough	Big		Small
	Peak	Big		Small
	Curvature	Sharp	Flat	Irregular
FLEX	*Transition*		-	

3.2.2 Symbols Extraction Method (SEM)

ISA will be used to get symbolic sequences from numerical temporal sequences. The Symbols Extraction Method (SEM), whose architecture is shown in Fig. 7, was designed to make this transformation. SEM is divided into two parts. The first one is domain independent (DIM) and, therefore, can be applied and reused for any domain. The second part is domain dependent (DDM) and is the part that contains the expert knowledge about the symbols needed to analyze a particular sequence.

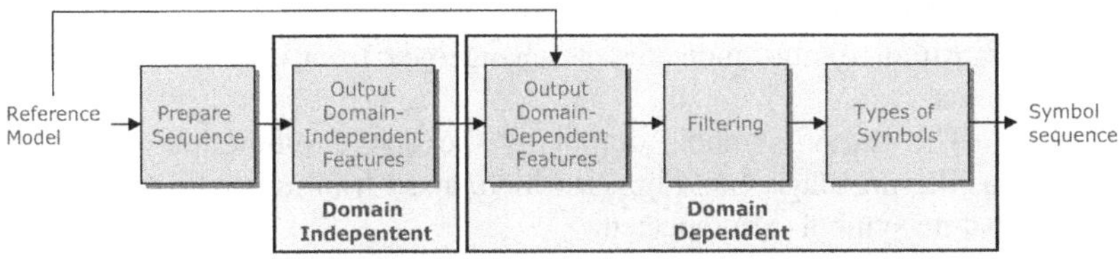

Fig. 7. Architecture of SEM

The I4 application contains a database of isokinetics exercises done by all sorts of patients. A particular exercise, done at a speed of 60 radians per seconds is used as input for the SEM. The DIM is made up of a submodule that outputs a set of domain independent features: peaks and troughs, which, after some domain-dependent filtering, will be matched to symbols. Both the features output by the DIM (or simple features) and the domain-dependent data will be used as input for the DDM, which is divided into two submodules: extraction of the ISA symbols and characterization of each symbol by type and region. The DDM output will be the symbolic sequence.

3.2.3 Domain-Independent Module (DIM)

The DIM sequentially scans the whole time series and extracts a series of simple features (peaks and troughs) that can be found in any sequence irrespective of the domain. These features are actually the point at which the peak or trough has been located and data related to its surroundings.

This module has been also tested with sequences from domains other than isokinetics (stock market, electrocardiograms, and so on) providing outcomes that demonstrate its validity.

3.2.4 Domain-Independent Module (DIM)

This module consists of three components:

1. *Output of domain-dependent symbols*:
   - Peaks and troughs: at first glance, it would appear that all the features supplied by the DIM would result in a peak/trough output by the DDM. However, this is out of the question, because, if we did it like this, all the peaks and troughs, no matter how insignificant they were, would be taken as symbols. The expert only analyzes some peaks or troughs, disregarding irrelevant ones. Therefore, the peaks/troughs supplied by the DIM need to be filtered by means of a condition (i.e. amplitude/relation > threshold) that assesses whether a peak, or a trough, can be considered as a symbol. The values of the thresholds were determined by an iterative procedure.

- The ascent and descent symbols were determined similarly to the peaks and troughs extraction. To avoid confusion between ascents/descents and peaks/troughs, ascents or descents must fulfill a condition based on gradient, duration and amplitude (i.e. (gradient >= slope_threshold) and ((duration >= dur_threshold) or (amplitude>= ampl_threshold))).
- Regarding curvatures, the objective was to locate the section of the region where a curvature could be found, irrespective of whether the region was an extension or a flexion. It was estimated that the curvature accounted for around 20% of the upper section of each region.
- The transition symbol indicates the changeover from extension to flexion and vice versa.

2. *Filtering*. The set of symbols output by the above submodule would be put through a filtering stage (see Fig. 7), which, apart from other filtering processes, checks that no symbols are repeated.
3. *Symbol types*. The goal of this submodule is to label each symbol with a type. This will provide more precise information about the original temporal sequence. Remember also that the expert instinctively uses a symbol typology based on his expertise. This classification is done using a set of thresholds that define the symbol type for each case.

4 Results and Evaluation of the Semantic Reference Model

A graphical user interface has been designed to ease the use of the SEM (Fig. 8). This interface was designed for the purpose of evaluating the system in conjunction with the expert. The final user interface will highlight the presentation of the symbolic series output, as the goal of the system is for the user to compare models and exercises on the basis of their symbolic features.

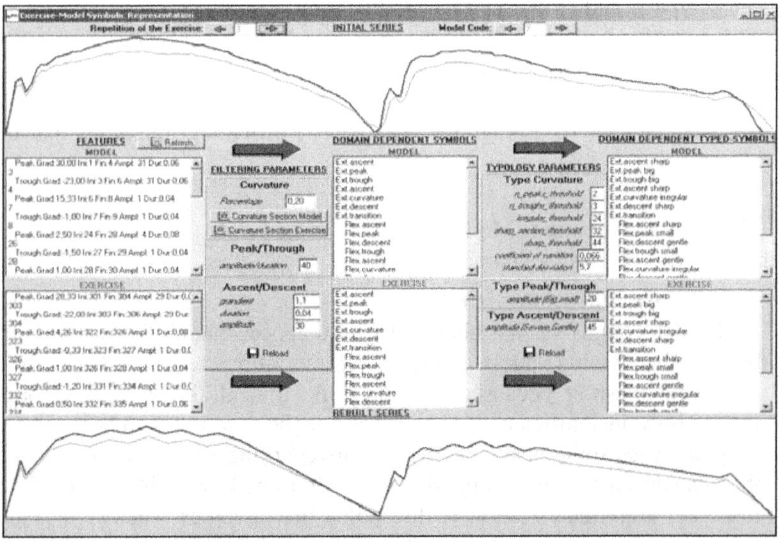

Fig. 8. Symbolic representation interface

An isokinetic model and an exercise are selected as input for the SEM. The original temporal sequence of the model (darker line) and the exercise (lighter line) are displayed at the top of the interface. The central part displays the translation of the temporal sequences into symbols, illustrating all the SEM stages. The first stage outputs the domain-independent features ("Features"). The next stage is to output the "domain-dependent symbols". The parameters used to output these symbols are listed under "Filtering parameters". The result of the last stage of the SEM is set out on the right-hand side of the interface ("Domain-dependent typed symbols") and is the type characterization of each symbol. The threshold parameters used are shown as "Typology parameters". The curves reconstructed from the symbols are shown at the bottom.

As stated by the expert, SEM is an important aid for physicians in writing reports, examining the evolution of an athlete's joint, diagnosing injuries or controlling the treatment of a medical diagnosis.

The results evaluation process was divided into several different testing phases designed for three purposes: to verify the correctness of the results from a technical point of view, to empirically validate their fitness for achieving the established goals and to evaluate their acceptability as a new tool for routine practice.

Details of the results of the reference models evaluation are given in [6]. In this paper, we will focus on the results of the SEM-based evaluation.

The idea of SEM emerged, interestingly, in view of the results of applying the reference models directly, without any semantic transformation. These results were validated using a Turing test-based approach. Although system accuracy was excellent (achieving a success rate of over 0.9), we observed a circumstance related to the similarity within the population calculated by the system as opposed to what was estimated by the expert. We took a set of cases that had been classed within a given population (Table 2 shows an example), and the expert was asked to list these cases in decreasing order of similarity to the reference model. When the expert's classification was compared with the system's, we found that there were some differences. These variations were due to the fact that while the system compared the full curves, the expert only focused on particular aspects of the curves, aspects that can be associated with semantic criteria.

This discovery was the seed of SEM. Indeed, when we repeated the same experiment using the distances between the symbolic transformations, the two calculations were still slightly different, but we found that they tended to be more similar. There are two reasons for this:

- By discretizing the curve using semantic factors, we remove the influence of fairly insignificant parts on the distance from the system.
- The expert is obliged to run a more thorough analysis of the curve, taking into account aspects of the curve that were overlooked beforehand.

5 Conclusions

In this paper, we have presented a DM process for creating reference models for population groups from numerical time series and we have designed a method (SEM) that transforms a numerical sequence into a symbolic sequence with semantic content in a specific domain. This work has been included in the I4 project, which provides a set of tools to analyze isokinetics strength curves of sports people or other patients.

Table 2. Classifications achieved by the system and by the expert for a population of uninjured men

	System (direct)	Expert (direct)	System (SEM)	Expert (SEM)
More similar	Case #16	Case #10	Case #10	Case #10
to ref. model	Case #10	Case #21	Case #16	Case #16
	Case #21	Case #16	Case #21	Case #21
	Case #15	Case #12	Case #13	Case #12
	Case #13	Case #13	Case #12	Case #13
	Case #14	Case #7	Case #15	Case #7
	Case #12	Case #25	Case #14	Case #15
	Case #7	Case #15	Case #7	Case #25
Less similar	Case #25	Case #14	Case #25	Case #14
to ref. model	Case #9	Case #9	Case #9	Case #9

While the reference models built from the numerical series are highly accurate as compared with the expert's diagnosis, the inclusion of the automated SEM method that extracts the same set of symbols from a time series as the expert would have inferred naturally has substantially improved these results. SEM includes a domain-independent and domain-dependent module. The domain-dependent module was necessary because the process followed by the expert suggested that the method needed to include domain-dependent information to assure that the system would emulate the expert. And this information, due to the circumstances of this domain, needed to be expert knowledge.

Additionally, it should be noted that the extraction of symbols for subsequent temporal sequence analysis is an important part of the expert's job of writing reports on patient strength based on such concepts/symbols. The transformation process is very useful for isokinetics domain experts, since they no longer have to perform a task that requires a lot of calculations, but it is more useful still for the non-specialist medical user, because it provides knowledge that they would find it hard to extract from the numerical sequence.

Although SEM is undergoing further tests, we have conducted a field study, introducing a set of cases to the isokinetics expert, where each case is composed of the original temporal sequences of the model and the isokinetic exercise, the symbolic sequences and the rebuilt sequences (providing the expert with a graphical view of the transformation). In addition, the detailed examination of each specific case showed that the rebuilt curves mostly include the essential features that will allow an accurate diagnosis of the patient.

References

1. Alonso, F., Lopez-Chavarrías, I., Caraça-Valente, JP., & Montes, C. Knowledge Discovery in Time Series Using Expert Knowledge. In K. J. Cios, Medical Data Mining and Knowledge Discovery. Heidelberg: Physica-Verlag 2001.
2. Agrawal R, Faloutsos C, and Swam A N. Efficient Similarity Search In Sequence Databases. In D. Lomet, editor, Proceedings of the 4th International Conference of Foundations of Data Organization and Algorithms (FODO), pages 69-84, Chicago, Illinois, 1993. Springer Verlag.

3. Faloutsos C, Ranganathan M, Manolopoulos Y (1994b) Fast subsequence matching in time series databases. In Proceedings of SIGMOD'94, Minneapolis, MN, pp 419-429.
4. Rafei D, Mendelzo A. ·Similarity-Based Queries for Time Series Data. In Proceedings of SIGMOD, Arizona, 1997.
5. Han J, Dong G, Yin Y (1998) Efficient mining of partial periodic patterns in time series database. In Proceedings of the 4th international conference on knowledge discovery and data mining. AAAI Press, Menlo Park, CA, pp 214-218.
6. Alonso F, Valente J P, Martínez L and Montes C. Discovering Patterns and Reference Models in the Medical Domain of Isokinetics. In: J. M. Zurada, editor, New Generations of Data Mining Applications, IEEE Press/Wiley, 2004 (in press).

Control of Artificial Hand via Recognition of EMG Signals

Andrzej Wolczowski and Marek Kurzynski

Wroclaw University of Technology, Faculty of Electronics,
Wyb. Wyspianskiego 27, 50-370 Wroclaw, Poland
{andrzej.wolczowski,marek.kurzynski}@pwr.wroc.pl

Abstract. The paper presents a concept of bioprosthesis control via recognition of user intent on the basis of myopotentials acquired from his body. The EMG signals characteristics and the problems of their measurement have been discussed. The contextual recognition has been considered and three description method for such approach (respecting 1st and 2nd -order context), using: Markov chains, fuzzy rules, neural networks, as well as the involved decision algorithms have been described. The algorithms have been experimentally tested as far as the decision quality is concerned.

1 Introduction

The activity of human organisms is accompanied by physical quantities variation which can be registered with measuring instruments and applied to control the work of technical devices. Electrical potentials accompanying skeleton muscles' activity (called EMG signals) belong to this type of biosignals. They can be detected through the skin using surface electrodes located above selected muscles [3]. They are made by ion movements in the sarcoplasma of activated muscle fibres. Since a single fibre works in a binary way, contracting according to all-or-nothing principle, the gradation of the range and the force of muscle contraction is obtained physiologically by separate recruitment of the muscle fibre groups. The group of fibres stimulated simultaneously by the same moto-neuron (along with the neuron) is called a motor unit [9].

EMG signals measured on skin are the superposition of electrical potentials generated by recruited motor units of contracting muscles. Various movements are related to the recruitment of distinct motor units, different spatial location of these units in relation to the measuring points leads to the formation of EMG signals of differing features, e.g. with different *rms* values and different frequency spectrum. The features depend on the type of executed or (in the case of an amputated limb) only imagined movement so they provide the information about the user's intention [4], [5].

A particular kind of biologically controlled machines are limb prostheses which give the disabled a chance to regain lost motion functions: artificial hands, legs or wheelchairs [9], [11], [12]. Bioprostheses can utilize the EMG signals measured on the handicapped person's body (on the stump of a hand or a leg) to control the actuators of artificial hand's fingers, the knee and the foot of an artificial leg or the wheels of a wheelchair. If this kind of prostheses are to significantly help to regain the lost motion functions, they should be characterised by dexterity (the ability to perform diverse grasps) in the case of a hand and agility (the ability to manoeuvre in dynamic environment) in the case of a leg or a wheelchair. Such properties require the control

J.M. Barreiro et al. (Eds.): ISBMDA 2004, LNCS 3337, pp. 356–367, 2004.

process to be able to recognize a large range of patterns in EMG signals, which is essential for the independent control of prosthesis with a lot of degrees of freedom, in a way which enables forming the motion dynamic for each individual actuator. On the other hand prosthesis control should follow the movement imagined by the user and expressed by the activation of their muscles. Excessive delay in prosthesis movement is confusing for the user and significantly decreases operation accuracy, this especially affects prosthesis agility. Therefore the algorithm of EMG signal analysis must be fast enough to prevent any significant delay caused by its execution in a microprocessor system.

The paper presents the concept of a bioprosthesis control system which in principle consists in the recognition of a prosthesis user's intention (i.e. patient's intention) based on adequately selected parameters of EMG signal and then on the realisation of the control procedure which had previously been unambiguously determined by a recognised state. The paper arrangement is as follows. In chapter 2 we provide an insight into the nature of myopotentials, which are the source of information exploited in the recognition and control procedure. Chapter 3 includes the concept of prosthesis control system based on the recognition of "patient intention". Chapter 4 describes variants of the key recognition algorithm. Chapter 5 in turn presents a specific example of the described concept and its practical application for the control of dexterous hand bioprothesis.

2 Myopotentials and the Problem of Their Measurement

As it has already been mentioned in the introduction the activity of skeleton muscles is accompanied by the generation of electrical potentials which can be detected on skin surface by surface electrodes located above the selected muscles [3], [9], [12]. A signal measured in this way is a superposition of electrical potentials generated by recruited motor units of all muscle groups contracting in a given movement.

The activity of individual motor units in a contracting muscle changes randomly at time. They are activated and relieved in turns. (However, the number of recruited units remains constant and is proportional to the muscle activation level). In addition to that, the surrounding tissue suppresses individual components of the original signal to a varying degree – this results in the *spatial filtration* effect. Thus the amplitude of the resulting EMG signal is characterised by stochastic nature with distribution similar to Gauss distribution [3], [4]. The signal *rms* value clearly depends on the degree of contracting muscles activation and, depending on the location of measurement electrodes in relation to the muscles, it assumes values in the range 0-1.5 mV. The effective energy of EMG signal from human skeleton muscles falls into 0-500 Hz band, where it assumes the highest values in the range of 50-150 Hz.

The measurement of EMG signals is accompanied by electric noise [3], [12]. It can significantly distort the information carried by the signal thus decreasing its usefulness for control purposes. These are some sources of interference:

- external electromagnetic field, especially if generated by equipment using 50Hz power supply;
- varying impedance of electrode/skin contact and accompanying chemical reactions;
- movements of electrodes and the cable connecting them to the amplifier.

The electric noise can be effectively eliminated using a differential measurement system with two active electrodes placed directly above the examined muscle and one reference electrode placed as far as possible above electrically neutral tissue (directly above a bone or a joint, etc.). Signals obtained from active electrodes are subtracted from each other and amplified. The common components of the signals, including surrounding noise, are thus excluded and the useful signal included in the difference is amplified. The ability to suppress the common components of subtracted signals is measured by the Common Mode Rejection Ratio (CMMR). The remaining above mentioned interference (resulting from the skin/electrode contacts and the movements of cables) can be significantly limited by the application of high impedance amplifier located near the electrodes. Thus the concept of *active* electrode appears, i.e. the electrode integrated with the amplifier, it gives a signal resistant to external disturbances [12].

In the case of myoelectrical control of limb prostheses there is one more significant factor, namely that a large part of muscles driving the amputated elements of a limb are situated in its part above the amputation level, for example most of muscles initiating the movement of fingers are located in a forearm. As a result, following a hand amputation (the palm segment) these muscles remain in the stump and can still be used for bioprosthesis control. Contemporary bioprostheses of a hand usually use quite distinct amplitude changes in EMG signals, generated by antagonistic muscle groups of a forearm, for closing and opening a prosthesis grip (and frequently also the movement speed and grip strength) [5], [12]. However, such information is insufficient for the control of a differentiated movement of fingers [11].

New opportunities appear with application of multi-point measurement (numerous electrodes are placed over particular muscles). However, there is one significant problem in this approach, i.e. the crosstalk effect – a signal generated by an examined muscle is overlapped by signals from neighbouring muscles. In effect it is necessary to use sophisticated methods of signal recognition.

3 Control System of Bioprosthesis

In the considered control concept we assume that each prosthesis operation (irrespective of prosthesis type) consists of specific sequence of elementary actions, and the patient intention means its will to perform a specific elementary action.

Thus prosthesis control is a discrete process where at the *n*-th stage (*n*=1,2,..., *N*) occurs successively:

- the measurement of EMG signal parameters x_n, ($x_n \in \mathcal{X} \subseteq \mathcal{R}^d$), that represent patient's will j_n ($j_n \in \mathcal{M} = \{1,2,...,M\}$) (the intention to take a particular action),
- the recognition of this intention (the result of recognition at the n-th stage will be denoted by $i_n \in \mathcal{M}$) and
- the realisation of an elementary action $a_n \in \mathcal{A}$, uniquely defined as a recognized intention.

This means that there is *M* number of elementary actions $\mathcal{A} = \{a^{(1)}, 2^{(2)}, ..., a^{(M)}\}$ (an exemplary meaning of elementary actions in relation to a dextrous hand prosthesis is defined in chapter 5).

The assumed character of control decisions (performing an elementary action) means that the task of bioprosthesis control is reduced to the recognition of patient's intent in successive stages on the basis of available measurement information, thus the determination of the recognition algorithm is equivalent to the determination of prosthesis control algorithm.

For the purpose of determining patient's intent recognition algorithm, we will apply the concept of the so-called sequence recognition. The essence of sequence recognition in relation to the issue we are examining is the assumption that the intention at a given stage depends on earlier intentions. This assumption seems relevant since particular elementary actions of a prosthesis must compose a defined logical entity. This means that not all sequences of elementary actions are acceptable, only those which contribute to the activities which can be performed by a prosthesis. Examples of such actions (sequences of elementary actions) are presented in chapter 5.

Since the patient's current intention depends on history, generally the decision (recognition) algorithm must take into account the whole sequence of the preceding feature values (parameters of EMG signal), $\bar{x}_n = (x_1, x_2, ..., x_n)$. It must be stressed, however, that sometimes it may be difficult to include all the available data, especially for bigger n. In such cases we have to allow various simplifications (e.g. make allowance for only several recent values in the $\bar{x}_n$ vectors), or compromises (e.g. substituting the whole activity history segment that spreads as far back as the k-th instant, i.e. the $\bar{x}_k$ values, with data processed in the form of a decision established at that instant, say i_k).

Apart from the data measured for a specific patient we need some more general information to take a valid recognition decision, namely the *a priori* information (knowledge) concerning the general associations that hold between decisions (patient's intentions) and features (EMG signal parameters). This knowledge may have multifarious forms and various origin. From now on we assume that it has the form of a so-called training set, which – in the considered decision problem – consists of training sequences:

$$S = \{S_1, S_2, S_3, ..., S_m\} \tag{1}$$

A single sequence:

$$S_k = ((x_{1,k}, j_{1,k}), (x_{2,k}, j_{2,k}), ..., (x_{N,k}, j_{N,k})) \tag{2}$$

denotes a single-patient sequence of prosthesis activity that comprises N EMG signal observation instants, and the patient's intentions.

An analysis of the sequential diagnosis task implies that, when considered in its most general form, the explored decision algorithm can in the n-th step make use of the whole available measurement data, as well as the knowledge included in the training set. In consequence, the algorithm is of the following form:

$$\psi_n(\bar{x}_n, S) = i_n \tag{3}$$

Fig. 1 shows the block diagram of the dynamic process of prosthesis control.

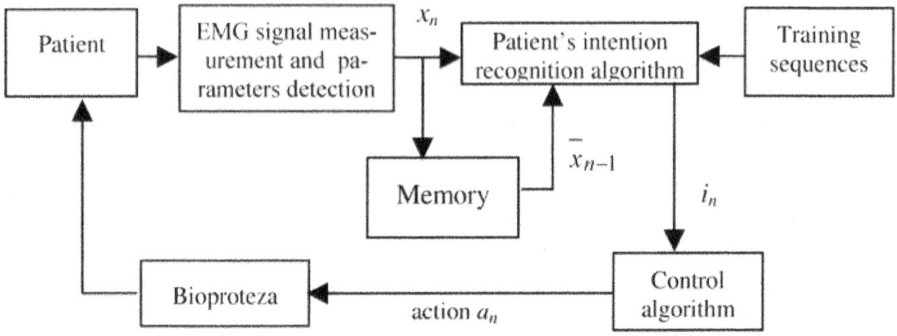

Fig. 1. System of bioprosthesis control via sequential recognition of patient's intentions

4 Pattern Recognition Algorithms

The form of sequential recognition algorithm (3.3) depends on the mathematical model of a recognition task. As it results from the analysis presented in the chapter 2, object features (parameters of EMG signal) do not inform us explicitly about patient's intention, therefore an appropriate mathematical model should be considered in the uncertainty terms. Now let us consider several cases.

4.1 The Probabilistic Algorithm

From probabilistic model of the sequential diagnosis problem there ensues the assumption that x_n and j_n are observations of a pair of random variables $\boldsymbol{X_n}$ and $\boldsymbol{J_n}$ given by class-conditional probability density functions (CPDFs) of features in classes (independent of n):

$$f(x/j) = f_j(x), \; x \in \mathcal{X}, \; j \in \mathcal{M} \tag{4}$$

and relevant probability characteristics that formulate the dependencies between random variables $\boldsymbol{J_n}$ for different n. We will now examine two description methods using first and second order Markov chains and the involved decision algorithms [4].

The Algorithm for First Order Markov Chains – The Markov I Algorithm
First we will assume that patient's intentions at given instant depends only on that at the preceding instant. The probabilistic formalism for such a dependence is the first order Markov chain given by the initial probabilities:

$$p_j = P(\boldsymbol{J_1} = j), \; j \in \mathcal{M} \tag{5}$$

and by the transition probabilities:

$$p_{j_n, j_{n-1}} = P(\boldsymbol{J_n} = j_n / \boldsymbol{J_{n-1}} = j_{n-1}), \; j_n, j_{n-1} \in \mathcal{M}, \; n = 2,3,... \tag{6}$$

Under the assumed description we obtain the following diagnostic algorithm for the n-th instant using the Bayes decision theory methods:

$$\Psi^*(\bar{x}_n) = i_n \,, \text{ if } \; p(i_n / \bar{x}_n) = \max_{k \in \mathcal{M}} p(k / \bar{x}_n), \tag{7}$$

where the *a posteriori* probabilities

$$p(i_n/\bar{x}_n) = \frac{p(i_n, \bar{x}_n)}{\sum_{i_n \in \mathcal{M}} p(i_n, \bar{x}_n)} \tag{8}$$

are recursively determined:

$$p(i_n, \bar{x}_n) = f_{i_n}(x_n) \sum_{j_{n-1}=1}^{M} p_{i_n, j_{n-1}} p(j_{n-1}, \bar{x}_{n-1}), \tag{9}$$

with the following initial condition:

$$p(i_1, x_1) = p_{i_1} f_{i_1}(x_1). \tag{10}$$

In the examined problem we determine the empirical approximations for the probability distributions (4), (5) and (6) on the basis of the training set, using the well-known non-parametric estimation methods (e.g. Parzen estimation method) [7] and the following probability estimations:

- the initial probabilities:

$$p_j^{(S)} = \frac{m_j}{m}, \tag{11}$$

where m_j denotes the number of cases for which $j_{k,1} = j$ ($k = 1,2,...,m,\ j \in \mathcal{M}$),

- the transition probabilities:

$$p_{j,i}^{(S)} = \frac{m_{j,i}}{m_i}, \tag{12}$$

where $m_{j,i}$ denotes the number of pairs $(j_{k,n-1}, j_{k,n})$ for which $j_{k,n-1} = i$ $j_{k,n} = j$; now m_i is the number of situations where $j_{k,n-1} = i$, ($k = 1,2,...,m$, $n = 2,3,...,N, i, j \in \mathcal{M}$). The constructive algorithm (7) will be obtained by substituting the unknown real probability distributions with their empirical estimations.

The Algorithm for Second Order Markov Chains – The Markov II Algorithm

Now we regard the second order Markov chain which nevertheless fully show the procedure imposed by the examined model's specificity. This procedure can be readily generalized for higher order chains.

Thus let us assume that a random variable sequence $\{\boldsymbol{J_n}\}$ constitutes a second order Markov chain given by the following transition probabilities:

$$p_{j_n, j_{n-1}, j_{n-2}} = P(\boldsymbol{J_n} = j_n / \boldsymbol{J_{n-1}} = j_{n-1}, \boldsymbol{J_{n-2}} = j_{n-2}) \tag{13}$$

and initial probabilities:

$$p_{i,j} = P(\boldsymbol{J_1} = i, \boldsymbol{J_2} = j) \tag{14}$$

where $j_n, j_{n-1}, j_{n-2} \in \mathcal{M},\ n = 3,4,...$

We introduce the following denotation:

$$g_n(j_n, j_{n-1}, \bar{x}_n) = p^{(n)}_{j_n, j_{n-1}} f(\bar{x}_n / j_n, j_{n-1}), \tag{15}$$

where

$$p^{(n)}_{j_n, j_{n-1}} = P(\boldsymbol{J_n} = j_n, \boldsymbol{J_{n-1}} = j_{n-1}), \tag{16}$$

and let us further notice that the following holds:

$$g_n(j_n, j_{n-1}, \bar{x}_n) = f_{j_n}(x_n) \sum_{j_{n-2} \in \mathcal{M}} p_{j_n, j_{n-1}, j_{n-2}} g_{n-1}(j_{n-1}, j_{n-2}, \bar{x}_{n-1}), \tag{17}$$

with the initial condition:

$$g_2(j_2, j_1, \bar{x}_2) = f_{j_1}(x_1) f_{j_2}(x_2) p_{j_1, j_2} \tag{18}$$

The *a posteriori* probabilities that appear in (7) are determined according to the following formula:

$$p(j_n / \bar{x}_n) = \sum_{j_{n-1} \in \mathcal{M}} g_n(j_n, j_{n-1}, \bar{x}_n) / \sum_{j_n \in \mathcal{M}} \sum_{j_{n-1} \in \mathcal{M}} g_n(j_n, j_{n-1}, \bar{x}_n). \tag{19}$$

The unknown probability distributions are estimated based on the training set, in a manner similar to the former one.

The explored task of sequential diagnosis can be treated as a sequence of single independent tasks without taking into account the associations that may occur between them. So, if we stick to the probabilistic model, the sequential diagnosis can also apply the well-known Bayes decision algorithm formulated for an independent object sequence [8]. Such an algorithm (henceforth called the **Markov 0 algorithm**) will be applied in the next chapter that depicts experimental comparative analysis of decision algorithms. This algorithm will enable us to answer the question whether it is profitable (i.e. whether it leads to higher operational quality of an algorithm) to include the inter-state dependencies and, consequently, apply more complex decision rules.

4.2 The Fuzzy Methods

Now we take to decision algorithms for the sequential diagnosis task using the inference engine that makes inferences on a fuzzy rule system. For all the algorithms presented below there is a common rule form for rules that associate an observation vector $c = (c^{(1)}, c^{(2)}, ..., c^{(L)})$ with a diagnosis. Further, we assume the following general form of the k-th rule in the system ($k = 1, 2, ..., K$):

$$IF\ c^{(1)} is\ C_{1,k}\ AND\ c^{(2)}\ is\ C_{2,k}\ AND ... AND\ c^{(L)}\ is\ C_{L,k}\ THEN\ D_k \tag{20}$$

where $C_{i,k}$ are fuzzy sets (whose membership functions are designated by $\mu_{C_{i,k}}$) that correspond to the nature of particular observations (for simplicity we assume the sets to be triangular fuzzy numbers) whereas D is a discrete fuzzy set defined on the diagnosis set $\mathcal{M}$, with the μ_{D_k} membership function.

The particular decision algorithms to be used in sequential diagnosis have in common both the inference engine and the procedure for rule system (20) derivation from the learning sets (1). As recognition algorithm the Mamdani fuzzy inference system has been applied [7]. In this system we use the minimum t-norm as AND connection in premises, product operation as interpretation of conjuctive implication in rules, the maximum t-conorm as aggregation operation, and finally the maximum defuzzification method. One of the best known method of rules generating from the given training patterns, is the method proposed by Wang and Mendel [10].

The Algorithm without Context – Fuzzy 0
The algorithm includes neither inter-state dependences nor the influence the applied therapy has exerted on a state but it utilizes only the current symptom values instead. Thus it will be obtained by assuming $a = x_n$ for the n-instant. Now, rule derivation is performed based on the whole training set S for which neither the division into sequences S_i nor element succession in the sequence is pertinent.

The Algorithm with First-Order Context – Fuzzy 1A
This algorithm makes allowance for the one-instant-backwards dependence using full bulk of the measurement data. In effect, we have two kinds of rules:

- initial rules for the first instant i.e. those for which $a = x_1$. They are derived from the first elements of sequences S_i, $i = 1,2,...,m$.
- rules for the subsequent instants — now $a = (x_n, x_{n-1})$; rule derivation is achieved based on the whole training set S, taking into account the succession of particular element pairs in sequences S_i.

The Reduced Algorithm with First-Order Context – Fuzzy 1B
As above, this algorithm includes one-instant-backwards dependence. However, use is now made of the immediately preceding state (for rule derivation) or the immediately preceding decision (for decision-making), rather than the symptom values from the preceding instant. Thus, now for the subsequent-instant rules the following holds $a = (x_n, i_{n-1})$ whilst rule derivation is achieved in a manner identical as above, with the reservation that now the real state j_{n-1} is utilized, instead of the preceding state i_{n-1} diagnosis.

The Algorithm with Second-Order Context – Fuzzy 2A
This time we make allowance for the two-instant-backwards dependence with full measurement data. Rules for the first instant as in the Fuzzy 1A algorithm, for the second-instant rules $a = (x_2, x_1)$ are derived from the two first elements of particular sequences S_i; finally, for subsequent-instant rules $a = (x_n, x_{n-1}, x_{n-2})$.

The Reduced Algorithm with Second-Order Context – Fuzzy 2B
We include the two-instant-backwards dependence using the previous diagnoses in lieu of the previous symptom values. So for the subsequent instant rules $a = (x_n, i_{n-1}, i_{n-2})$, and rule derivation utilizes real values of the previous states that are contained in the training set.

4.3 The Neural Network Approach

Similarly to the fuzzy approach, applying artificial neural networks as an implementation of the decision algorithm for control procedure is concerned exclusively with the relevant selection of input data. The Back Propagation (BP) neural network has been accepted for the needs of a comparative analysis [2], [7].

Data Presentation Methods

The input data sets are just the same as those for the fuzzy-approach algorithms. Thus the ***NN-BP-0*** designation corresponds to BP networks, with data that comprise only the x_n vector i.e. the features characteristic for the intention that is now being recognized. This case implies that we do not take into account the dependences between patient's intentions and that the successive decision tasks are treated as independent ones.

Further, the ***NN-BP-1A*** algorithm designation denotes the relevant network used with the (x_n, x_{n-1}) data, the ***NN-BP-1B*** designation — those used with the (x_n, i_{n-1}) data, and, finally, the ***NN-BP-2A*** designation as well as the ***NN-BP-2B*** ones denote the BP networks used with the (x_n, x_{n-1}, x_{n-2}) or (x_n, i_{n-1}, i_{n-2}) input data, respectively.

All the decision algorithms that are depicted in this chapter have been experimenttally tested as far as the decision quality is concerned. Measure for the decision quality is the frequency of correct decisions for real data that are concerned with recognition of patient's intention on the base of parameters of EMG signal.

5 Experimental Investigations – Comparative Analysis of Methods

The presented above sequence recognition algorithms have been tested experimentally on real data, on an example of the task of controlling a hand prosthesis model. It was assumed that such model has a mechanic structure of r degree of freedom (articulated joints). Prosthesis links can assume particular geometric configurations.

An elementary action now will mean a movement in prosthesis joints resulting in a particular type of fingers' configuration change. During the tests we distinguished elementary actions (patient's intentions) connected with realisation stages of selected grasp movements: (***a***) **palm**, (***b***) **spherical**, (***c***) **lateral**.

The number of analysed elementary actions was limited to 10: 1. preparation for ***a*** grasp; 2. preparation for ***b*** grasp; 3. preparation for ***c*** grasp; 4. closing ***a*** grasp (grasping); 5. grasping type ***b***; 6. grasping type ***c***; 7. opening ***a*** grasp; 8. opening ***b*** grasp; 9. opening ***c*** grasp; 10. assuming a rest position.

Hand (palm) configurations completing the three selected grasping movements (i.e. the final stages of elementary actions: $a^{(4)}$, $a^{(5)}$, $a^{(6)}$) are illustrated in Fig. 2.

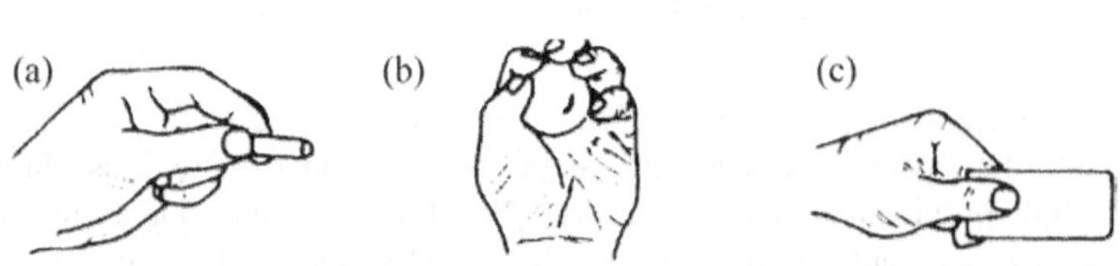

Fig. 2. Grasping movements: (***a***) palm, (***b***) spherical, (***c***) lateral

For the purpose of simplifying our considerations, the constant time of 256ms for each action was adopted. This means that a movement of a given type, e.g. closing a spherical grasp (5), is represented by a sequence of the same elementary actions, e.g.: $<a^{(5)}_{k+1}, a^{(5)}_{k+2}, \ldots a^{(5)}_{k+n}>$, with a variable number of elements proportional to movement duration.

EMG signals registered in a multi-point system [12] on a forearm of a healthy man were used for the recognition of elementary actions. The measurements were taken by means of 6 electrodes at the frequency of 10^3 samples/s. The *rms* values of signals in 256-sample windows (1 feature/channel) and selected harmonics of an averaged frequency spectrum in these windows (8 features/channel) were considered as potential features. This gives a total of 54 features. Finally the *rms* values of 3 EMG signals, coming from electrodes 2, 4 and 5, were accepted as a feature vector x.

The electrodes were respectively located above the following muscles:

2 – the wrist extensor (*extensor carpi radialis brevis*);
4 – wrist flexor (*flexor carpi ulnaris*);
5 – thumb extensor (*extensor pollicis brevis*).

The algorithms were constructed on the basis of the collected learning sequences (2) of the length encompassing from 6 to 20 elementary actions. The tests were conducted on 100 subsequent sequences.

Table 1. Frequency of correct decisions in per cent versus the number of learning sets for various recognition algorithms

	The number of learning sets							
Algorithm	30	40	50	60	70	80	90	100
Markov 0	63.4	65.6	66.2	68.2	70.6	71.6	72.4	74.8
Markov I	80.4	87.6	90.2	90.8	91.8	92.6	93.2	93.4
MarkovII	84.6	90.8	93.6	94.2	94.4	95.2	95.8	96.8
Fuzzy 0	43.2	46.8	56.2	59.6	62.4	66.2	68.0	69.2
Fuzzy 1A	69.6	74.2	77.0	78.8	82.8	84.2	85.6	87.6
Fuzzy 1B	61.2	66.0	70.6	72.2	76.4	77.8	79.6	82.4
Fuzzy 2A	70.2	74.4	77.8	80.6	84.0	85.2	86.8	88.2
Fuzzy 2B	63.6	66.8	71.0	73.8	77.4	78.8	80.8	82.6
NN-BP-0	67.2	68.8	70.2	71.8	72.6	74.2	75.8	77.4
NN-BP-1A	85.4	92.6	96.0	97.8	98.4	98.4	98.6	99.0
NN-BP-1B	72.4	77.6	82.6	84.4	86.8	89.6	90.4	93.6
NN-BP-2A	86.0	93.2	97.2	98.4	98.8	99.0	99.2	99.4
NN-BP-2B	73.6	78.4	84.8	85.6	87.4	90.2	91.0	94.4

The outcome is shown in Table 1. It includes the frequency of correct decisions for the investigated algorithms depending on the number of training sets. These results imply the following conclusions:

1. Out of all the above-mentioned approaches to sequential recognition, the best outcome is the one achieved as a result of using the Back Propagation neural network type with data including both the current- and preceding instant- EMG signal parameters. The probabilistic algorithm using the complex second order Markov model yields a little worse results. The fuzzy logic algorithms undoubtedly turn out to be the worst ones.

2. There occurs a common effect within each algorithm group: algorithms that do not include the inter-state dependences and treat the sequence of intentions as independent objects (Markov 0, Fuzzy 0, NN-BP-0) are always worse than those that were purposefully designed for the sequential decision task, even for the least effective selection of input data. This confirms the effectiveness and usefulness of the concepts and algorithm construction principles presented above for the needs of sequential recognition.
3. In the probabilistic algorithm case the model of higher complexity (i.e. Markov 2) turns out to be more effective than the first order Markov dependence (Markov 1) algorithm.
4. In the fuzzy algorithm and neural network case, algorithms that utilize the original data (i.e. EMG signal parameters) always yield better results than those which substitute the data with decisions.
5. In both the fuzzy algorithm and neural network cases, there is no essential difference between the one-instant-backwards and two-instant-backwards approaches.

6 Conclusions

The presented concept of bioprosthesis control has a character of a study. We assumed that the recognition result $i_n \in \mathcal{M}$ is equivalent to the directive controlling action realisation. In more general terms such directive may initiate the whole control procedure which takes into consideration the situation information in which a given action is performed. Such information may originate from the prosthesis sensory system [11].

The introduced approach is general and can be applied for the control of a dextrous hand and an agile wheelchair as well as other types of prostheses, exoskeletons, etc. This, however, requires a further study, mainly in the experimental phase, which would allow to assess and verify the effectiveness of the adopted concept.

References

1. Chan, A., Englehart, K., Hudgins, B., Lovely, D.F.: Hidden Markov model based classification of myoelectric signals in speech. 23rd Annual International Conference of the IEEE Engineering in Medicine and Biology Society, Istanbul. (2001)
2. Czogala, E., Leski, J.: Fuzzy and Neuro-Fuzzy Intelligent Systems. Physica Verlag, New York. (2000)
3. De Luca, C. J.: The use of Surface Electromyography in Biomechanics. Journal of Applied Biomechanics, Vol. 13, No 2. (1997)
4. Englehart, K., Hudgins, B., Parker, P.A., Stevenson, M.: Classification of the Myoelectric Signal using Time-Frequency Based Representations. Medical Eng. and Physics, Special Issue: Intelligent Data Analysis in Electromyography and Electroneurography. (1999)
5. Krysztoforski, K., Wolczowski, A., Bedzinski, R., Helt, K.: Recognition of Palm Finger Movements on the Basis of EMG Signals with Application of Wavelets. TASK Quarterly, vol. 8, No 2. (2004)
6. Kurzynski, M.: Pattern Recognition - Statistical Approach. Publisher: Wroclaw Univ. of Technol. (1997) (in Polish)
7. Kurzynski, M.: Benchmark of Approaches to Sequential Diagnosis. Artificial Neural Networks In Biomedicine. P. Lisboa, Springer Verlag. (1999) 129-140

8. Kurzynski, M., Zolnierek, A.: A Recursive Classifying Decision Rule for Second-Order Markov Chain. Control and Cybernetics, vol. 9. (1980) 141-147
9. Morecki, A.: Control aspects of artificial hand. IFAC Control Aspect of Biomedical Engineering. Pergamon Press. (1987)
10. Wang, L-X., Mendel, J.M.: Generating Fuzzy Rules by Learning from Examples. IEEE Trans. On Systems, Man and Cybernetics, vol. 22. (1992) 1414-1427
11. Wolczowski, A.: Smart Hand: The Concept of Sensor based Control. Proc. of 7th IEEE Int. Symp. on 'Methods and Models in Automation and Robotics', Międzyzdroje. (2001)
12. Wolczowski, A., Krysztoforski K.: Control-measurement circuit of myoelectric prosthesis hand. Proc. of 13th Conf. of the European Society of Biomechanics, Acta of Bioengineering and Biomechanics, Vol.4, Supplement 1, Wrocław. (2002) 576-577

SEQPACKER: A Biologist-Friendly User Interface to Manipulate Nucleotide Sequences in Genomic Epidemiology

Oscar Coltell[1], Miguel Arregui[1], Larry Parnell[2], Dolores Corella[3], Ricardo Chalmeta[1], and Jose M. Ordovas[2]

[1] Systems Integration and Re-Engineering Research Group (IRIS), Universitat Jaume I, Avda. Vicent Sos Baynat, s/n, 12071-Castellón, Spain
{coltell,rchalmet}@lsi.uji.es, marregui@sg.uji.es
http://www.iris.uji.es

[2] Nutrition and Genetics Laboratory (NUTRIGEN), Human Nutrition Research Center on Aging, Tufts University, 711, Washington Street, Boston, MA, 02111, USA
{Larry.Parnell,Jose.Ordovas}@tufts.edu
http://www.hnrc.tufts.edu

[3] Genomic and Molecular Epidemiology Unit (EPIGEM). Universitat de València, Avda. Vicente Blasco Ibañez, 15, 46009-Valencia, Spain
dolores.corella@uv.es
http://www.uv.es

Abstract. The aim of this paper is to present a new integrated bioinformatics tool for manipulating nucleotide sequences with a user-friendly graphical interface. This tool is named "SeqPacker" because it uses DNA/RNA sequences. In addition, SeqPacker can be seen as a kind of nucleotide chain editor using standardized technologies, nucleotide representation standards, and high platform portability in support of research in Genomic Epidemiology. SeqPacker is written in JAVA as free and stand-alone software for several computer platforms.

Keywords: Bioinformatics tool, visual editor for DNA sequences, nucleotide representation standards, JAVA stand-alone interface, Genomic Epidemiology research support.

1 Introduction

DNA and RNA sequence manipulation is now an ordinary task in Molecular Biology and Genomic research, for example, when it is necessary to extract primer `subsequences from a longer DNA/RNA sequence, or to search something in forward and reverse modes. It is also hard to manage nucleotide chains in raw lines of the computer screen, or in Genbank or FASTA formats. But, it is better to see them in 5-block or 10-block columns, particularly when the sequences are long. On the other part, the standard nucleotide color set, applied to DNA/RNA chains in graphical interfaces, could be useful for color blind people. In addition, the standard size of the nucleotide letters could be difficult to see for eye handicapped people [1].

IRIS and EPIGEM groups are working together under the scientific framework of a Spanish cooperative research network in Biomedical Informatics [2] named INBIOMED. This network is developing a technological platform for storage, integration and analysis of clinical, genetic and epidemiological data and images support-

J.M. Barreiro et al. (Eds.): ISBMDA 2004, LNCS 3337, pp. 368–377, 2004.

ing the research on human pathologies. The main areas INBIOMED is studying are cardiovascular diseases, cancer, and neuropsychiatry syndromes. Part of the tasks IRIS develops to help the EPIGEM research is to build bioinformatics tools to manipulate nucleotide chains for identifying new polymorphisms associated to cardiovascular and lipid abnormalities [3]. One of the results of this collaboration is the tool presented here.

The standard LIMS software to visualize and manage nucleotide chains, for example to obtain the corresponding primers, is not much flexible to adapt displaying features with the capability of the user. For example, tools of ABI-PRISM [4], Qiagen [5], Affymetrix [6], etc. are complex software systems designed to match the management and control requirements of the corresponding laboratory instruments. These tools usually run in a server with a small number of authorized users, and their use is restricted to existing licenses. In most of the cases, fast and simple utilities as SeqPacker are missing in LIMS. On the other hand, there are simplex tools too old and less powered [7]. Other tools are designed for specific tasks, as sequence alignments [8], representation of exon-intron gene structure [9], or are most neither algorithms nor visual tools [10]. There are visual tools for analysis and visualization of DNA genes but more focused on microarray or SAGE experiments, as SeqExpress [11], which includes also support in statistical analysis with R. But SeqExpress runs only under the .NET framework and for Windows platforms. Finally, we found PCR primer design packages with similar features of SeqPacker, but some of them are Web-based programs, as PROBEmer [12], or some are commercial packages, as it is mentioned in [13]. Amplicon [13] is another PCR primer design presented as stand-alone software, but it is written in Python 2.3 and should run as script.

The aim of this paper is to present a new integrated bioinformatics tool for manipulating nucleotide sequences with a friendly graphical interface. This tool is named "SeqPacker" because it uses DNA/RNA sequences. In addition, SeqPacker can be seen as a kind of nucleotide chain editor using standardized technologies [14], nucleotide representation standards as FASTA [15] in support of research in Genomic Epidemiology. SeqPacker is written in JAVA as free and stand-alone software for several computer platforms.

In the following, we will introduce the main features of SeqPacker. Section C is an introduction to the ABI files management. Section D is a short description of SeqPacker internal functionality. Section E is a description of how it works. Next, we will comment future improvements of the tool.

2 Features of Seqpacker

Broadly classified, the current version of SeqPacker (version 2.0) has the following features:

1. Representation of nucleotide sequences in fancy Format: 5-nucleotide or 10-nucleotide columns, numbered or non numbered lines, each nucleotide character is represented under the standard color set (NBI SNPSHOT system); or in FASTA format. The nucleotide font size and type can be also changed.
2. A graphical interface with high usability features: panel division, quick access buttons attached to the main actions of each panel, and panel automatic reconfiguration when the size of the tool window.

3. It can read and write sequence files in FASTA, plain text, and ABI formats. The ABI format is a binary format in which the files of ABI PRISM laboratory instruments are produced.
4. It allows to translate sequences obtained from Internet directly to the tool window using the clipboard.
5. There is a search engine working in a exact match fashion. The main sequence is located in the upper panel, and the search sequence is located in the lower panel. The search mode is case non-sensitive by default, but there is a checkbox to change to case sensitive mode. The search sequence can be read from a file or handwritten directly in the lower panel.
6. It can works with forward and reverse chains. Each panel (main and search) clearly shows the sense of the corresponding sequence. This allows to combine forward to forward, forward to reverse, and reverse to forward searches.
7. Extreme portability as a Java application.

The aim in developing SeqPacker is to supply a nucleotide sequence manipulation editor with standardized technology for every computer platform, so that benefits as many users as possible. The main standardized features that SeqPacker supports are in "graphical notation" and "application integration environment".

Currently, the SeqPacker version 2.0 MS Windows executable file is freely available from [16]. However, provided that SeqPacker is implemented in Java, it can be compiled and executed for the platforms that support the Java Runtime Environment (JRE). For example: MS Windows family (98SE, 2000, and XP), Linux family (RedHat 8.0, SUSE 9.0, etc.), and MacOS X. In addition, provided that the SeqPacker source code is available, it is easy to migrate to other platform (as UNIX platforms) with the proper compiler and make tools.

3 The ABI Format for Nucleotide Files

When writing software for nucleotide manipulation, the first challenge one encounters is the decoding of ABI-like formats. The ABI file format is probably one of the most confusing formats ever designed. It consists of a set of heterogeneous records containing the complete list of nucleotides in a sequence, amongst several other pieces of information, as obtained from a sequencing device (usually an ABI PRISM sequencer).

The sequencing devices we work with, irradiate the fluorescent marked material to be sequenced with a laser beam and then read the light reflection separating it in four tracks, one per each type of nucleotide (A, C, G and T). The reads represent the probability of each nucleotide to be of either type. As the sequencing advances, the device applies a proprietary algorithm to the tracks and deduces which nucleotide type had the highest probability, for each and all of the nucleotides, thus including at the end of the run the complete sequence as part of the data within the file. We inspected the proprietary decision-making algorithm and found that output sequences have an average error rate of only 0.5%. For example, in the chromatogram shown by the Chromas program there exist 5 mistaken bases in every 1000 bases. In this sense, we believe there was no further need to improve the precision of the proprietary decision making algorithm.

Amongst the data contained in the ABI file there is the complete nucleotide sequence as decided by the ABI PRISM sequencer. We have considered it important to provide a simple algorithm which permits to go through the file's contents and read the sequence of nucleotides. For practical reasons we have coded it in JAVA instead of using a more generic pseudo language. The Figure 1 shows the object submodel representing the ABI format information structure using UML representation [3, 17].

In addition, we did find a need to improve the representational level of the products we were using, due to several causes such as user-friendly interfaces, color blindness of the users, forward and reverse representations of nucleotide chains, sequence display format, and many other features to be improved. That was the main reason we based our decision to develop SeqPacker.

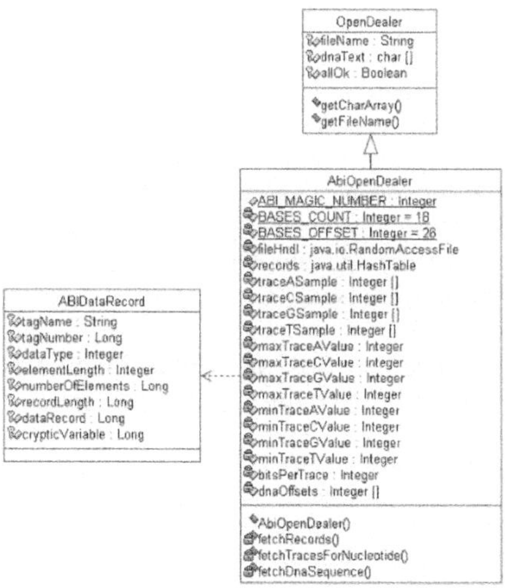

Fig. 1. The ABI format object submodel in UML notation (class diagram). The *ABIDataRecord* class represents all different registers (structure and length) which compose an ABI file. The *OpenDealer* class is a generic file manager. The *AbiOpenDealer* class is a subclass of *OpenDealer* specialized for managing ABI files. Note attributes "ABI_MAGIC_NUMBER" "BASES_COUNT" and "BASES_OFFSET". The first one is to save the number corresponding to the specific register type. The rest are parameters with a fixed value to work properly with ABI files. See ABI specifications for more information

4 Seqpacker Internals

SeqPacker was designed initially for managing ABI format files produced by the Chromas software. But it was extended to deal with other DNA file formats as FASTA and Genbank formats. Currently, SeqPacker offers the functionality shown in the Figure 2.

The user has the choice to either open a brand new file, be it in the ABI flummoxing format or in plain FASTA formatted text, or to load it by pasting it from the clipboard. This latter option permits the copying of sequences from arbitrary sources, such as the Internet (for example, copied from a Genbank HTML page), because the parsing algorithm is clever enough so as to filter out everything other than the nucleotide sequence of interest.

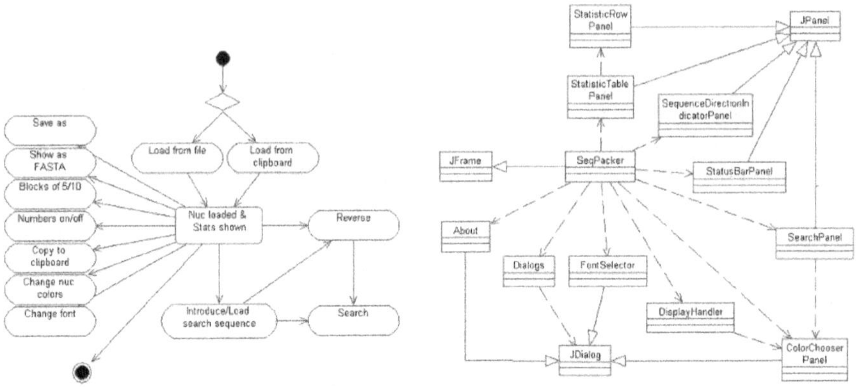

Fig. 2. The SeqPacker functionality in UML notation. A. The workflow represented with an activity diagram. The *Nuc loaded & Stats shown* state represents the usual state of the program when it has been launched and some data has been loaded. Activities *Save as*, *Show as FASTA*, etc. represent all different auxiliary operations to be applied to sequences contained in the work areas. B. The the class hierarchy of the graphical interface. The *JPanel* class is an abstract class for representing all kind of panels used in the interface. The SeqPacker class is the process class which uses each interface class (doted arrows)

Once the sequence has been opened, the application allows one to perform several displaying transformations over the sequence (Figure 3).

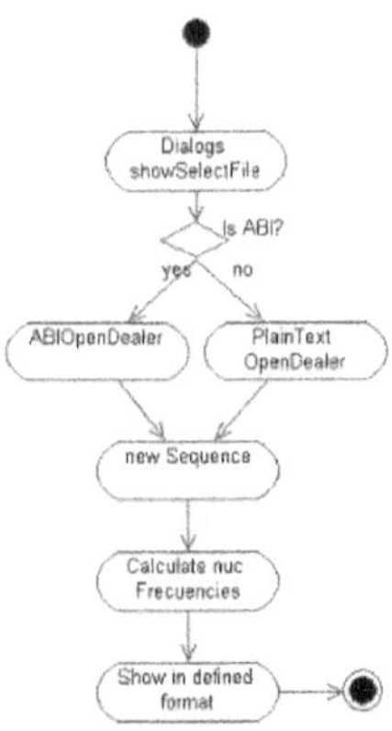

Fig. 3. The SeqPacker partial workflow in UML notation (activity diagram) to represent how the program allows the user to apply several displaying transformations over a previously loaded sequence. For example, it can format the input sequence into FASTA representation, or group it in blocks of 5/10 nucleotides. In addition, it also can show or hide the nucleotide count per line at the end of each line and change the color, size and face of the font

SeqPacker computes the reverse complementary of the sequence very quickly at a click of the mouse and offers the possibility to perform simple searches of exact match over the sequence, detecting whether the user is attempting to search uneven couples, such as RNA with DNA and vice-versa.

When the user has finished transforming the sequence, it is also possible to save it for future use, always in the very same format as shown in the main window, adding a first line with the typical FASTA headers (file name and comments). The Figure 4 shows the classes involved in the file read workflow composing the main object model using classes of the ABI format object submodel shown in the Figure 1.

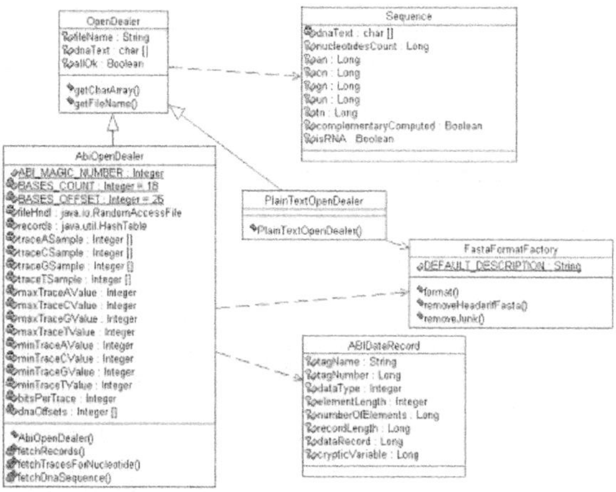

Fig. 4. The SeqPacker object flow in UML notation (class diagram). Classes *AbiOpenDealer* and *PlainTextOpenDealer* are specializations of OpenDealer. The attribute *dnaText* of *OpenDealer* is a data of the abstract object type *Sequence*. The class *PlainTextOpenDealer* only can work with registers of the abstract object type *Sequence*. But the class *AbiOpenDealer* also works with registers of the abstract object type *ABIDataRecord*

5 How to Install and Use the Tool

Using chain manipulation is quite straightforward. For example, in MS Windows, the current version (2.0) is an "*.exe" file with only 149 KB of size named, of course, "SeqPacker.exe". This file is coming inside a compressed Winzip file [18]. It can be copied to any folder without having to run an install tool.

Once the application is launched, the integrated window is opened as it is shown in the Figure 5. The user can read the main sequence from a FASTA, ABI or text file, and the tool shows it in the Main area. Next, the user can read the search sequence from another file, and the tool shows it in the Search area (Figure 6).

In the integrated window, the user has several choices to change chain directions ("Original" and "Reversal"), or representation mode (FASTA, 5-nucl. columns, 10-nucl. columns, line numbers), or the color set (change the standard colors assigned to A, C, G, T, and U), or the nucleotide fonts (letter type and size). It is also useful to know how many A, C, G, T, and U nucleotides are included in the sequence, and their respective frequencies. This is shown in one of the subpanels of the Main Area (Figure 7).

The user can activate the search pressing (clicking) the "Find" button in the Search area. If there is not match, a dialog window notices it to the user. On the contrary, SeqPacker highlights the matched nucleotides in the main sequence. If there are more than sequence matching, in the window appears highlighted each subsequence. The user can also highlight any subsequence in both areas and copy or cut them to the clipboard as it is shown in the Figure 8. This is useful to extract small nucleotide sequences.

The rest of Seqpacker features can be accessed by means of the main menu options and their respective suboptions. For example, the user can change representation features of nucleotide letters: type, size and color (taking in account color blind persons).

The program only includes a subset of adequate letter types, as Courier new, Microsoft Sans Serif, Monospaced, etc., because not all types can combine with the nucleotide column formats in the interface.

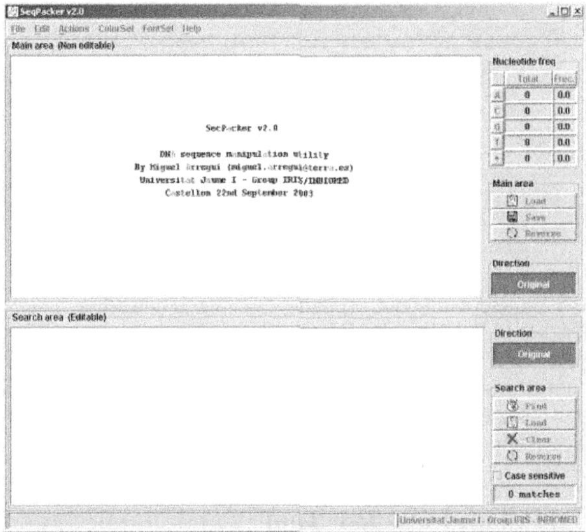

Fig. 5. The integrated window of SeqPacker. The window is divided into two main panels called "Main area" and "Search area", and two minor panels called "Title area" and "Menu area". The menu area shows six main menus: "File", "Edit", "Actions", "ColorSet", "FontSet", and "Help". Each panel is divided into four subpanels. The "Main area" panel has a sequence subpanel (to work with DNA/RNA chains), a "Nucleotide frequency" panel (statistical data about the current chain), a button subpanel (to load, save and reverse chains), and a "Direction" subpanel (to show the direction of the current chain). The "Search area" panel has a sequence subpanel (to work with DNA/RNA chains), a match counter panel, a button subpanel (to find, load, clear and reverse chains), and a "Direction" subpanel (to show the direction of the current chain). There is also a "Case sensitive" button to change the search mode

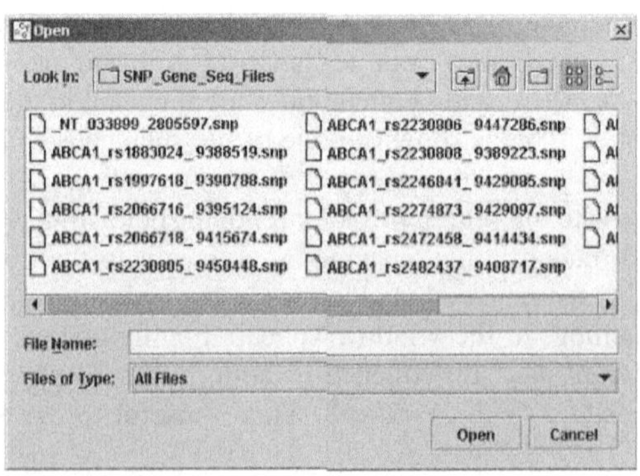

Fig. 6. The Load window of SeqPacker. This is a window designed in standard form which allows to select a file from a list, to change the file path, to change the file type, or to change the view format (list, details, etc.)

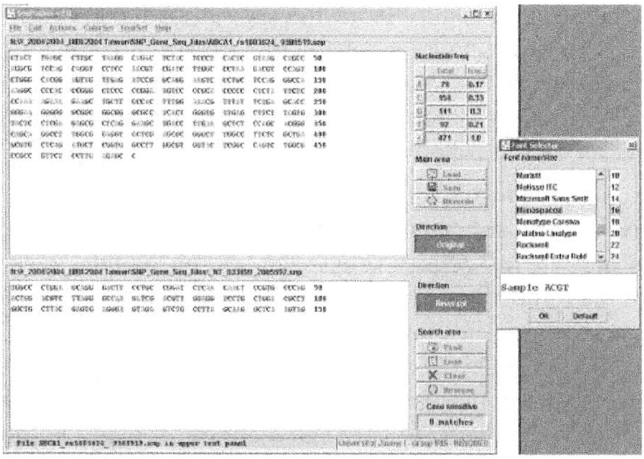

Fig. 7. Format and chain features of the SeqPacker interface. Both main and query sequences are displayed in 5-nucleotide columns format. To avoid uncontrolled offsets in columns, only are allowed letter types with fixed width (Courier new, Microsoft Sans Serif, Monospaced, etc.)

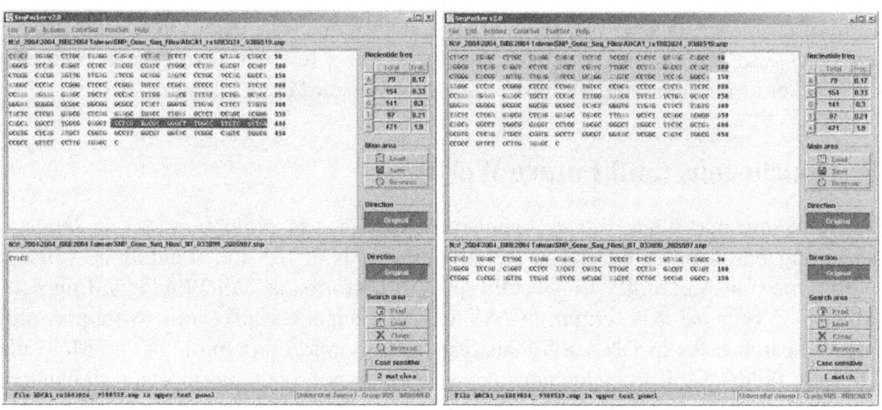

Fig. 8. Search process results. A. The query sequence is "CTACT" in the lower panel. SeqPacker has found two matches in the main sequence (positions 1-5 and 27-31) independently of the sequence display format because it works with the background contents: the whole chain. B. A case with a larger query sequence

Seqpacker can deal easily nucleotide files up to 4 MB size. Therefore, the program is also useful to extract relatively large nucleotide sequences. This limit is not inherent to the program but a default parameter value set by the Java virtual machine to avoid executing errors of the type "null pointer" or violations of the virtual memory space assigned to the program. Any experienced user in systems administration can change that value to a bigger one.

6 Future Improvements

SeqPacker is a simple tool to be used by those who are not familiar with computer complex DNA tools, and he/she needs a powerful support to avoid prune tasks in the research. Therefore, we designed it to be as user-friendly as possible. But the tool is not closed or concluded related to the features it can be incorporate. Dr. Parnell, one of the authors, has been testing each version of SeqPacker against his data files in the NutriGenomics Lab and he has suggested some improvements which could extend the tool functionality to other research areas. The most important suggestions to be developed in the program are the following:

1. Allowing to mix main and query sequences and, at the same time, avoiding matches between forward and reverse chains.
2. Allowing to insert a full sequence between two nucleotides of other sequence as "selection of the insertion site". This could be useful to simulate the gene insertion in a plasmid to DNA replication [19, 20].
3. Managing restriction enzymes: a background mechanism based on specific features of each enzyme to make automatic searches in the main sequence [21].
4. Managing protein sequences: to apply all features of Seqpacker to display, format and search protein sequences (in one letter or three letter code).

We think some of these improvements are really new and different tools. Therefore, we changed our development strategy, following the approach in [22], and we decided to build an integrated toolbox with specialized tools to deal with different kind of problems: DNA/RNA sequences, protein sequences, insertion sites, restriction enzymes, etc. We are working to implement these features in the next version of SeqPacker as an integrated toolbox with OMG standard design languages [23].

7 Conclusions (and Future Work)

We have introduced Seqpacker, a nucleotide sequence manipulation tool for sequence searching based on standardized technologies. It is a free and stand-alone software with wide transportability to several types of platforms as MS Windows, Linux and MacOS X because it is written in JAVA code. Seqpacker also aims to support ordinary research tasks in DNA/RNA analysis in Genomic Epidemiology and Molecular Biology fields. SeqPacker includes some features not available in other similar programs and, in a near future, some powerful functions will be added to built an integrated toolbox. A MS Windows executable file is freely available from http://www.iris.uji.es/ocoltell/seqpacker.html.

Acknowledgements

This research is part supported by the Spanish research network "INBIOMED. Plataforma de almacenamiento, integración y análisis de datos clínicos, genéticos, epidemiológicos e imágenes orientada a la investigación sobre patologías", the Ministerio de Educación y Ciencia de España, grants PR2004-0054 (D. Corella), and Ministerio de Ciencia y Tecnología de España (DPI2003-02515).

References

1. Fischer, C., Schweigert, S., Spreckelsen, C., Vogel, F. "Programs, databases, and expert systems for human geneticists-a survey". Hum. Genet. (1997), 97:129-137.
2. INBIOMED Home page. http://www.inbiomed.retics.net/. Accessed July 2004.

3. Ordovas, J.M., Corella, D., Cupples, L.A., Demissie, S., Kelleher, A., Coltell. O., Wilson, P.W., Schaefer, E.J., Tucker, K. "Polyunsaturated fatty acids modulate the effects of the APOA1 G-A polymorphism on HDL-cholesterol concentrations in a sex-specific manner: the Framingham Study".Am J Clin Nutr., Jan;75(1); 2002: 38-46.".
4. Applied Biosystems. Life Science LIMS software. http://www.appliedbiosystems.com/catalog/myab/StoreCatalog/products/CategoryDetails.jsp?hierarchyID=101&category1st=111765&category2nd=111784&category3rd=112004&parts=none. Accessed July 2004.
5. Qiagen Instruments Home page. http://www.qiageninstruments.com/. Accessed July 2004.
6. Affymetrix. LIMS Server Software and Computer Packages. http://www.affymetrix.com/products/software/specific/lims_softpacks.affx. Accessed July 2004.
7. Nilsson, M.T., Klein, G.O. "SEQ-ED: an interactive computer program for editing, analysis and storage of long DNA sequences". Bioinformatics, Vol 1; 1985: 29-34.
8. DeSantis, T.Z., Dubosarsky, I., Murray, S.R., Andersen, G.L. "Comprehensive aligned sequence construction for automated design of effective probes (CASCADE-P) using 16S rDNA". Bioinformatics, Vol 19(12); 2003: 1461-1468.
9. Hill, A., Sorscher, E. "Common structural patterns in human genes". Bioinformatics, Vol 20(10); 2003: 16321-1635.
10. Vinga, S., Almeida, J. "Aligment-free sequence comparison-review". Bioinformatics, Vol 19(12); 2003: 1461-1468.
11. Boyle, J. "SeqExpress: desktop analysis and visualization tool for gene expression experiments". Bioinformatics, Vol 20(10); 20043: 1649-1650.
12. Emrich, S.J., Lowe, M., Delcher, A.L. PROBEmer: a webbased software tool for selecting optimal DNA oligos. NucleicAcids Res., 31: 2003: 3746–3750.
13. Jarman, S.N. "Amplicon: software for designing PCR primers on aligned DNA sequences". Bioinformatics, Vol 20(10); 20043: 1644-1645.
14. Object Management Organization Home page. http://www.omg.org. Accessed July 2004.
15. http://www.ncbi.nlm.nih.gov/Genbank/index.html.
16. SeqPacker in MS Windows executable version. http://www.iris.uji.es/ocoltell/seqpacker.html.
17. Booch G., Rumbaugh J., Jacobson I. The Unified Modeling Language User Guide. Addison-Wesley, Reading, MA, 1999.
18. Winzip compress program. http://www.winzip.com. Accessed July 2004.
19. R PLASMID. In Madigan, M., Martinko, J.M., Parker, J. Brock. Biology of Microorganisms. 10th Ed. Prentice Hall. Upper Saddle River, 2003. http://www.arches.uga.edu/~lace52/rplasmid.html. Accessed July 2004.
20. Plasmid Maker Stack. http://iubio.bio.indiana.edu/soft/molbio/mac/plasmid-maker.html. Accessed July 2004.
21. Restriction Enzymes. Background Paper. Access Excellence Classic Collection. The National Health Museum. http://www.accessexcellence.org/AE/AEC/CC/restriction.html. Accessed July 2004.
22. Boyle, J. "A visual environment for the manipulation and integration of JAVA Beans". Bioinformatics, Vol 19(12); 2003: 1461-1468.
23. OMG-UMLSpec. "OMG Unified Modeling Language Specification. March 2003. Version 1.5. formal/03-03-01". An Adopted Formal Specification of the Object Management Group, Inc., 2003. (http://www.omg.org/technology/documents/. Accessed July 2004.

Performing Ontology-Driven Gene Prediction Queries in a Multi-agent Environment

Vassilis Koutkias, Andigoni Malousi, and Nicos Maglaveras

Aristotle University of Thessaloniki, Medical School, Lab. of Medical Informatics, P.O. BOX 323, 54124, Thessaloniki, Greece
{bikout,andigoni,nicmag}@med.auth.gr

Abstract. Gene prediction is one of the most challenging problems in Computational Biology. Motivated by the strengths and limitations of the currently available Web-based gene predictors, a Knowledge Base was constructed that conceptualizes the functionalities and requirements of each tool, following an ontology-based approach. According to this classification, a Multi-Agent System was developed that exploits the potential of the underlying semantic representation, in order to provide transparent and efficient query services based on user-implied criteria. Given a query, a broker agent searches for matches in the Knowledge Base, and coordinates correspondingly the submission/retrieval tasks via a set of wrapper agents. This approach is intended to enable efficient query processing in a resource-sharing environment by embodying a meta-search mechanism that maps queries to the appropriate gene prediction tools and obtains the overall prediction outcome.

1 Introduction

Identifying protein-coding regions within genomic sequences is one of the most challenging problems in Computational Biology [1]. During the last decade, several computational techniques have been developed trying to identify potential gene structures by examining uncharacterized DNA sequences. The majority of these techniques incorporate sophisticated methods and, even though they cannot guarantee accurate results, they can effectively support biological evidence in conjunction with experimental methods.

Most computational techniques are currently available on-line through Web interfaces. Typically, gene prediction tools require several input parameters to be set by the user and support different formatted output representations. Moreover, the underlying computational methods are trained on species-specific datasets for which they provide highly accurate predictions, and usually emerge lower accuracy levels on other genesets [2]. Considering the wide variety of the available gene identifiers and their functional heterogeneity, it is difficult for a researcher to select the tool that can meet his/her expectations in each case.

In this paper, an approach for semantic selection and transparent access to gene prediction tools is presented, which is based on a) a conceptual classification of tools, and b) a Multi-Agent System responsible for knowledge management and task coordination [3]. The classification of tools involves the definition of a domain ontology, which semantically describes and associates essential input-output parameters, providing the schema for the construction of a Knowledge Base [4]. Accordingly, user requests for gene prediction are served by an agent-based brokering protocol, in order

J.M. Barreiro et al. (Eds.): ISBMDA 2004, LNCS 3337, pp. 378–387, 2004.

to identify which tools, described in the Knowledge Base, fulfill the functional requirements of each request. The set of tools obtained are transparently accessed via wrapper agents and the extracted results are provided to the end-user [5].

The main objective of this work is to provide a resource-sharing environment that enables automated query executions without requiring prior knowledge of the tools' technical details and functional specifications.

2 Motivation – Rationale

2.1 Gene Prediction Techniques

Computational gene identification is typically implemented either by similarity-based approaches, or by ab-initio techniques [6]. Similarity-based gene prediction exploits the information derived by matching a query DNA sequence against a database of annotated proteins, cDNA libraries, or databases of Expressed Sequence Tags (ESTs). Alternatively, several hybrid gene prediction methods have been developed that consolidate accuracy levels by combining the evidence coming from comparisons against a user-defined set of sequences that is known to be homologous to the query DNA sequence [7].

Ab-initio methods attempt to locate specific content-based and signal-based features that have been proven to contribute in the protein-coding mechanism, such as promoter elements, donor and acceptor sites, polyadenylation sites, and so forth [1]. Currently available tools involve various probabilistic algorithms that computationally detect and locate potential gene features. This means that the reported features come with associated probabilities reflecting the reliability of a prediction, as it is estimated by the underlying probabilistic model.

Regardless of the computational approach followed, the majority of the existing Web-based techniques are limited by a set of functional constraints and requirements. Accordingly, an abstract set of classification criteria follows:

1. Each tool performs predictions against gene models of specific organisms. Typically, the organisms of interest together with other input parameters have to be defined in the submission form.
2. A query is submitted and processed, only if the sequence length does not exceed the specified limitations.
3. Similarity-based gene identifiers are classified according to whether they perform matches against protein databases, cDNA/EST databases, or a group of user-defined protein sequences that is known to be homologous to the query sequence.
4. Restrictions related to the input sequence format and the capability of making predictions in both DNA strands must be taken into account before submitting a query sequence.
5. Some gene identifiers can predict multiple and partial genes within a single DNA sequence submission, while others are capable of performing only single gene predictions [8].
6. The output features of ab-initio gene predictors diverge. For example, some tools' outputs include only the identification of the predicted coding regions, while others provide additional information, such as the amino acid sequence of the predicted peptide(s), and/or the type and position of the signal sensors detected.

7. Results are encoded in different formatted outputs that can be either displayed in Web pages or delivered to a user-defined e-mail address.

Considering the aforementioned issues, we developed a query processing mechanism, which selects the suitable tools and transparently executes queries, based on a semantic representation, enabling advanced access to existing gene prediction methods.

2.2 Related Work

Agent technology is a rapidly evolving interdisciplinary field that is favorable in the development of complex and distributed systems, and emerges considerable acceptance in the Bioinformatics community [9]. During the last decade, several agent-based systems have been developed to address various types of domain problems, focusing basically on integrating biological databases. Research projects such as BioMAS [10] and GeneWeaver [11] worked towards integrated genomic annotation, with extensions related to efficient query processing mechanisms.

In general, integrated approaches gain increasing interest in gene prediction research. Relevant to the proposed system, GENEMACHINE is an application that allows query submissions to multiple gene prediction tools through a common user interface [12]. Users are prompted to select a tool from a list of available gene predictors and the results are provided via e-mail in various textual or graphical formats. METAGENE[1] is another combinatorial application that enables multiple submissions simultaneously to a set of gene prediction resources and displays a comprehensive report on the sequence features. Both GENEMACHINE and METAGENE have the prerequisite that target users have prior knowledge of each tool's capabilities and requirements, to avoid random selection.

In comparison with the approaches referred above, this work is intended to serve requests made by users who are not necessarily aware of the functionality supplied by each tool or it is out of their interest to familiarize with their technical details. This is accomplished by adopting a component-based architecture, via software agents, described below.

3 System Description

3.1 Agent-Based Architecture

The proposed Multi-Agent architecture relies on the broker/wrapper paradigm [13], [14]. Fig. 1 illustrates the incorporated modules, which are described below:

- A *User Agent* acquires the gene finding query parameters from the user (via a user interface) and submits an appropriate request to the *Broker Agent*. It also receives the outcome of the gene prediction procedure by the *Broker Agent*.
- The *Broker Agent* has the key-role to control access to gene prediction tools upon request of a *User Agent*. It cooperates with the *Knowledge-Base Wrapper Agent* to map queries into selection of tools. It also coordinates access to gene prediction tools and compiles the corresponding outcome in a transparent way.

[1] http://rgd.mcw.edu/METAGENE/

- The *Knowledge Base* module contains a semantic classification of tools as well as their functional descriptions. This approach enables the execution of the matching procedure between user-implied requirements and the functional specification of tools, constituting a meta-search mechanism. Knowledge is retrieved/acquired from/to the *Knowledge Base* via the *Knowledge-Base Wrapper Agent.*
- The *Knowledge-Base Wrapper Agent* applies the matching procedure between the gene query parameters and the tools that fulfill the underlying requirements by accessing the *Knowledge Base.* In addition, it registers gene prediction tools to the *Knowledge Base* upon request of a *Wrapper Agent.*
- A *Wrapper Agent* is delegated the task to receive requests for gene prediction from the *Broker Agent* and translates them to the appropriate format, which is specific to each gene prediction tool. Accordingly, it submits the query to its associated tool and returns the results to the *Broker Agent.* As it is depicted in Fig. 1, the design followed is one *Wrapper Agent* for each prediction tool available. It has to be noted, that prior to utilizing a gene tool, the relevant *Wrapper Agent* has to register the tool's description to the *Knowledge Base* via the *Broker Agent.*

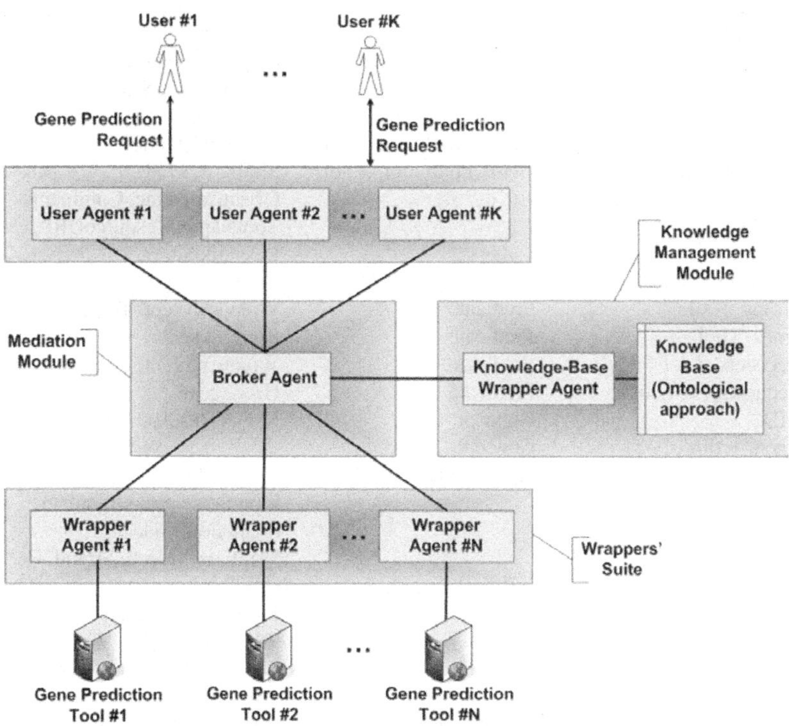

Fig. 1. The proposed agent-based architecture

3.2 Classification of Tools – Ontology Description

In order to provide a mechanism for matching user requirements with the appropriate tools, we constructed a *Knowledge Base* that enables meta-searches on user-implied criteria. The *Knowledge Base* is ontology-driven. Typically, an ontology defines the common terms and concepts used to describe an area of knowledge and encodes their meaning in groups of classes, properties, and relationships among classes [4], [15]. In our scenario, the domain ontology was constructed to facilitate data exchange among agents by conceptualizing the information related to the prediction resources.

The defined classes and their corresponding attributes provide the essential description regarding the specifications of each tool and the services of the relevant agents. In Table 1, the classification of the basic concepts, together with their assigned attributes, is provided. The left column lists the basic classes of the ontology along with their parent classes shown in the middle, and the corresponding properties on the right column. For each attribute, an appropriate set of range values and constraints was defined.

Table 1. Classes and properties of the domain ontology

Class	Subclass of	Attributes
Concept		
Gene_Prediction_Tool	Concept	ToolName, Description, SequenceLength, ResultsType, Strand, Organism
Ab_Initio	Gene_Prediction_Tool	PredictionMode
Similarity_Based	Gene_Prediction_Tool	SimilarityMode
Organism		OrganismName, Comments
Availability		ToolName, ResourceURL, ResourceScript
Predicate		
Wraps_Tool	Predicate	WrapperAgent, ToolName
Finds_Tool	Predicate	SearchAgent
Registers_Tool	Predicate	WrapperAgent, ToolName
Requests_Prediction	Predicate	UserAgent
AID	Concept	Name, Resolvers, Addresses
AgentAction	Concept	
Wrap_Tool	AgentAction	ToolToWrap, InputSequence, Organism, PredictionMode, SimilaritySearch, Strand, ResultsType
Find_Tool	AgentAction	InputSequence, Organism, PredictionMode, SimilaritySearch, Strand, ResultsType
Register_Tool	AgentAction	Description, Organism, SequenceLength PredictionMode, SimilaritySearch, ResultsType, Strand
Request_Prediction	AgentAction	Organism, PredictionMode, SimilaritySearch, ResultsType, Strand

Two groups of concepts can be distinguished in the domain ontology:

- Concepts related to the functionalities and constraints of the gene prediction tools: This kind of information is structured under the *Gene_Prediction_Tools* class, which classifies the resources according to the type of the prediction performed and the outcome provided. Moreover, a set of subclasses was defined in order to capture additional functional parameters, such as sequence length limitations, supported organism-specific gene models, etc.
- Concepts that describe agent tasks: Specifically, *Agent_Action* class corresponds to concepts that indicate actions that can be performed by system's agents, e.g., *Find_Tool*, or *Wrap_Tool*. *Predicates* class contains expressions that claim something about the status of our "agent-system world" and can be true or false, thus, relevant classes are defined, such as *Finds_Tool*, or *Registers_Tool*.

3.3 Agent Interactions

Coordination among agents is achieved by exchanging messages, which encapsulate the domain ontology described above [16]. To illustrate agent interactions, we provide AUML sequence diagrams [17] presenting the registration of a new tool to the *Knowledge Base* (Fig. 2 (a)) and the brokering protocol that is implemented for gene finder selection and execution (Fig. 2 (b)).

Regarding the registration of a new gene prediction tool, the corresponding *Wrapper Agent* provides information to the *Broker Agent*, relevant to the functional description of the tool. The *Broker Agent* forwards this request to the *Knowledge-Base Wrapper Agent*, which registers the tool's description to the *Knowledge Base*. Finally, the *Wrapper Agent* is informed about the outcome of the registration procedure by the *Broker Agent*. Finally, the *Broker Agent* informs the *Wrapper Agent* about the outcome of the registration procedure.

The gene finder selection and execution procedure corresponds to a brokering protocol [13], which is initiated and controlled by the *Broker Agent*. Specifically, upon a request for gene prediction by a *User Agent*, the *Broker Agent* formulates another request containing the user-defined criteria for tool selection to the *Knowledge-Base Wrapper Agent*, in order to search the *Knowledge Base*. This matching procedure results in a set of providers (if there is a match) that fulfills the query and then, each tool's *Wrapper Agent* address is sent to the *Broker Agent* by the *Knowledge-Base Wrapper Agent*. In the following, the *Broker Agent* generates gene prediction requests to each specific *Wrapper Agent*, which wraps the corresponding gene finder. Finally, the *Broker Agent* compiles the total outcome and provides it to the user via the *User Agent*. Alternatively, only the results of the fastest gene finder could be sent to the user, taking into account that some tools require several minutes to serve a request, depending on their underlying prediction algorithm, as well as their current workload.

3.4 Implementation Issues

Software agents of the proposed system were constructed using JADE (Java Agent DEvelopment Framework) [18]. JADE is compliant with the interoperability specifications of FIPA[2] (Foundation of Intelligent Physical Agents) and provides both an

[2] http://www.fipa.org

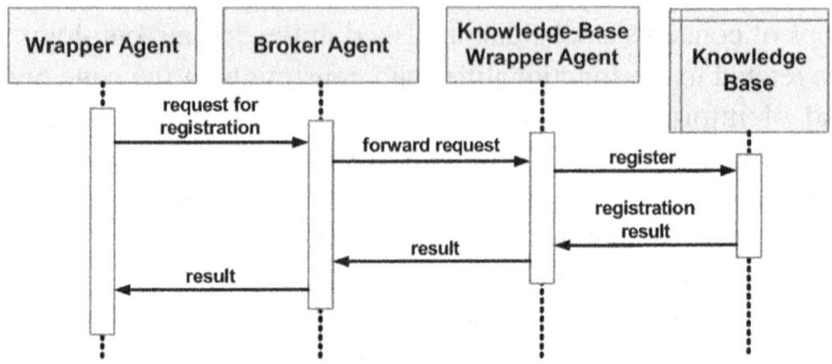

(a)

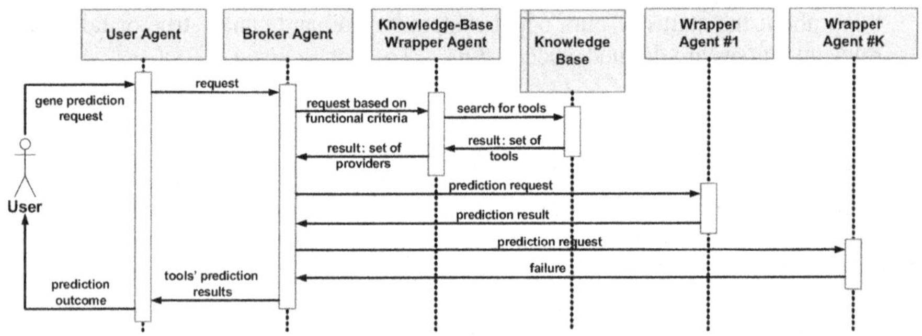

(b)

Fig. 2. (a) Registration of a gene finder tool to the *Knowledge Base*, and (b) the brokering protocol for gene finder selection and query execution

agent execution environment and an agent-application programming interface. Furthermore, it enables the embodiment of user-defined ontologies, in order to support effective domain-oriented agent communication acts.

The application ontology and the relevant *Knowledge Base* were developed in Protégé, an integrated software environment used to implement knowledge-based systems [19]. The meta-search mechanism incorporated between user-implied requirements and the *Knowledge Base* corresponds to queries expressed in the Protégé Axiom Language (PAL). PAL extends the Protégé knowledge-modeling environment with support for writing and storing logical constraints and queries about frames in a *Knowledge Base*.

The messages exchanged among agents are encoded in the FIPA ACL agent communication language [16]. Aiming to provide a generic solution and to meet scalability concerns, all the agents of the Multi-Agent System register their services with the *Directory Facilitator* of the JADE platform, which provides "yellow page" services to the agents of the framework. The *Directory Facilitator* was not included in the agent interactions described for simplicity reasons.

4 Examples of Use

To illustrate the application of the proposed system, a set of 12 widely known gene prediction tools was described according to the domain ontology. The basic decision factor in selecting the specific tools was to construct a representative group of re-

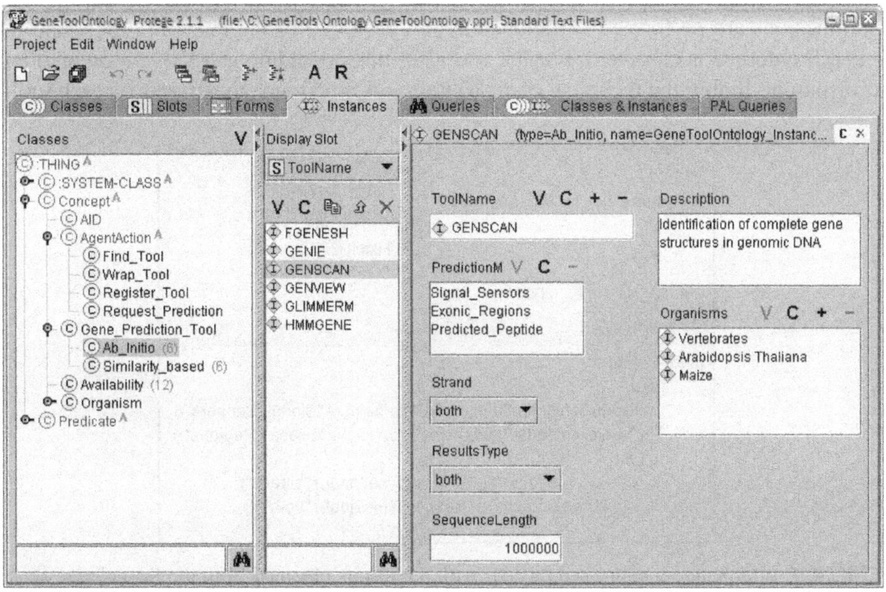

Fig. 3. A screenshot of the domain-ontology in Protégé that illustrates the class hierarchy on the left panel, the instances of the Ab_Initio subclass in the middle, and the properties of the "GENSCAN" instance on the right

sources that covers a wide range of functionalities and can give answers to multiple types of requests. The major difficulty in describing those tools under a controlled vocabulary was the diversity of the parameters and the terms used. As a consequence, during this process various modifications had to be made to the structural elements of the ontology, in order to avoid inconsistencies and extend functional capabilities. Fig. 3 depicts a screenshot of Protégé that contains the class hierarchy and the values of an example instance.

To clarify the capabilities of the query processing mechanism, a set of example queries follows. Given a query DNA sequence, a researcher could perform requests such as:

- *Query 1*: Display on screen the results of all the ab-initio gene finding tools that can predict both the exonic regions and the incorporated signal features. Fig. 4 illustrates the relevant query represented in PAL language and the list of tools that can serve this request.
- *Query 2*: Submit the query DNA sequence to all the similarity-based gene finders that perform predictions for Homo sapiens and send results by e-mail.
- *Query 3*: Is there any tool that can predict features for genomic sequences larger than 1 MB?

Initially, the system processes each request by querying the Knowledge Base to search for matching tools. If there is no tool that accomplishes the defined criteria, a relevant notification is generated. In case of one match, the system submits the query to the corresponding gene predictor and obtains the results in the tool's specific formatted output. When more than one tool fulfills the user implied criteria, multiple submissions are performed simultaneously to each one of the matching tools and the overall outcome is compiled. For the end user, this procedure is totally automated and transparent, hiding the technical complexities and functional constraints of each tool.

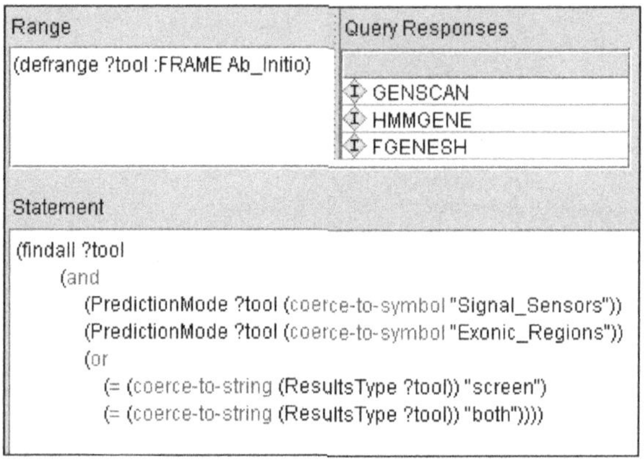

Fig. 4. A sample query expressed in PAL with the results obtained from the Knowledge Base

5 Conclusions – Future Work

One of the most active areas in Bioinformatics research is the implementation of computational gene prediction techniques. Several techniques have been developed so far, most of them being publicly available over the Internet. However, their diversity and heterogeneity, regarding functional characteristics and requirements of use, makes their utilization difficult at least for non-experienced users. In this paper, we presented a classification schema, according to which computational tools are categorized based on the aforementioned criteria. The corresponding information is stored in a Knowledge Base, designed as a domain ontology, which is managed through a Multi-Agent System. Upon a user request for gene prediction, an agent-based brokering interaction protocol is initiated, involving a meta-search applied to the Knowledge Base for tools that match the implied user requirements. In case of successful match(es), appropriate wrapper agents access the corresponding gene prediction tool(s) and provide the final outcome to the end-user.

As a next step, we plan to embody in our system an XML-based module to uniformly represent gene prediction outputs, which relies on the General Feature Format (GFF)[3] specifications [20]. Thus, in cases where the matching procedure results in a set of tools that fulfill the user's request, a common-structured report of predictions will be generated, enabling comparative analysis and evaluation of tools.

Moreover, we plan to incorporate additional Web-based gene finders, a direction which is facilitated by the component-based agent design and the reusability of the domain ontology. During this procedure, we will be able to examine potential re-engineering issues, in order to include descriptive features that are currently not taken into account in the knowledge model.

---

[3] http://www.sanger.ac.uk/Software/formats/GFF/GFF_Spec.shtml

References

1. Mathé, C., Sagot, M.F., Schiex, T., Rouzé, P.: Current Methods of Gene Prediction, their Strengths and Weaknesses. Nucleic Acids Research 30 (2002) 4103-4117
2. Rogic, S., Mackworth, A.K., Ouellette, F.: Evaluation of Gene-Finding Programs on Mammalian Sequences. Genomic Research Vol. 11 (2001) 817-832
3. Sycara, K.: Multiagent Systems. AI Magazine Vol. 10 (2) (1998) 79-93
4. Devedzic, V.: Knowledge Modeling - State of the Art. Integrated Computer-Aided Engineering Vol. 8 (3) (2001) 257-281
5. Tork Roth, M., Schwarz, P.: Don't Scrap it, Wrap it! A Wrapper Architecture for Legacy Sources. Proceedings of the 23rd VLDB Conference Athens Greece (1997) 266-275
6. Mount, D.W.: Bionformatics: Sequence and Genome Analysis. CSHL Press New York (2001) 337-373
7. Rogic, S., Ouellette, F., Mackworth, A.K.: Improving Gene Recognition Accuracy by Combining predictions from two gene-finding programs. Bioinformatics Vol. 18 (8) (2002) 1034-1045
8. Zhang, M.Q.: Computational Prediction of Eukaryotic Protein-coding Genes. Nature Vol. 3 (2002) 698-709
9. Karasavvas, K., Baldock, R., Burger, A.: Bioinformatics System Integration and Agent Technology. Journal of Biomedical Informatics Vol. 37 (3) (2004) 205-219
10. Decker, K., Khan, S., Schmidt, C., Situ, G., Makkena, R., Michaud, D.: BioMAS: A Multi-agent System for Genomic Annotation. International Journal of Cooperative Information Systems Vol. 11 (3-4) (2002) 265-292
11. Bryson, K., Luck, M., Joy, M., Jones, D.T.: Applying Agents to Bioinformatics in GeneWeaver. Cooperative Information Agents IV. Lecture Notes in Artificial Intelligence Vol. 1860 Springer-Verlag Berlin Heidelberg New York (2000) 60-71
12. Makalowska, I., Ryan, J.F., Baxevanis, A.D.: GeneMachine: Gene Prediction and Sequence Annotation. Bioinformatics Vol. 17 (9) (2001) 843-844
13. Wong, C., Sycara, K.: A Taxonomy of Middle Agents for the Internet. Proceedings of the Fourth International Conference on Multiagent Systems Boston MA. (2000) 465-466
14. Aldana, J.F., Roldan, M., Navas, I., Perez, A.J., Trelles, O.: Integrating Biological Data Sources and Data Analysis Tools through Mediators. Proceedings of the 2004 ACM Symposium on Applied Computing Nicosia Cyprus (2004) 127
15. Baker, P.G., Goble, C.A., Bechhofer, S., Paton, N.W., Stevens, R., Brass, A.: An Ontology for Bioinformatics Applications. Bioinformatics Vol. 15 (6) (1999) 510-520
16. Labrou, Y., Finin, T., Peng, Y.: Agent communication languages: The current landscape, IEEE Intelligent Systems Vol. 14 (2) (1999) 45-52
17. Odell, J., van Dyke Parunak, H., Bauer, B.: Representing Agent Interaction Protocols in UML. In: Ciancarini, P., Wooldridge, M., (eds): Agent-Oriented Software Engineering, Springer-Verlag Berlin Heidelberg New York (2001) 121- 140
18. Bellifimine, F., Poggi, A., Rimassa, G.: JADE – A FIPA-compliant Agent Framework. In: Proceedings of the 4th International Conference and Exhibition on the Practical Application of Intelligent Agents and Multi-Agents (1999) 97-108
19. Noy, N.F., Sintek, M., Decker, S., Crubezy, M., Fergerson, R.W., Musen, M.A.: Creating Semantic Web Contents with Protégé 2000. IEEE Intelligent Systems 16 (2) (2001) 60-71
20. Malousi, A., Koutkias, V., Maglaveras, N.: A Unified XML-based Output Representation of Ab-initio Gene Prediction Tools. Proceedings of the Fourth European Symposium on Biomedical Engineering Patras Greece (2004)

Protein Folding in 2-Dimensional Lattices with Estimation of Distribution Algorithms

Roberto Santana, Pedro Larrañaga, and José A. Lozano

Intelligent System Group
Department of Computer Science and Artificial Intelligence
University of the Basque Country
P.O. Box 649, 20080 San Sebastián - Donostia, Spain
{rsantana,ccplamup,lozano}@si.ehu.es

Abstract. This paper introduces a new type of evolutionary computation algorithm based on probability distributions for the solution of two simplified protein folding models. The relationship of the introduced algorithm with previous evolutionary methods used for protein folding is discussed. A number of experiments for difficult instances of the models under analysis is presented. For the instances considered, the algorithm is shown to outperform previous evolutionary optimization methods.

Keywords: Estimation of Distribution Algorithms, protein folding, HP model.

1 Introduction

Searching for the minimum conformation structure of a protein given its sequence is a difficult problem in computational biology. Even for a small number of amino acids, the conformational space of proteins is huge. This fact has led to the need of using simplified models that can help to find approximate structures of proteins. Lattice models are an example, where each amino acid of a protein can be represented as a bead, and connecting bonds are represented by lines, which follow the geometry of the chosen background lattice [10]. The problem consists in finding the structure in the lattice that minimizes a predefined fitness function associated with protein structure stability. These problems can be dealt with using search algorithms that try to optimize the fitness function. In these simplified models, the dimension of the search space remains huge. Therefore, the efficiency of the optimization algorithm is critical for the success of the search.

Several different heuristics [1, 3, 8, 11, 14, 19] have been applied to a simplified version of the protein folding problem called the Hydrophobic-Polar (HP) model [4]. The HP model is based on the fact that hydrophobic interactions are a dominant force in protein folding. Although simple, this model has proven to be useful as a test bed for folding algorithms.

In this paper, to solve the HP model we propose a new type of evolutionary computation algorithm that belongs to the class of Estimation of Distribution Algorithms (EDAs) [13, 17]. The EDA is also applied to a version of the HP

J.M. Barreiro et al. (Eds.): ISBMDA 2004, LNCS 3337, pp. 388–398, 2004.

model called the functional model protein [6], which has a unique native state (i.e. a unique global optimum), and thus difficult to solve with optimization algorithms. We show that the results achieved with the EDA are better than those obtained with other evolutionary optimization techniques [9, 12, 19], and are also competitive with other approaches.

The paper is organized as follows. In the next section, we introduce the HP model and present the problem representation. Section 3 briefly reviews a number of previous approaches to the solution of simplified models. Section 4 presents the class of EDAs, and introduces the EDA used for protein folding. Section 5 presents the experimental benchmark and the numerical results of our experiments. In section 6, the conclusions of our work are given, and possible extensions of EDAs for dealing with the protein folding problem are discussed.

2 The Hydrophobic-Polar Model

In the HP model a sequence comprises residues of only two types: hydrophobic (H) and hydrophilic or polar (P). Residues are located in regular lattice models forming self-avoided paths. There is a zero contact energy between P-P and H-P pairs. Different values can be taken to measure the interaction between hydrophobic non-consecutive residues; a common choice that we use in this paper is -1. The energy interactions can be represented by the following matrix:

$$E = \begin{pmatrix} -1 & 0 \\ 0 & 0 \end{pmatrix}$$

The function evaluation of a given configuration or protein conformation is simplified to the sum of every two hydrophobic residues that are non-consecutive nearest neighbors on the lattice.

In this paper, we consider the 2-dimensional regular lattice. In the linear representation of the sequence, hydrophobic residues are represented with the letter H and polar ones with P. In the graphical representation, hydrophobic proteins are represented by black beads and polar proteins by white beads. Figure 1 shows an optimal folding for the sequence $S1 = HPHPPHHPHPPHPHHPPHPH$. The optimal energy corresponding to this sequence is -9.

2.1 Functional Model Protein

The functional model protein is a 'shifted' HP model. The name comes from the fact that the model supports a significant number of proteins that can be characterized as functional. This model has native states, some of which are not maximally compact. Thus, in some cases, they have cavities or potential binding sites, a key property that is required in order to investigate ligand binding using these models [6]. The energy matrix associated with the model contains both attractive and repulsive interactions. Its representation is as follows:

$$E = \begin{pmatrix} -2 & 1 \\ 1 & 1 \end{pmatrix}$$

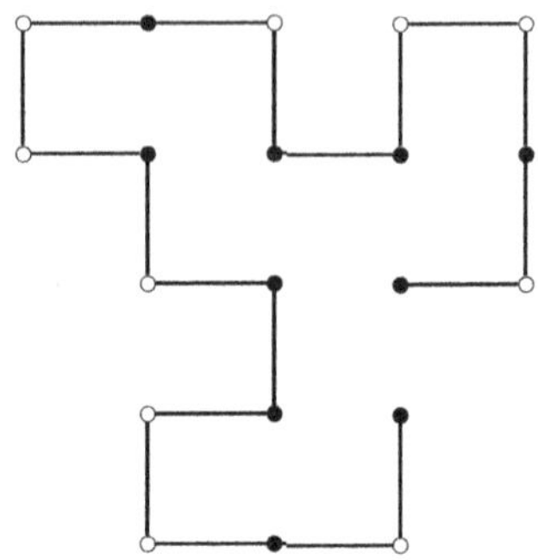

Fig. 1. Best solution found for the sequence $S1$.

2.2 Problem Representation

We use X_i to represent a discrete random variable. A possible instance of X_i is denoted x_i. Similarly, we use $\mathbf{X} = (X_1, \ldots, X_n)$ to represent an n-dimensional random variable and $\mathbf{x} = (x_1, \ldots, x_n)$ to represent one of its possible instances. For a given sequence on the lattice, X_i will represent the relative move of residue i in relation to the previous two residues. Taking as a reference the location of the previous two residues in the lattice, X_i takes values in $\{0, 1, 2\}$. These values respectively mean that the new residue will be located on the left, forward or on the right with respect to the previous locations. Therefore, values for X_1 and X_2 are meaningless. The locations of these two residues are fixed as positions $(0, 0)$ and $(1, 0)$. The representation corresponding to the sequence shown in figure 1 is $\mathbf{x} = (0, 0, 0, 1, 0, 0, 2, 2, 0, 1, 0, 0, 2, 0, 2, 2, 0, 0, 1, 0)$.

3 Previous Approaches to the Solution of Simplified Protein Models

We focus on approaches to simplified protein folding based on Genetic Algorithms (GAs) [7] and Monte Carlo (MC) methods [16]. Some versions of these methods are compared with EDAs in the experiment section.

A pioneer work in the use of population based optimization algorithms for the simplified protein folding problem is [19]. In this paper, the authors proposed a GA that used heuristic based crossover and mutation operators. The GA outperformed a number of variants of MC methods at different sequences. In [11], a search strategy called pioneer search was used together with a simple GA. Although the algorithm improved some of the results achieved in [19], it was unable to find the optimal solutions for the longest instances considered.

In [3] and [9] evolutionary algorithms for the 3-D HP problem are proposed. While in [9] a simple GA shows no better results than those achieved in [19], a more sophisticated approach is presented in [3]. By using a backtracking based repairing procedure, the latter algorithm guarantees that the search is constrained to the space of legal solutions. Since the number of self-avoided paths on square lattices is exponential in the legth of the sequence [19], generating legal solutions with a backtracking algorithm is a feasible alternative.

The MultiMeme Algorithm (MMA) for protein structure prediction [12] is a GA combined with a set of local searches. From this set, the algorithm self-adaptively selects which local search algorithm to use for different instances, states of the search, or individuals in the population. The results achieved for a number of instances were better than those reported in [19], but in some of the most difficult instances the algorithm failed to reach the optimal solution.

Traditional MC methods sample from the protein folding space one point at the time. However, and due to the rugged landscape, traditional MC methods tend to get trapped in local minima. Two alternatives to avoid this problem are either to use chain growth algorithms [1], or to sample the space with a population of Markov chains in which a different temperature is attached to each chain [15]. A common and remarkable characteristic of these methods is that they employ problem information to improve the results of the optimization algorithms.

4 Estimation of Distribution Algorithms

We study the suitability of EDAs as a non-deterministic search procedure for the HP model. A main difference between EDAs and GAs is that the former constructs an explicit probability model of the solutions selected. This model can capture, by means of probabilistic dependencies, relevant interactions among the variables of the problem. The model can be conveniently used to generate new promising solutions. The main scheme of the EDA approach is shown in algorithm 1. Although the introduction of EDAs is relatively new, there already exists a number of succesful applications of EDAs in computational biology [2, 18].

EDAs differ in the type of models that they use and the corresponding factorizations of the probability that these models determine. For the protein folding problem, we define a probability model that assumes that proteins adjacent in the sequence are related in their lattice positions. The probability model then encodes the dependencies between the move of a residue and the moves of the previous residues in the sequence. This information is used in the generation of solutions.

Let $p(\mathbf{x})$ be the probability distribution of random variable $\mathbf{X}$. Our probability model considers that the configuration of variable X_i depends on the configuration of the previous k variables, where $k \geq 0$ is a parameter of the model. $p(\mathbf{x})$ can be factorized as follows:

$$p(\mathbf{x}) = p(x_1, \ldots, x_{k+1}) \prod_{i=k+2}^{n} p(x_i \mid x_{i-1}, x_{i-2}, \ldots, x_{i-k}) \tag{1}$$

The learning phase of our EDA will only comprise a parametric learning of the parameters in contrast to some state-of-the-art EDAs that make structural

Algorithm 1: Main scheme of the EDA approach

$D_0 \leftarrow$ Generate M individuals (the initial population) randomly
$l = 1$
do {
  $D^s_{l-1} \leftarrow$ Select $N \leq M$ individuals from D_{l-1} according to a selection method
  $p_l(\boldsymbol{x}) = p(\boldsymbol{x}|D^s_{l-1}) \leftarrow$ Estimate the joint probability of selected individuals
  $D_l \leftarrow$ Sample M individuals (the new population) from $p_l(\boldsymbol{x})$
} **until** A stop criterion is met

and parametric learning of the model. Therefore, the computational complexity of the algorithm is reduced, and it can be faster than sophisticated GAs that incorporate complex local search procedures. In addition to the probabilistic model, there are two particular features that characterize our EDA approach to the protein folding problem. The first one is the inclusion of a restart step in the EDA. The restart step tries to avoid early convergence of the population. The other feature added to our EDA is a method to ensure that all the vectors evaluated are valid (i.e. self-avoided) paths. We describe these two additions to the EDA scheme shown above in detail. It should also be noted that none of these changes use knowledge about the problem.

Every time that the diversity of solutions in the population goes under a predefined threshold, all solutions except the best are randomly modified with a given probability value in the same way mutation operators are applied in GAs, but with a higher mutation probability. Diversity is measured by calculating the number of different vectors in the selected population divided by N. Restart tries to avoid the early convergence of the population.

In the representation that we used, not all vectors correspond to self-avoiding sequences. Our search procedure organizes the search within the space of valid solutions. To enforce the validity of the solutions, we employ the backtracking method proposed in [3]. This method can be used in two different ways: as a generator procedure or as a repairing algorithm. In the first case, a solution is incrementally constructed in such a way that the self-avoidance constraint is fulfilled. At position i, the backtracking call is invoked only if self-avoidance cannot be fulfilled with any of the three possible assignments to X_i.

Used as a repairing method, the algorithm inspects every sampled solution. It checks whether the current vector position assignments violates the self-avoidance constraint. If such is the case, another value is assigned to the position and tested. The order of the assignment of variables is random. If all the three possible values have been checked, and self-avoidance is not fulfilled yet, backtracking is invoked. Further details about the backtracking algorithm, originally proposed for the 3-D HP model, can be found in [3].

The repairing procedure destroys some of the statistical dependencies generated from the model. However, the effect of this step is beneficial because solutions will be altered only if their current assignment violates the constraint.

There exist EDAs that are able to generate solutions that consider the fulfillment of constraints at the generation step [13]. A similar approach could be applied to the protein folding problem. Nevertheless, this procedure has an additional computational cost because the fulfillment of the constraints must be checked at each step of the solution generation.

5 Experiments

We compare the results achieved by the EDA approach to results obtained with previous GAs and other MC heuristics. First, we present the set of instances used for the experiments. The algorithms compared are later presented. Finally, the results of the experiments are shown and discussed.

5.1 Function Benchmark

Two different sets of instances are used in our experiments. Table 1 shows HP sequences $S1$-$S7$, which were originally proposed in [19]. The optima corresponding to some of these sequences were incorrectly determined in [19]. Optimal values shown in table 1 have been taken from [15]. These sequences have been used as a benchmark for different algorithms [1, 11, 14, 15, 19].

Table 1. HP instances used in the experiments.

name	size	opt.	sequence
$S1$	20	−9	$HPHPPHHPHHPHPHHPPHPH$
$S2$	25	−8	$PPHPPHHP^4HHP^4HHP^4HH$
$S3$	36	−14	$P^3HHPPHHP^5H^7PPHHP^4HHPPHPP$
$S4$	48	−23	$PPHPPHHPPHHP^5H^{10}P^6HHPPHHPPHPPH^5$
$S5$	50	−21	$HHPHPHPHPH^4PHP^3HP^3HP^4HP^3HP^3HPH^4\{PH\}^4H$
$S6$	60	−36	$PPH^3PH^8P^3H^{10}PHP^3H^{12}P^4H^6PHHPHP$
$S7$	64	−42	$H^{12}PHPH\{PPHH\}^2PPH\{PPHH\}^2PPH\{PPHH\}^2PPHPHPH^{12}$

Table 2 shows sequences $S8$-$S18$ that belong to the functional model protein and they were previously used as a benchmark in [12]. All these intances have size 23. They are an example of a challenging set of problems with only one solution.

5.2 Design of the Experiments

To evaluate the behavior of the EDA introduced in this paper, we compare its results with the results achieved by the GA and MC algorithms presented in [19] and MMA [12]. In the case of the HP model, results of the MMA are available only for some of the sequences shown in table 1. On the other hand, experiments

Table 2. Two dimensional functional model protein instances.

name	opt.	sequence
$S8$	-20	$PHPPHPPHHHHPPHPPHPHPPHH$
$S9$	-17	$PHPPHPPHHHHHPPPPHPPHPPH$
$S10$	-16	$HPHPHPHHHPPHPPPHPHHPPHH$
$S11$	-20	$HHHPHHHPPHHPPPHPHPPHHHH$
$S12$	-17	$PHPPPPPPHPHHPHPHHHHPHPH$
$S13$	-13	$HHPHPPHPPPPHPPPPHPPPHHH$
$S14$	-26	$PHPHHPHHHHHHPPHHHPHHHHH$
$S15$	-16	$HPHPPPHHHHPHPPPPHPHPHHH$
$S16$	-15	$PHPHHPHHPHHPHPHPHPPPPPH$
$S17$	-14	$HPHPHPPPPPHHPPPHPHPHPHH$
$S18$	-15	$PHPPHHHPHPPHPHHPHPPPPPH$

for the instances of the functional model shown in table 2 were not provided in [19], and results are only available for MMA.

The GA population size used in [19] was $M = 200$ and the maximal number of generations was $g = 300$. The MC algorithms performed 50000000 steps. MMA uses tournament selection, crossover probability 0.8, mutation probability 0.3 and replacement strategies with different population sizes. The main criteria that we used to compare the algorithms were their effectiveness to find the optimum, and the number of evaluations needed to reach the optimum.

In all of the experiments done in this paper, the EDA uses truncation selection of parameter $T = 0.1$. We use best elitism, a replacement strategy where the population selected at generation t is incorporated into the population of generation $t+1$. Let M be the population size, only $M - T * M$ individuals are generated at each generation except the first one. The threshold used for the restart process was 0.5. The probability of modifying the value at every position is 0.9. Although better results can be achieved by tuning the EDA parameters for each sequence, we kept all the parameters except population size fixed.

5.3 Results of the Experiments

Table 3 presents the results achieved by the different algorithms for sequences $S1$-$S7$. The results of EDAs are the average of ten experiments for the given parameters. The results of GA, MC and MMA are the best taken as the most efficient run in five, so the comparison gives only an idea of the relative performance of the algorithms. In the table, B is the energy of the best solution found when it was not the optimal one. Optimal values of the energies for the sequences are shown in table 1.

We calculate the number of times that the best solution was found (S) and the average number of function evaluations ($\bar{e}$) needed by the EDA to find the this solution. $k = 2$ was the choice for parameter k. We use parameter $k = 3$ only when the optimum was not found with $k = 2$. When the results are improved

Table 3. Results achieved by the different algorithms for the HP instances.

		EDA				GA		MC		MMA	
inst.	k	B	M	S	$\bar{e}$	B	$\bar{e}$	B	$\bar{e}$	B	$\bar{e}$
$S1$	2		1000	10	4510		30492		292443		14621
$S2$	2		4000	10	13880		20400		2694572		18736
$S3$	2		5000	1	113000		301339	−13	6557189		208233
$S4$	2		5000	2	53995	−22	126547	−20	9201755	−22	1155656
$S5$	2		10000	10	118000		592887		15151203		
$S6$	2	−35	10000	2	473500	−34	208781	−33	8262338		
$S7$	2	−41	10000	7	595900	−37	187393	−35	7848952		
$S7$	3		10000	1	154000						

using this value, they are shown. In the table, we include the best results achieved by the GA and MC algorithms presented in [19] and MMA [12].

The first conclusion of our experiments is that the EDA is able to find the best known optimum for all instances except instance $S6$, where nevertheless it achieves better results than the other algorithms. For the instances where all the algorithms find the optima, the average number of evaluations needed by the EDA is smaller than the best result achieved by the experiments conducted with the three other algorithms. $S6$ and $S7$ are the most difficult instances among those shown in table 1. For $S7$, the best result achieved with one of the best MC algorithms [1] that uses information about the problem structure was −40. The EDA has been able to find more than one optimal solution for this instance. In figure 2, the configurations corresponding to two optimal solutions found by the EDA are shown. As far as we know, only two methods have been able to deal with this instance successfully [14, 15].

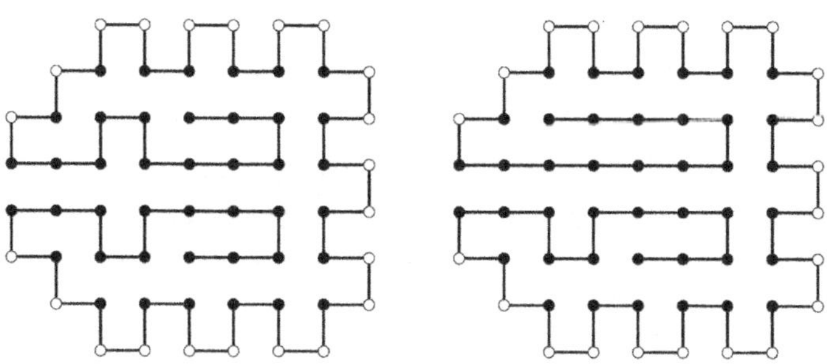

Fig. 2. Two optimal solutions found for the $S7$ sequence.

Now we evaluate the EDA for the functional model protein instances. The number of evaluations needed by MMA to optimize the functional model protein instances are shown in table 4. The results correspond to the best out of five experiments where the optimum has been reached at least once. To make a fair comparison, we run our algorithm in similar conditions. We find the population size (M) for which the EDA finds the optimum in at least one of the five experiments. Additionally, we present the number of times (S) the optimum was found with the given population size and the number of evaluations (e) for the best run where it was found.

For the functional model protein instances, we found that the simple EDA with $k = 1$ was able to improve the results achieved by MMA. In table 4, it can be appreciated that the EDA is able to find the optimum for all the instances with a number of evaluations that is, in all cases, lower than the number needed by MMA. Another observation is that, for eight of the eleven instances treated, the optimum could be found with the minimum population size tested, i.e. $M = 500$.

Table 4. Results for the two dimensional functional model protein instances.

	EDA				MMA
inst.	k	S	M	e	e
$S8$	1	4	500	12650	15170
$S9$	1	5	500	2750	61940
$S10$	1	1	1000	35900	132898
$S11$	1	3	1000	15900	66774
$S12$	1	4	500	20950	53600
$S13$	1	5	500	5420	32619
$S14$	1	1	500	19450	114930
$S15$	1	1	1500	10350	28425
$S16$	1	1	500	4950	25545
$S17$	1	2	500	8950	111046
$S18$	1	5	500	2950	52005

6 Conclusions

The probability models used by the EDA introduced in this paper can be regarded as Markovian models where the parameter k determines the extent of the dependency on previous variables. Markovian models have been used in computational biology to identify coding regions in genes and in sequence alignment. However, the authors are not acquainted with any previous application of these models in the context of population based search algorithms applied to computational biology problems.

On the other hand, while most of current EDA applications consider structural learning algorithms, our proposal emphasizes the convenience of using the dependencies determined by the sequence ordering to construct the model structure. This strategy reduces the computational cost of the EDA learning phase. Even so, the use of the parameter k gives some flexibility to the model learning step without the need of the more costly structural learning.

The experimental results have proven the effectiveness of the EDA approach and the fact that it is a usable search algorithm. The EDA approach can be extended in many ways. We enumerate some of these possible developments:

1. The structure of the probability model does not have to be fixed and can be learned from the data.
2. Off-lattice HP problems [8], where continuous variables represent the angles between contiguous residues, can be dealt with using EDAs that store probability models for continuous variables [13].
3. Problem information can be added by incorporating structural and parametric priors in the probabilistic models.
4. The algorithm can be combined with local optimizers in different ways.
5. EDAs could be applied to less simplified versions of the protein folding problem. In this area, a number of GA applications have been proposed [5].

Acknowledgments

This work was supported in part by the Spanish Ministerio de Ciencia y Tecnología under grant TIC2001-2973-C05-03, by Etortek-Genmodis and Etortek-Biolan projects from the Basque Government, and by the University of the Basque Country under grant 9/UPV 00140.226-15334/2003.

References

1. U. Bastolla, H. Frauenkron, E. Gerstner, P. Grassberger, and W. Nadler. Testing a new Monte Carlo algorithm for protein folding. *Proteins: Structure, Function, and Genetics*, 32:52–66, 1998.
2. R. Blanco, P. Larrañaga, I. Inza, and B. Sierra. Selection of highly accurate genes for cancer classification by Estimation of Distribution Algorithms. In *Proceedings of the Workshop 'Bayesian Models in Medicine' held within AIME 2001*, pages 29–34, 2001.
3. C. Cotta. Protein structure prediction using evolutionary algorithms hybridized with backtracking. In J. Mira and J. R. Alvarez, editors, *Artificial Neural Nets Problem Solving Methods*, volume 2687 of *Lecture Notes in Computer Science*, pages 321–328. Springer Verlag, 2003.
4. K. A. Dill. Theory for the folding and stability of globular proteins. *Biochemistry*, 24(6):1501–1509, 1985.
5. W. Garrison, W. Greenwood, and J.-M. Shin. *Evolutionary Computation in Bioinformatics*, chapter On the Evolutionary Search for Solutions to the Protein Folding Problem, pages 115–136. Morgan Kaufmann, 2002.
6. J. D. Hirst. The evolutionary landscape of functional model proteins. *Protein Engineering*, 12:721–726, 1999.
7. J. H. Holland. *Adaptation in Natural and Artificial Systems*. University of Michigan Press, Ann Arbor, MI, 1975.
8. H.-P. Hsu, V. Mehra, and P. Grassberger. Structure optimization in an off-lattice protein model. *Physical Review E*, 68(2):4 pages, 2003.

9. M. Khimasia and P. Coveney. Protein structure prediction as a hard optimization problem: The genetic algorithm approach. *Molecular Simulation*, 19:205–226, 1997.
10. P. Koehl and M. Delarue. Building protein lattice models using self consistent mean field theory. *Journal of Chemical Physics*, 108:9540–9549, 1998.
11. R. König and T. Dandekar. Improving genetic algorithms for protein folding simulations by systematic crossover. *Biosystems*, 50:17–25, 1999.
12. N. Krasnogor, B. Blackburne, E. K. Burke, and J. D. Hirst. Algorithms for protein structure prediction. In J. M. Guervos, P. Adamidis, H.-G. Beyer, J.-L. Fernandez-Villacañas, and H.-P. Schwefel, editors, *Parallel Problem Solving from Nature - PPSN VII*, pages 769–778, Paris, France, 2002. Springer Verlag. LNCS 2439.
13. P. Larrañaga and J. A. Lozano. *Estimation of Distribution Algorithms. A New Tool for Evolutionary Optimization.* Kluwer Academic Publishers, Boston/Dordrecht/London, 2002.
14. N. Lesh, M. Mitzenmacher, and S. Whitesides. A complete and effective move set for simplified protein folding. Technical Report TR-2003-03, Mitsubishi Electric Research Laboratories, February 2003.
15. S. Liang and W. H. Wong. Evolutionary Monte Carlo for protein folding simulation. *Journal of Chemical Physics*, 115:3374–3380, 2001.
16. N. Metropolis, A. Rosenbluth, A. Teller, and E. Teller. Equations of state calculations by fast computing machines. *Journal of Chemical Physics*, 21:1087–1091, 1953.
17. H. Mühlenbein and G. Paaß. From recombination of genes to the estimation of distributions I. Binary parameters. In A. Eiben, T. Bäck, M. Schoenauer, and H. Schwefel, editors, *Parallel Problem Solving from Nature - PPSN IV*, pages 178–187, Berlin, 1996. Springer Verlag.
18. Y. Saeys, S. Degroeve, D. Aeyels, P. Rouzé, and Y. VandePeer. Feature selection for splice site prediction: A new method using EDA-based feature ranking. *BMC Bioinformatics*, 4:5–64, 2004.
19. R. Unger and J. Moult. Genetic algorithms for protein folding simulations. *Journal of Molecular Biology*, (231):75–81, 1993.

Quantitative Evaluation of Established Clustering Methods for Gene Expression Data

Dörte Radke and Ulrich Möller

Jena Centre for Bioinformatics
Hans Knöll Institute for Natural Products Research,
Junior Research Group "Pattern Recognition",
Beutenbergstr. 11a, 07745 Jena, Germany
+49-3641-656832
{doerte.radke,ulrich.moeller}@hki-jena.de

Abstract. Analysis of gene expression data generated by microarray techniques often includes clustering. Although more reliable methods are available, hierarchical algorithms are still frequently employed. We clustered several data sets and quantitatively compared the performance of an agglomerative hierarchical approach using the average-linkage method with two partitioning procedures, k-means and fuzzy c-means. Investigation of the results revealed the superiority of the partitioning algorithms: the compactness of the clusters was markedly increased and the arrangement of the profiles into clusters more closely resembled biological categories. Therefore, we encourage analysts to critically scrutinize the results obtained by clustering.

1 Introduction

The introduction of high-throughput techniques such as microarrays into the Life Sciences over the past decade produces rapidly increasing amounts of data. Their analysis not only requires the modification and improvement of established as well as the development of new pattern recognition methods, but also necessitates the communication of their strengths and pitfalls to the practitioners generating and frequently evaluating the microarray data. Complete packages for analysis available commercially or free from the scientific community often result in an overestimation of the correctness of the obtained output by the analyst.

Unsupervised learning is employed, if no or only very few information about the data is available. Clustering methods are widely applied tools to find groups in large data sets generated by microarray analyses. Hierarchical algorithms are emphasized in recent biomedical reviews [1, 2] and still frequently employed for the clustering of samples [3–5] or gene profiles [6–9]. However, hierarchical clustering of microarray data has been criticized for a number of years [10–12] because of several shortcomings. A major problem is the hierarchy artificially imposed on the data – patterns joined into one cluster can not be separated and assigned to different clusters in later steps of the algorithm, thereby leading to misclassification.

J.M. Barreiro et al. (Eds.): ISBMDA 2004, LNCS 3337, pp. 399–408, 2004.

Alternative methods include model-based clustering strategies. This approach is relatively new to gene expression analysis, currently several algorithms are being developed [10, 13] and investigated for their performance. In addition a variety of partitioning methods have been used for some time for microarray data analysis, the most prominent are k-means and fuzzy c-means (FCM). They have been thoroughly tested [14, 15] and are robust and flexible. Therefore, we chose these two methods for comparison with hierarchical clustering. Self-organizing maps (SOM) also were applied to microarray data [16, 17]. They require the choice of a two-dimensional map size prior to clustering and present a good tool for visualizing the data. Newer methods employ larger map sizes and hierarchically cluster the map nodes in a second step (SOM clustering) [18, 19]. Application of SOM clustering [19] to our data collection in most cases yielded diverse results depending on the map topology. Thus, we did not include this algorithm in our investigation.

Most studies criticizing hierarchical and recommending other methods focus on the theoretical background and employ one or two datasets only. To present more practical evidence and to encourage practitioners to switch to more reliable procedures we quantitatively demonstrate for several biological and two simulated data sets the better performance of the partitioning methods over the widely applied average-linkage hierarchical algorithm.

2 Methods

Clustering algorithms use a dissimilarity measure to cluster the data. The objective functions employed in partitioning algorithms as well as the agglomeration of profiles in hierarchical clustering focus on the compactness of clusters based on this dissimilarity measure. To compare the different methods we defined an average dissimilarity D_c for a partition (grouping of profiles into clusters) with c clusters and n_k profiles in cluster k ($k = 1, ..., c$) as

$$D_c = \frac{\sum_{k=1}^{c} s_k}{\sum_{k=1}^{c} n_k\,(n_k - 1)} \,. \tag{1}$$

s_k is the sum of pairwise dissimilarities for cluster k calculated with

$$s_k = \sum_{\substack{i,j \\ i \neq j}}^{n_k} d\,(x_i, x_j) \tag{2}$$

for all members x_i and x_j of cluster k where $d(x_i, x_j)$ represents the pairwise dissimilarity between x_i and x_j. The calculation accounts for the different cluster sizes to avoid overestimation of very compact, but small clusters.

Some partitions, especially in hierarchical and k-means algorithms, include clusters with only one profile (singleton). There is no pairwise dissimilarity in these clusters and D_c can not be obtained. We chose to omit these clusters from the partition thus reducing the effective number of clusters.

Two different measures of dissimilarity were employed: (i) (Squared) euclidean distances were used for hierarchical and partitioning methods. These applications are available in most clustering software packages. (ii) Clustering applying a correlation measure was performed with $d(x_i, x_j) = 1 - cc(x_i, x_j)$ [20] where $cc(x_i, x_j)$ is the correlation coefficient introduced as 'uncentered correlation' in the widely used tool 'Cluster' by Eisen [21].

Clustering algorithms do not calculate the number of clusters present in the data. Partitioning methods require its selection prior to the actual clustering process. In hierarchical clustering the tree is cut into a certain number of clusters or at a given height according to some criterion defined by the analyst. To estimate the correct number of clusters the data are frequently investigated at different preset cluster numbers and the results are analyzed by additional procedures, e.g. cluster validity indices [22]. We decided not to rely on this non-trivial process and not to explore results at a potentially false number of clusters, but to compare the partitions obtained from the different clustering algorithms over a range of cluster numbers.

Hierarchical as well as k-means and FCM algorithms are explained in detail and with possible variations in [23, 24]. Briefly, we used the agglomerative hierarchical approach with the average-linkage method as described by Eisen et al. [21] and employed by many researchers [3, 7]. The correlation was transformed into a dissimilarity measure with $d = 1 - cc$ (see above). The resulting tree was cut at different heights to yield partitions with increasing numbers of clusters. FCM with fuzzy exponent 1.3 (pbmc 1.5) and k-means were employed over a range of preset cluster numbers depending on the size of the data set. In order to avoid poor results produced by unfavorable initialization of these local optimization algorithms we repeated the clustering at least 75 times with random starting values at every number of clusters and chose the partition showing the best value for the objective function [25].

All calculations were performed with build-in or custom-made functions in MatLab 6.5.1 or 7.0 (The Mathworks).

3 Data

3.1 E. Coli Treated PBMC (pbmc)

The time profile data used were obtained by stimulation of PBMC with heat killed E. coli [26]. We used a subset of the data downloaded via the supplementary web site (http://genome-www.stanford.edu/hostresponse/; data files no. 6205, 6208, 6210, 6213, 6214). Log ratios of the data were preprocessed by zero time point subtraction, feature selection, normalization and missing value imputation resulting in a data set of 1336 genes at 4 time points (excluding $t = 0$) – the procedure is detailed in [27]. For correlation-based clustering the zero time point was included yielding 1336 genes at 5 time points.

3.2 Yeast Cell Cycle (Yeast)

The widely used yeast sporulation data [28] were retrieved from the supplementary web site (http://yscdp.stanford.edu/yeast_cell_cycle/cellcycle.html), the 90 minute time point was excluded [11, 29] for all subsequent steps. Three datasets were constructed from the original data comprising 507, 214 or 208 genes, respectively. For clustering with the euclidean dissimilarity measure each gene was normalized by subtracting its mean and dividing by its standard deviation.

Yeast-507. Genes selected showed an absolute value of expression at all times of not less than 100 and at least a 3-fold change in expression level over the complete profile.

Yeast-214. Based on Table 1 from Cho et al. [28] we selected all genes listed in one cell cycle phase only.

Yeast-208. Starting with the k-means clustering result of yeast-214 (correlation dissimilarity measure) a cluster showing very high intra-cluster dissimilarity was inspected to find genes contributing chiefly to this aberrant result. Briefly, pairwise dissimilarities between any two profiles in the cluster were calculated and the genes involved in the twenty highest values identified. Six genes found more than twice and up to eight times in this analysis were removed from the yeast-214 data set to result in yeast-208.

3.3 Response of Human Fibroblasts to Serum (fibro)

Time course data for the response of human fibroblasts to serum stimulation were described by Iyer et al. [30], we used the 517 genes selected by the authors and available from the internet (http://genome-www.stanford.edu/serum/; data for Figure 2 cluster). The data containing ratios versus $t = 0$ of the mRNA levels at each time point were logarithmized. For clustering with the euclidean dissimilarity measure each gene was normalized as described in 3.2.

3.4 Simulated Data (sim)

Two data sets comprising 450 and 600 profiles respectively were randomly generated. Normalization for both data sets was performed as detailed in 3.2.

Sim-450. FCM clustering of the fibro data set and cluster validation revealed six clusters [22, 31]. Based on the cluster mean and standard deviation values at each time point of this result six clusters of 50, 150, 60, 80, 40 and 70 random profiles with 12 dimensions were simulated.

Sim-600. 600 profiles with 8 points each were artificially generated by selecting 5 mean time profiles and randomly creating 100, 120, 150, 50 and 180 profiles with a minimal correlation of 0.5, 0.6, 0.35, 0.95, 0.4 to the respective mean profile.

4 Results

We compared the hierarchical agglomerative average-linkage algorithm with two partitioning methods using equal measures of dissimilarity and clustering objectives. To quantitatively evaluate the performance of the different procedures we introduced the average dissimilarity, a value decreasing with increasing cluster compactness. Therefore, the average dissimilarity curves (Fig. 1) are expected to decline with growing numbers of clusters. Our analysis revealed three major results:

First, the partitioning algorithms performed better for all data sets and almost all numbers of clusters (Fig. 1). In general, the difference between hierarchical and partitioning procedures most prominently was seen in results obtained with the euclidean dissimilarity measure. Comparing the partitions over a range of increasing cluster numbers the average dissimilarity decreased much stronger for FCM and k-means than for the hierarchical method – the values for the pbmc data analysis using euclidean dissimilarity improved more than twice as much for the partitioning algorithms as for the hierarchical clustering.

The only exception was seen after application of the k-means procedure employing a correlation dissimilarity measure to the yeast-507 and yeast-214 data sets (Fig. 1B). The curves for yeast-507 are not presented; the FCM and k-means results were similar to yeast-214, the hierarchical methods showed a lower performance. Removal of six genes from yeast-214 and clustering of the new data set yeast-208 improved the k-means clustering result, while the FCM performed equally well as for yeast-214. The hierarchical result improved for some numbers of clusters, while it was impaired for others.

Second, the average dissimilarity obtained with hierarchical clustering at larger numbers of clusters was higher than the value received with the partitioning algorithms at much lower cluster numbers. For example, comparing the average dissimilarities of the fibro data set (Fig. 1B) the values for the hierarchical analysis calculated over the range of cluster numbers presented here always were greater than the value for the FCM and k-means 7-cluster partitions.

Finally, the arrangement of the gene profiles into clusters (cluster memberships) differed between the clustering algorithms to a high extend. The 5-cluster partition of yeast-214 suggested by the cell cycle phases [28] most closely was matched by the results of the partitioning algorithms (Fig. 2). The hierarchical clustering result did not reflect the biology as seen most prominently at the aberrant cluster sizes. Clear differences in cluster memberships between the partitioning and hierarchical algorithms were observed for all data sets; the degree depended on data set, method and number of clusters. In most data sets hierarchical results deviated from the FCM cluster memberships more than 15% for $c > 2$ (data not shown), e.g. for the 6-cluster partition of fibro the relative difference was greater than 35% corresponding to 180 out of 517 genes.

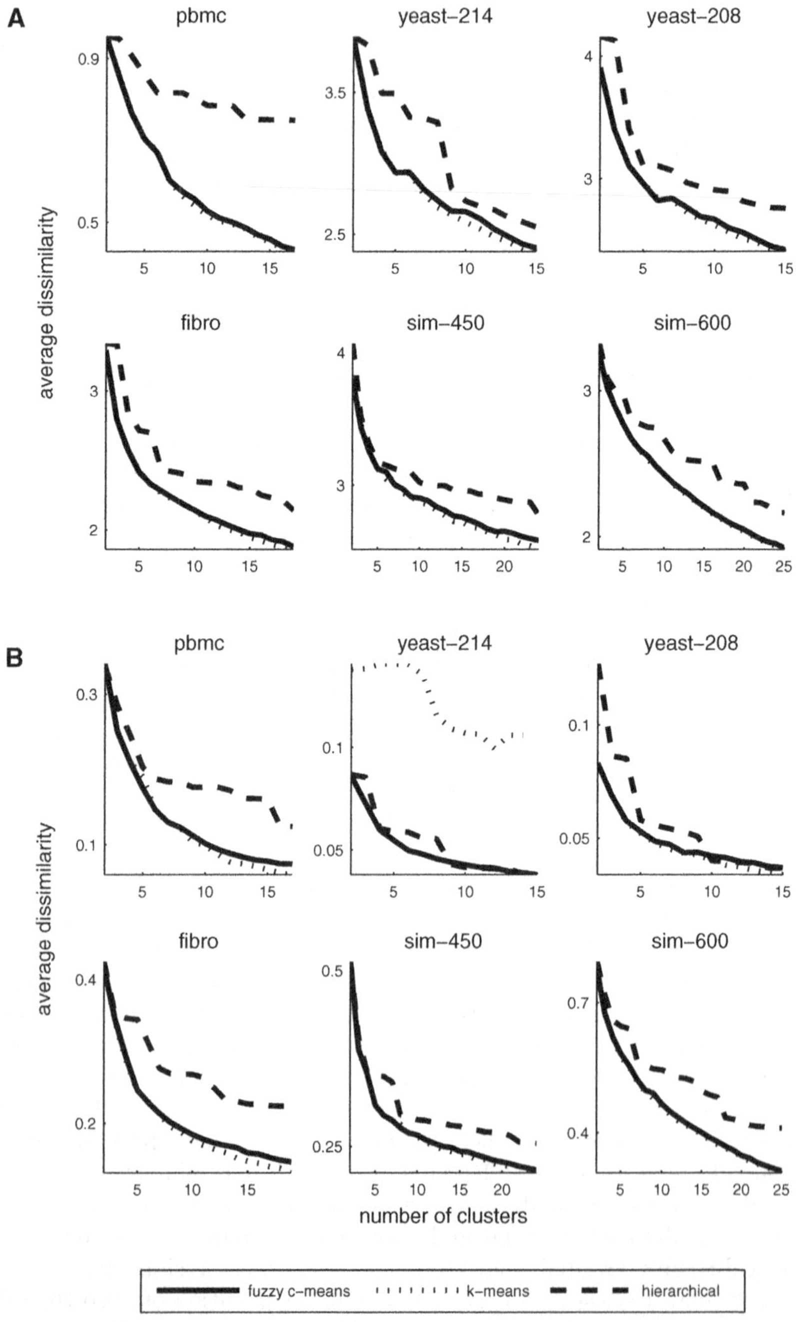

Fig. 1. The average dissimilarity plotted for different data sets and algorithms. (A) (Squared) euclidean and (B) correlation dissimilarity measure.

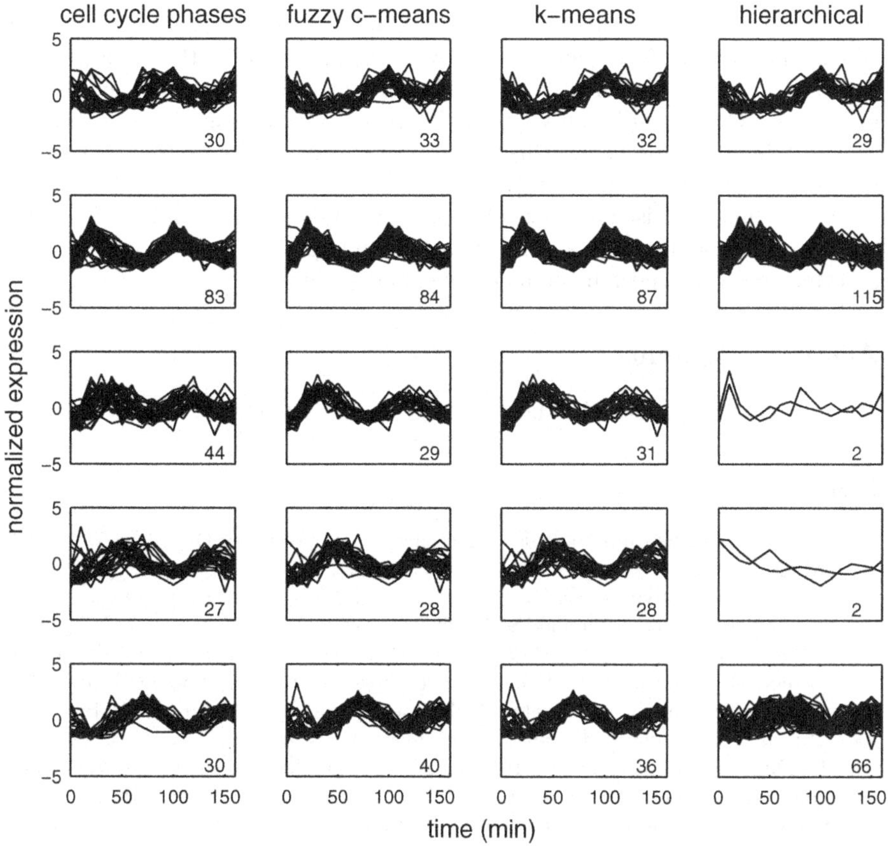

Fig. 2. Gene profiles of yeast-214. Column 1: the five yeast cell cycle phases from Cho et al. [28]. Columns 2 to 4: profiles clustered with a (squared) euclidean distance measure ($c = 5$). The number of genes per phase or cluster is indicated in the lower right corner.

5 Discussion

We have presented practical evidence for the problems arising in the application of hierarchical clustering algorithms to gene expression profiles. Partitioning methods achieved better results in optimizing the compactness of the generated clusters, an objective common to all procedures investigated. Examination of the corresponding partitions showed marked discrepancies in the arrangement of gene profiles into clusters. The superior performance of the partitioning algorithms is confirmed by the analysis of the cluster memberships in comparison with the functional information available for genes expressed in different yeast cell cycle phases [28].

The gene profiles discussed all represent one type of data set: large numbers of patterns with relatively low dimensionality. The other group of data frequently clustered with the algorithms investigated comprise data sets with relatively few samples and high dimensionality, e.g. tumor tissues. We analyzed genome profiles of cancer cell lines [32] with the presented methods, but did not detect a major improvement with partitioning algorithms over the hierarchical procedures. Other studies suggest that there are general difficulties in discriminating different tissue types; this also concerns other unsupervised methods as well as supervised classification [10].

For the unsupervised analysis of gene expression data we emphasize the possibility of misclassification and recommend the application of a procedure with a better performance than the hierarchical algorithms.

Acknowledgment

This work was supported by the BMBF (FKZ 0312704D).

References

1. Butte, A.: The use and analysis of microarray data. Nat Rev Drug Discov **1** (2002) 951–60
2. Shannon, W., Culverhouse, R., Duncan, J.: Analyzing microarray data using cluster analysis. Pharmacogenomics **4** (2003) 41–52
3. Bullinger, L., Dohner, K., Bair, E., Frohling, S., Schlenk, R.F., Tibshirani, R., Dohner, H., Pollack, J.R.: Use of gene-expression profiling to identify prognostic subclasses in adult acute myeloid leukemia. N Engl J Med **350** (2004) 1605–16
4. Murata, Y., Watanabe, T., Sato, M., Momose, Y., Nakahara, T., Oka, S., Iwahashi, H.: Dimethyl sulfoxide exposure facilitates phospholipid biosynthesis and cellular membrane proliferation in yeast cells. J Biol Chem **278** (2003) 33185–93
5. Shimoji, T., Kanda, H., Kitagawa, T., Kadota, K., Asai, R., Takahashi, K., Kawaguchi, N., Matsumoto, S., Hayashizaki, Y., Okazaki, Y., Shinomiya, K.: Clinico-molecular study of dedifferentiation in well-differentiated liposarcoma. Biochem Biophys Res Commun **314** (2004) 1133–40
6. Amatschek, S., Koenig, U., Auer, H., Steinlein, P., Pacher, M., Gruenfelder, A., Dekan, G., Vogl, S., Kubista, E., Heider, K.H., Stratowa, C., Schreiber, M., Sommergruber, W.: Tissue-wide expression profiling using cdna subtraction and microarrays to identify tumor-specific genes. Cancer Res **64** (2004) 844–56
7. Kawahara, N., Wang, Y., Mukasa, A., Furuya, K., Shimizu, T., Hamakubo, T., Aburatani, H., Kodama, T., Kirino, T.: Genome-wide gene expression analysis for induced ischemic tolerance and delayed neuronal death following transient global ischemia in rats. J Cereb Blood Flow Metab **24** (2004) 212–23
8. Mirza, A., Wu, Q., Wang, L., McClanahan, T., Bishop, W.R., Gheyas, F., Ding, W., Hutchins, B., Hockenberry, T., Kirschmeier, P., Greene, J.R., Liu, S.: Global transcriptional program of p53 target genes during the process of apoptosis and cell cycle progression. Oncogene **22** (2003) 3645–54
9. Weinberg, E.O., Mirotsou, M., Gannon, J., Dzau, V.J., Lee, R.T., Pratt, R.E.: Sex dependence and temporal dependence of the left ventricular genomic response to pressure overload. Physiol Genomics **12** (2003) 113–27
10. Mar, J.C., McLachlan, G.J.: Model-based clustering in gene expression microarrays: an application to breast cancer data. In: Proceedings of the First Asia-Pacific bioinformatics conference on Bioinformatics 2003, Australian Computer Society, Inc. (2003) 139–144

11. Tamayo, P., Slonim, D., Mesirov, J., Zhu, Q., Kitareewan, S., Dmitrovsky, E., Lander, E.S., Golub, T.R.: Interpreting patterns of gene expression with self-organizing maps: methods and application to hematopoietic differentiation. Proc Natl Acad Sci U S A **96** (1999) 2907–12
12. Morgan, B.J.T., Ray, A.P.G.: Non-uniqueness and inversions in cluster analysis. Appl. Statist. **44** (1995) 117–134
13. Yeung, K.Y., Fraley, C., Murua, A., Raftery, A.E., Ruzzo, W.L.: Model-based clustering and data transformations for gene expression data. Bioinformatics **17** (2001) 977–87
14. Dougherty, E.R., Barrera, J., Brun, M., Kim, S., Cesar, R.M., Chen, Y., Bittner, M., Trent, J.M.: Inference from clustering with application to gene-expression microarrays. J Comput Biol **9** (2002) 105–26
15. Granzow, M., Berrar, D., Dubitzky, W., Schuster, A., Azuaje, F.J., Eils, R.: Tumor classification by gene expression profiling: Comparison and validation of five clustering methods. SIGBIO Newsletter Special Interest Group on Biomedical Computing of the ACM **21** (2001) 16–22
16. Harris, T.M., Childs, G.: Global gene expression patterns during differentiation of f9 embryonal carcinoma cells into parietal endoderm. Funct Integr Genomics **2** (2002) 105–19
17. Xiao, L., Wang, K., Teng, Y., Zhang, J.: Component plane presentation integrated self-organizing map for microarray data analysis. FEBS Lett **538** (2003) 117–24
18. Wang, J., Delabie, J., Aasheim, H., Smeland, E., Myklebost, O.: Clustering of the SOM easily reveals distinct gene expression patterns: results of a reanalysis of lymphoma study. BMC Bioinformatics **3** (2002) 36
19. Wu, S., Chow, T.W.S.: Clustering of the self-organizing map using a clustering validity index based on inter-cluster and intra-cluster density. Pattern Recognition **37** (2004) 175–188
20. Golay, X., Kollias, S., Stoll, G., Meier, D., Valavanis, A., Boesiger, P.: A new correlation-based fuzzy logic clustering algorithm for fMRI. Magnetic Resonance in Medicine **40** (1998) 249–260
21. Eisen, M.B., Spellman, P.T., Brown, P.O., Botstein, D.: Cluster analysis and display of genome-wide expression patterns. Proc Natl Acad Sci U S A **95** (1998) 14863–8
22. Bezdek, J.C., Pal, N.R.: Some new indexes of cluster validity. IEEE Trans. SMC, Part B Cybernet. **28** (1998) 301–315 ISSN: 1083-4419.
23. Duda, R.O., Hart, P.E., Stork, D.G.: Pattern Classification. 2nd ed. edn. John Wiley & Sons (2001)
24. Theodoridis, S., Koutroumbas, K.: Pattern Recognition. Academic Press (1999)
25. Möller, U., Ligges, M., Grunling, C., Georgiewa, P., Kaiser, W.A., Witte, H., Blanz, B.: Pitfalls in the clustering of neuroimage data and improvements by global optimization strategies. Neuroimage **14** (2001) 206–18
26. Boldrick, J.C., Alizadeh, A.A., Diehn, M., Dudoit, S., Liu, C.L., Belcher, C.E., Botstein, D., Staudt, L.M., Brown, P.O., Relman, D.A.: Stereotyped and specific gene expression programs in human innate immune responses to bacteria. Proc Natl Acad Sci U S A **99** (2002) 972–7
27. Guthke, R., Thies, F., Moeller, U.: Data- and knowledge-driven dynamic modeling of the immune response to bacterial infection. In Dounias, G.D., ed.: Hybrid and adaptive computational intelligence in medicine and bio-informatics., EUNITE (2003) 33–39

28. Cho, R.J., Campbell, M.J., Winzeler, E.A., Steinmetz, L., Conway, A., Wodicka, L., Wolfsberg, T.G., Gabrielian, A.E., Landsman, D., Lockhart, D.J., Davis, R.W.: A genome-wide transcriptional analysis of the mitotic cell cycle. Mol Cell **2** (1998) 65–73
29. Sharan, R., Maron-Katz, A., Shamir, R.: Click and expander: a system for clustering and visualizing gene expression data. Bioinformatics **19** (2003) 1787–99
30. Iyer, V.R., Eisen, M.B., Ross, D.T., Schuler, G., Moore, T., Lee, J.C., Trent, J.M., Staudt, L.M., Hudson, Jr, J., Boguski, M.S., Lashkari, D., Shalon, D., Botstein, D., Brown, P.O.: The transcriptional program in the response of human fibroblasts to serum. Science **283** (1999) 83–7
31. Radke, D., Thies, F., Dvinge, H., Möller, U.: Improved clustering methods for the analysis of microarray data. In: German Conference on Bioinformatics. (2003)
32. Scherf, U., Ross, D.T., Waltham, M., Smith, L.H., Lee, J.K., Tanabe, L., Kohn, K.W., Reinhold, W.C., Myers, T.G., Andrews, D.T., Scudiero, D.A., Eisen, M.B., Sausville, E.A., Pommier, Y., Botstein, D., Brown, P.O., Weinstein, J.N.: A gene expression database for the molecular pharmacology of cancer. Nat Genet **24** (2000) 236–44

DiseaseCard: A Web-Based Tool for the Collaborative Integration of Genetic and Medical Information

José Luís Oliveira[1,*], Gaspar Dias[1], Ilídio Oliveira[1], Patrícia Rocha[1], Isabel Hermosilla[2], Javier Vicente[2], Inmaculada Spiteri[2], Fernando Martin-Sánchez[2], and António Sousa Pereira[1]

[1] Universidade de Aveiro, IEETA/DET, 3810 193 Aveiro, Portugal
[2] Instituto de Salud Carlos III (ISCIII), Madrid, Spain

Abstract. The recent advances on genomics and proteomics research bring up a significant grow on the information that is publicly available. However, navigating through genetic and bioinformatics databases can be a too complex and unproductive task for a primary care physician. Moreover, considering the rare genetic diseases field, we verify that the knowledge about a specific disease is commonly disseminated over a small group of experts. The capture, maintenance and sharing of this knowledge over user-friendly interfaces will introduce new insights in the understanding of some rare genetic diseases. In this paper we present DiseaseCard, a web available collaborative service that aims to integrate and disseminate genetic and medical information on rare genetic diseases.

Keywords: Biomedical databases, Biomedicine, Rare genetic diseases
Paper Domain: Methods and systems for database integration Biological and medical data visualization Health bioinformatics and genomics

1 Introduction

The recent advances in the field of molecular biology have raised the expectations concerning the use of this new knowledge in medicine [1]. The Human Genome Project [2], in particular, is providing a major contribution to the understanding of genetic level implications to the human health. This information promises to foster our current understanding of diseases and health and to change the way medicine is practiced [3, 4]. As human genes are progressively unraveled, both in their sequence and function, there will be a transition from a genomic to a post-genomic era. The latter will involve a wide range of applications and a new agenda in health research, education and care. However, despite the massive amounts of genetic data that has being produced and the world-wide investment on genomics and proteomics, a significant and direct impact on medicine has not yet been achieved. Bioinformatics is playing a key role on molecular biology advances, not only by enabling new methods of research, as to manage the huge amounts of relevant information and make it available worldwide. State of the art methods on bioinformatics include the use of public databases, often accessible through a standard web browser, to publish the scientific break-

* Contact Author: José Luís Oliveira , Universidade de Aveiro, IEETA/DET,3810 193 Aveiro, Portugal, Email: jlo@det.ua.pt, Tel : +351 234 370 523

J.M. Barreiro et al. (Eds.): ISBMDA 2004, LNCS 3337, pp. 409–417, 2004.

throughs. According to [5] there are today more than 500 molecular biology databases available. A major hindrance to the seamless use of these sources, besides the quantity, is the use of *ad-hoc* structures, providing different access modes and using different terminologies for the same entities. The specificity of these resources and the knowledge that is required to navigate across them leave its plain usage just to a small group of skilled researchers. These databases are not only relevant for the basic research in biology, as they provide valuable knowledge for the medical practice, providing details on patient conditions, diagnostic laboratories, current pharmacogenetic research, related clinical trials, metabolic disorders, bibliographic references, to name but a few. Given their specificity and heterogeneity, one cannot expect the medical practitioners to include their use in routine investigations. To obtain a real benefic from them, the clinician need integrated views over the vast amount of knowledge sources, enabling a seamless querying and navigation. In this paper we present DiseaseCard, a collaborative web-based framework that aims to integrate and disseminate experts' knowledge on rare genetic diseases from phenotype to genotype.

2 The INFOGENMED Project

Project Overview

The INFOGENMED project [6] is an EU funded project that aims to fulfill some of the gaps identified in the BIOINFOMED study [7], namely the need for new methods to integrate medical and genomic information. The main objective of the project is to build a virtual laboratory for accessing and integrating genetic and medical information for health applications [8]. For example, starting from patients' symptoms and diseases, medical and related genetic information can easily be accessed, retrieved and presented in an unified and user-friendly way. On the application side, the project has focused on the field of rare genetic diseases, since few efforts have been dedicated to them, compared to other pathologies.

Work Approaches and Results

The *virtual laboratory* concept was pursued by applying several complementary strategies, specially resorting to vocabulary unification, shared ontologies and virtual database integration. The main results of the project are summarized below:

1. Determination of the needs of genetic and medical information in health practice environments for several pathologies (considered as "rare genetic diseases"). This required an understanding of health practitioners' requirements, an endeavor started at the very beginning of the project. A twofold approach was applied to characterize user needs, including interviews to a restricted expert panel and a questionnaire distributed to a wider prospective target [6, 11, 12].
2. Design of the methods and development of tools for the integration of heterogeneous databases over the Internet. A first prototype of a mediator, agent-based system for biomedical information sources integration was developed. The system builds on the abstraction of Virtual Repositories, which integrate fragmented data, and addresses the unification of private medical and genetic databases that frequently cannot be accessed over Internet [9, 10].

3. Design and implementation of a friendly user interface to help users to search, find and retrieve the contents of remote databases, assisted by a vocabulary server that integrates medical and genetic terms and concepts.
4. Development of an assistant to help health practitioners to seamless navigate over local and remote internet resources related to genetic disease, from the phenotype to the genotype. A navigation protocol (a workflow for access public databases available on the *web*) was created by skilled users, familiar in retrieving information associated to rare diseases, over medical and genomic data. Based upon this protocol we have developed a web-based portal (DiseaseCard) that optimizes the execution of the information gathering tasks specified on the protocol. The DiseaseCard and its navigation protocol are the main results discussed on this paper, detailed in the next sections.

3 The DiseaseCard Portal

DiseaseCard is a web portal publicly available [13] that provides an integrated view over medical and genetic information with respect to genetic diseases, in many aspects similar to the approach found in GeneCards with respect to genes.

The system enables a group of experts to cooperate on-line to elaborate a card to study a given disease. These users will define the relevant information retrieval tasks, resorting to on-line information sources providers (web links relevant for the study of a genetic disease). The end-user will typically start the investigation by searching for a disease, providing its name. Upon the identification of the disease, the DiseaseCard will present a structured, intuitive report, containing the details of the pathology and providing entry points to further details/resources ("data zooming"), either on the clinical and genetic domains.

Objectives

The first goal that was behind the conception of DiseaseCard was the development of a collaborative application where a group of experts could collaborate on-line in order to share, store and disseminate their knowledge about diseases. The field of rare genetics diseases will be the main target for this tool.

Second, we did not want to replicate information that already exist in several public or private databases. The system must be supported by a metaphor and by an information model that allow sharing this data.

Third, we want to support the system on a navigation protocol that allows to guide users in the process of retrieving rare diseases information from the Internet. This protocol could be used both as the user interface and as a base structure for the system information model.

Navigation Protocol

The selection of the sources for biomedical information is crucial for DiseaseCard. Nucleic Acids Research (NAR), for instance, publishes "The Molecular Biology Database Collection" annually, a list of the most important databases hierarchically classified by areas [5]. Guaranteed scientific reliability, exact and frequently updated data and public and free access are common characteristics shared by these databases.

Each database has its own domain, its own architecture, its own interface and its own way of making queries, reasons why that these resources are considered heterogeneous and distributed [14]. In the 2004 update, there were 548 databases registered in the journal, a number clearly unmanageable by a primary care physician.

To achieve the previously mentioned objectives we select twenty databases registered in NAR and we built a navigation protocol linking these databases. This navigation model provides also the user interface metaphor for DiseaseCard. It follows logical rules from both the clinical and genetic perspective (Figure 1). The pathology (*Pathology*) is the starting point of the protocol. In here, several centers of reference for the pathology are available. A disease is due to a disorder or mutation in the genetic make up of the patient (*Disorder & Mutation*), like a polymorphism (*Polymorphism*) for instance. This is due to a change in the sequence of nucleotides (*Nucleotide sequence*) causing a change in the corresponding protein (*Protein: sequence*) with a domain and belonging to a family (*Domain & Families*). As a result the 3D structure of the protein is altered (*Protein: 3D structure*) and therefore its biological function (*Protein: function*). The protein takes part in a metabolic pathway (metabolic pathway), carrying out enzymatic reactions (*Enzyme*). It is at this level where the drugs act, if available (*Drug*). Clinical trials (*Clinical Trials*) are carried out with the drugs in Europe and the USA and also pharmacogenetics and pharmacogenomics research (*Pharmacogenomics & Pharmacogenetics research*). There is bibliography about the disease (*Bibliography*) and there are centers where the genetic diagnosis is made (*Genetic Test Lab*). There is also genetic information relevant for R&D such as the exact location in the chromosome (*Chromosome location*), official name of the affected gene (*Official name*), genetic data integrated in an individual card for each gene (*Gene*) and information relative to the 'Molecular function, Biologic process and Cellular component' in which the gene(s) is (are) involved, included in Gene Ontology.

From the clinical perspective, we have divided the protocol into user profiles fitting the different types of users, according to their information needs. In the top part of the protocol, area 1 (in white), there are the resources that provide information useful to primary care physicians such as information about bibliography, centers for genetic diagnosis and available treatments. The patient asks the primary care physician for the information about the disease and the doctor gets the information by querying DiseaseCard from his own office PC connected to the Internet.

Generally, the hospital specialist, to whom the patient was referred by the primary care physician, does the follow up in this type of pathologies. The specialist looks for more specific and detailed information than the primary care doctor, the areas 1 and 4.

Next to the specialist is the hospital genetician, which uses the information available in the areas 2 and 3 of the protocol.

Methods and Design Approaches

The DiseaseCard portal manages *cards*. A card is a structured report documenting a disease, which obtains its content from a net of web pages, as defined by the card developer(s). Each card can have its own structure of information but, for convenience, the cards are usually built on a predefined template, tailored to the genetic diseases field. The basic template provided is a direct mapping of the protocol previously discussed.

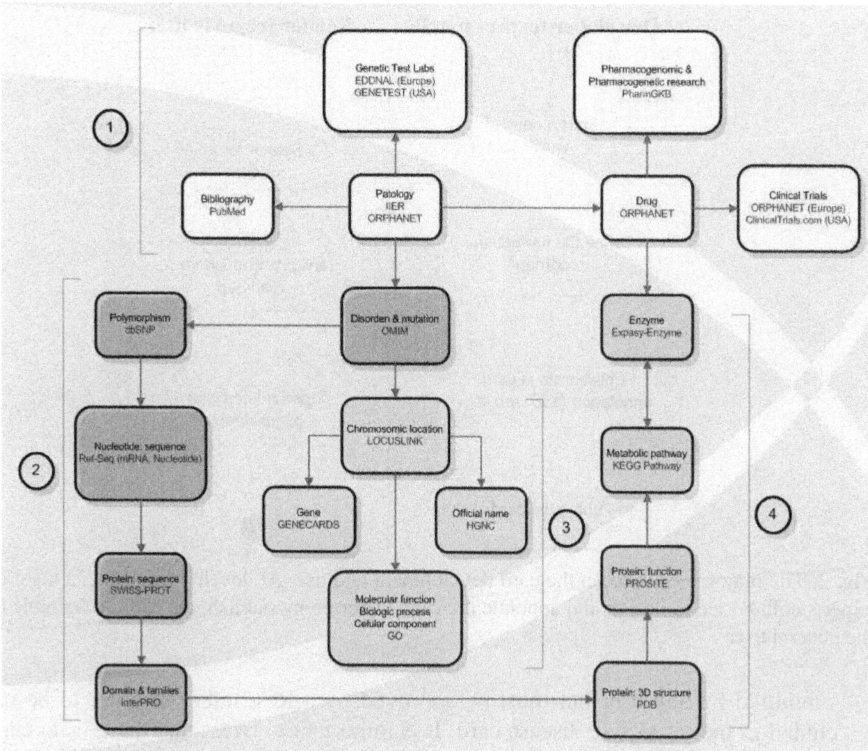

Fig. 1. Navigation protocol. Different areas are associated with different clinical users

A card holds a network of biomedical concepts and the navigation map the user may follow to go from one to another (Figure 2). For example: the card could start by providing the "Pathology" as the entry concept; from here, the user would advance to disorders and mutations, drugs, polymorphisms or snp, protein structure, genetic tests, genes, protein sequences, etc.

The DiseaseCard system allows the following user roles:

- Card manager Is the author (owner) of a card. He can nominate a set of users (researchers) to share his card's development. Card manager can give to his researchers/developers different views and permissions, according to each one responsibility.
- Researcher Is a person who have clinical or genetic knowledge and who wants to grab information about a rare disease and put them into a card. This user is allowed to create new cards and edit existing ones.
- Reader This type of user can be general clinicians, geneticists, pharmacologists, etc, who want to view and consult relevant information about a rare disease. In this profile the user does not have permission to modify existing cards. Each Reader may choose different views of the card to restrict the navigation protocol according to its own expertise. Readers can give suggestions, corrections, new links and some guidelines about existing disease cards. This information can be

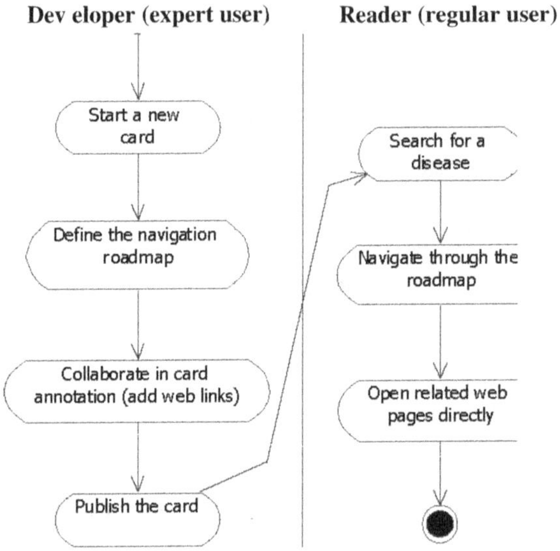

Fig. 2. The major workflow on the card development and use. At development time, a team of experts collaborate to design and annotate the card. After being publish, the card is available to the general user

submitted by any user but must be approved by a Researcher in order to be included in the respective disease card. It is important to stress that there is no centralized control access in DiseaseCard. The security policies are user-centered, i.e. each card manager decide about these policies for there own cards. They can provide for instance free read/write access to everyone.

The DiseaseCard user interface is based on two main windows (Figure 3). The left one is a tree-based navigation model that mirrors the pathway protocol. Through this tree the user can select the different disease domains and retrieve the information that is available for each, at that moment, in the Internet. The second window is used to display the data that is successively being downloaded by the user. Moreover, it can be used to show a graphical view of the navigation protocol allowing to select the navigation paths through this interface.

We can summarize the DiseaseCard current features as:

- The system is freely available through a Web interface.
- The entry point is the disease name.
- Anonymous user can navigate into the diseases information.
- Any user can register in the system though a simple process.
- Registered users are allowed to create cards and invite other users to help building their cards.
- Each card follows a common template in order to enhance readiness.
- The card visualization is supported both on tree-like view and on a map view.
- For each point in the protocol multiple links to information are available.
- The construction of the protocol is simple and intuitive (for instance, using directly URL from the browser, allow direct browsing and capture…).

- The user can create its own map according to a base plan of top concepts (Disease, Drugs, Gene…). For instance adding Bibliography, Case studies, Notes, Experts …).

Methodology

DiseaseCard is a web application developed with Java technology (Java Server Pages and Jakarta Struts), running on Tomcat 4.1 web server. All system and users information is stored and managed in a MS SQL Server database. The navigation map was built upon the SVG toolkit.

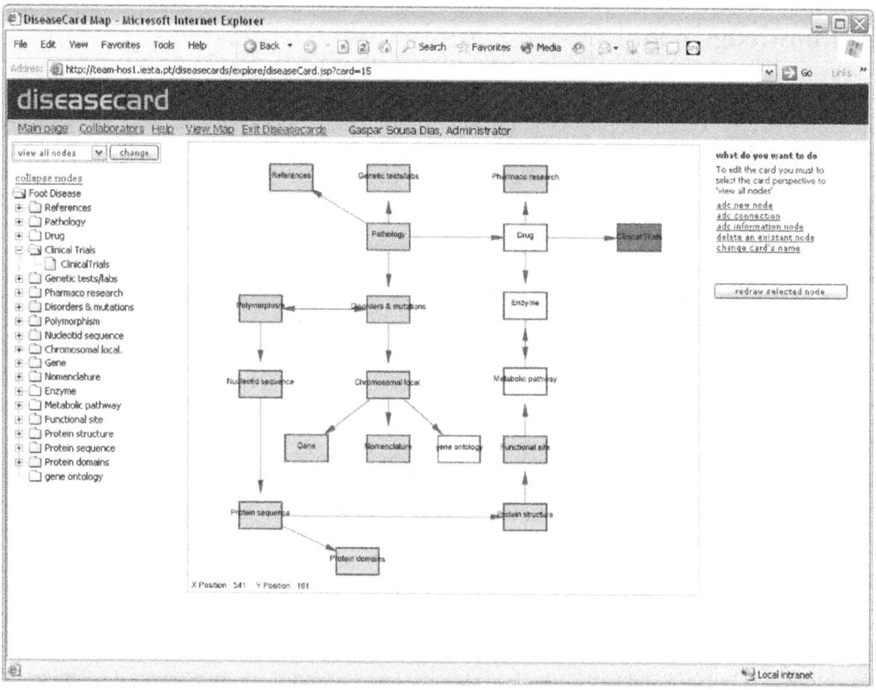

Fig. 3. After selecting a disease a conceptual navigation map is displayed, showing the user the information available

4 Assessment

The system was tested by a group of skilled users, clinicians with a strong experience on rare genetic diseases and, although done through non formal procedures, the first evaluation was very positive. Beside, the consensual agreement on the main focus of the system, users also highlighted the great potential of diseasecard on health education. Moreover, the automatization of several tasks was also a point that was identified in this assessment. Currently we are working on an automatic version of DiseaseCard from which we expect to create, on the fly, the overall navigation map for a selected disease.

5 Conclusions

The main objective of the presented work is the integration of clinical and genetic information from heterogeneous databases through a protocol management system. The DiseaseCard system allows capturing the knowledge of molecular biologists and biomedical experts available in the Internet about rare genetic diseases. With this system medical doctors can access genetic knowledge without the need to master biological databases, teachers can illustrate the network of resources build modern biomedical information landscape and general citizen can learn and benefit from cards developed and published by experts.

Acknowledgement

The INFOGENMED project is funded by the European Community, under the Information Society Technologies (IST) programme, Key Action 1 Systems & Services for the Citizen/Health.

References

1. A. E. Guttmacher and F. S. Collins, "Genomic Medicine - A Primer", *The New England Journal of Medicine*, vol. 347, no. 19, pp. 1512-1520, 2002.
2. I. Consortium, "Initial sequencing and analysis of the human genome", *Nature*, vol. 409, pp. 860-921, 2001.
3. A. Bayat, "Science, medicine, and the future: Bioinformatics", *British Medical Journal*, vol. 324, pp. 1018-22, 2002.
4. F. S. Collins and V. A. McKusick, "Implications of the Human Genome Project for Medical Science", *JAMA*, vol. 285, no. 5, pp. 540-544, 2001.
5. M. Galperin, "The Molecular Biology Database Collection: 2004 update", *Nucleic Acids Res*, 2004.
6. *The INFOGENMED project homepage,* www.infogenmed.net
7. Martin-Sanchez, I. Iakovidis, S. Norager, V. Maojo, P. de Groen, J. Van der Lei, T. Jones, K. Abraham-Fuchs, R. Apweiler, A. Babic, R. Baud, V. Breton, P. Cinquin, P. Doupi, M. Dugas, R. Eils, R. Engelbrecht, P. Ghazal, P. Jehenson, C. Kulikowski, K. Lampe, G. De Moor, S. Orphanoudakis, N. Rossing, B. Sarachan, A. Sousa, G. Spekowius, G. Thireos, G. Zahlmann, J. Zvarova, I. Hermosilla, and F. J. Vicente, "Synergy between medical informatics and bioinformatics: facilitating", *J Biomed Inform*, vol. 37, no. 1, pp. 30-42., 2004.
8. A. S. Pereira, V. Maojo, F. Martin-Sanchez, A. Babic, and S. Goes, "The Infogenmed Project", in *Int. Congress on Biological and Medical Engineering (ICBME02)*, Singapure, 2002.
9. M. García-Remesal, V. Maojo, H. Billhardt, J. Crespo, R. Alonso-Calvo, D. Pérez, F. Martin-Sanchez, J. Sánchez, F. J. Vicente, M. García-Rojo, A. Gómez de la Cámara, A. S. Pereira, J. L. Oliveira, I. Oliveira, M. Santos, and A. Babic, "Designing New Methodologies for Integrating Biomedical Information in Clinical Trials", in *IMIA Working Conference on Statistical Methodology in Bioinformatics and Clinical Trials (EuroMISE2004)*, Prague, Czech Republic, 2004.
10. M. García-Remesal, V. Maojo, H. Billhardt, J. Crespo, R. Alonso-Calvo, D. PérezRey, A. S. Pereira, and F. Martin-Sanchez, "ARMEDA II: Supporting Genomic Medicine through the Integration of Medical and Genetic Databases", in *Fourth IEEE Symposium on Bioinformatics and Bioengineering (BIBE'04)*, Taichung, Taiwan, ROC, 2004.

11. I. Oliveira, J. L. Oliveira, M. Santos, F. Martin-Sanchez, and A. S. Pereira, "On the requirements of biomedical information tools for health applications: the INFOGENMED case study", in *7th Portuguese Conference on Biomedical Engineering (BioEng'2003)*, Lisbon, Portugal, 2003.
12. *The infogemed Project homepage,* http://www.infogenmed.net
13. *The DiseaseCard homepage,* http://team-hos1.ieeta.pt/diseasecard/index.jsp
14. W. Sujansky, "Heterogeneous database integration in biomedicine", *J Biomed Inform.*, vol. 34, no. 4, pp. 285-98, 2001.

Biomedical Informatics: From Past Experiences to the Infobiomed Network of Excellence

Victor Maojo[1], Fernando Martin-Sánchez[2], José María Barreiro[1], Carlos Diaz[3], and Ferran Sanz[3]

[1] Biomedical Informatics Group, Artificial Intelligence Lab, Polytechnical University of Madrid, Spain
[2] Bioinformatics Unit, Institute of Health Carlos III, Majadahonda, Madrid, Spain
[3] Biomedical Informatics Research Group, Municipal Institue of Medical Research – IMIM, Barcelona, Spain

Abstract. Medical Informatics (MI) and Bioinformatics (BI) are now facing, after various decades of ongoing research and activities, a crucial time, where both disciplines could merge, increase collaboration or follow separate roads. In this paper, we provide a vision of past experiences in both areas, pointing out significant achievements in both fields. Then, scientific and technological aspects are considered, following an ACM report on computing. Following this approach, both MI and BI are analyzed, from three perspectives: design, abstraction, and theories, showing differences between them. An overview of training experiences in Biomedical Informatics is also included, showing current trends. In this regard, we present the INFOBIOMED network of excellence, funded by the European Commission, as an example of a systematic effort to support a synergy between both disciplines, in the new area of Biomedical Informatics.

1 Introduction

Medical Informatics (MI) is a discipline, which was academically established during the 70s. Some pioneers already suggested at the end of the 50s that physicians could use computers for clinical applications, including complex calculations or diagnosis (1). Later, the discipline was consolidated and evolved towards various research and practical objectives. Among these, the development of AI-based methods for medical diagnosis and care reached a considerable academic impact [2]. In general, the development of "practical" tools for routine care has led the course of the discipline [3]. During the last years, the impact of Bioinformatics has introduced a debate about the future of MI, in which the authors have participated [4,5,6,7].

Bioinformatics (BI) was developed before the beginning of the Human Genome Project, which accelerated BI development and recognition [8]. BI professionals aimed to create the informatics methods and tools needed to advance genomic research. The success of the Human Genome Project and the interest of industry have recently motivated a shortage of BI professionals, addressed by an increasing number of academic institutions. Some of these institutions offer independent training programs and academic degrees in both MI and BI, held at different departments.

The impact of the Human Genome Project has encouraged people to look forward to apply genomic findings to clinical medicine. Novel diagnostic tools and pharmaceutical products should reach patient care soon according to these views. Whereas

J.M. Barreiro et al. (Eds.): ISBMDA 2004, LNCS 3337, pp. 418–426, 2004.

BI professionals still focus, in general, their goals within the "omics" areas, some of them are beginning to envision that genomic findings will be available for clinicians. This approach might reduce, for instance, the period of time that is needed to transfer basic scientific results to patient settings.

For this purpose, an increasing number of BI professionals look forward to build applications that might lead to results that will applied in clinical routine, not only in clinical genetics labs. If this vision were fulfilled, we could imagine that BI professionals might need a fast training in customer satisfaction techniques to deal with average medical practitioners, given the special characteristics of the work carried out by these professionals. This kind of expertise has been obtained and developed by MI professionals over four decades of practice and interaction with clinicians. Thus, some exchange between MI and BI could be helpful to build computer applications of genomic results for patient care.

2 Lessons Learned from the Past

It has been previously reported that too many medical computer applications have been built without a clear sense of which was the state of the art in the area, therefore continuosly "reinventing the wheel" [9]. A contribution of professionals with MI training and background should have helped to build better system applications in many cases. The main problems of the discipline are more difficult than it was expected decades ago and many remain unsolved. Meanwhile, it seems that many BI professionals are looking forward to develop clinical applications without recognizing the importance of the lessons learned during many years of hard work within MI. Thus, some collaborative efforts between MI and BI could give a deeper insight of the real problems that the clinical applications of genomic research face.

MI has decisively contributed to improve healthcare during the last decades of the discipline. At the same time, it is experiencing some kind of lack of definition on its agenda for future research and activities. Many MI projects have gotten academic recognition but have lacked the clinical impact that their developers expected. MI journals do not get, either, the impact that should be expected according to the importance of computer applications in current biomedical research. Thus, many debates have been carried out during the last years in conferences and scientific journals to debate the future of MI.

The development of genomics and related research has favoured the development of new methods and applications, ranging from diagnostic tests to new pharmaceuticals. Discussing these issues with many genomic and BI professionals it seems that there is a feeling that the transfer of different laboratory achievements to patient care is a logical step that will follow soon. But the history of medicine has showed that results in basic sciences cannot be immediately and easily applied to patient care.

As suggested above, physicians are a difficult target for computer system developers. Medical reasoning is radically different from how engineers solve problems and build computer programs and devices [10]. The specific circumstances of medical practice – for instance, different vocabulary, lack of technical training, reduced time, stressful situations, environmental factors – can make the creation of computer applications for medical tasks a nightmare for untrained engineers.

MI professionals have suffered that difficult exchange with physicians for some decades. The latter are commonly difficult computing customers, shifting from indifference to anger quickly. It is not unsual, al all, that clinicians change rapidly their perceptions of a computerized system, suggesting changes impossible to carry out once the application is completed. Only when clinicians realize that the application improves their tasks or they observe that their colleagues accept and succesfully use some informatics systems they will be willing to incorporate these systems into their routines.

In this regard, a deeper analysis of MI and BI as computing disciplines should provide some clues.

3 Medical Informatics and Bioinformatics as Computing Disciplines

The 1989 ACM report on computing [11] introduced a framework for a curriculum in computer science that the authors of this paper have used to analyse the scientific and engineering characteristics of MI [12]. This framework could be also useful for a joint analysis of MI-BI, based on three perspectives: design, abstraction and theories.

A. From a *design* perspective, some of the methods and tools used in both MI and BI are quite similar. For instance, algorithms for data mining, image processing techniques, knowledge representation approaches or probabilistic tools in MI and BI are based on similar assumptions and techniques. From this view, some methods, tools and educational approaches could be easily shared or exchanged. For instance, the current last version of the UMLS includes the specifications of Gene Ontology. Yet, although pure engineering aspects are similar there are other aspects such as ethical issues, human and cognitive factors, different terminologies and assumptions, environmental factors or evaluation requirements, that are different. These factors have affected MI applications throughout its history and should affect BI is the latter enters the clinical areas.

MI professionals have dealt with the complexities of medicine and many health care scenarios. To succeed in their work, they have learned specific approaches that are not taught in textbooks. For instance, clinical approaches to manage the same patients might change from one hospital to another one located around the corner. These approaches will include some implicit information and clinical reasoning that are surely imposible to understand for people lacking clinical experience. Similarly, no comprehensive textbooks are available to learn the difficulties that appear when implementing hospitals information systems (HIS), diagnostic systems or computerized medical records. Thus, getting the participation of experienced MI professionals will be fundamental to develop genomic applications in medicine, where most BI professionals have no background and training.

B. From an *abstraction* perspective, researchers in MI and BI construct models, based on scientific hypothesis, that can be experimentally tested. Following this view, differences between both disciplines are significant. MI have concentrated, since the pioneering experiences of the first medical expert systems, in developing top-down models to justify the pathophysiological processes of diseases. Developers of systems such as CASNET [13] suffered the lack of medical knowledge of the fundamental mechanisms underlying diseases. These models only captured a narrow and superficial vision of the causal processes of diseases.

BI has concentrated on a bottom-up approach, trying to understand physiology from its molecular and cellular basis. Building models in BI to explain the mechanisms of diseases from current knowledge is an impossible task at this moment, given the lack of scientific knowledge in medicine. MI and BI professionals may create a synergy, carrying out a collaborative effort to contribute to fill the intermediate knowledge gaps existing at the pathophysiological level of most diseases [4].

C. From a *theoretical* perspective, MI and BI should hypothesize relationships between the objects of study and determine their truth in various experimental contexts (11,12). From its beginning, work in MI concentrated on building practical systems. Developers, coming from a wide variety of fields, created practical applications to get immediate results rather than scientific developments. Some kind of trial and error approach has dominated the discipline, also determined by the lack of established scientific theories in medicine. Thus, theoretical research has not dominated and launched the discipline.

In contrast, BI has been centered in tasks around one of the most challenging scientific projects of the last century, the Human Genome Project. Thus, BI has been more focused and had obtained clear benefits from the scientific theoretical basis that dominate biology. In this regard, BI should provide theoretical and methodological approaches that could be fundamental to give a scientific basis to MI.

Both MI and BI have experienced serious problems in gaining academic and professional recognition. Many computer scientists consider MI or BI – and many others, such as law informatics, chemoinformatics or neuroinformatics – as just the application of informatics to medicine and biology, respectively. In the other hand, many clinicians view medical informaticians as technology professionals that just build software programs – such as databases – to help them. Similar arguments can be given to explain the relationship between biologists and bioinformaticians [4].

MI and BI scholars have fought to establish their own independent fields, departments, conferences and journals, gaining scientific recognition In both cases, most pioneers had a technical background in fields such as computer science or engineering. This scenario changed after some time, most remarkably in MI – which is in fact an older discipline –, and physicians joined MI training programs. Later, a similar phenomenon occurred within BI. These new professionals could get a greater recognition from professionals from their related domains of interest – medicine and biology –, acting as promoters or leaders of both fields among their peers.

To justify the difficulties that MI research faces, it has been suggested that medical information is more complex than information in other areas. According to previous research reports (12,14), we can consider several information levels in medicine. There is a surface or clinical level, where physicians examine, for instance, symptoms, signs and results of different tests. At deeper levels, they analyze, for instance, pathophysiological processes, metabolic networks, biochemical alterations or genetic mutations. Since most of these processes are still unknown, they are difficult to model.

Medicine is also influenced by other factors, which we have discussed elsewhere (12). These include, among others, emotional, environmental and ethical factors. A medical researcher cannot study patients in the laboratory, isolated from their surroundings and circumstances, and disect them, as biologists can routinely do. By contrast, biological research can be more easily isolated from other external factors, although biologists and bioinformaticians have put forward similar arguments about the inner complexity of information in biology (8).

Maybe because of the above difficulties, there has been a lack of exploratory research of basic concepts in MI. Almost from its beginning, the field of MI focused on the development of applications that could reward the original funding invested. Developing solutions for practical issues was immediately funded, and therefore, this direction was preferred to searching a "big-bang" in the discipline, as has been pointed out before (3). It was common during the 60s, when the field of MI was just starting up, that most hospitals wanted applications that could be immediately used for patient care or cost management.

As an example of directions in the research agenda, the table below reports the main milestones in MI as seen by two distinguished MI scholars:

Table 1. Main achievements in MI during the last decades

Unified Medical Language System (UMLS)	Clinical reasoning processes
Health Level Seven (HL7)	Reminder systems
Human Visible Project	Uncertain reasoning (Bayes, rules, neural networks)
Clinical Decision Support System (e.g., HELP, CARE)	Computerized patient records (CPRs)
Diagnostic systems (e.g., QMR, DxPlain)	Elucidating patients' information needs
MEDLINE	

On the left side of the table, Sittig suggested the main MI achievements, more related to application design. On the right, Buchanan suggested that MI success was more related to the processes underlying patient care, as cited elsewhere (15).

Funding for basic research in "human information systems" – which can be classed as the study of human physiology and pathology from an informatics perspective – was rare within MI. This was a kind of research that was usually left "for tomorrow" in MI research, as has been suggested elsewhere (3).

Given this scenario, it is clear that training in both MI and BI is fundamental to develop the skills needed to understand the specific particularities of informatics and its relationships with medicine and biology, respectively. In this regard, new approaches are also being taken to shorten the distances and differences between both disciplines in the novel framework of BMI.

As expanded below, this analysis is also one of the goals of the INFOBIOMED European Research Network of Excellence in Biomedical Informatics, funded by the European Commission, where the authors participate.

4 Training in MI and BI

MI programs have been available since the beginning of the 70s. In 1972, the US National Library of Medicine funded 13 programs – most of them offering postdoctoral positions only – through a program that ended in 1984, because of qualitative and economic factors. Soon later a new support initiative provided funding for five of those training programs, which were later expanded until present. In Europe, national initiatives were launched by MI pioneers at different academic institutions and hospitals. The European Commission also funded later different initiatives to foster education in MI, including projects to enhance distance learning in MI by using multimedia applications and Internet-based courses.

BI is a much younger discipline and academic programs were established during the 90s at different institutions. There is currently a large list of academic settings offering BI degrees at various levels, from undergraduate to PhDs. Since the needs of industry and research groups are larger than the number of trainees enrolled in these programs, recent initiatives have promoted the use of Internet as the basis for distance learning, where students can get on-line courses and degrees. The US National Institute of Health and the European Commission are also supporting various initiatives to foster and promote experiences for teaching BI and grants for student training and exchanges.

MI and BI programs have been traditionally separated. Only a few examples could be cited to show some kind of exchange between professionals from both sides. For instance, a recognized program is the Biomedical Informatics Training Program at Stanford University –currently directed by Russ Altman, a bioinformatician, with a medical degree–, which offers a common program for both disciplines. This program, established in 1982, was primarily centered on MI, including courses in five areas: Medical Informatics, Computer Science, Decision Theory and Statistics, Biomedicine, Health Policy/Social Issues. In recent years the program has shifted towards a larger focus on bioinformatics courses and issues, while the title has also changed – the former degree was awarded on "Medical Information Sciences".

Another recent interesting approach has been taken in Europe, at the Karolinska Institute in Sweden, where a Ph.D. Programme in Medical Bioinformatics has been launched. The purpose is "to build up competence in bioinformatics with special emphasis on biomedical and clinical applications". The interest of some BI professionals to build clinical applications supports this new approach.

The Stanford University and Karolinska Institute programs show these recent trends in the field. In one hand, some MI and BI professionals are establishing common activities disciplines and opportunities for exchange. This interaction has already led to combined training programs and interdisciplinary research projects. In the other hand, the success of the Human Genome Project has created significant expectations that results may be applied to generate clinical applications which may be personalized for specific groups of patients.

Young – in this case, medical – students use a reasoning approach based on simple principles. Later, there is some lack of coordination in clinical reasoning at the resident level – where they use a mixture of art and basic science. Finally, the experienced clinicians automate the problem solving strategies they use but frequently cannot verbalize them (16). It has been proposed that clinicians used to reason and teach medicine in terms of "art" and practice rather than in terms of scientific principles (17). Therefore, there is a gap between the initial training of medical students, based on scientific teaching, such as biology, biochemistry, physics or genetics and the clinical practice that they experience later.

Since the times of Galen, clinical medicine has been taught at the bedside. Physicians learn a knowledge of basic sciences such as biology, physics or chemistry at medical schools but they shift their practice to a more "practical" view later. Many practitioners have learned through clinical practice and experience – correctly? – that basic scientific theories cannot support by themselves the whole rationale needed to diagnose and treat many patients. It has been suggested that physicians may be misled in patient management by adopting a pure scientific approach (17), given our current gaps in the basic principles of medicine. Thus, they use a variable combination of their scientific knowledge, obtained from books and scientific journals, and the lessons learned in their practice and subjective judgment. There may be a gap between two stages, one at the beginning of the education of medical students, with basic scientific principles – from biology, biochemistry, physics or genetics – and the more practical, "clinical" approach that the real practice impose on them. At the latter stage, many heads of clinical units can be even proud to acknowledge that they do not use purely scientific approaches to clinical care.

Similarly, MI students must acquire the foundations and methods of the discipline while learning to reason and use the rules of thumb inherent to MI. They do not need to reason strictly like experienced doctors or engineers but they should know the cognitive characteristics of medical and computer science reasoning. A similar approach could be applied to BI with respect to biology.

A problem may appear if BI professionals tried to develop clinical applications. To succeed in this task they should be able to understand the mechanisms of medical reasoning and the characteristics of health care and routines or collaborate with experts in the field, i.e. MI professionals. Developing by themselves these clinical applications may mean to repeat the history and failures of MI in the past, forgetting the lessons learned by MI professionals.

5 New Trends in Biomedical Informatics and Genomic Medicine

The idea that transfer discoveries obtained in basic sciences into patient care is immediate has been generally unsuccessful until now. The history of medicine is plenty of negative examples, including diseases such as diabetes, tuberculosis, bacterial infections, and many more. In most of these examples, it took a long period of time between the discovery of the agents or mechanisms that cause a disease and the emerging of a therapeutic procedure. Distinguished scholars [17] have expressed their views that the introduction of basic scientific achievements – particularly in genetics – in medicine would not be easy. The success of the Human Genome Project has risen high expectations for outstanding breakthroughs in medical care and research but they need to be fulfilled.

One of the important constraints to advance towards molecular medicine is the shift in education that will be required for physicians to learn how to interpret and manage genomic and genetic information in their clinical routines. The knowledge and reasoning methods that will be needed in this new concept of medicine may be provided by informatics tools. Physicians should learn how to use these tools but it does not sound reasonable to make them understand, for instance, how to interpret microarray results or SNPs (single nucleotide polymorphisms) information, without a thorough shift in medical education and training.

A different issue is to create the methods and build the informatics tools that will be needed to facilitate the work of practitioners. For that purpose, different backgrounds and expertises will be needed. Figure 1 shows an example of the kind of environment and relationships that this purpose could create.

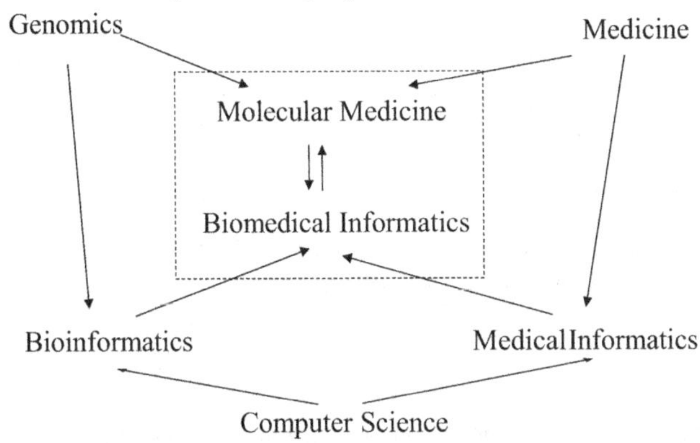

Fig. 1. Different interactions betwwen informatics-related disciplines and biomedicine

These perspectives may provide a foundation for an interaction between both disciplines. They could give also clues to advance research and determine the educational needs of both MI and BI to address issues surrounding molecular medicine.

In this regard, the European INFOBIOMED Network of Excellence has envisioned a series of activities designed to cover significant challenges, relevant to both MI and BI, in areas such as: (1) Data interoperability and management, including data characteristics and ontologies, integrating approaches, and ethics and confidentiality issues, (2) Methods, technologies and tools, including data analysis and information retrieval, image visualisation and analysis, and nformation systems and decision support tools. Finally, this horizontal approach is linked to four pilot applications, in the areas o pharmainformatics, genomics and microbiology, genomics and chronic inflammation, and genomics and colon cancer.

These research-centered activities are linked to various exchange, dissemination and mobility activities, aiming to create the infrastructure for supporting further activities in Biomedical Informatics at the European level. In this regard, one of the main issues of the network will be the analysis and proposal of specific actions for BMI training, that could be adopted by other stakeholders. For this vision to become real, the analysis provided in this paper should be expanded.

6 Conclusions

One might wonder what kind of emphasis and skills will be needed to develop informatics tools to address genomic applications in medicine. May BI professionals be able to develop by themselves these applications? We have pointed out that, without collaborative efforts, BI professionals could miss the lessons learned in four decades of building clinical applications in MI. A number of MI projects failed because the intrinsic difficulties of the field. This acquired expertise could avoid the "reinvention of the wheel" and many future failures in future genomic-based clinical systems. Similarly, if MI professionals tried to build a novel "genetic medical record" or launch research projects in modelling pathophysiological mechanisms, without the BI expertise in managing genomic data and modelling physiological processes, the effort may lead to an unsuccessful end.

In this regard, novel approaches such as the European Network of Excellence in Biomedical Informatics and various local initiatives in the European countries, the USA and others, will prove fundamental to address these issues.

Acknowledgments

The work presented in this paper has been funded by the European Commission thorugh the IST INFOBIOMED Network of Excellence.

References

1. Ledley, R.S. and Lusted, L. Reasoning Foundations of Medical Diagnosis. Science 1959. 130 (3366): 9-21.
2. Clancey, W. and E.H. Shortliffe (Eds). Readings in Medical Artificial Intelligence: The First Decade. Reading: Addison Wesley. 1984
3. Blum, B. and K. Duncan. (Eds). 1990. A History of Medical Informatics. Reading: Addison Wesley Pub.
4. Maojo, V. and Kulikowski, CA. Bioinformatics and Medical Informatics: Collaborations on the Road to Genomic Medicine? J Am Med Inform Assoc. 2003 Nov-Dec;10(6):515-522
5. Maojo V, Crespo J. Challenges for future intelligent systems in biomedicine. Journal of Intelligent and Fuzzy Systems 2002; 12 (1): 1-3.
6. Altman, R. 2000. The Interactions Between Clinical Informatics and Bioinformatics. JAMIA Vol 7, 5: 439-443
7. Martín-Sanchez, F.; Maojo, V. and López-Campos, G. 2002. Integrating genomics into health information systems. Methods of Information in Medicine, 41:25-30.
8. Hagen, J. 2000. The origins of bioinformatics. Nat. Rev. Genetics, 1: 231-236
9. Shortiffe, E.H., L. Perreault, L. Fagan, and G. Wiederhold (Eds). Medical Informatics. Computer Applications in Health Care. 2001. 2nd Edition. New York: Springer Verlag.
10. Kassirer, J. and R. Kopelman. Learning Clinical Reasoning. Baltimore: Williams and Wilkins. 1991.
11. Denning P, Comer D, Gries D, Mulder, Tucker A and Young P. "Computing as a discipline". Communications of the ACM 1989. Vol 32, 1, pp. 9-23.
12. Maojo, V., F. Martín-Sanchez, J. Crespo, and H. Billhardt. 2002. Theory, Abstraction and Design in Medical Informatics. Methods of Information in Medicine, 41: 44-50.
13. Kulikowski, C. and Weiss, S. 1971. Computer-based Models of Glaucoma. Report no. 3, Department of Computer Science, Computers in Biomedicine, Rutgers University.
14. Blois M. Information and Medicine : The Nature of Medical Descriptions. Berkeley CA: Univ. of California Press, 1984.
15. Musen, 2001. Presentation given at the IMIA Satellite Working Conference. Challenges in Medical Informatics. Successes and Failures. March 29-31. Madrid.
16. Anderson J. Cognitive Psychology and Its Implications (5th Ed). Worth Publishing. 1999.

Network Analysis of the Kinetics of Amino Acid Metabolism in a Liver Cell Bioreactor

Wolfgang Schmidt-Heck[1], Katrin Zeilinger[2], Michael Pfaff[3], Susanne Toepfer[3], Dominik Driesch[3], Gesine Pless[2], Peter Neuhaus[2], Joerg Gerlach[2], and Reinhard Guthke[1]

[1] Hans Knoell Institute for Natural Products Research, Beutenbergstr. 11a, 07745 Jena, Germany
{wolfgang.schmidt-heck,reinhard.guthke}@hki-jena.de
http://www.hki-jena.de

[2] Charité Campus Virchow, University Medicine Berlin, Augustenburger Platz 1, 13353 Berlin, Germany
{katrin.zeilinger,joerg.gerlach}@charite.de

[3] BioControl Jena GmbH, Wildenbruchstr. 15, 07745 Jena, Germany
{michael.pfaff,susanne.toepfer,dominik.driesch}@biocontrol-jena.com

Abstract. The correlation of the kinetics of 18 amino acids, ammonia and urea in 18 liver cell bioreactor runs was analyzed and described by network structures. Three kinds of networks were investigated: i) correlation networks, ii) Bayesian networks, and iii) dynamic networks that obtain their structure from systems of differential equations. Three groups of liver cell bioreactor runs with low, medium and high performance, respectively, were investigated. The aim of this study was to identify patterns and structures of the amino acid metabolism that can characterize different performance levels of the bioreactor.

1 Introduction

Hybrid liver support systems are being developed for temporary extracorporeal liver support [1]. The human liver cell bioreactor investigated here as part of such a system consists of a three-dimensional system of interwoven capillaries within a housing that serve medium inflow and outflow as well as oxygenation and carbon dioxide removal. The liver cells are cultivated in the inter-capillary space. They reconstitute to liver tissue-like structures after inoculation of the bioreactor with cell suspensions obtained from discarded human livers explanted but not suitable for transplantation. This bioreactor mimics conditions close to those in the natural organ. Not only can this bioreactor be used as part of a therapeutic system but also as a valuable tool to analyze the dynamics and network structures of the physiological and molecular interactions of hepatocytes and other liver cells under different yet standardized conditions.

Recently, data from this bioreactor system has been analyzed by fuzzy cluster and rule based data mining and pattern recognition methods in order to identify early performance predictors for the bioreactor's long-term performance based on the kinetics of biochemical variables not including the amino acids [2].

J.M. Barreiro et al. (Eds.): ISBMDA 2004, LNCS 3337, pp. 427–438, 2004.

In order to discover and understand the complex molecular interactions in living systems, such as the human liver organ, network reconstruction by reverse engineering is a valuable approach. Several such methods have for instance been established for gene expression data analysis to reconstruct gene regulatory networks [3,4].

The focus of this paper is on pattern recognition and network modeling of amino acid metabolism in terms of kinetic behavior [5]. A particular point of attention was on continuously valued models to consider concentration profiles of the amino acids and related nitrogen-containing molecules. Three different modeling paradigms were investigated in this context: i) correlation networks, ii) Bayesian networks and also iii) systems of differential equations.

Correlation analysis performs a pairwise comparison of the amino acid time series. *Correlation networks* provide a graphical representation of the correlation analysis results obtained and, more specifically, allow to visualize groups that are characterized by similar temporal behavior [6]. Correlation networks, however, are unable to map the causality of putative interactions in the sense of cause-and-effect relationships. In order to reconstruct such relationships from experimental data more complex model structures with corresponding inferring methods such as Bayesian networks or systems of differential equations are required.

Bayesian networks are graph-based models of joint probability distributions that describe complex stochastic dependencies [7]. The liver cell bioreactor behavior is characterized by a considerable amount of variability that is not understood in detail. The individuality of the donor liver organs appears to be a major general reason for this. This individuality with respect to liver cell functionality is highly complex and insufficiently characterized. Bayesian networks therefore allow to deal with this unpredictability and individual variability in a stochastic way. However, most Bayesian network approaches are restricted to static and acyclic structures. They do not allow to directly model the inherent dynamic behavior. Furthermore, in the presence of feedback loops in biological systems, acyclic model structures cannot be assumed to reconstruct the true relationships between the variables of such systems.

In order to describe the dynamic cause-and-effect relationships within the liver cell bioreactor system from a systems biological point of view [8], *systems of ordinary differential equations* can be employed. They are widely used to model for instance biochemical systems or gene regulatory networks [9]. These deterministic model structures express the temporal change of variables as linear or nonlinear functions of other time-dependent variables. They are capable of reconstructing highly complex nonlinear dynamic interactions from experimental data and they are also very well suited to incorporate different types of prior knowledge. These networks, however, are deterministic, i.e. they do not allow to reflect inherent biological variability.

In the present work it will be demonstrated that the joint use of different network reconstruction methods has the potential to generate complementary information about the structure and the dynamics of the liver cell bioreactor system investigated here.

2 Material and Methods

2.1 Bioreactor and Data

This paper focuses on the amino acid metabolism as quantified by the measured time series of the concentrations $c(t)$ of 18 amino acids (ASP, GLU, ASN, SER, GLN, HIS, GLY, THR, ARG, ALA, TYR, MET, VAL, TRP, PHE, ILE, LEU, LYS) as well as of ammonia (NH3) and urea. These concentrations were measured daily in the outflow (waste) of the liver cell bioreactor system, the amino acid concentrations up to the third day daily and every third day afterwards.

The bioreactor was continuously supplied with medium containing the 18 amino acids among other compounds. This was done at different flow rates depending on the bioreactor's mode of operation during the cell recovery phase (up to 3 days) and the stand-by phase (up to 34 days) prior to clinical application. This study focuses on the operation of the bioreactor prior to clinical application only. Therefore, the kinetics over the first 6 days were analyzed here.

The bioreactor system consists of the actual bioreactor (volume $V_2 = 600\,\mathrm{ml}$) that contains the liver cells in the inter-capillary space and a perfusion system (volume $V_1 = 900\,\mathrm{ml}$) that supplies a stream through the inside of the capillaries. This perfusion stream carries the concentrations of the compounds that are supplied to or removed from the actual bioreactor. These compounds cross either way via diffusion through the capillary membranes between these two compartments. Due to the high flow rate of the perfusion stream ($F = 250\,\mathrm{ml\,min}^{-1}$), an almost ideal mixing within this compartment can be assumed. To this perfusion stream the below explained inflow streams are added and the equivalent volumes of these streams are run to waste via the outflow stream. Due to the almost ideal mixing, the concentrations $c_{0i}(t)$ in the perfusion stream are the same as in the outflow stream. The measurements are taken from the waste after accumulation of the outflow stream over 24 hours.

Depending on the mode of operation, there are two time-variant inflow streams that are added to the perfusion stream with the flow rates $F_A(t)$ and $F_B(t)$ as defined by (1). $F_A(t)$ follows a step function from $F_{A1} = 150\,\mathrm{ml} \cdot \mathrm{h}^{-1}$ down to $F_{A2} = 50\,\mathrm{ml} \cdot \mathrm{h}^{-1}$ switching at the first day of operation and $F_B(t)$ one from $F_{B1} = 0$ up to $F_{B2} = 1\,\mathrm{ml} \cdot \mathrm{h}^{-1}$ switching at the third day, respectively. The outflow rate $F_0(t)$ equals the sum of both inflow rates.

$$
\begin{aligned}
F_A(t) &= \begin{cases} F_{A1} & \text{for } t < 1d \\ F_{A2} & \text{for } t \geq 1d \end{cases}, \\
F_B(t) &= \begin{cases} F_{B1} & \text{for } t < 3d \\ F_{B2} & \text{for } t \geq 3d \end{cases}, \\
F_0(t) &= F_A(t) + F_B(t).
\end{aligned} \tag{1}
$$

The inflow rate $F_A(t)$ provides the 18 amino acids and ammonia at the concentrations c_{Ai} (see Table 1 for the c_{Ai} of the $i = 1, \ldots, 8$ selected compounds used in Sect. 3.3). The inflow rate $F_B(t)$ provides only the amino acid aspartate (ASP) at the concentration $c_{B3} = 200\,\mathrm{mg/ml}$, i.e. $c_{Bi} = 0$ for all $i \neq 3$.

Table 1. Concentrations c_{Ai} of the 6 selected amino acids (methionine, leucine, aspartate, asparagine, glutamate, glutamine) as well as of ammonia (NH3) and urea in the inflow stream fed with the flow rate $F_A(t)$ as used in Sect. 3.3 for modeling.

Index i	Symbol	Concentration c_{Ai} (μmol $\cdot$ L^{-1})
1	MET	258.8
2	LEU	2258.2
3	ASP	283.9
4	ASN	167.9
5	GLU	265.1
6	GLN	687.0
7	NH3	41.5
8	UREA	0.0

The time courses of the concentrations $c_{Oi}(t)$ in the outflow stream may be considered to describe the response of the medium to the inoculation of the actual bioreactor with liver cells. These concentrations are in steady-state at $c_{Oi}(0) = c_{Ai}$ due to the perfusion of the technical system prior to inoculation. The available time series data for the time $t = 0$ therefore also represent both concentrations since the ones in the inflow equal those measured in the outflow at this particular time just before inoculation under steady-state conditions.

A data set C with the elements $c_{i,j,k}$ $(i = 1, \ldots, I; j = 1, \ldots, J; k = 1, \ldots, K)$ for $I = 20$ kinetic variables, $J = 18$ bioreactor runs and $K = 7$ time-points t_k was analyzed. Each run was labeled by $L_j \in \{$'low', 'medium', 'high'$\}$ describing the performance with respect to the long-term maintenance of the functionality of the liver cells within the bioreactor. 4, 7 and 7 runs were labeled 'low', 'medium' and 'high', respectively. This performance labeling was provided by an expert based on his assessment of altogether 99 variables that were measured to quantitatively characterize the system.

2.2 Correlation Networks

Correlation coefficients $r_{i,i',j} = corrcoef_k(\{c_{i,j,k}\}, \{c_{i',j,k}\})$ were calculated for all pairs of time series of two different variables i and i'. This was done for each bioreactor run j separately. Two networks N_{low} and N_{high} were generated and drawn separately for the $n = 4$ bioreactor runs with low performance and the $n = 7$ runs with high performance. The nodes of the networks symbolize the respective variables. A connection was drawn between the nodes i and i' if the correlation coefficient exceeded a certain threshold R ($|r_{i,i',j}| > R$) for at least $n - 1$ runs. A node i was only drawn if there was any connection to this node at all.

2.3 Bayesian Networks

Preceding the Bayesian network generation, the 18 bioreactor runs were clustered into 3 clusters for each individual variable i separately using the fuzzy C-means algorithm (with the fuzzy exponent 2). As distance measure for the clustering the squared difference between the $c_{i,j,k}$ and $c_{i,j',k}$ of two runs j and j' averaged over the time-points k was used. The membership degrees $M_{i,j,l}$ obtained for the clusters ($l = 1, \ldots, 3$), the variables ($i = 1, \ldots, 20$) and the runs ($j = 1, \ldots, 18$) together with the 3 performance labels L_j were then used as input data for the Bayesian network generation by a publicly available tool [10].

2.4 Differential Equation Systems

A semi-mechanistic model (2) for the description of the amino acid metabolism within the liver cell bioreactor was developed taking into account the inflow rates $F_A(t)$ and $F_B(t)$ and the outflow rate $F_0(t)$ of the system according to the operation mode (see Sect. 2.1). The diffusion across the capillary membrane system between the compartment containing the liver cells and the perfusion compartment as explained in Sect. 2.1 was modelled using the parameter p_1 that was identified as part of the parameter fitting procedure. The structure of the interactions of the amino acids, ammonia and urea was defined based on physiological knowledge of amino acid metabolism including ammonia assimilation.

The simulated kinetics obtained from the model were averaged over 24 hours and then compared to the measured data since the measured data from the waste constitute concentrations accumulated over one day of operation from the outflow of the bioreactor system.

The differential equations were solved using a Runge-Kutta 4th order algorithm and the model parameters were fitted minimizing the scaled mean square error (*mse*, scaled by the square of the maximum of the respective variable). The parameter optimization was performed using a simplex search method.

3 Results and Discussion

3.1 Correlation Networks

Figure 1 shows the correlation network obtained from the 7 high performance runs. The kinetics of 11 amino acids (7 of them essential ones) are correlated in the way shown. They form a large group in the network while the two amino acids ASP and GLU are only correlated with themselves without any connections to the others. The urea kinetics (node in the center of the large group in Figure 1) is negatively correlated ($r_{i,i',j} < -0.8$) to 10 of the 11 amino acids in the large group. For these three groups in the network, Figure 2 shows the mean kinetics averaged over the 7 runs and the respective compounds. The kinetics of the 11 amino acids in the large group are decreasing whereas that of urea is increasing. The kinetics of ASP and GLU are decreasing up the 3rd day before they are strongly increasing up to the 6th day. Altogether, the high performance runs are characterized by a large number of amino acids with decreasing kinetics (Figure 2a). This however is not the case for the low performance runs.

The correlation networks obtained from the low and the medium performance runs were very sparse. The kinetics of the low performance runs were found to

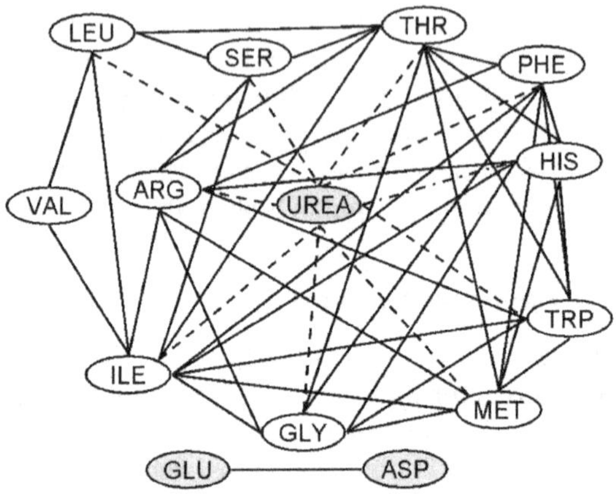

Fig. 1. Correlation network obtained from the kinetics of the 7 high performance runs. Full lines between nodes i and i' represent correlation coefficients $r_{i,i',j} > 0.8$ and dotted lines correlation coefficients $r_{i,i',j} < -0.8$, all for at least 6 runs j.

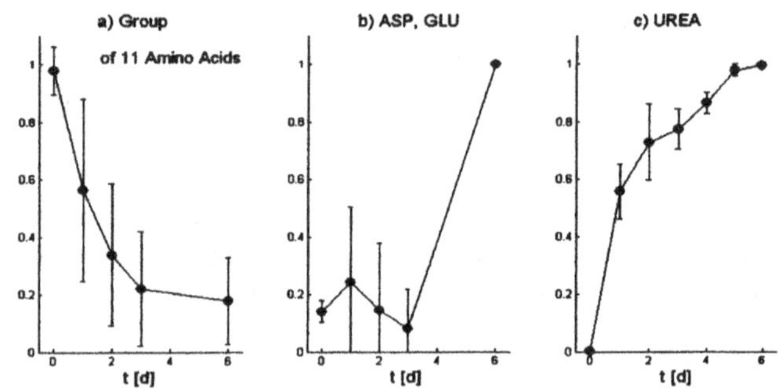

Fig. 2. Mean kinetics (± standard deviations) averaged over the kinetics of the 7 high performance runs as well as over (*a*) MET, SER, THR, ARG, HIS, GLY, TRP, LEU, VAL, PHE, ILE, (*b*) ASP and GLU, and (*c*) UREA after scaling by the respective maximum value.

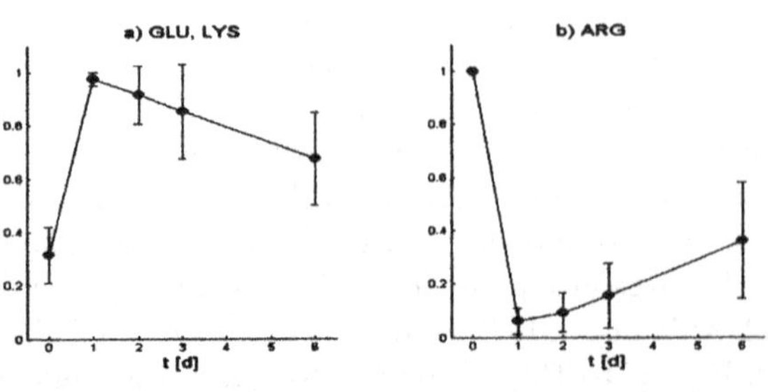

Fig. 3. Mean kinetics (± standard deviations) averaged over the kinetics of the 4 low performance runs as well as over (*a*) GLU and LYS, and (*b*) ARG after scaling by the respective maximum value.

be very heterogeneous with only 2 correlation coefficients greater than 0.8 and 2 smaller than −0.8 whereas the kinetics of the high performance runs were much more homogeneous with many higher correlations leading to the network with 49 connections shown in Figure 1. The correlation of the kinetics of the low performance runs proved low, i.e. these runs are more individual. The network for the low performance runs consists only of 3 nodes, where GLU and LYS were solely found to be positively correlated and both these amino acids were negatively correlated with ARG. The kinetic patterns of GLU and ARG differ for the high and low performance runs: The profile of GLU after 3 days is increasing in high performance runs (Figure 2b) but decreasing in low performance runs (Figure 3a). The profile of ARG after 1 day is decreasing in high performance runs (Figure 2a) but increasing in low performance runs (Figure 3b).

3.2 Bayesian Networks

Figure 4 shows the results of the clustering of the 18 runs for the kinetics of MET and LEU. This kind of result was calculated for all 20 variables studied here. For each variable i, each run j and each cluster l a membership degree $M_{i,j,l}$ was calculated and used together with the performance labels L_j to generate the Bayesian network shown in Figure 5. It illustrates that the five amino acids LEU, SER, MET, THR and VAL are correlated directly with the bioreactor's performance. The performance is high when the kinetics of the five amino acids belong to the respective cluster 1. Two of them, MET and LEU, can already sufficiently predict the performance as shown in Table 2.

3.3 Differential Equation Systems

The kinetic patterns of high performance runs that were found to be highly correlated (see Sect. 3.1) were described by a dynamic model (2) as follows. The time profiles of the individual 18 amino acids each averaged over the 7 high performance runs were grouped with respect to their qualitative behavior into 6

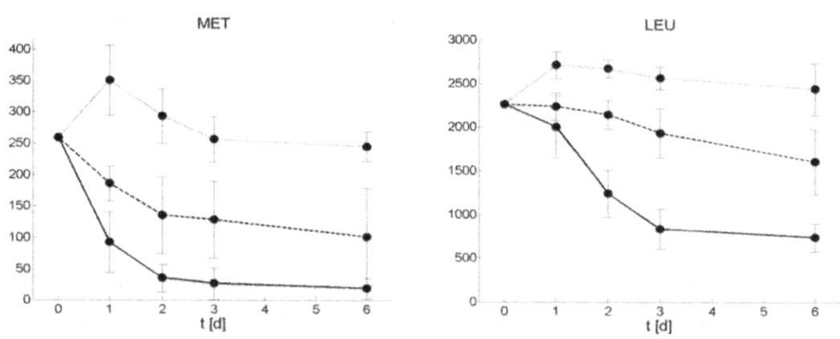

Fig. 4. Mean kinetics (± standard deviations) of (*a*) MET and (*b*) LEU averaged over the runs that were assigned to the respective cluster out of the three clusters with a membership degree greater than 50% (*full lines*: cluster 1, *dashed lines*: cluster 2, *dotted lines*: cluster 3).

Table 2. Probability of 'high', 'medium' and 'low' bioreactor performance under the condition that the amino acids MET and LEU belong to the clusters 1, 2 or 3, respectively (mean kinetics in Figure 4), as calculated by the Bayesian network shown in Figure 5.

MET	LEU	Performance		
		Low	Medium	High
Cluster 1	Cluster 1			0.939
Cluster 2	Cluster 2		0.977	
Cluster 3	Cluster 3	0.954		

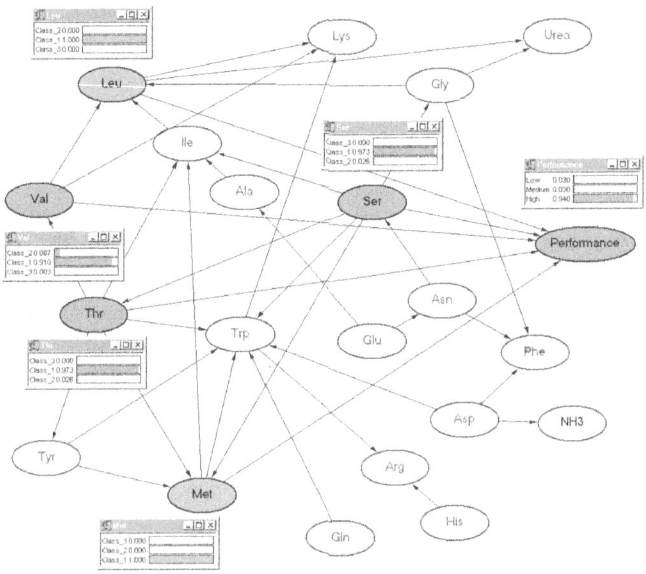

Fig. 5. Bayesian network obtained from the kinetics of 20 variables and 18 runs as well as the labels that characterize the performance of the runs. The conditional probabilities for the variables LEU, SER, MET, THR and VAL (*highlighted*) are directly connected to the performance (also highlighted). The conditional probabilities with values and horizontal bars for the respective three clusters (named Class 1, 2, 3) of these variables with respect to the conclusion 'performance high' (with its probability and bar) are shown next to the variables.

groups as listed in Table 3. The 11 amino acids in groups 1 and 2 are the same as found by the correlation network analysis (see Sect. 3.1).

The groups 1, 2, 4 and 6 contain more than one amino acid. From these groups representative amino acids were selected for the subsequent modeling. MET and LEU were used as representatives for groups 1 and 2, respectively, due to the results of the Bayesian network analysis (see Sect. 3.2). The amino acids ASP, ASN, GLU and GLN were selected due to their physiological role in

Table 3. Number n of amino acids grouped according to the qualitative behavior of their time courses averaged over the 7 high performance runs. Group representatives shown in Figure 6.

Group	n	Amino Acids	Qualitative Behavior
1	7	MET, SER, THR, ARG, HIS, GLY, TRP	Decreasing fast
2	4	LEU, VAL, PHE, ILE	Decreasing retarded
3	1	ASP	Temporal minimum low
4	3	ASN, GLU, ALA	Temporal minimum high
5	1	LYS	Temporal maximum
6	2	GLN, TYR	Almost constant

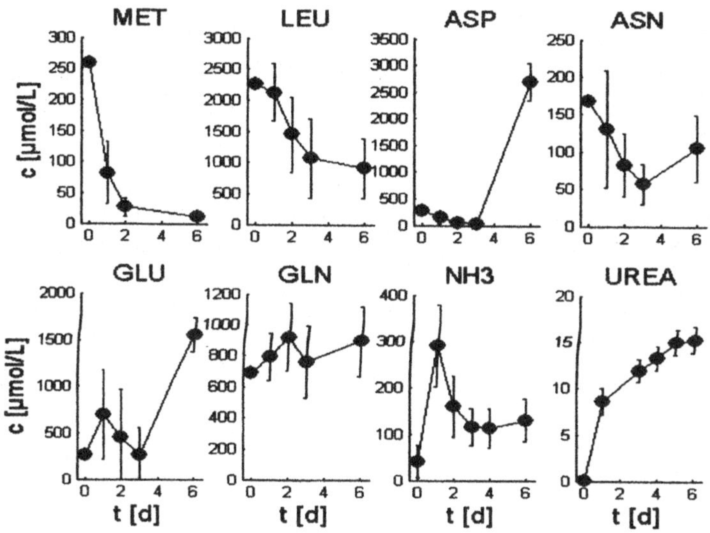

Fig. 6. Mean kinetics (±standard deviations) averaged over the 7 high performance runs for the 6 representative amino acids as well as for ammonia (NH3) and urea.

ammonia metabolism. ASP had to be included in the modeling also due to its feeding with the inflow rate $F_B(t)$.

The mean kinetics $c_{0i}(t)$ (indices i in Table 1, data in Figure 6) averaged over the high performance runs were simulated using the dynamic model (2) whose structure is graphically shown in Figure 7. It describes the ammonia assimilation via glutamine synthetase (model parameters p_8 and p_9) and via glutamate dehydrogenase (model parameter p_7; the co-substrate alpha-ketoglutarate was not measured and therefore not included in the model). The conversion of ammonia into urea was modeled in a simplified way by the reaction quantified by the model parameter p_{10} in (2). The role of ASP for urea formation from ammonia was not considered here for simplicity reasons. The asparagine synthetase was represented by the parameters p_5 and p_6 in (2). The catabolism of the essential amino acids (represented by MET and LEU) was modeled using the parameters p_2 and p_3. The efflux of amino acids (e.g. into amino acids not measured or pro-

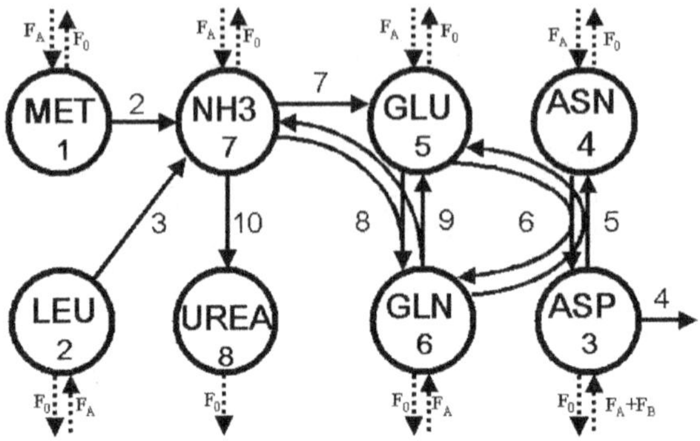

Fig. 7. Structure of model (2). The numbers within the circles denote the indices i of the corresponding concentrations c_i and the numbers at the arrows the indices m of the corresponding parameters p_m in model (2). (The diffusion process modeled by parameter p_1 is not shown).

tein biosynthesis) was postulated in the way represented by parameter p_4 taking into account the nitrogen balance in order to improve the model fit.

$$
\begin{aligned}
\frac{dc_{0i}}{dt} &= F_A(t)/V_1 \cdot c_{Ai} + F_B(t)/V_1 \cdot c_{Bi} - F_0(t)/V_1 \cdot c_{0i} - p_1/V_1 \cdot (c_{0i} - c_i) \qquad (2)\\
\frac{dc_1}{dt} &= p_1/V_2 \cdot (c_{01} - c_1) - p_2 \cdot c_1,\\
\frac{dc_2}{dt} &= p_1/V_2 \cdot (c_{02} - c_2) - p_3 \cdot c_2,\\
\frac{dc_3}{dt} &= p_1/V_2 \cdot (c_{03} - c_3) - p_4 \cdot c_3 - p_5 \cdot c_3 \cdot c_6 + p_6 \cdot c_4 \cdot c_5,\\
\frac{dc_4}{dt} &= p_1/V_2 \cdot (c_{04} - c_4) + p_5 \cdot c_3 \cdot c_6 - p_c \cdot c_4 \cdot c_5,\\
\frac{dc_5}{dt} &= p_1/V_2 \cdot (c_{05} - c_5) + p_5 \cdot c_3 \cdot c_6 - p_6 \cdot c_4 \cdot c_5 + p_7 \cdot c_7 - p_8 \cdot c_5 \cdot c_7 + p_9 \cdot c_6,\\
\frac{dc_6}{dt} &= p_1/V_2 \cdot (c_{06} - c_6) - p_5 \cdot c_3 \cdot c_6 + p_6 \cdot c_4 \cdot c_5 + p_8 \cdot c_5 \cdot c_7 - p_9 \cdot c_6,\\
\frac{dc_7}{dt} &= p_1/V_2 \cdot (c_{07} - c_7) + p_2 \cdot c_1 + p_3 \cdot c_2 - p_7 \cdot c_7 - p_8 \cdot c_5 \cdot c_7 + p_9 \cdot c_6 - 2 \cdot p_{10} \cdot c_7,\\
\frac{dc_8}{dt} &= p_1/V_2 \cdot (c_{08} - c_8) + p_{10} \cdot c_7.
\end{aligned}
$$

The biochemical reactions were assumed to be either of linear or bilinear nature (1st or 2nd order). The diffusion process of the compounds across the capillary membranes between the actual bioreactor (i.e. the reaction compartment) and the perfusion system (i.e. the supply and removal compartment) (see Sect. 2.1) was modeled for all compounds in the same way according to the first equation in (2) using the parameter p_1. The inflow and outflow rates, the volumes and concentrations are those explained in Sect. 2.1. The results of the model fit to the mean kinetics measured in the waste (Figure 6) are shown in Table 3 and Figure 8.

Table 4. Model parameters p_m identified by fitting the model (2) to the measured data.

Index m	Parameter Value for p_m	Index m	Parameter Value for p_m
1	$49.628\ d^{-1} \cdot ml$	6	$0.0050\,d^{-1} \cdot \mu mol^{-1} \cdot L$
2	$34.5261\,d^{-1}$	7	$13.8254\,d^{-1}$
3	$1.8155\,d^{-1}$	8	$0.0312\,d^{-1} \cdot \mu mol^{-1} \cdot L$
4	$26.7968\,d^{-1}$	9	$4.5403\,d^{-1}$
5	$0.0002\,d^{-1} \cdot \mu mol^{-1} \cdot L$	10	$0.2002\,d^{-1}$

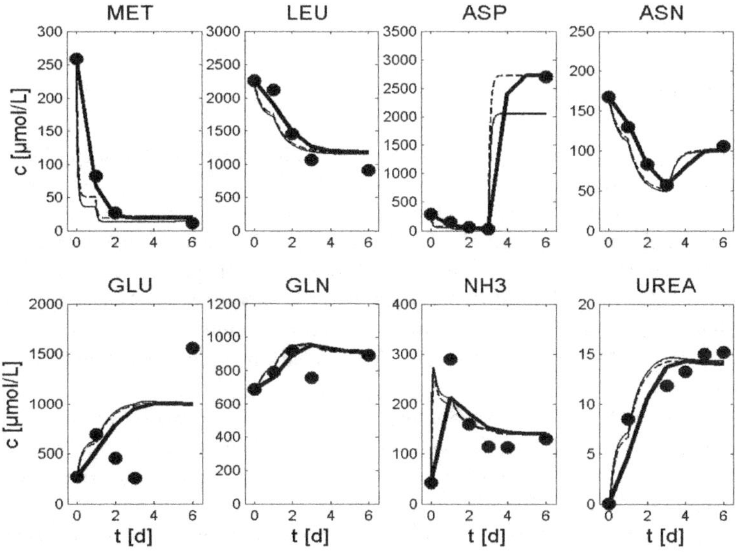

Fig. 8. Measured and simulated kinetics of the 6 representative amino acids, ammonia and urea. The measured kinetics (*dots*) are those of the mean profiles in Figure 6. The simulated kinetics ($c_i(t)$: *thin full lines*; $c_{0i}(t)$: *thin dashed lines*) are those obtained from the model (2). The simulated kinetics $c_{0i}(t)$ were averaged over the past 24 hours (*thick lines*) in order to use them to fit the model to the measurements taken from the waste (outflow accumulated over 24 h).

4 Conclusion

The kinetics of amino acids and related nitrogen-containing compounds in a liver cell bioreactor were analyzed and described using correlation networks, Bayesian networks and differential equation systems. Correlation analysis was used to identify kinetic patterns, in particular those for glutamine and arginine, that can discriminate between low and high performance bioreactor runs. Bayesian networks were applied to identify relevant compounds, such as methionine and leucine, that are suitable to predict bioreactor performance. An initial nitrogen balancing model in the form of a differential equation system has to be further improved by the inclusion of additional amino acids and proteins. The submodel developed here however represents already several aspects of metabolic interaction, such as the catabolism of amino acids to ammonia as well as the assimilation and elimination of ammonia to urea.

Acknowledgement

This work was supported by the German Federal Ministry for Education and Research BMBF within the Programme 'Systems of Life – Systems Biology' (FKZ 0313079B).

References

1. Sauer, I.M., Obermayer, N., Kardassis, D., Theruvath, T., Gerlach, J.C.: Development of a Hybrid Liver Support System. Ann. N.Y. Acad. Sci. 944 (2001) 308–319
2. Pfaff, M., Toepfer, S., Woetzel, D., Driesch, D., Zeilinger, K., Pless, G., Neuhaus, P., Gerlach, J.C., Schmidt-Heck, W., Guthke, R.: Fuzzy Cluster and Rule Based Analysis of the System Dynamics of a Bioartificial 3D Human Liver Cell Bioreactor for Liver Support Therapy. In: Dounias, G., Magoulas, G., Linkens, D. (eds.): Intelligent Technologies in Bioinformatics and Medicine. Special Session Proceedings of the EUNITE 2004 Symposium. A Publication of the University of the Aegean (2004) 57
3. D'haeseleer, P., Liang, S., Somogyi, R.: Genetic Network Inference: From Co-Expression Clustering to Reverse Engineering. Bioinformatics 16 (2000) 707–726
4. De Jong, H.: Modeling and Simulation of Genetic Regulatory Systems: A Literature Review. J. Comput. Biol. 9 (2002) 69–105
5. Pless, G., Obermayer, N., Sauer, I.M., Zeilinger, K., Buentemeyer, H., Lehmann, J., Gerlach, J.C., Neuhaus, P.: Aminosäurestoffwechselmuster humaner Leberzellen in 3-D-Hochdichtekultur. 19. Jahrestagung der Deutschen Arbeitsgemeinschaft zum Studium der Leber, Berlin (2003)
6. Arkin, A., Shen, P., Ross, J.: A Test Case of Correlation Metric Construction of a Reaction Pathway from Measurements. Science 277 (1997) 1275–1279
7. Cooper, G.F., Herskovits, E.: A Bayesian Method for the Induction of Probabilistic Networks from Data. Machine Learning 9 (1992) 309–347
8. Kitano, H. (ed.): Foundations of Systems Biology. MIT Press, Cambridge, MA (2001)
9. Schmidt-Heck, W., Guthke, R., Toepfer, S., Reischer, H., Duerrschmid, K., Bayer, K.: Reverse Engineering of the Stress Response during Expression of a Recombinant Protein. Proceedings of the EUNITE 2004 Symposiumé Verlag Mainz, Aachen (2004) 407–412
10. Ramoni, M., Sebastiani, P.: Bayesian Methods. In: Intelligent Data Analysis. An Introduction. Physica Verlag, Heidelberg (1999) 129–166. www.bayesware.com

Model Selection and Adaptation for Biochemical Pathways

Rüdiger W. Brause

J.W. Goethe-University, Computer Science Dept., 60054 Frankfurt a. M., Germany
RBrause@Informatik.uni-frankfurt.de

Abstract. In bioinformatics, biochemical signal pathways can be modeled by many differential equations. It is still an open problem how to fit the huge amount of parameters of the equations to the available data. Here, the approach of systematically obtaining the most appropriate model and learning its parameters is extremely interesting.
One of the most often used approaches for model selection is to choose the least complex model which "fits the needs". For noisy measurements, the model with the smallest mean squared error of the observed data results in a model which fits too accurately to the data – it is overfitting. Such a model will perform good on the training data, but worse on unknown data.
This paper proposes as model selection criterion the least complex description of the observed data by the model, the minimum description length MDL. For the small, but important example of inflammation modeling the performance of the approach is evaluated.

1 Introduction

In living organisms many metabolisms and immune reactions depend on specific, location-dependent interactions. Since the interactions occur in a timed transport of matter and molecules, this can be termed as a network of biochemical pathways of molecules. In Bioinformatics, these pathways or signal interactions are modeled by many differential equations. For complicated systems, differential equations systems (DES) with up to 7,000 equations and 20,000 associated parameters exist and model reality. The motivation for life science industry to use such systems is evident: A prediction of reactions and influences by simulated models helps avoiding time-consuming, expensive animal and laboratory experiments, decrease the high costs for developing new drugs and therefore may save millions of Euros. For small signal transduction networks, this has already been done by estimating the parameters by data-driven modeling of expression profiles of DNA microarrays, see e.g. [2–4]. Interestingly, no problems were reported fitting the models to the data.

Although the basic idea is quite seducing, the practical problems associated with the simulation approach are difficult to solve: How do we know that our selected model is valid and how can all parameters be set to the correct values? And if all parameters are different for each individual, how can they be adapted to the real values based only on a small set of measured data per organism?

In this paper we will try to answer some of theses questions for the example of the small but important problem of inflammation and septic shock.

J.M. Barreiro et al. (Eds.): ISBMDA 2004, LNCS 3337, pp. 439–449, 2004.

2 The Differential Equation Neural Network of Inflammation and Septic Shock

The symptoms of septic shock contain low blood pressure, high ventilation and high heart rates and may occur after an infection or a trauma (damage of tissue). The septic shock research has no convincing results yet; there is still a high mortality of about 50% on the intensive care units (ICU) and nobody knows why. It is only possible to predict the outcome for a patient in advance just for 3 days, see [5]. In 1999, about 250,000 death were associated with sepsis in the USA.

The septic shock state is produced by a confusing myriad of immune pathways and molecules. For studying the basic problems we restrict ourselves first to a simplified but still functional version of the model which uses only three variables and 12 constant parameters [6]. Let *P* be the pathogen influence, *M* the immunological response, e.g. the macrophages involved and *D* the obtained cell damage. Then, using some basic assumptions [7], we might combine them into a coupled system of three first order differential equations:

$$P'(t) = a_1(1-P)P + a_2MP \qquad \alpha_i>0 \tag{1}$$

$$M'(t) = a_3M + a_4M(1-M)P + a_5M(1-M)D \qquad \beta_i>0 \tag{2}$$

$$D'(t) = a_6D + a_7\,h(\,(M-a_9)/a_8) \qquad \chi_i>0 \tag{3}$$

The plot of the time course for the three outputs (three variables) for the set of parameters shown in is shown in Fig. 1. For this, the differential equations were numerically integrated using the Runge-Kutta method.

Table 1. The constant parameter values

$a_1 =\ 0.054$	$a_3 = -1.0$	$a_6 = -0.01$
$a_2 = -0.2155$	$a_4 =\ 5.0$	$a_7 = 0.00384$
$a_9 = 0.2018$	$a_5 = 1.0$	$a_8 = 0.1644$

It can be concluded that an infection (P) causes cell damage (D) and a delayed activity of the macrophages (M). The infection is defeated by the macrophages which decrease to a sufficient level afterwards. In this case (parameter regime), the infection remains chronically and the cell damage reaches a stable level.

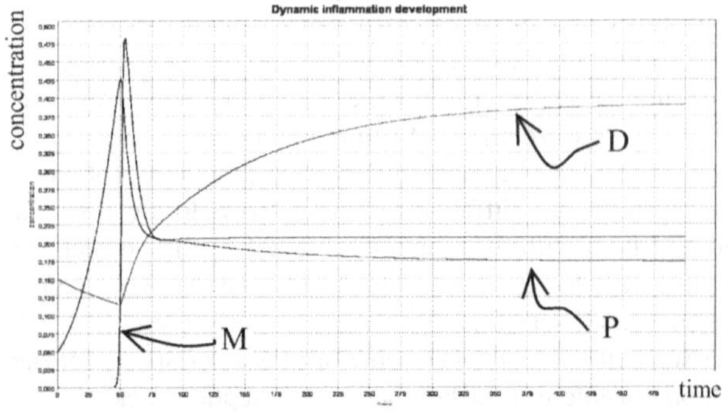

Fig. 1. The time dynamics of the equations (4),(5) and (6)

Now, how can the parameters, which correspond to the weights of the second layer, be learned? It is well known that the non-linear transfer function of deterministic chaotic systems can be efficiently be learned in order to predict a chaotic time series, see for instance [8]. Therefore, all dynamics which evolve by recurrent influence may be modeled by recurrent neural nets containing delayed signals, implemented e.g. in the discrete case by delay elements like tapped delay lines. In this case, the learning can be done by simple error reducing algorithms.

In the next section let us regard the adaptation of the parameters more closely.

3 Learning the Parameters

Generally, the biochemical pathways are very complex. It is not clear, which influences are important and which are not important. For the analytical description by equations this means that the number of terms ("model selection") and the values of its parameters ("model adaptation") are not given *a priori*, but have to be estimated ("learned") by the real observed data. How can this be done?

First, we are troubled by the fact that we do not have the full data set of Fig. 1 but only the small set of observed data given in Table 3.

This situation is different from the previous one of learning the unknown parameters: the time scales of the observed training data and of the iteration cycles are different. For instance, the dynamics of inflammation might be in the reach of hours, whereas the observed data is taken once each day.

Table 2. The observed sparse data

Time step	P	M	D
0	0.050000	0.001000	0.150000
100	0.201215	0.206079	0.254347
200	0.183751	0.206844	0.342027
300	0.177270	0.206750	0.374282
400	0.174876	0.206680	0.386141
500	0.173995	0.206649	0.390500

In Fig. 2 this situation is shown. Here, the variable y(t) changes after each time tick, but it is only measured at time points t_i.

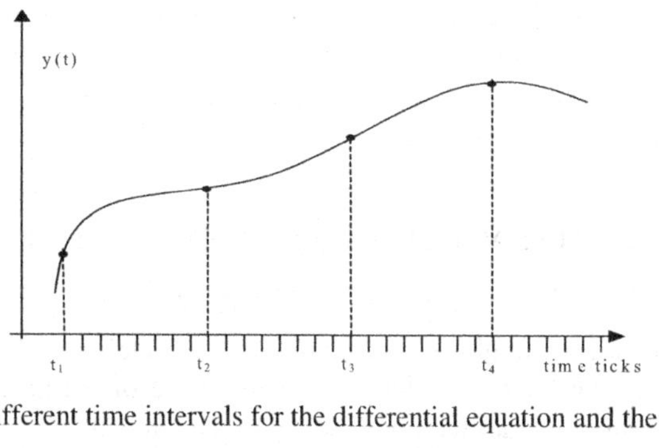

Fig. 2. The different time intervals for the differential equation and the observations

The different time scales will change heavily the approximated coefficients and difference equations, see [7]. Therefore, if we ignore the time steps between the observations and assume that system iterates once for one observation we will not be able to predict the best fitting parameters ai for the difference equations that have several time steps between the observations.

Now, how can we proceed to approximate the unknown parameters from sparse observations? Obviously, the direct approach of a gradient descend for reducing the mean squared error between a simulated time sequence and an observed one used for instance in chaotic time sequence parameter estimation [8] is not possible here because we have no knowledge of the intermediate samples.

Instead, let us consider a variant of the classical evolutionary approach as it was introduced by Rechenberg 1973 [7], see [10].

- Generate a new set of random weights numerically by incrementing the old value with a random number, e.g. a Gaussian deviation.
- test it: does it decrease the objective function?
- If no, inverse the sign of the increment and test it: does it decrease the objective function?
- If no, take the old weight values and choose another weight set.
- Continue until the error has sufficiently decreased or the number of iterations has exceeded a predefined maximum.

In order to avoid getting stuck in a suboptimum, the whole process might be repeated several times using different random starts.

The advantage of this approach is its independency of the complexity of the objective function. The disadvantage is its high computational burden: we have to recompute the objective function each time we change only one parameter, and we can not adapt the step width in advance. Nevertheless, for a given DES and given observed data this approach shows good performance, see [7].

For a given model, this is fine. If the model is not given we are in trouble: How should we select the model and adapt the parameters at the same time? The initial idea of first adapting the parameters and then selecting the model by pruning all terms that has very small parameter values might work. Consider for instance our model of eqs. (1),(2),(3). We might add the following ideas:

- If the pathogen influence (microbes) is present at the location where cell damage occurs, the pathogen influence will be increased: $P' \sim PD$
- Macrophages will die due to toxic influence of microbes, proportional to the co-occurrence probability and the microbe concentration : $M' \sim -P^2M$

These two possible extensions of the model will be translated into the modified differential equations

$$P'(t) = a_1(1-P)P + a_2MP + a_{10}PD \tag{4}$$

$$M'(t) = a_3M + a_4M(1-M)P + a_5M(1-M)D + a_{11}P^2M \tag{5}$$

$$D'(t) = a_6D + a_7\,h((M-a_9)/a_8) \tag{6}$$

On the other hand, we might have a more simple model in reality than we expect. For instance, we might have a model without influence of variable D to variable M, i.e. $a_5 = 0$, or a changed model with both $a_{10},a_{11}\neq 0$ and $a_5 = 0$.

With these ideas, we have now four different possible models. How can we decide which model is implemented by reality? How can we choose the best model?

4 Model Selection

The choice of the model is important for all diagnosis and therapies of the septic process. First, we have to discuss several possibilities for selecting the appropriate model and then we will select one strategy of our choice.

4.1 Model Selection by Parameter Pruning

As the first, naïve approach let us consider the case where we have the pure differential equations (1),(2),(3) or (4),(5),(6) encountering no noise and we have recorded observation samples. How do we know which model is the right one for the observations? In this case, we might expect that the additional terms produce an error in modeling the observations. In the other way, reducing the error in the parameter adaptation process might result in setting the unnecessary parameters to zero, if they exist: the describing model is automatically tailored to the observed data.

Strategy 1: Adapt the parameters of the most complex model. All unnecessary parameters will automatically become zero and can be pruned.

Let us make an experiment to review this approach. For a time series produced by equations (1),(2),(3) we start the adaptation process, once for the small model of equations (1),(2),(3) and once for the augmented model of or equations (4),(5),(6). Now, what parameter values will we encounter for the new parameters a_{10} and a_{11}? We expect them to become zero. For good starting points and short approximation runs, this is true. Even for k = 1000 cycles the deviations are not huge: in Table 3 the mean squared error is shown for a certain number of cycles, once with the additional terms clamped to zero (i.e. without the terms) and once with the terms.

Table 3. The modeling error and the development of additional parameter terms

k	MSE	a_{10}	a_{11}
1,000	2.4633 **E-7**	0.0	0.0
	7.6321 **E-7**	0,006796	0,645184
10,000	2.2348 **E-9**	0.0	0.0
	3.9750 **E-7**	0,004453	0,549848

We observe that in the long run the approximation with additional terms does not improve while the correct model does. How can this be explained? The additional interactions that are caused by the additional parameters a_{10} and a_{11} in the augmented model will produce small disturbances that will deviate the approximation process: the approximation will slow down in relation to the non-augmented model which fits well to the observed data. This is shown in Fig. 3.

This might inspire us to the second strategy:

Strategy 2: Adapt the parameters of all models. Select the model, which converges best.

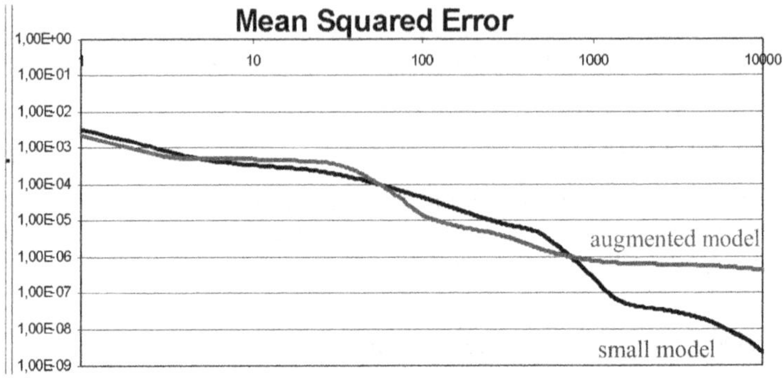

Fig. 3. The error development with and without additional terms

Do we have discovered a good selection criterion for the model? The answer is no: the additional interactions slow the convergence down, but the inverse is also true for too simple models which can not approximate the observed samples well, but initially converge faster than the true model.

Additionally, in nearly almost all natural systems we encounter noise that is not considered in this approach. So, we have to relay on other approaches.

4.2 Model Selection by Minimum Description Length

In the previous section we have seen that the convergence of the parameters cannot automatically replace the model selection process. Instead, we have to evaluate the performance of each model, i.e. each form of DES separately related to the observed time course samples. What kind of performance measure should we choose? We know that the deviation of the samples to the predicted values, the mean squared error, is not a good approach: by the additional parameters the more complex models will tend to overfit on adapting to the observed values perfectly whereas the best model will produce sample differences within the variance of the samples. This leads to our

Strategy 3: Adapt the parameters of all models to fit the observed data. Select the model which gives the shortest description of the observed data, on average and asymptotically.

So, we are looking for a model which neither fits too good nor too bad and needs only a small amount of information to describe the observations. How do we evaluate this?

Let us formalize our problem: For each of the *k* subjects and each variable, we observe values at different time steps t_1, t_2, …,t_n. For example as shown in Fig. 4, we might measure the dynamics at four times. All the four samples of one subject might be grouped together in one set. The set of observations for one subject is called a sample $\mathbf{x} = (x_1,\ldots,x_n)$ of all possible observations $\{\mathbf{x}\}$. Each model m which has been fit to the sample also produces by simulation a sample $\mathbf{f} = (f_1,\ldots,f_n)$ for the designated *n* time steps.

The deviation of the i-th observed sample $\mathbf{x}(i)$ from its adapted model $\mathbf{f}(i)$ of the same type is for all time steps $t = 1\ldots N$ its empirical variance [11]

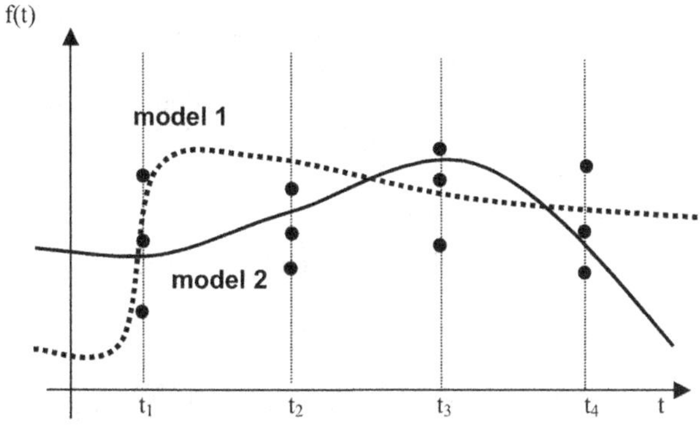

Fig. 4. Selecting the best fitting model

$$\sigma_i^2 = \frac{1}{N-1}\sum_{t=1}^{N}(x_t(i) - f_t(i))^2 = \frac{1}{N-1}(x(i) - f(i))^2 . \tag{7}$$

Observing S subjects, the variance for all subjects from their approximated models is

$$\sigma^2 = \sum_{i=1}^{S}\sigma_i^2 . \tag{8}$$

Since each sample of each subject contain measurements at the same time period, we might draw these samples together in one chart as it is done in Fig. 4.

Assuming that the deviations at each time step are differently distributed, i.e. time dependent, we might compute the variance for one time step *t* for the set of all observed subjects to all models *i* by

$$\sigma_t^2 = \frac{1}{S-1}\sum_{i=1}^{S}(x_t(i) - f_t(i))^2 \text{ and } \sigma^2 = \sum_{t=1}^{N}\sigma_t^2 . \tag{9}$$

Now, we might analyze the system by two different approaches:

- Either we have only one model for all subjects. Then, all samples are random deviations of the true model sample **f**. We select as best model the one which best "fits the data ". Biologically, the approach of only one fixed model is improbable.
- Or we assume a different model **f**(i) for each subject *i*. This means that either the parameters of m are different or even the basic model type m might be different. Then, each observed sample **x**(i) deviate slightly from the best fitting model sample **f**(i). As best model m* we might select the one which, after the individual parameter adaptation, "fits best" for all subjects.

Now, in order to evaluate the fitting of the model we have to compute the description length L of the data, given the model. This is the average information of the data. It can be shown that the description length L, is bounded below by the entropy of the probability distribution of the data set X

$$L \geq H(X)$$

Thus, the minimal description length of the data is obtained for the model which provides the smallest entropy of the observed data. For normally distributed data according to [13], we know that for the compound random variable X we have

$$H(X) = \ln \sqrt{(2\pi e)^n \det C_{XX}} \ .$$

For uncorrelated samples **x** we have

$$\det C_{XX} \approx \prod_t \sigma_t^2$$

and therefore

$$H(X,m) = \tfrac{1}{2} \ln (2\pi e)^n + \tfrac{1}{2} \ln \prod_t \sigma_t^2(m) = A + \tfrac{1}{2} \sum_{t=1}^{n} \ln \sigma_t^2(m) \ . \tag{10}$$

Therefore, the best model m* is the one which minimizes H(X,m), i.e. which has the smallest variances for all time steps.

The information can be measured for two cases: the situation for training and the situation for testing. For training, we have the mean squared error between the observations of the training sample and those of the model sample, averaged over all variables *v* and all models *k* of the same type

$$MSE_{train} = \frac{1}{S \cdot m \cdot N} \sum_{k=1}^{S} \sum_{v=1}^{m} \sum_{t=1}^{N} \left(x_t(k,v) - f_t(k,v)\right)^2 \ . \tag{11}$$

For the test case, we compare the model sample with all other possible observations, i.e. the rest of the training set, also averaged over all variables and all models of the same type

$$MSE_{test} = \frac{1}{S \cdot m \cdot N \cdot (S-1)} \sum_{k=1}^{S} \sum_{v=1}^{m} \sum_{t=1}^{N} \sum_{j \neq k} \left(x_t(j) - f_t(k)\right)^2 \ . \tag{12}$$

For the two cases, the information of eq.(10) is averaged over all models *k* of same type m and variables *v* and becomes

$$H(m) = \langle H(k,v) \rangle_{k,v} = \frac{1}{S} \sum_{k=1}^{S} \frac{1}{m} \sum_{v=1}^{m} \left(\tfrac{1}{2} N \cdot \ln (2\pi e) + \tfrac{1}{2} \sum_{t=1}^{n} \ln \sigma_t^2(k,v) \right)$$

with $$\sigma_t^2(k,v) = \left(x_t(k,v) - f_t(k,v) \right)^2 \qquad \textit{for training} \tag{13}$$

or $$\sigma_t^2(k,v) = \frac{1}{S-2} \sum_{j \neq k}^{S} \left(x_t(j,v) - f_t(k,v) \right)^2 \qquad \textit{for testing} \ . \tag{14}$$

Therefore, we get for the averaged information *H* of a model of type m

$$H(m) = \frac{1}{S \cdot m \cdot N} \sum_{k=1}^{S} \sum_{v=1}^{m} \sum_{t=1}^{N} \ln(\sigma_t^2(k,v)) + \frac{N}{2} \ln(2\pi e) \ . \tag{15}$$

5 Evaluating the Data Simulations

For the simulation, we generated four data files for two different model types and *M* = 10 subjects. The *M* individually generated time courses start with the same initial values, but differentiate in the following aspects:

- All subjects have the same standard model parameters and all observations are the same.
- All subjects have the same standard model parameters, but the observations have random deviations (N(0,0.02) distribution) of the true values.
- All subjects have individual, different model parameters (N(0,0.001) distribution); the observations are the true values.
- All subjects have individual, different model parameters; but the observations have random deviations of the true values.

These four model assumptions are used to generate four observation files. Each set of observations contain n = 5 sampled values of all three variables for each of the M = 10 subjects.

The four data files of observations are analyzed by four different model types:

m_1) The smaller model with $a_5 = 0$.

m_2) The "standard" model with $a_5 \neq 0$ and $a_{10}, a_{11} = 0$.

m_3) The augmented model with $a_5, a_{10}, a_{11} \neq 0$.

m_4) The changed (dropped and added terms) model with $a_{10}, a_{11} \neq 0$ and $a_5 = 0$.

Each of the four observation files is used to adapt the parameters of each of the M = 10 subjects of the same model type to the observations by the evolutionary method described in section 3. So, we get 16 result sets for 10 subjects each.

For each adaptation try we use 100 cycles of adapting all parameters in order to minimize the mean squared error R between the model prediction and the observations. For each subject, 10 tries are performed and the one with the smallest R is recorded in order to avoid getting stuck in a suboptimum. After adaptation, the performance of the models was evaluated by computing the minimum description length, i.e. entropy H for the model adaptations. The evaluated values for the entropy H for the four model types m_1, m_2, m_3, m_4 adapting to the data of the four observed situations a),b),c) and d) are presented in table 1. The results of the standard model is shown in bold face.

What can we conclude by these results?

Keeping in mind that m_2 is the standard model type that was used to produce all data, we see that this model type has the smallest entropy of all other models in the context of cases a) and b) – it turns out as the best model to select. Therefore, our model selection criterion is valid in our example.

For cases c) and d) of different parameter regimes and random deviations the smaller model fits slightly better to the data. Why? The reason behind is that the random deviations and the systematic deviations are in the same range; for only a small number of observations for one individual (N = 6) the difference becomes hard to detect: the proposed method reaches its limits.

Here we encounter a fundamental problem of data modeling: how do we know that for a given observation variance the number of observed data points are sufficient to select a model properly? What difference of complexity should be taken as argument for a model to be more valid than another one? Theses questions are still open for research.

Table 4. The evaluated observations for N = 6 samples

Simulation	Model	MSE train	MSE test	H train	H test
a) 1	1	1.4686 E-4	1.4686 E-4	3.3993	3.2162
2	**2**	**4.6640 E-4**	**4.6640 E-4**	**3.5141**	**3.3310**
3	3	2.4891 E-3	2.4891 E-3	4.5359	4.3528
4	4	4.8081 E-2	4.8081 E-2	5.4169	5.2338
b) 5	1	2.0826 E-3	2.2171 E-3	4.3146	4.2963
6	**2**	**8.2153 E-4**	**1.0491 E-3**	**4.2346**	**4.2163**
7	3	4.2131 E-2	4.2006 E-2	4.7925	4.7742
8	4	1.0672 E-2	1.0916 E-2	4.9448	4.9264
c) 9	1	2.7123 E-4	5.3854 E-3	3.5523	3.3692
10	**2**	**2.5080 E-3**	**7.5664 E-3**	**3.7953**	**3.6122**
11	3	3.5737 E-3	8.4245 E-3	4.2872	4.1041
12	4	3.0380 E-2	3.3430 E-2	5.1236	4.9405
d) 13	1	1.3788 E-2	2.3057 E-2	5.4111	5.3744
14	**2**	**1.3771 E-2**	**2.3096 E-2**	**5.4219**	**5.3853**
15	3	4.9014 E-2	5.9496 E-2	5.3382	5.3016
16	4	6.9419 E-2	7.7748 E-2	5.5937	5.5571

6 Discussion

Data driven modeling is an important attempt to rationalize the efforts of creating models guided not by assumptions but by reality. The paper shows some of the problems involved in this kind of modeling and proposes the minimum description length of the observed data as selection criterion.

For the small but important problem of inflammation and septic shock differential equations we consider four different models types: a standard model, the model with one term dropped, the model with two additional terms and a changed model. These four models are confronted with synthetic data, generated by random versions of the standard model. Here, all four possible model types converge more or less fast to fit the data; no terms can be pruned due to small parameter values; an automatic tailoring of the model to the data is not possible.

Thus, the model selection can neither be based on the convergence speed nor on the "complexity" of the formulas (is a multiplication more complex than an addition?) but have to be based on another criterion. In this paper we chose the minimum description length MDL of the data using the model as performance criterion. Assuming normally distributed deviations we computed the entropy as lower limit of the MDL by using the observed variance between the adapted models and the observed data. The simulation results validated our approach: The analyzing model describes the data with the lowest MDL if data generation model type and analyzing model type coincide.

Nevertheless, for a small amount of observed data, many different parameter regimes of the same model type and many random deviations the difference between the models cannot be detected by the MDL criterion any more. Here, more problem-specific information is needed.

References

1. Brause R., Hanisch E., Paetz J., Arlt B.: The MEDAN project: results and practical meanings, 3. Int. Symposium "*Sepsis, SIRS, Immune Response - Concepts, Diagnostics and Therapy*", A. Nierhaus, J. Schulte am Esch (Eds.), PABST Science Publishers, Lengerich, Germany, pp.122-129, (2003)
2. D'haeseleer, P.; Liang, S.; Somogyi, R. *Genetic network inference: from co-expression clustering to reverse engineering*. Bioinformatics 16, 707-26. (2000)
3. Steffen, M., Petti, A., D'haeseleer, P., Aach, J., and Church, G.M. *Automated Modeling of Signal Transduction Networks*. BMC Bioinformatics 3:34-44. (2002)
4. Yeung, M.K.; Tegner J.; Collins, J.J. *Reverse engineering gene networks using singular value decomposition and robust regression*. Proc Natl Acad Sci USA. 99, 6163-8. (2002)
5. Paetz J., Brause R.: "A Frequent Patterns Tree Approach for Rule Generation with Categorical Septic Shock Patient Data"; in: J. Crespo, V. Maojo, F. Martin, *Medical Data Analysis*, Springer Verlag Berlin Heidelberg, pp.207-212, (2001)
6. Chow C.: Development of a Dynamical Systems Model of Acute Inflammation, E. Neugebauer: 2nd workshop on complex systems: *Analysis in Shock and Trauma Research*, University of Cologne, (2003)
7. Brause R.: *Adaptive modeling of biochemical pathways*. IEEE 15th Int. Conf on Tools with Art. Intell. ICTAI-2003, IEEE Press 2003, pp.62-68, (2003)
8. Lapedes A., Farber R.: "How Neural Nets Work"; Report LA-UR-88-418, Los Alamos Nat. Lab. 1988; and in Y.C. Lee (Ed.): *Evolution, Learning and Cognition*; World Scientific, Singapore, New Jersey, London (1988)
9. Rechenberg I.: *Evolutionsstrategie*; problemata frommann-holzboog, (1973)
10. Schwefel H.-P.: *Evolution and Optimum Seeking*, J.Wiley, (1995)
11. Bronstein I.N. et al., *Handbook of Mathematics*, Van Nostrand Reinhold; 3rd edition (1991)
12. Hansen M., Yu B.: *Model selection and the principle of Minimum Description Length*, Journal of the American Statistical Association, Vol.96 (454),pp. 746-774, (2001)
13. Cover T., Thomas J.: *Elements of Information Theory*, John Wiley, New York (1991)

NeoScreen: A Software Application for MS/MS Newborn Screening Analysis

Miguel Pinheiro[1], José Luís Oliveira[1,*], Manuel A.S. Santos[1], Hugo Rocha[2], M. Luis Cardoso[2], and Laura Vilarinho[2]

[1] Universidade de Aveiro, IEETA/DET, 3810 193 Aveiro, Portugal
[2] Instituto de Genética Médica Jacinto de Magalhães, Porto, Portugal

Abstract. The introduction of the Tandem Mass Spectrometry (MS/MS), in neonatal screening laboratories, has opened the doors to innovative newborn screening analysis. With this technology the number of metabolic disorders, that can be detected, from dried blood-spot species, increases significantly. However, the amount of information obtained with this technique and the pressure for quick and accurate diagnostics raises serious difficulties in the daily data analysis. To face this challenge we developed a software system, NeoScreen, which simplifies and allow speeding up newborn screening diagnostics.

Keywords: Newborn Screening Software, MS/MS
Paper Domain: Health bioinformatics and genomics Statistical methods and tools for biological and medical data analysis

1 Introduction

In the last few years the advances in Tandem Mass Spectrometry (MS/MS) technology had led to its introduction in neonatal screening laboratories [1, 2] . This screening is intended to detect inborn disorders that can result in early mortality or lifelong disability. Significant challenges still remain since it implies a significant financial effort, a change in the way of thinking the diagnosis of inborn errors of metabolism (IEM) and the need to manage and process a massive amount of data.

The introduction of MS/MS in the Portuguese national neonatal screening lab (with over 110.000 samples/year) has led to the development of a new application, NeoScreen, that can help technicians to handle the large amount of data involved (with more than 80 parameters/sample) and can assist in the implementation of a reliable quality control procedure.

The application consists of an information system supported by mathematical and statistical tools that automate the evaluation data procedure. These processing tools allow a daily update of marker cut-offs through the use of percentile scores of valid historical data. It is possible to define mathematical expressions over existing markers, allowing to check combinations that are responsible for specific diseases [3]. The user interface is constructed upon familiar paradigms simplifying the usage of the application.

Concerning results validity, NeoScreen software guarantees an effective control of internal standards intensities as well as quality control (QC) samples values. This

* Contact Author: José Luís Oliveira, Universidade de Aveiro, IEETA/DET, 3810 193 Aveiro, Portugal, Email: jlo@det.ua.pt, Tel : +351 234 370 523.

J.M. Barreiro et al. (Eds.): ISBMDA 2004, LNCS 3337, pp. 450–457, 2004.

automatic facility can be yet complemented by the construction of longitudinal histograms, with the values of QC samples and average values of all daily sample markers, allowing a better understand of their evolution over time.

2 MS/MS Screening of Inherited Metabolic Diseases

Tandem Mass Spectrometry

Tandem mass spectrometers allow the rapid analysis of individual compounds in complex mixtures [4, 5]. MS/MS systems are composed by two analytical quadrupoles (MS1 and MS2) joined by a collision cell (Figure 1).

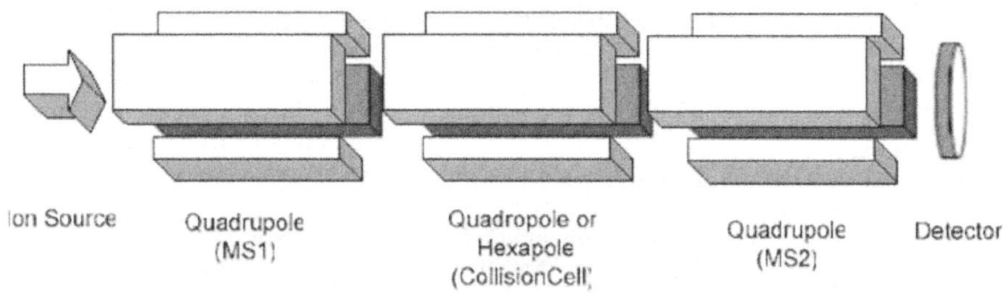

Fig. 1. Schematic representation of a triple quadrupole Tandem Mass Spectrometer

First, the injection projects the elements that will be analyzed. Both analytical quadrupoles can be configured independently, either to scan a mass range or to select/reject ions of a specific mass-to-charge ratio (m/z). After the MS1 selection the collision cell is used to further breakdown the ions, using a neutral gas (e.g., nitrogen), and transmit them to second analytical quadrupole (MS2). Finally, the detector gathers the spectra ions spectrum according to two axes (mass-to-charge ratio versus number of ions).

For acylcarnitine profiling, for instance, MS1 scans a defined mass range and MS2 is set to transmit only fragment ions with a specific m/z value, 85, following collision-activated fragmentation. This way, the data system correlates each detected ion to its respective precursor scanned in MS1 (precursor or parent ion scan).

In a neutral loss experiment spectrum includes only those compounds that fragment with a common neutral loss (a behavior that indicates they belong to a family of structurally related compounds). This mode of operation is used for the generation of amino acid profiles.

However, the concentrations of a few selected amino acids are more accurately measured when taking advantage of a MS/MS analysis in selected reaction monitoring (SRM) mode, where the selection of a parent ion in MS1 is followed by a similar process for a specific fragment ion in MS2. The resulting signal corresponds, exclusively, to the transition from parent to product ion, a process virtually free of any interference regardless of the specimen analyzed [6].

Newborn Screening

The first newborn screening test was developed by Dr. Robert Guthrie aiming the detection of elevated levels of phenylalanine using a bacterial inhibition assay, best known as the Guthrie Test [7]. While still in use in a few laboratories, most testing is done today using immuno-and enzymatic assays [8]. In the 1980s, MS/MS was initially introduced in clinical laboratories for the selective screening for inborn errors of fatty acid and organic acid metabolism. Over the last decade, this technology has been applied to newborn screening because it is open to population-wide testing for a large number of disorders of fatty acid, organic acid and amino acid metabolism [9, 10].

Table 1. Diagnosed diseases using technology MS/MS with effectiveness of early treatment [8].

Disorders of amino acid metabolism	Disorders of organic acid metabolism	Disorders of fatty acid transport &mitochondrial oxidation
Phenylketonuria	GlutaricAcidemia-1 (GA-1)	Carnitine transport defect
Maple Syrup Urine Disease (MSUD)	Propionic Acidemia	medium-chain acyl-CoA dehydrogenase (MCAD) deficiency
Tyrosinemia type I	Methylmalonic Acidemias	short-chain 3-ketoacyl-CoA thiolase (SKAT) deficiency
Tyrosinemia type II	Isovaleric Acidemia	Riboflavin responsive form(s) (GA2)
Citrullinemia	3-Methylcrotonyl-CoA carboxylase (3MCC)	deficiency
Argininosuccinic aciduria (ASA)	Multiple Carboxylase deficiency	
Argininemia		

Newborn testing with MS/MS starts with the same steps used in more traditional methods. A small amount of blood is taken from a newborn within the first 2 - 6 postnatal days and is absorbed onto a piece of filter paper. This sample is sent to the laboratory, where a small disk is punched out from the spot and loaded into a multiwell plate, where it is extracted with various solvents.

The QC samples (as for example CDC controls[1]), which contain known concentrations of metabolites, are introduced in the plates. Besides QC samples it is also usual to monitor the intensity of the internal standards. This information is of great importance to validate sample analysis.

Once the molecules in the sample are injected into the triple quadrupole MS/MS they are analyzed in 2.5 minute runs. The ion patterns are then analyzed by comparing the intensities of sample peaks with those of the internal standards using peak identification and pattern recognition software. This information is then saved in tabular files for later analyses.

The Portuguese Scenario

The national newborn diagnosis program started in Portugal in May 1979 with the screening of the Phenylketonuria, followed in 1981 by the congenital hypothyroidism

1 The Centers for Disease Control and Prevention (CDC), in partnership with the Association of Public Health Laboratories (APHL), operates the Newborn Screening Quality Assurance Program (NSQAP) [11, 12]. Their program continually strives to produce certified dried-blood-spot materials for reference and quality control analysis, to improve the quality of the analyzes, and to provide consultative assistance [11]. They produce dried blood-spot materials for amino acids and acylcarnitines quality control and proficiency testing purposes.

[13]. Between 1987 and 1995 they were performed pilot tests of the Congenital adrenal hyperplasia, Biotinidase deficiency and Cystic fibrosis, which were later abandoned because they did not offer new advantages to the population.

Until now, there were more than 2 million newborn screened and more than 1000 cases detected.

Presently 99.5% on Portuguese newborns are screened and the average time of the starting of the treatment is of 12,5 days, which represents a solid implementation of the screening at a national level [13].

With the recent introduction of MS/MS (Two API2000 from Applied Biosystems) in the Portuguese national neonatal screening program, it will be possible, in a short time, diagnose twenty new metabolic diseases, decreasing morbidity and mortality associated to these disorders due to presymptomatic diagnosis or even proceed to an in time genetic advice. However, the usage of this new technology brings problems at an information management level. The use of this technology in Portugal with more than 110.000 samples per year, containing each sample more than 80 parameters, has culminated in the development of a innovative application that reprocesses the data generated by ChemoViewNT (PE Sciex). NeoScreen helps technicians handling not only the huge amount of data involved but also helps to assure the effective quality control of the data.

3 NeoScreen – A Software Application for Screening of Inherited of Metabolic Diseases

Due to the necessity of managing a huge amount of information produced by the MS/MS, to assist the technicians in the diagnostic, and to speed up the screening processes, we have developed the NeoScreen application. The software architecture is based upon four main blocks: Acquisition, Processing, Visualization and Configuration (Figure 2).

The Acquisition, reads the data presented in data files (generated by ChemoView – PE Sciex), tests whether the markers are present in the database (DB), tests if individuals standards intensities are within the limits and confirms and presents the QC samples.

The Processing compares values of the markers in each individual with the limits for each marker and defines if the marker is in or out the established range. Later it analyses individual samples, testing for the presence of possible diseases, keeping all the information in the NeoScreen DB. It also performs a control test, in which all the average values of all daily sample markers and QC samples are analysed in different perspectives: daily evolution, average and standard deviation. Any significant deviation from normal historical values will triggers an alarm to the user.

The Visualization block allows different representations of the data recorded in the DB. The user can verify the diagnosis for each individual, confirming the suspicious and non-suspicious diseases and navigating throughout the markers reported for a newborn. One also has the possibility of consulting the evolution of the daily averages of the concentrations of the markers and QC samples, using histogram specially constructed for each marker and controls.

Within the Configuration block the user has the possibility to define the laboratory spectrometers (since for different systems we can have different results), define markers, algorithms for identification of diseases and QC samples used. This facility provides a dynamic adaptation of NeoScreen to new markers, controls and new screening diseases, according to the state of the art.

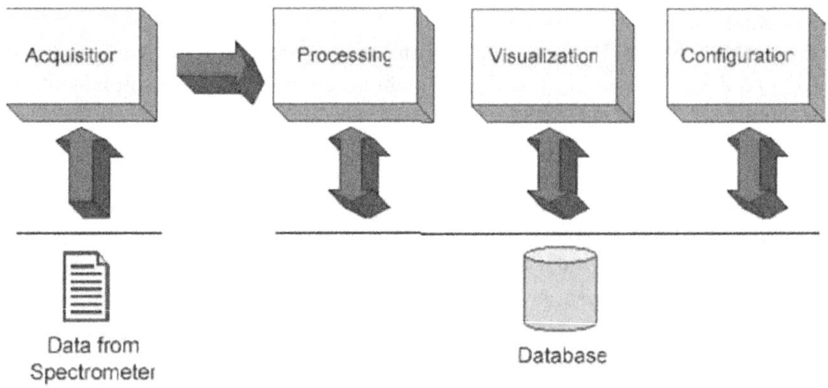

Fig. 2. Architecture of the NeoScreen software

One of the main objectives for developing this application was the simplification of technician's daily procedures. So, the user interaction was the primary priority in the design of this system. We have adopted a well know and used paradigm – the File Explorer interface (Figure 3) – and improved it with a rich set of graphical views.

Considering the program main window (Figure 3), in the left frame, it is presented a tree showing the results from a specific search in the database (date range). In this view, the individuals are separated in several diagnostic categories, such as "very suspicious", "suspicious", "not suspicious", etc. Some of these categories represent individuals with markers out of the established limits, but that are not associated with any known disease. Within this box, the user can also have access to several histograms to visualize the average evolution and the standard deviation of the QC samples and markers.

The middle frame represents the marker values from the selected sample and is synchronized with the navigation performed in the left window.

In the right frame it is displayed the relevant information that was extracted and processed by the software for each individual, like: plate information, markers concentrations, and suspicious diseases. With this information the technician can make the diagnosis, confirming the suspicion of one or several diseases (the final decision is always from the user) and printing reports resulting from this analysis.

A sample of the application functionalities is shown in Figure 4 in particular the ones related with configuration tasks. The A window shows the interface that allows to create new markers. The application already has a set of pre-defined markers of acilcarnitynes and amino acids. The markers concentrations cut-offs may be defined in one of two ways: with absolute scores or with percentile scores, obtained from valid historical data. The intensity check box assures that a minimum intensity of standards is needed in order to considerer this sample in the evaluation process. During this process, a signal will be activated if the concentration, during the data acquisition, is inferior to the established minimum. In this case the user will have to repeat the analysis of this individual in the MS/MS due to a control of intensity failure.

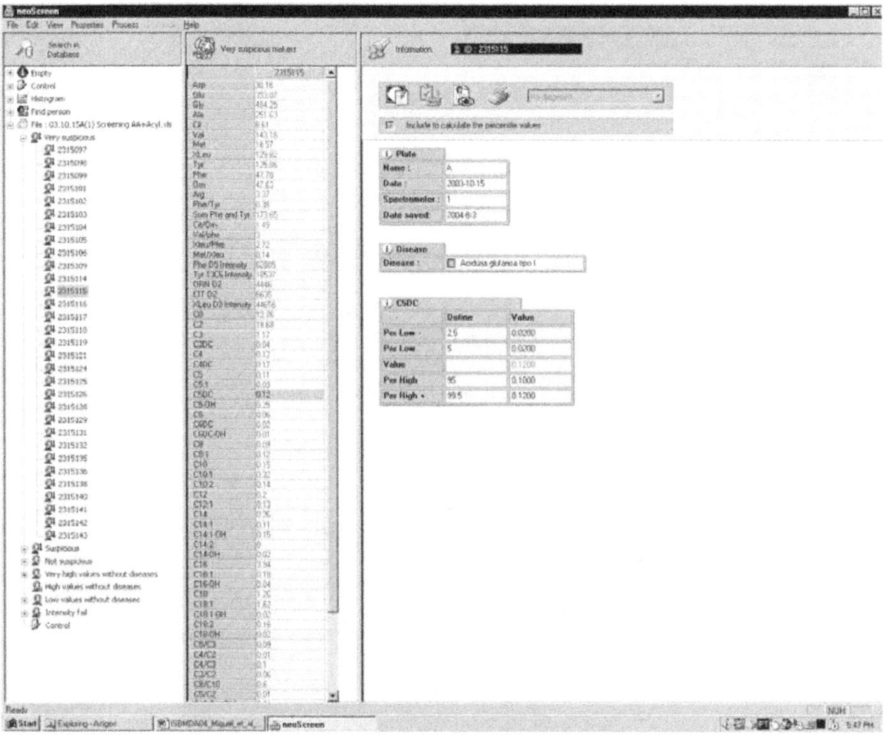

Fig. 3. NeoScreen main window

In Figure 4B window the user can define the diseases to search for as well as the markers algorithms for each one. It is possible to specify the marker limits (upper, lower or both) that indicate when a disease is probably present.

The interface represented in C provides a mathematical expressions editor that allow to create new expression markers ((C16+C18)/C0, for instance). These expressions will be then automatically processed by the system and will be available for subsequent analysis.

In the Figure 4D interface the user has the possibility of building rules for reference ranges, which later will be confronted with the data imported from ChemoView. The rules are built by the markers present in the system. The user defines the values for the percentile if the marker is defined as such. Defines the cutoffs of a marker if this is defined as having pre set values or a minimum value in case of the standards intensities.

The user can define as many rules as he/she finds necessary. The cut-offs of percentile are diary calculated for all the set rules, according to valid historical data.

4 Results

The system is being tested at Portuguese national newborn screening laboratory, located at Unidade de Biologia Clínica of Instituto de Genética Médica Jacinto de Magalhães.

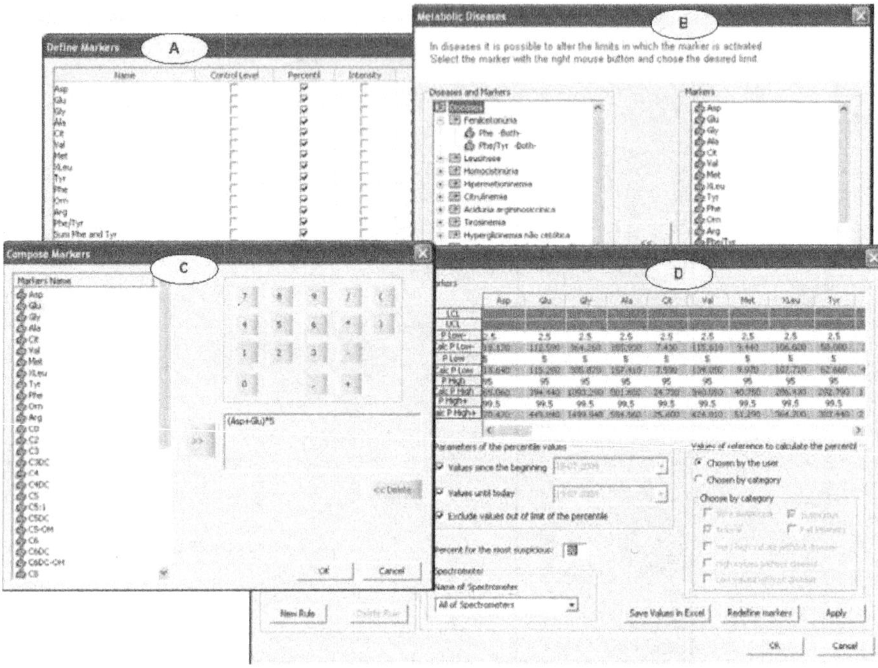

Fig. 4. Multiple overlapped windows that show some of the NeoScreen facilites

The tests made to the NeoScreen performance involve the retrospective analyses of thousands of normal newborn screening samples as well as pathological ones. From the tests preformed so far it is clear the user friendliness of the system as well as it great flexibility.

Regarding the identification of possible pathological samples, the system revealed to be precise and robust, being the accuracy obviously dependent on the user ability in defining the disease algorithms and types of cut off limits. The analyses of huge amounts of samples revealed to be quick, but always controlled by the operator.

From the quality control point of view this application revealed to be very useful in controlling all the parameters to assure the quality of the results.

5 Conclusions

The introduction of Tandem Mass Spectrometry technology in neonatal screening programs allows an enhanced detection of inborn disorders and will result in a decrease mortality and disability, if a treatment is promptly initiated. However, the massive amount of data that is generated and the need for accurate and expeditious diagnostics raises significant challenges to laboratories experts. The NeoScreen application provides an integrated solution to manage the data gathered in such labs and assist the technicians in the screening process. The application imports data files into a database, organizes and maintains this information through the time and provides a set of statistical, mathematical and graphical tools that allows the automation of the newborn diagnosis. The system is completely reconfigurable to assure that new markers, new diseases, and new parameters can be created when necessary. The system is starting being used in the Portuguese neonatal screening program (in the IGM, Porto) and we expect that, during the next months, others centers will benefit from its functionalities.

References

1. S. A. Banta-Wright and R. D. Steiner, "Tandem Mass Spectrometry in Newborn Screening: A Primer for Neonatal and Perinatal Nurses", *Journal of Perinatal and Neonatal Nursing*, vol. 18, no. 1, pp. 41-60, 2004.
2. K. H. Carpenter and V. Wiley, "Application of tandem mass spectrometry to biochemical genetics and newborn screening", *Clinica Chimica Acta, Elsevier Science*, vol. 322, pp. 1-10, 2002.
3. D. H. Chace, J. E. Sherwin, S. L. Hillman, F. Lorey, and G. C. Cunningham, "Use of phenylalanine-to-tyrosine ratio determined by tandem mass spectrometry to improve newborn screening for phenylketonuria of early discharge specimens collected in the first 24 hours", *Clinical Chemistry*, vol. 12, no. 44, pp. 2405–2409, 1998.
4. E. W. Naylor, H. Donald, and D. H. Chace, "Automated Tandem Mass Spectrometry for Mass Newborn Screening for Disorders in Fatty Acid, Organic Acid and Amino Acid Metabolism", *Child Neurol*, vol. 14, pp. S1S4, 1999.
5. ACMG/ASHG Working Group, "Tandem mass spectrometry in newborn screening", vol. 2, no. 4, pp. 267-269, 2002.
6. D. Matern and M. J. Magera, "Mass Spectrometry Methods for Metabolic and Health Assessment", *American Society for Nutritional Sciences*, vol. 131, pp. 1615S-20S, 2001.
7. R. Guthrie, "The introduction of newborn screening for phenylketonuria. A personal history." *Eur J Pediatr.*, vol. 155 Suppl 1, pp. S4-5, 1996.
8. D. Matern and P. Rinaldo, "Opportunities and Challenges of Tandem Mass Spectrometry", *Clinical Laboratory News*, vol. 185, pp. 12-15, 2003.
9. D. H. Chace and E. W. Naylor, "Expantion of newborn screening programs using automated tandem mass spectrometry", *Mental retardation and developmental disabilities research reviews*, vol. 5, pp. 150-154, 1999.
10. M. Marble and F. P. Hooper, "Expanded Newborn Screening for Metabolic Disease", *A Pratical Review of Advances in Pediatrics From Children's Hospital*, vol. 8, no. 6, 2004.
11. CDC, "Using tandem mass spectrometry for metabolic disease screening among newborns", *MMWR*, vol. 50, pp. 1-22, 2001.
12. *Centers of Disease Control and Prevention (CDC),* http://www.cdc.gov/nceh/dls/newborn_screening.htm
13. R. V. Osório, "Twenty five years of newborn screening in Portugal", in *XL Conferências de Genética (in Portuguese)*, Porto, Portugal, 2004.

Technological Platform to Aid the Exchange of Information and Applications Using Web Services

Antonio Estruch and José Antonio Heredia

Dep. Tecnología, Universitat Jaume I, Castellón, Spain

Abstract. Motivation: This article describes a technological platform that allows sharing not only the access to information sources, but also the use of processing data algorithms through Web Services.
Results: This architecture has been applied in the Thematic Network of Cooperative Investigation named INBIOMED. In this network, several groups of biomedical research can harness their results by accessing to the information of other groups, and besides, to be able to analyze this information using processes developed by other groups specialized in the development of analysis algorithms.
Additional information: http://www.inbiomed.uji.es
Contact: estruch@sg.uji.es

1 Introduction

Nowadays, the research groups involved in tasks related with the bioinformatics have diverse problems when they have to cooperate with other research groups to cover their needs and to present the results of their investigations.

One of the main problems is the management of the information generated in the laboratories or the collection of clinical data. The volume of these data raises problems in the storing and analysis of them.

In addition, the Internet provides a massive public amount of relevant information. However, the great variety of formats available to represent the information, the duplicity of information among databases and the update of theses databases make difficult the election of the sources used to get and to relate the information needed for the research.

The same problem occurs with the analysis and the data processing tools. There are available proprietary tools of public domain that use different representation formats, with different methodologies for different platforms.

The solution for these problems happens to use an IT infrastructure that makes easy the access to your own data sources, to the public data stores, and besides, that helps to connect with analysis and processing data tools allowing to store the results obtained for future use.

2 Used Technologies

The starting of a platform like this one, required to work in several directions. By a side, it worked to facilitate the access to the information sources wished to arrange in the platform, adapting their structures when it was needed. On the other side, an infrastructure was developed that lets the communication among the Network nodes.

J.M. Barreiro et al. (Eds.): ISBMDA 2004, LNCS 3337, pp. 458–467, 2004.

To adapt the information originated in the local information systems or in the public data sources, the more practical option is to use ETL (Extraction, Transformation and Load) Data Warehousing techniques, with the intention of building a data store with all the information required, consolidated and oriented to be queried. The existence of a replica of the information lets to the researchers of a group, to keep working with their original data sources, without worrying that someone else will access directly to their data sources meanwhile they are working with them. The content of the store will be updated whenever it is considered necessary.

It is worked with the Data Transformation Services (DTS) available in Microsoft SQL Server 2000, through which, have been created the data stores in a very intuitive and productive way, using the available design information flow tools. The connection among the several technological platforms used by the researcher groups is the access through the Internet. To take advantage of this connection, the best option is to use Web Services using the SOAP protocol, which uses HTTP as transfer protocol and uses XML to exchange the information, avoiding any problem with the actual firewalls.

From the actual development environments, we can emphasize two of them, Sun J2EE and Microsoft .NET, as the most suitable to implement this platform.

In our case, the option selected is .NET because of several reasons. The availability of a development environment, Visual Studio .NET, aids a lot in the development of the Web Services, as it can generate automatically the WSDL documents. However, the main reason has been the possibility to take profit from the use of the Class DataSet available in ADO.NET (Access Data Objects .NET) that has been the core Class in the design of the platform.

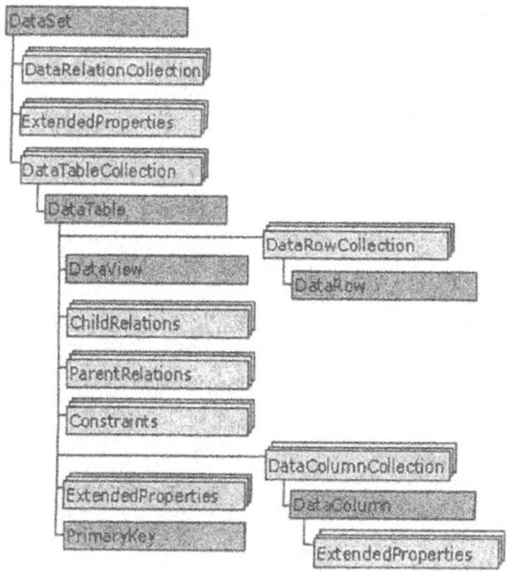

Fig. 1. DataSet Object Model

A DataSet is a data structure that holds in memory the basic elements of a Relational Database, including tables (DataTables), with the columns definition (DataColumns) and their data rows (DataRows), besides, it stores the relations between tables (DataRelations). The DataSet structure can be manipulated, allowing creating, modifying and deleting the elements in memory. Another interesting thing is that the DataSet, allows to work with the data stored in the structure without being connected to the origin data source. The DataSet manages the changes and can, later, consolidate the changes with the Source or reverse them in a very easy way.

This data structure is serializable in XML, what makes easy the transfer through the Internet. It is ideal to use in Web Services or to exchange with external applications.

Regarding the portability among platforms, it was considered interesting allowing the execution of the server layers and the data access of the platform in Linux using Novell Mono 1.0. The client side is not supported yet by Novell.

3 INBIOMED Platform

The technological infrastructure needed to achieve the targets raised is materialized in the INBIOMED platform. This platform is based in the development of three layers:

a) Data Sources Layer (Storage)

In this layer are located the database servers that contain the information sources accessible through the platform. The Datawarehouse technology plays a fundamental role, guaranteeing that the information stored in the databases is well consolidated and oriented to be queried, and is obtained from the internal data sources or the public externals.

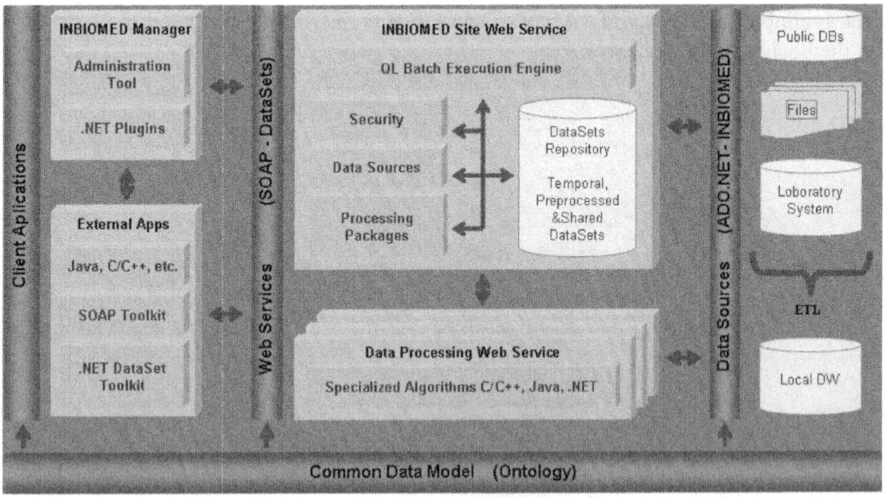

Fig. 2. INBIOMED Platform Architecture

b) Web Services Layer (Logic)

Once the access to the information is solved, it has to be provided an easy way to query and process the information. The Web Services technology guarantees an independent platform access interface, easy to use in any actual development environment.

Two types of Web Services are defined: Net Site Service and Data Process Service.

Data Process Services

The Data Process Services are responsible to implement the logic necessary to analyze the data, process them and generate the results. The implementation of the necessary algorithms can be made in the programming language most suitable for the resolution of the problem.

To comprise in the platform, it needs to build at the top of these services a common Web Service interface with some methods pre-established that fulfill all these type of services. So, it can be achieved a black box approach with data and parameters as inputs and an output that will be the results after applying the algorithms.

The objective that is trying to achieve is to make available a wide catalog of services of this type that implement the mathematical treatment and statistics algorithms most suitable to the needs of the researchers groups.

Net Site Service

The Net Site Service is a point of entry in the platform to the client applications. It receives the query and processing requests in a language oriented to the batch execution called IQL (INBIOMED Query Language).

This language allows, apart from throw classic queries to get the data about the defined sources, to manage the several elements needed for the proper work of the system, as the definition of the data source connections, the Data Process Services Catalog, the users, the roles and the privileges or rights to access or execute data and processes.

Every request that is sent to the Net Site Service is made by calling a unique method, where must be specified, at least, the sentences that have to be executed, in a string format. In that way, it is consolidated a basic communication interface that will not be modified by the inclusion of more functionality in the IQL language, as it does not affect the definition of the Web Service and only affects to the execution engine that is responsible to process the requests.

Every request received is executed in a separated thread, so that can be controlled its execution separately. The sentences are executed in a sequential way, allowing in one request ask for data from several data sources and call a Data Process Service that processes the data obtained, delegating all the processing load in the server.

Input data can be included as part of the request, they are provided by the client applications and are sent to the server with the query sentences that reference these input data as parameters.

To make easy the data manipulation, during the execution of the IQL sentences, variables can be defined to store temporally partial results and be reused during the execution of a sequence of instructions. Once the sentences execution is finished, the variables are removed.

In case that you want to store the results to use them later, there is a Persistent Data Repository, which has an analog structure to a conventional file system with directories and subdirectories and with documents that store the DataSets result of the execution of IQL sentences. This sentences can be saved and load whenever, whether the user has the proper rights.

As the execution of a sequence of IQL sentences can take a long time, the system can leave running the query in the server and return an ID to the client, that can be used by the client to interrogate to the system about the state of the query, and when the query is finished to recover the result. When the client waits until the end of the execution the result is returned to the client that made the request.

c) Client Applications (User Interface)

The philosophy of the platform is to try to minimize the load of the processing in the client applications in favor of the conversion of the algorithms used in processes on where will be built Web Services that fulfill the specifications of the Process Data Services.

So, the platform applications only have to implement the User Interface with their input forms and the presentation results, delegating in the platform the responsibility to query, store and process the information as much as possible.

The communication between the client applications and the Site Web Service must be made using the SOAP protocol, so the applications have to be implemented using a programming language that is able to consume Web Services.

The communication between the application and the platform will be done using IQL sentences, sending and receiving DataSets.

The common Data Model will establish the data structures used in the data flows between the several layers.

As part of the platform development, among others, an administrative tool has been developed named INBIOMED Manager, that allows to connect to the platform, throw the execution of IQL sentences and has the necessary options to manage all the elements in the platform, as users, roles, datasource connections, Data Process Services Catalog, etc.

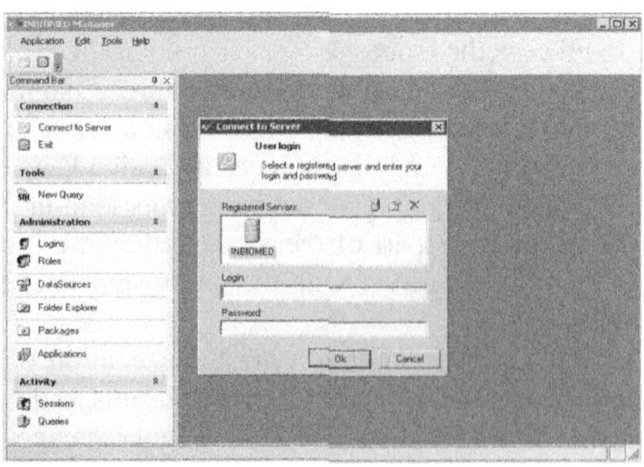

Fig. 3. INBIOMED Manager

4 Cooperative Model

Every network node collaborates with the other nodes in, at least, one of the following ways:

a) Develops Its Own Net Site Service.
   In this way, it facilitates the sharing data access. Every node keeps its own Site independently. Every node provides a user to the other nodes; this user is used to send requests and will have the proper rights or privileges to access to the data sources, Data Process Services Catalog and data Repository.
b) Develop Data Processes.
   A node in the net, may not have information by itself, but can provide the development of a Data Processing Web Service implementing algorithms to analyze information for the other nodes.
c) Develop Client Applications.
   Using the resources available in the platform (datasources, processes, etc.) can be implemented applications that solve complex problems and provide support to advance in the researches made by the members of the INBIOMED net.
   So, the topology of the net can vary from models completely centralized where there is only one Net Site Service in a node, and all the other nodes receive and send data from and to this node, to models decentralized, where every node keeps its own information independently.

5 Conclusions

The problems that have been solved are the general issues that appear in any system that tries to give a response to the changing needs of its users. The platform has been equipped with the maximum possible flexibility, creating a live system, where every group that belongs to any Network node enriches collaborating with data or processes.

The inclusion of new processes or data raises the need to agree its content adding new concepts, attributes and relations to the data model.

The more processes available in the platform, the more attractive will be the implementation of applications that use them. This effect is harnessed as INBIOMED is a multidiscipline network, where every node contributes with its own methodology in the study, research and analysis of the knowledge area.

ANNEX A: Description of the Web Services Methods

a) Site Web Service

DataSet Login(String a_sUsuario, String a_sPassword)

Starts a new session, the arguments are the user identification and the password for authentication.

Returns a DataSet, with a table, with only one column and one row with the global unique id that represents the new session (128 bits).

DataSet Logout(Guid a_guidSesion)

Close the session identified by the global unique identifier. Returns an empty DataSet named "OK" if return successfully.

DataSet ExecuteQuery(Guid a_guidSesion, String a_sQuery, DataSet[] a_dsArguments, bool a_bWait)

Throws a request for an specific session of the IQL sentences in the server, using the specified arguments as input. The returned Dataset depends on whether the client waits for the end of the full execution, in that case, the result is the DataSet result, or the client does not wait, in that case the return is a DataSet with only one table, with one column and one row with the unique identifier of the query; so that can be interrogated the state of the query and obtain the result once is finished using IQL.

b) Data Processing Web Services

Independently of the functionality that each service provide, all these services have to fulfill the interface to be integrated in the platform and allow to be called during the execution of an IQL sentence by the Net Site Service.

DataSet Execute(String a_sMethod,
DataSet[] a_dsArguments)

Throws the execution of a method, with an array of datasets specified as input argument. It returns the DataSet result of the execution.

If there is any error during the execution of a Web Service method, it will return a DataSet named "EXCEPTION", with only one table and three columns and only one row with the error identifier (integer), an error message and context additional information (string).

ANNEX B: Batch Execution Language IQL (INBIOMED Query Language).

Execution of Multiple Queries

Executes in sequential form the sentences of the query separated by ';'.

The Basic Type of Data is a DataSet of ADO.NET

Contains several Tables, with their Fields, Data Rows and the Relations between them. An scalar value is a DataSet with only one table, with one column and one data row that contains the scalar value.

Expressions and Identifiers

The expressions can be of any type and can generate any type of result. All the operations are executed with the stored data in DataSets, although it can be a unique value.

An identifier is written in Upper Case, or in any case delimited with [ ].

If the suffix '*!table*' is used, an specific table from the Dataset is accessed.

A path in the Data Repository is specified in the following way:

- The folders are separated with '.': *Root.Folder.SubFolder*
- The resource (stored DataSets) with '!': *Root.Folder.SubFolder!Resource1*

Variables Assign

SET var = expr.

It can be defined a DataSet variable during the execution with the sentence SET where var is an identifier with the prefix '@'

Values Return

RETURN expr;

To return a result the command RETURN is used.

Management Sentences

CREATE | ALTER
USER *username* PASSWORD '*password*' COMMENT '*description*';
ROLE *rolename* COMMENT '*description*';
DATASOURCE *connectionname* TYPE OLEDB | ODBC | INBIOMED
USING '*connectionstring*' COMMENT '*description*';
PACKAGE *packagename* URL '*url*' COMMENT '*description*';
FOLDER *foldername* AT *parentfolderpath*;

Create or modify an element of the platform.

DROP
USER *username*;
ROLE *rolename*;
DATASOURCE *datasourcename*;
PACKAGES *packagename*;
FOLDER *folderpath*;

Delete elements of the platform.

GRANT | REVOKE PRIVILEGE *privilegename* TO *rolename* IN
DATASOURCE *datasourcename*;
PACKAGE *packagename*;
FOLDER *folderpath*;
RESOURCE *resourcepath*;

Grant or revoke privileges over platform elements.

Query Functions over DataSources

= QUERY *fd* { *sql1* } AS *t1*, { *sql2* } AS *t2*, ...;

They can be used as part of an expression to obtain a DataSet which content has been extracted of a DataSource.

Query Functions over DataSets

= SELECT
ALL | { *column1, column2* }
FROM
dataset1
INNER | OUTER | CROSS JOIN
dataset2
ON
{ *col_of_dataset1 = col_of_dataset2* }
WHERE
{ *boolexpr* }

They can be used as part of an expression to relate several DataSets to obtain only the data that fulfill the relation.

Sentences of Modification over Variables that Contain DataSet Tables

INSERT INTO *variable|variable!table*

{ *column1, column2, ...* }
VALUES
{ *value1, value2, ...* }
Insert values into a DataSet table.
UPDATE *variable|variable!table*
SET { *column1 = value1, ...* }
WHERE {*boolexpr* }
Updates data into a DataSet table over the rows that fulfill the filtering expression.
DELETE *variable|variable!table*
WHERE { *boolexpr* }
Deletes data from a DataSet table over the rows that fulfill the filtering expression.

Execution of a Method in a Data Process Service
= CALL *pkg!name (ds1, ds2, ...)*
It can be used as part of an expression to invoke the execution of a method of a Data Process Service and operate with the result.

Access to the Data Repository
WRITE *ds* TO *folder1.subfolder1!resource*
Sentence that allows to save the content of a DataSet in a folder of the Data Repository with an specific name.
= READ *folder1.subfolder1!resource*
It can be used as part of an expression to obtain the content of a DataSet stored into an specific folder.

Result of a Not Waiting Query
= RESULT QUERY '*queryguid*'
It can be used as part of an expression to obtain the result of a query that was thrown previously without waiting.

Special Sentences
KILL SESSION '*sessionguid*';
Close the session identified by the specified unique session global identifier.
KILL QUERY '*queryguid*';
Cancel the execution of the query identified by the specified unique query global identifier.

Examples
/* Create a user */
CREATE USER guest PASSWORD 'guest';

/* Create a Data Source */
CREATE DATASOURCE pubs TYPE OLEDB USING '....';

/* Grant Read privileges to the guest user */
GRANT PRIVILEGE READ TO guest IN DATASOURCE pubs;

/* Obtain a DataSet with 2 tables from the Data Source Pubs */
SET @a = QUERY pubs

```
        { SELECT * FROM authors } As [Autores],
        { SELECT * FROM titles} AS [Titulos];

/* Save the DataSet in a folder with the name Ejemplo */
WRITE @a TO [ROOT].[My Folder]![Ejemplo];

/* Get the DataSet from the Data Repository */
SET @b = READ [ROOT].[My Folder]![Ejemplo];

/* Get a DataSet table*/
SET @c = @b![Titulos];

/* Delete from @c the rows of the first table where nombre = 'A' */
DELETE FROM @c WHERE { name = 'A' };

/* Call the method of an external process using the content of the variable @c as ar-
gument */
SET @d = CALL [PackageName]![Metodo](@c);

/* Return the content of a variable */
RETURN @c;
```

References

http://www.microsoft.com/sql/
Microsoft SQL Server 2000

http://www.w3.org/TR/soap/
Simple Object Access Protocol (SOAP) W3C Recommendation Documents

http://msdn.microsoft.com/netframework/
Developer Center for Microsoft .NET Framework

http://www.mono-project.com
Novell Mono OpenSource Project

http://msdn.microsoft.com/library/default.asp?url=/library/en_us/cpref/html/frlrfSystemDataDataSetClassTopic.asp
MSDN Library ADO.NET DataSet Class information.

http://www.inbiomed.retics.es
Thematic Network INBIOMED

Visualization of Biological Information with Circular Drawings*

Alkiviadis Symeonidis[1,2] and Ioannis G. Tollis[1,2]

[1] Forth, Foundation Of Research and Technology Heraklion
Vassilika Vouton, P.O Box 1385 Heraklion, Crete GR-71110 Greece
{tollis,asimeon}@ics.forth.gr
http://www.ics.forth.gr

[2] University of Crete, Computer Science Department,
University of Crete, P.O. Box 2208, Heraklion, Crete, Greece
{tollis,asimeon}@csd.uoc.gr
http://www.csd.uoc.gr

Abstract. Being able to clearly visualize clusters of genes provided by gene expressions over a set of samples is of high importance. It gives researchers the ability to create an image of the structure, and connections of the information examined. In this paper we present a tool for visualizing such information, with respect to clusters trying to produce an aesthetic, Symmetrie image, which allows the user to interact with the application and query for specific information.

1 Introduction

The expression of genes over a set of patients is of major interest since we can find clusters of genes with similar expression profile and consequently predict those responsible for a specific disease. The need for visualizing such information urged scientists to build such tools. Many applications have been developed. Cytoscape [1] is a well known tool which has integrated many different visualization algorithms, and allows for different types of visualization with respect to the information needed. Geneplacer [2], provides a different approach and uses treemaps [3] in order to visualize tree-structured information. Here, we try to provide an algorithm for visualizing genes and clusters more clearly giving the user the ability to interact and try to find relationships not offered by the clustering algorithm.

1.1 Gene Expressions

A gene expression is an arithmetic value associated with a gene and may vary significantly between different individuals [4]. Given the expression of many genes

* This work was supported in part by INFOBIOMED code: IST-2002-507585 and the Greek General Secretariat for Research and Technology under Program "ARISTEIA", Code 1308/B1/3.3.1/317/12.04.2002.

J.M. Barreiro et al. (Eds.): ISBMDA 2004, LNCS 3337, pp. 468–478, 2004.

over a set of samples, we can obtain useful biomedical information [4,6]. Using knowledge about a patient's medical Status, we can find genes with similar behavior over our data, and thus expect them to be related to the object of investigation, usually a disease.

A typical way to obtain this information is using DNA-microarray technology [5]. A microarray is a chip containing hundreds to thousands of probes (DNA fragments) corresponding to unique genes and allows a researcher to perform an expression analysis of these genes under specific conditions [7]. The results obtained from this analysis form a two dimensional matrix with genes as rows and samples (patients) as columns. The value of each cell is the respective gene ex-Pression. Many tools have been developed in order to visualize this information. In Fig. 1 appears a screenshot of a new tool under development in our lab. Here, we introduce a visualization tool which emphasizes on the possible relations between genes and their strength. We try to visualize clearly clusters of genes with similar behavior, while we also want the final image to be comprehensive and easy to interact with. In order to achieve this, we need some transformations.

First, let us consider every gene as a node. These nodes can be connected in two ways. The first case appears when two or more genes belong to the same cluster. What is important here is that every cluster can be described as the set of genes it consists of. The second case occurs when the correlation between two genes is very strong according to some set criteria. The correlation between any pair of genes (u, v) is noted as r_{uv} We consider two genes-nodes to be strongly connected

- if u, v belong to the same cluster and for the correlation r_{uv} between them holds that

$$r_{uv} > threshold \cdot mean\{r_{ij} | i, j \in group(u)\} \tag{1}$$

- or if they belong to different clusters and satisfy

$$r_{uv} > threshold - (mean\{r_{ij} | i, j \in group(u)\} + mean\{r_{kl} | k, l \in group(w)\}) \tag{2}$$

For every such pair of genes, a link is added in order to indicate this property. The model described so far, is called a graph. A graph $G(V, E)$ is a set of vertices-nodes (genes) V and a set of edges-links (the links inserted) E is a subset of $V * V$. Every cluster is a subset of vertices-genes and forms a super-node. This is a subgraph, a part of the graph that consists of the selected genes- vertices and any links that exist between these genes. At this point it is important to notice the use of the links added. Links between genes that belong to the same cluster, indicate that their correlation is very strong, and by increasing the value of the thresholds we can ask for an even stronger correlation. If for a subset of the genes in a cluster a lot of such links exist, we expect their behavior to be very similar and they possibly form a smaller but probably more important cluster. We would like our visualization to make such dense subgroups easily identifiable by eye. For genes that have been placed in different clusters, a link that indicates strong correlation (as strong as we want if we modify the threshold) can be translated as a sign of two genes with very similar expression even if they are not placed in the same cluster. This should draw the attention of the user as a fact that possibly requires searching or even perhaps as a sign of miss-classification.

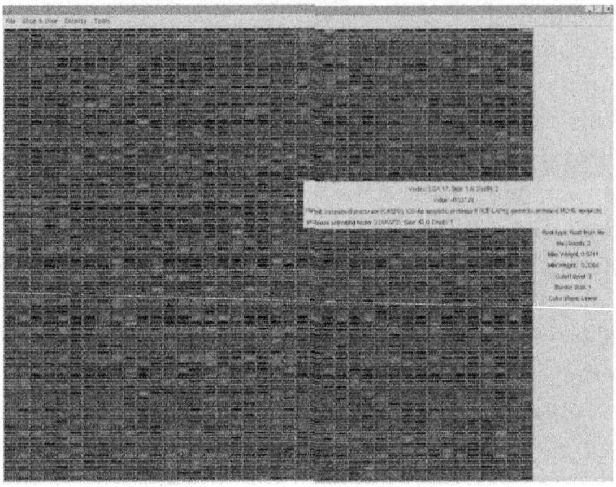

Fig. 1. A way to visualize the results of a microarry.

At this point we know that our needs from the graph drawing algorithm are

- clusters should be highly visible, allowing a clear image of the connections
- dense subgraphs should be easily identifiable
- links must be clear, not cutting other links
- the Overall drawing should be aesthetically pleasing.

2 Gene Selection

Our data consist of thousands of genes but only a small portion of them is expected to be of interest for a specific search. In an attempt to reduce the data size and -more important- keep only useful information we filter our data and keep only the genes that seem to have different behaviour between healthy people and patients who suffer from a specific disease. In order to achieve this, we compute a signal to noise score for every gene, and concentrate on those that provide the biggest values. We separate the expressions of a gene in two categories. One includes the values for all the healthy people in our data set, while the other consists of the expressions measured over patients. For the first category C_1 we compute the mean value m_1 and the Standard deviation sd_1. For the second category C_2 we get m_2 and sd_2 respectively. The signal-to-noise score for every gene is calculated by the following formula:

$$\textit{signal-to-noise} = \frac{|m_1 - m_2|}{sd_1 + sd_2} \qquad (3)$$

After the score is calculated for every gene we keep only the genes with the highest scores, and work on this subset.

3 Clustering

In order to search for similarities and relations between the genes under process, some clustering is needed. A huge variety of such algorithms exist. In [6], [8] and [9] many different clustering algorithms are described. Hierarchical, k-means and other clustering algorithm are implemented in our lab, but for experimental reasons a simple, fast but ineffective algorithm has been integrated in the application. Pearson's correlation coefficient r_{ij} is calculated for every pair i, j of genes. Let X, Y be the vectors that have the gene expressions for genes i, j respectively. Then

$$r_{ij} = \frac{\sum XY - \frac{\sum X \cdot \sum Y}{N}}{\sqrt{\left(\sum X^2 - \frac{(\sum X)^2}{N}\right)\left(\sum Y^2 - \frac{(\sum Y)^2}{N}\right)}} \tag{4}$$

The clustering algorithm picks a gene i at random and creates a cluster in which all non-clustered genes j with r_{ij} greater than a threshold are included. The procedure is repeated until no unclustered genes are left. The results of the algorithm clearly depend on the order of the chosen genes, which means that in successive repetitions the results will be different if the gene picked is not the same.

Furthermore, we expect big clusters to be created in the first iterations and small or even Single-element clusters will appear towards the end . In the first case, smaller, higher correlated subsets of genes can be found as dense subgraphs while in the second case, edges towards other clusters could indicate a probably better classification for the genes.

4 Description of the Visualization Algorithm

The visual representation of a graph is given in the most common way: Vertices are represented as circles, and edges as straight lines joining the respective vertices. In crder to further discriminate between the two categories of edges (intracluster and inter-cluster)the former are coloured blue, while the later green. In addition to this the brightness of an edge reflects the Pearson's coefficient value for the pair of genes it links. Groups-clusters are considered to be circles, on whose periphery must be placed the vertices-genes they consist of. Our main interest is to pay attention to the visualization of clusters. So what we want to do first is to determine the position of the center of each cluster-circle. The radius of each cluster is proportional to the number of its elements. After all clusters are placed, the next step is to determine the ordering of the genes of a cluster, on the embedding circle. The criterion we follow is minimization of crossings that appear between edges in a cluster. A crossing appears when two lines-edges that link genes intersect. A final step follows in order to minimize the crossings that appear between edges that link genes of different clusters. We attempt to minimize the crossings in order to simplify the final image. The algorithm we use is a Variation of the algorithm proposed by Six and Tollis [10]. It combines a graph theoretic approach for the positioning of the genes in a group and a forte-directed drawing method for the placement of the groups.

4.1 Determine Groups' Positions

The need for a globally aesthetic drawing urged us to use a forte-directed algorithm.The main advantage of such algorithms is that they are simple to implement and show symmetries allowing nice visualization. Force directed algorithms in general, set a number of criteria and try to minimize a value that combines them. The one we chose was inspired by the way a spring system behaves [11].

One super-vertex is created for each cluster. For each inter-group edge(u, v), we add an edge in the super-graph with ends in group(u) and group(v). The force directed algorithm is as follows.

- Consider every super-vertex to be an electric load. The load of each group is analogous to its radius.
- Let every edge represent a spring.
- Initialize the position of every super-vertex at random and let the system converge.

In order to guarantee that the algorithm will terminate within acceptable time limit a threshold is set for the number of iterations. The final positioning will have the following properties:

- Big clusters will be far away from each other so the picture will not be confusing.This is due to stronger electrical forces between such clusters since the loads are bigger.
- Genes connected with links will not appear far apart since there will be a spring trying to bring the two groups close.
- the result will be Symmetrie and thus nice-looking. This comes as a property of the simulated natural system.

4.2 Determine Vertices Position

This is the most challenging task. In order to efficiently (in terms of a low number of crossings) place vertices on the periphery of a circle the graph is placed in one of the following categories: tree, biconnected, non-biconnected. Since our goal is to reduce the number of crossings we are not interested in the exact position of a vertex but only in their ordering on the embedding circle. According to the type of the graph the ordering can be determined using a different approach. This is based on algorithms from Six and Tollis [12,13].

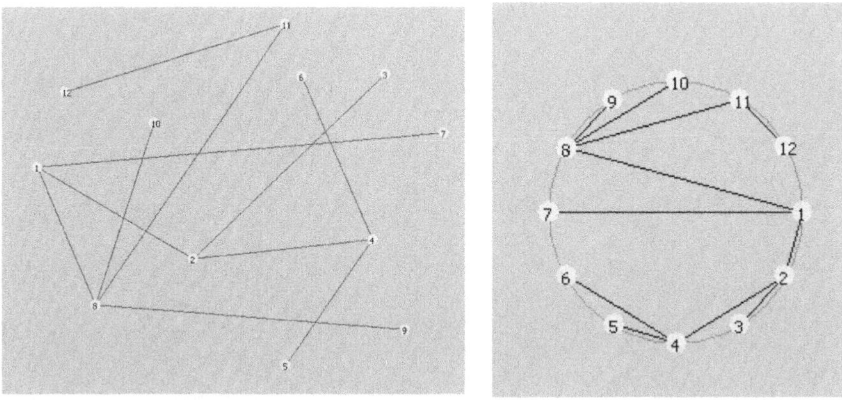

Fig. 2. A randomly generated visualization algorithm tree with $V = 12$, and the crossing-free result of the visualization algorithm.

Tree

The easiest case one might face is that of a tree. If the group we want to visualize on an embedding circle is a tree, applying a depth first search on it provides us with the discovery time for each vertex. This number denotes the order of the vertex on the circle, This procedure guarantees that the visualization will have no crossings. An example appears in Fig. 2.

Biconnected Graph

The second case is that of a biconnected graph. A graph is called biconnected if there exist two distinct paths that join every pair of vertices. The problem of minimizing the crossings in such a graph is NP-complete. However, Six and Tollis presented an efficient heuristic algorithm [12].

The main idea behind the algorithm is that of identifying triangles, that is triples of vertices u, v, w such that edges (u, v), (v, w) and (w, u) all appear in E. In case of lack of a triangle, an edge is added in order to create one. This action is integrated in a technique that visits all nodes in a wave-like fashion. At the end of this graph-exploring step all added edges together with pair edges (edges incident to two nodes which share at least one neighbor)are removed and a depth first search algorithm is applied. The longest path is drawn and the rest of the vertices are placed next to as many neighbors (two,one,zero) as possible. A detailed description of the algorithm can be found in [12].

The algorithm described above has three main advantages. The first is its low complexity, since it is linear to the number of the edges. The second property, which in this application is the most useful, is that the algorithm tries to place as many edges as possible towards the periphery of the circle, thus dense subgraphs are expected to appear uninterrupted in an arc and consequently be easily identifiable by eye. As we have already seen dense subgraphs are of high importance

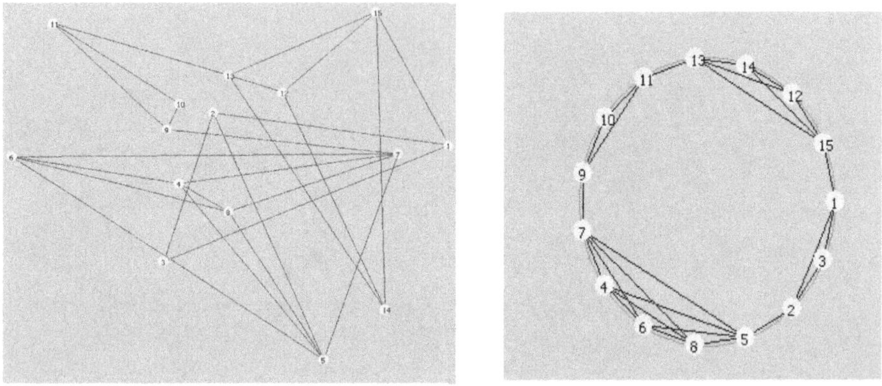

Fig. 3. A randomly placed visualization algorithm biconnected graph with $V = 15, E = 26$, and the result of thevisualization algorithm.

since they imply strong correlation between the members of the subgroup and thus possibly a smaller but more interesting cluster. The third advantage, which deals with the demand for few crossing is that if the group can be drawn without crossings this algorithm always achieves this goal. In any other case the number of crossings still remains low, since our attempt to place vertices next to neighbors at least guarantees that some edges will not produce crossings. Fig. 3 shows an example.

Non-biconnected Graph

A connected graph that is not biconnected is called 1-connected. For such graphs, or non-connected graphs, we identify all biconnected components and build a block cut point-tree, which is a tree with one vertex for every component and one for every cut-point. We draw this graph on the embedding circle using the depth first search algorithm and replace every vertex with the respective component ordered as described in the previous section.

What is important, is that O(E) time is still enough for the algorithm to execute. A low number of crossings is expected and the important need of easily identifiable dense subgraphs is again fulfilled. Fig. 4 shows an example.

4.3 Deal with Low Inter-group Crossings

Since the previous algorithms among others satisfy our need for a small number of intra-group crossings, the next goal is to minimize inter-group crossings.

An energy model, similar to the one described in 4.1 is adopted. The main difference is that instead of global cartesian coordinates this time we use polar coordinates, with point of reference the center of the embedding circle of the group a node belongs to. The total energy of the system is calculated as

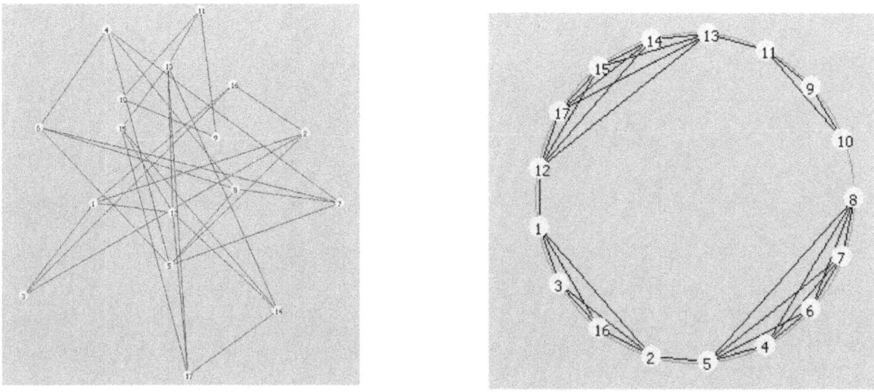

Fig. 4. A randomly placed non-biconnected graph with $V = 17, E = 32$, and the result of the visualization algorithm.

$$V = \sum_{(i,j)\in E} k_{ij} \cdot f_{ij} + \sum_{(i,j)\in V\times V} \frac{g_{ij}}{f_{ij}} \quad (5)$$

where f_{ij} is a force acting between vertices i, j:

$$f_{ij} = [(x_a + r_a \cdot \cos\theta_i) - (x_b + r_b \cdot \cos\theta_j)]^2 + [(y_a + r_a \cdot \sin\theta_i) - (y_b + r_b \cdot \sin\theta_j)]^2 \quad (6)$$

with x_a, y_a, r_a and x_b, y_b, r_b being the cartesian coordinates and radius of group a and b respectively to which genes i and j belong. It can be seen that the square root of the value of this force is equal to the distance between the respective vertices. The constants g and k are very important. Since we want a low number of crossings we want the distances to be as small as possible, so the k constant should be high. In practice, trying to minimize the sum of the distances provides most of the times the same solution, and is preferred due to its reduced computational complexity. The radii are analogous to the number of vertices in a group, thus fixed and the angles of all vertices with the center of their group needs to be determined. We use the ordering computed earlier and place the vertices on the periphery of the respective circle in that crder at equal distances. Next, we rotate all circles and compute the total energy. We then reverse the ordering and repeat the same procedure keeping the lowest energy Position. It is important to notice that reversing the ordering does not affect the intra-group state. The result of applying the algorithm on a random graph appears in Fig. 5.

5 Interactivity

The user can interact with the application in a number of ways. The most important feature, is the ability to alter the thresholds, and thus ask for more or less edges, or equivalently, stronger or weaker correlations to appear. The user can also gain access to more information about a gene, edge or cluster by clicking on

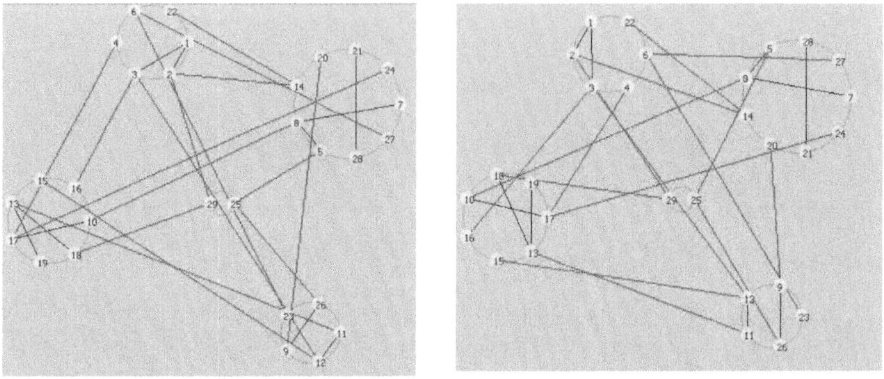

Fig. 5. Result of reducing inter-group crossings. Reduce from 36 to 31 crossings.

it. Another feature, is the ability to move a cluster, if the positioning computed by the algorithm does not match the user's needs. One can also move one gene from one cluster to another. This can be useful for a gene with many green edges going to genes in another cluster. Moving the gene to this cluster one can observe the behavior of edges. If less green (inter-cluster) and more blue (intra-cluster) edges appear, this could be a sign of a good classification. One more property, is the ability to hide genes, and view only groups and inter-group edges, so that one can see inter-cluster connections more clearly. Fig. 6 and Fig. 7, show the

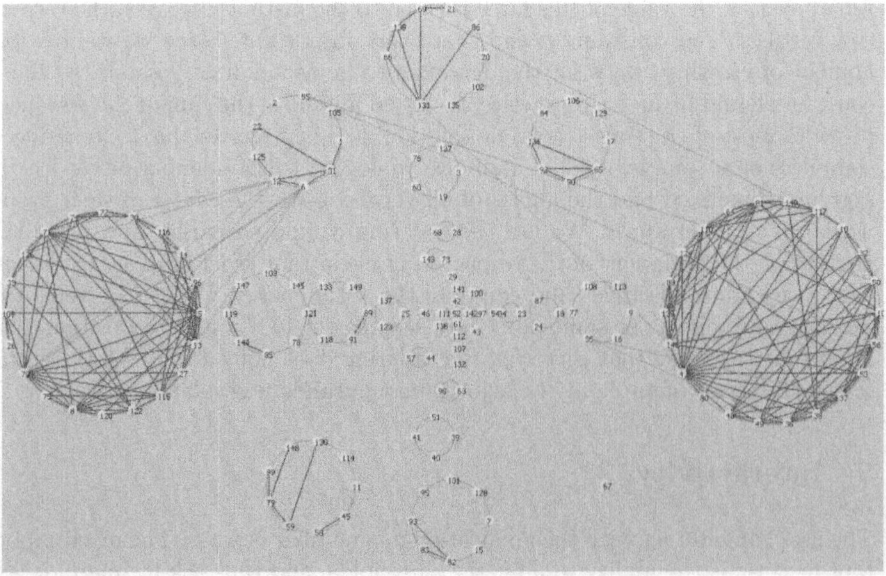

Fig. 6. Result on real data, 150 genes.

described scenario. In this mode, the user can still ask for information on a group by clicking on it, while detail about a specific gene can be still accessed. This can be seen in Fig. 8.

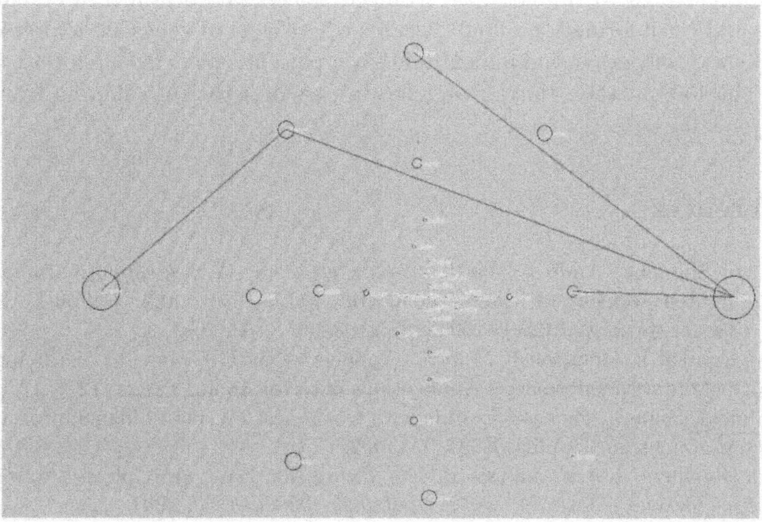

Fig. 7. The clusters of the previous graph.

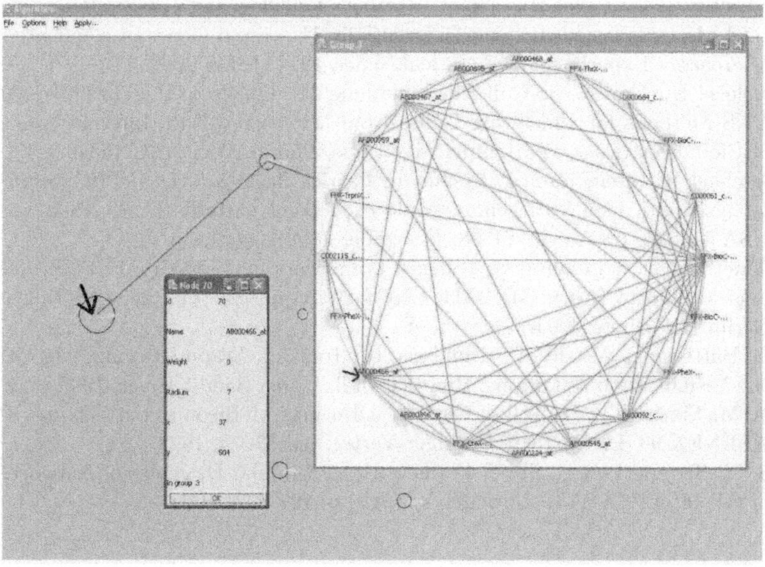

Fig. 8. Asking for more information on the previous figure.

6 Future Work

Another equally useful visualization would be that of patients suffering from different diseases. In that case a node represents a patient, a group a set of patients suffering from the same disease, while edges can link patients whose genes are expressed similarly, according to some statistical measure. This way, one could get information about diseases where a set of genes are expressed in a similar way, or perhaps an indication that a patient suffers from another disease, even clues about the behavior of genes in case of a patient suffering from more than one diseases.

References

1. Paul Shannon, Andrew Markiel, a.o.: Cytoscape: A Software Environment for Integrated Models of Biomolecular Interaction Networks. Genome Research (www.genome.org) 13:2498-2504. ISSN10889051 /03, 2003.
2. McConnell P., Johnson K., Lin S.: Application of Tree-Maps to hierarchical biological data. Bioinformatics Applications note vol. 18 no. 9 pages 1278–1279, 2002.
3. Shneiderman B: Tree visualization with tree-maps: 2-d space-filling approach. ACM Transactions on Graphics ll, 92–99, 1992.
4. E. Domany: Cluster Analysis of Gene Expression Data. arxiv:physics/02066056 vl *http://arziv.org/PScache/physics/pdf/0206/0206056.pdf*, 2001.
5. M. Gabig, G. Wegrzyn: An Intorduction to DNA Chips: Principles, Technology, Applications and Analysis. Acta Biochimical Polonica vol. 48 No. 3/2001 615–622.
6. Quackenbush: Computational Analysis of Microarray Data, Nature Reviews Genetics, vol. 2 June 2001, pp. 418–427.
7. Sandrine Dudoit, Yee Hwa Yang, Matthew J. Callow and Terence P. Speed: Statistical Methods for Identifying Differentially Expressed Genes in Replicated cDNA Microarray Experiments. Statistical Sinica 12, 111–139 2002.
8. Belacel N., Cuperlovic-Culf M., Laflamme M., Quellette R.: Fuzzy J-Means and VNS Methods for Clustering Genes from Microarray Data International Journal of Bioinformatics, Oxford University Press. March 2004. NRC 46546.
9. Michael B. Eisen, Paul T. Spellman, Patrick 0. Brown, David Botstein: Cluster analysis and display of genome-wide expression patterns Proc. Natl. Acad. Sci. USA Vol. 95, pp. 14863–14868, December 1998 Genetics.
10. Janet M. Six and Ioannis G. Tollis: A Framework for User-Grouped Circular Drawings. G. Liotta (Ed.): GD 2003, LNCS 2912, pp. 135–146, 2004. Springer-Verlag Berlin Heidelberg 2004.
11. Di Battista, G. , Eades, P., Tamassia, R., Tollis, I., Graph Drawing: Algorithms for the Visualization of Graphs, Prentice Hall, Upper Saddle River, 1999 p. 305–309.
12. J. M. Six and 1. G. Tollis: Circular Drawings of Biconnected Graphs, Proc. of ALENEX 99, LNCS 1619, Springer-Verlag, pp. 57–73, 1999.
13. J. M. Six and I. G. Tollis, A Framework for Circular Drawings of Networks, Proc. of GD 99, LNCS 1731, Springer-Verlag, pp. 107–116, 1999

Gene Selection Using Genetic Algorithms

Bruno Feres de Souza[1] and André C.P.L.F. de Carvalho[1]

Institute of Mathematical and Computer Sciences, University of Sao Paulo
Av. Trabalhador Sao-Carlense, 400, Sao Carlos, SP, Brazil
{bferes,andre}@icmc.usp.br

Abstract. Microarrays are emerging technologies that allow biologists to better understand the interactions between disease and normal states, at genes level. However, the amount of data generated by these tools becomes problematic when data are supposed to be automatically analyzed (e.g., for diagnostic purposes). In this work, the authors present a novel gene selection method based on Genetic Algorithms (GAs). The proposed method uses GAs to search for subsets of genes that optimize 2 measures of quality for the clusters presented in the domain. Thus, data are better represented and classification of unknown samples may become easier. In order to demonstrate the strength of the proposed approach, experimental results using 4 public available microarray datasets were carried out.

1 Introduction

With the matureness of the genomic sequencing programs, a wealth of biological data has become available, allowing a new understanding of the processes that conduct the living systems.

One of most benefited areas of the post-genomic research is medicine. The new achieved knowledge allows more accurate insights about the origin and evolution of several diseases, which can lead to the development of more specific treatments, as well as to the design of new drugs. In special, the combat to cancer has already achieved promising advances, mainly due to the introduction of new wide scale gene expression analysis technologies, such as microarrays.

Microarrays are hybridization-based methods that allow monitoring the expression levels of thousands of genes simultaneously [1]. This enables the measurement of the levels of mRNA molecules inside a cell and, consequently, the proteins being produced. Therefore, the role of the genes of a cell in a given moment and under some circumstances can be better understood by assessing their expression levels. In this context, the comparison between gene expression patterns through the measurement of the levels of mRNA in normal and disease cells can supply important indications on the development of determined pathological states, as well as information that can lead to earlier diagnosis and more efficient treatment.

Amongst the most trivial applications of microarrays, the classification of new tissue samples is an essential step for the assessment of severe diseases. However,

J.M. Barreiro et al. (Eds.): ISBMDA 2004, LNCS 3337, pp. 479–490, 2004.

when dealing with gene expression data, there is usually a disproportionate rate between the high number of features (genes) and the low number of training samples (tissues). Working with a compact subset of genes can be advantageous in the following aspects:

- there would be a higher chance to identify important genes for classification, in a biological perspective;
- the effects of noise in microarray experiments analysis would be minimized;
- the accuracy of classifiers could be improved, which is crucial for diagnosis purposes;
- by focusing only on a subset of genes, the microarrays technology would become more accessible, since they could be manufactured with fewer genes and thus become a common clinical tool for specific diseases.

In order to deal with this dimensionality problem, the authors employ Genetic Algorithms (GAs) [2] to perform feature selection. GAs have already been employed for the gene selection problem. Most of the approaches so far investigated can be regarded as wrappers [3], since they explicitly depend on classification methods to select genes. For example, Li et al [4] combined a K-Nearest Neighbor classifier and a GA to generate multiple subsets of genes and then assess the relative importance of the genes to the classification problem. Liu and Iba [5] studied the feasibility of Parallel GAs to discover informative genes. They employed the classifier proposed by Golub et al [6] to evaluate each subset. Souza et al [7] combined SVMs with GAs, which obtained a performance superior to a popular feature selection method for SVMs in the tissue classification problem. Finally, Ooi and Tan [8] applied GAs to multi-class prediction of microarray data by using a maximum likelihood classification method.

The main drawback of all the aforementioned methods is their very high computational burden, since the classifier embedded into the GA's fitness function has to be executed a large number of times. Another problem is that they are dependent of specific learning algorithms. Although one can argue that optimality (by classification point of view) of a subset of genes can only be inferred based on the classifier algorithm's performance, choosing the later can be very difficult on its own. Moreover, how to reliably measure the performance of an classifier when faced with a limited amount of training data (as it is the case with gene expression data) is still an open issue. The well known cross-validation technique has already been shown to be, in most cases, inadequate for that task [9].

To handle with all the previously mentioned difficulties, the authors propose in this work a simple and effective method to the problem of gene selection, which follows the filter approach [3]. It is called the GA-Filter method. It utilizes only the intrinsic characteristics of the training data to select a subset of genes. As a result, it is not limited to any classifier and its computation is very efficient. To evaluated how good a subset is, 2 measures of quality are employed: a validity index and an impurity measure. The idea is to use GAs to search for genes that better represent the domain. Thus, the classification complexity of the problem can the minimized and, at the same time, important genes to the studied pathology can be revealed.

This paper is organized as follows: in Section 2, the measures of quality are presented. In Section 3, the GA considered for gene selection is discussed. The experiments are carried out in Section 4. Finally, Section 5 contains the conclusions.

2 Cluster Quality Measures

Let $S = \{(\overrightarrow{x_1}, y_1), ..., (\overrightarrow{x_n}, y_n)\}$, where $\overrightarrow{x_i} \in X \subset R^m$ and $y_i \in \{0, 1, ..., c\}$, be a training dataset with n samples and c classes. Each $\overrightarrow{x_i}$ is a m-dimensional input vector and each y_i corresponds to the class associated to $\overrightarrow{x_i}$. In the microarray domain, $\overrightarrow{x_i}$ is the ith tissue sample, represented by a set of m genes and y_i can be, e.g., either normal or tumoral diagnosis, or different types of cancer.

Each class is represented by a group of samples in the dataset, named cluster. Clusters are formed by samples that share common characteristics with samples of the same group and are different of samples from other groups. The (dis)similarity between the samples of the clusters are heavily influenced by the subset of genes used to represent the domain. For example, genes $\{a, b, c\}$ can more suitable represent the clusters of the data than genes $\{d, e, f\}$. To determine to how extend a subset of genes is better than another, 2 measures are employed: a validity index and an impurity measure.

2.1 Validity Index

Validity indexes [10] are used in the clustering literature to evaluate the generated partitions regarding to how they fit the underlying data. Although no clustering is performed in this work, validity indexes can still be employed. Actually, they are used to evaluate how a given subset of genes compares with another subset accordingly to some criteria.

Two criteria widely accepted for evaluating a dataset regarding its clusters are their average compactness and separation [10]. The aim here is to favour subsets of genes that lead to clusters as far as possible from each other, while encouraging clusters to be compact.

In order to fulfill both criteria, the authors developed the COS-*index*, defined as:

$$\text{COS-}index = w * \frac{1}{n}\left(\sum_{i=1}^{c}\sum_{x\in C_i} D(\overrightarrow{x}, \overrightarrow{v_i})\right) + (1-w) * \left(1 - \min_{i,j=1, i\neq j}^{c} D(\overrightarrow{v_i}, \overrightarrow{v_j})\right) \quad (1)$$

where D is the distance between two elements, $\overrightarrow{v_i}$ are the cluster centroids, i. e., the most representative element of the cluster and w (stands for weight) is used to controls the relative influence of each term. It ranges from 0 to 1.

The first term of Eq. 1 assess the average compactness of the partition while the second one referrers to the separation between the clusters centers. The index ranges from 0 to 1, where low values indicate better clusters.

Recent studies [11] have shown that correlation-like distance measures are better suited for gene expression data as they focus on the relative shape of the profile and not on its magnitude. One such measure is the cosine of the angle between two tissue samples. In this study, the distance D is defined as:

$$D(\overrightarrow{x_i}, \overrightarrow{x_j}) = \frac{(1-\cos(\overrightarrow{x_i}, \overrightarrow{x_j}))}{2} \tag{2}$$

where values of D near to 0 indicates that the examples are close and values of D near to 1 indicates that the examples are far away.

When using the distance defined in Eq. 2, the cluster centroids v_j are calculated, provided that each example $\overrightarrow{x_i}$ is normalized such that $|\overrightarrow{x_i}|_1 = 1$, by:

$$v_j = \sum_{x_i \in C_j} x_i \tag{3}$$

2.2 Impurity Measure

The Gini Index has been commonly used to measure the impurity of a given split in decision trees [12]. In this work, it is used to measure how well a given subset of genes can represent the clusters. It achieves low values if the samples from one class are more similar to the samples of the cluster representing their class than to samples from clusters representing the other classes.

The Gini Index for a cluster C_j is defined as:

$$Gini_j = 1 - \sum_{i=1}^{c} \left(\frac{P_{ji}}{n_j}\right)^2, \ j = 1, ..., c \tag{4}$$

where P_{ji} is the number of examples assigned to the ith class in cluster j and n_j is the total number of examples in cluster j. The sample assignent is based on the NC scheme commented in Section 4.

The impurity of a data partition is:

$$Impurity = \frac{\sum_{j=1}^{c} T_{P_j} * Gini_j}{n} \tag{5}$$

where T_{P_j} is the probability of an example belonging to a cluster j and n is the total number of examples in the dataset.

3 Genetic Algorithms for Gene Selection

Genetic Algorithms (GAs) are search and optimization techniques inspired in the process of evolution of biological organisms [2]. A simple GA uses a population of individuals to solve a given problem. Each individual, or chromosome, of the population corresponds to an encoded possible solution for the problem. A reproduction based mechanism is applied on the current population, generating a new population. The population usually evolves through several generations until a suitable solution is reached. A GA starts generating an initial population formed by a random group of individuals, which can be seen as first guesses to solve the problem. The initial population is evaluated and for each chromosome a score (named fitness) is given, reflecting the quality of the solution associated to it.

The main aspects of the GA used here are discussed next.

- **Representation:** Each candidate solution can be encoded as a chromosome of length m, where m is the total number of genes of the domain. 1 or 0 at the ith position of the chromosome indicates the presence or absence of the ith gene at the sample.
- **Initialization:** In this work, all the chromosomes are initialized with few positions. The authors believe that only few genes are relevant for the tissue classification.
- **Mutation:** Mutation is the genetic operator responsible for keeping diversity in the population. Mutation operates by randomly "flipping" bits of the chromosome, accordingly to some probability. An usual mutation probability is $1/m$, where m is the chromosome's length.
- **Crossover:** This genetic operator is used to guide the evolutionary process through potentially better solutions. This is performed by interchanging genetic material of chromosomes in order to create individuals that can benefit of their parents' fitness. In the present work, the uniform crossover is used with a probability rate p empirically defined.
- **Replacement:** Replacement schemes determine how a new population is generated. The experiments performed in this work used the concept of overlapping populations, where parents and offspring are merged and the best individuals from this union will form the next population.
- **Selection:** It is the process of choosing parents for reproduction. Usually, it emphasizes the best solutions in the population. Here, the authors employed the tournament selection.
- **Random Immigrant:** It is a method that helps to keep diversity in the population, minimizing the risk of premature convergence [13]. It works by replacing the individuals whose fitness is under the mean by new randomly generated individuals. Random immigrant is invoked when the best individual does not change for a certain number of generations (here named re-start frequency).
- **Fitness:** A good function for gene selection should focusing on subsets of genes that produce good clusters of the data while punish subsets with many genes. The quality of the partition is measured by the impurity measure and the validity index presented in Section 2. The fitness function associated with a gene subset λ is expressed by:

$$fitness(\lambda) = b_1 * Impurity(\lambda) + b_2 * \text{COS-}index(\lambda) + b_3 * dim(\lambda) \quad (6)$$

  where $Impurity(\lambda)$ is the impurity measure defined by Eq. 5 with respect to gene subset λ, COS-$index(\lambda)$ is the validity index defined by Eq. 1 with respect to gene subset λ, $dim(\lambda)$ is the cardinality of λ and b_1, b_2 and b_3 are regularization terms.

4 Experimental Results

In this Section, the experiments carried out are presented. The principal aims of the experiments are three fold: first, the authors would like to compare the performance of the classifiers trained with the set of genes selected by the GA-Filter method and trained with the whole set of genes. Next, it is interesting to compare the proposed approach to others found in the literature, regarding both accuracy rate and dimensionality reduction. Finally, the authors give some insights about the misclassified samples.

4.1 Classification Methods

In this work, the authors employed 3 popular classification methods together with the GA-Filter method. The first one is the Nearest Centroid (NC) [14]. To apply this method, one has to compute a distance (e.g., the distance defined in Eq. 2) between the gene expression profile of each test sample and the cluster centroids (as calculated by Eq. 3). The predicted class is the one whose centroid is closest to the expression profile of the test sample. The second one is the K-Nearest Neighbors (KNN) [14]. To classify a test sample, its distances to the K nearest neighbors on the training set are calculated. The predicted class is determinated by a majority rule on the KNN samples. K was arbitrarily set to 3. Now on, this classifier is simply referred as 3NN. The third method is the Support Vector Machines (SVM) [15]. It works by constructing a hyperplane that maximizes the margin of separation between the examples of different classes. SVM looks for a compromise between training error and the so-called Vapnik-Chervonenkis dimension [15]. This way it minimizes a bound on test error. In this work, the linear kernel was used. The parameter C was set to 100.

Before applying any classification method, the samples in the datasets were normalized so that each sample has Euclidian length 1.

4.2 Parameters Setup

The parameters used by the GA were all empirically defined, as follows: population = 150, generations = 400, crossover probability = 0.8, re-start frequency = 25, $b_1 = 0.1$, $b_2 = 0.8$ and $b_3 = 0.1$.

Regarding the parameters for the fitness function, some aspects must be observed. Clearly, the most important term in Eq. 6 should be the COS-$index(\lambda)$, as it reflects the overall quality of the clusters. It works as a capacity control [15] for the GA-Filter method. The term $Impurity(\lambda)$ is used to assure that the evaluated subsets of genes do not badly represent the clusters, i.e., samples from one class being more similar to clusters from other classes. The term COS-$index(\lambda)$ reduces this problem but can not avoid its occurrence, so the term $Impurity(\lambda)$ is employed. Finally, small subsets of genes are preferred, provided that the other requirements are not affected. The chosen values for b_1, b_2, b_3 reflect all those observations.

The validity index itself has a tunable parameter that controls the tradeoff between the compactness and the separation of the clusters. The weight w in Eq. 1 was set to 0.05. This means that much more importance is given to the separation of the clusters than to the their compactness. Preliminary experiments suggested that this value is suitable for the obtainance of good clusters.

Since GAs are stochastic methods, there are no guarantees that the same subset of genes will be encountered in different runs. Actually, this is very unlike. Thus, in this Section, all the results of the proposed method are averaged over 10 runs. Mean and standard deviations are presented in the comparison tables or in the text in the form MEAN±STDV.

4.3 Datasets

Leukemia Dataset. The acute leukemia dataset has been extensively studied [6]. Commonly, it is used, together with the lymphoma and the colon datasets, as benchmark for new gene selection methods. It consists of 72 expression profiles obtained from Affymetrix high-density oligonocleotide microarrays containing probes for 6817 human genes. The task in hand is to discriminate acute myeloid leukemia (AML) from acute lymphoblastic leukemia (ALL). Originally, the data was splitted into training and testing sets. The former consists of 38 samples (27 ALL and 11 AML) and the later of 34 samples (20 ALL and 14 AML). Following standard pre-processing procedures [6], thresholding and filtering were applied to the dataset (to avoid any bias, these procedures were first applied to the training set. Next, the testing set was pre-processed accordingly). The final dataset comprises the expression values of 3051 genes.

With the whole set of genes, both NC and 3NN misclassified 1 sample on the testing set, while SVM made no error. Using gene selection methods, the best classification rate so far was obtained by Antonov et al [16]. Their Maximal Margin Linear Programming method achieved no errors using 132 genes. Before that, Fu and Youn [17] used a method based on SVM to select 5 genes and made just one misclassification. Other works also reported very good classification rates on this dataset. However, it must be noticed that some of them presented a methodology flaw, due to bias in feature selection or bias in normalization [17].

The GA-Filter method may lead to a promising tradeoff between dimensionality reduction and classification accuracy. Using, in average, 15 genes, both 3NN and NC makes perfect score over 9 runs. As can be seem in Figure 1(a), SVM systematically misclassifies sample number 30. This behavior is consistent with the results presented by Furey et al [18]. The sample number 16 was misclassifed once by the 3 classification methods. In the original Golub et al's work, this sample presented a very low prediction strength and was misclassified.

Lymphoma Dataset. B cell diffuse large cell lymphoma (DLBCL) is a heterogeneous group of tumors, based on significant variations in morphology, clinical presentation, and response to treatment [19]. Using cDNA microarrays, Alizadeh et al [19] have identified 2 molecularly distinct forms of DLBCL: germinal centre B-like DLBCL (GC B-like) and activated B-like DLBCL (activated B-like).

This dataset consists of 24 GC B-like samples and 23 activated B-like samples. Following the suggestion of Li et al [20], the data is splitted into training and testing sets. The former consists of 34 samples (20 GC B-like and 14 activated B-like) and the later of 13 samples (5 GC B-like and 8 activated B-like). Unlikely other studies, the expression values were not log-transformed.

With the whole set of genes, both SVM and NC made no errors on the testing set. The 3NN made 1 error. With 50 selected genes, Li et al [20] misclassified 2 samples, the same as Potamias et al [21] using 12 genes.

The GA-Filter method selects 10 genes, in average, and makes perfect classification for the 3 tested classifiers over many runs. The maximum number of misclassification per run was 2. The misclassified samples can be seem in Figure 1(b). The sample DLCL-0005 was also misclassified by the Li et al's method. There is no reference for the others misclassified samples in the literature.

Colon Dataset. The colon dataset comprises 62 Affymetrix oligonucleotide microarrays that measure the expression levels of 6500 human genes. There are 22 normal and 40 tumor colon samples. Alon et al [11] provided the dataset with 2000 genes, after the elimination of genes with low minimal intensite across the samples. In this work, the authors adopt the training/testing split suggested by Li et al. This split was also used by Potamias et al.

This dataset is one the most difficult to classify publicly available. Kadota et al [22] have recently developed a method that tries to identify outliers in microarray experiments. The application of their method over the colon dataset showed that heterogeneity and sample contamination can result in several outlier samples. They pointed out 7 samples as outliers. These were chosen from 31 outlier candidates. Most of those outliers has been misclassified in several studies.

Using all available genes, the 3 classifiers misclassified the same 5 samples (T30, T33, T36, N34 and N36). As can be seem in Figure 1(c), theses samples were frequently misclassified by the 3 classifiers when using the GA-Filter method. They also were amongst the 6 samples misclassified by Furey et al's SVM method and they were the exact samples misclassified by Li et al's approach [4].

A plausive explanation for this systematically misclassification is given by Alon et al. They conjecture that normal samples had high muscle index while tumors had low muscle index. The samples T30, T33, T36, N34 (and 4 more examples) present aberrant muscle indexes and can be regarded as true outliers. The sample N36 were considered as outlier by Kadota et al.

Two other samples (N32 and N39) were eventually misclassified by the 3 classifiers when using the GA-Filter method. They both were identified as outlier candidates by Kadota et al. The sample N39 was also misclassified by the Li and Wong's emerging patterns method [23].

It is worthy to mention that over all commented approaches, the GA-Filter method found out the smallest subsets of genes for the colon problem. It obtained good classification rates with only 17 genes, in average. Li and Wong's method required 35 genes. Li et al's method required 50 genes. Furey et al's method required 1000 genes.

SRBCT Dataset. The small round blue cell tumors of childhood (SRBCT) dataset was first analysed by Khan et al [24]. It consistes of the expression of 6567 genes measured over 88 samples. The technology employed was cDNA microarrays. After an initial filtering, Khan et al provide the dataset with 2308 genes. The tumors are classified as Burkitt lymphoma (BL), Ewing sarcoma (EWS), neuroblastoma (NB), or rhabdomyosarcoma (RMS). The dataset was slitted into a training set of 63 samples (23 EWS, 8 BL, 12 NB and 20 RMS) and a testing set of 25 examples (6 EWS, 3 BL, 6 NB, 5 RMS and 5 non-SRBCT).

Using 2308 genes, NC made 4 errors, 3NN made 1 error and SVM made no error. Using a complex neural network approach, Khan et al achieved a test error of 0 and identified 96 genes for the classification. With their nearest shrunken centroids method, Tibshirani et al [25], reduced the required number to makes a perfect classification to 43 genes.

Using 22.7 genes, in average, the GA-Filter method misclassified, in average, 1.3, 0.9 and 0.4 samples for the NC, the 3NN and the SVM, respectively. As can be seem in Figure 1(d), TEST-20 was the most misclassified sample. In Khan et al's work, it was corrected classifier but, due to its very small confidence, it was not diagnosed. There is no reference for the others misclassified samples in the literature.

Table 1 compares the classifiers' accuracies using the whole set of genes and the reduced set obtained by the GA-Filter method. The bold entries indicate that the difference between the accuracies of the classifier using the 2 sets of genes was statistical significant with 99% of certainty (applying a two-tailed t-test). When there is no bold entries for the 2 sets of genes, it means that the difference was not statistical significant. In most cases the classifiers trained with the reduced set of genes performed equally or better than those using the whole set of genes. The only exception was the SVM trained with the leukemia dataset.

Table 2 compares the GA-Filter method together with the best classifier and the best reference methods found in literature for each dataset. Using the same scheme as that for Table 1, bold entries means that the difference in accuracies is statistically significant. For the lymphoma dataset, the NC together with the GA-Filter performed significantly better than its competitor, using almost the same number of genes. For the other datasets, there were no significative differences, although the GA-Filter method greatly reduced the number of genes.

Table 1. Comparison between the classifiers' accuracies using the whole set of genes and the reduced set obtained by the GA-Filter method.

Classifiers	Gene Set	Datasets			
		Leukemia	Lymphoma	Colon	SRBCT
NC	Original	97.05/0.00	100.00/0.00	75.00/0.00	84.00/0.00
	Reduced	**99.70/0.88**	96.15/5.16	73.15/2.83	**94.80/4.23**
3NN	Original	97.05/0.00	92.30/0.00	75.00/0.00	96.00/0.00
	Reduced	**99.70/0.88**	93.07/7.25	74.21/1.57	96.40/2.95
SVM	Original	**100.00/0.00**	100.00/0.00	75.00/0.00	100.00/0.00
	Reduced	97.64/1.17	93.84/7.53	77.50/2.50	98.40/2.06

Table 2. Comparison between the GA-Filter method together with the best classifier and the best methods found in literature for each dataset.

Gene selection	Misc	Datasets			
		Leukemia	Lymphoma	Colon	SRBCT
Reference	#genes	132.00/0.00	12.00/0.00	50.00/0.00	43.00/0.00
	Method	Antonov et al [16]	Potamias et al [21]	Li et al [4]	Tibshirani et al [25]
	Accuracy	100.00/0.00	84.60/0.00	75.00/0.00	100.00/0.00
GA-Filter	#genes	15.10/2.30	10.20/2.82	17.10/4.57	22.70/5.78
	Method	NC	NC	SVM	SVM
	Accuracy	99.70/0.88	**96.15/5.16**	77.50/2.50	98.40/2.06

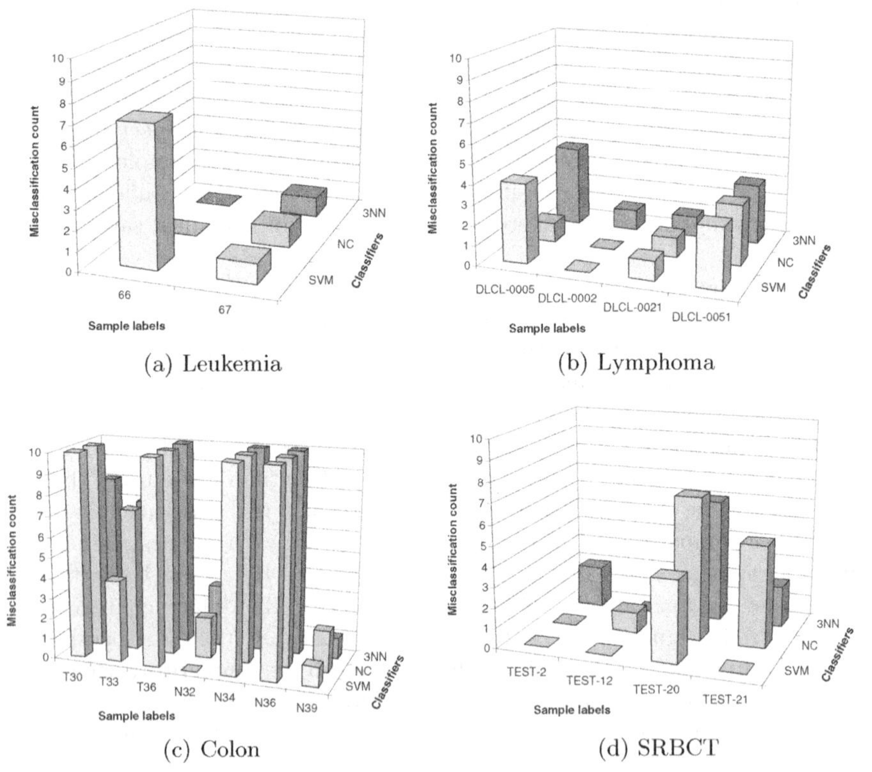

(a) Leukemia (b) Lymphoma

(c) Colon (d) SRBCT

Fig. 1. Misclassification samples for the 3 classifiers over 10 runs of the GA-Filter method for each datset.

5 Conclusion

In this work, the authors presented a novel gene selection method based on GAs. It was called GA-Filter, since it makes use of the intrinsic characteristics of the data to discover potentially optimal subsets of genes.

Due to space constrains, the selected genes were not shown here. They can be downloaded from http:://www.icmc.usp.br/~bferes. Most of the top selected genes is very likely to be biological relevant to the investigated phenomenons. By comparing these genes with those selected by other gene selection methods, on can see that there is a strong overlap between the sets. However, since the GA-Filter method selects much smaller subsets of genes, it may be more useful to researchers and biologists.

Although the selected subsets are small, they retained (and sometimes significatively improved) the classification accuracy of the tested classifiers, as can be seem in Tables 1 and 2.

A note on the computational costs of the GA-Filter should be taken. On an ordinary Pentium IV-like machine, it tooks, in average, only 5.06 seconds to select the subset of genes for the leukemia dataset. The average times for the lymphoma, colon and SRBCT datasets were 5.00 seconds, 4.61 seconds and 15.07 seconds, respectively.

As future works, the authors plan to test the proposed methods with other gene expression datasets and to deeply investigate the biological interpretation of the selected genes.

Acknowledgments

The authors would like to thank CAPES, FAPESP and CNPq, Brazilian Research Agencies, for their support.

References

1. Schena, M., Knudsen, S.: Guide to Analysis of DNA Microarray Data, 2nd Edition and Microarray Analysis Set. 2nd edition edn. Wiley Publishers, Canada (2004)
2. Goldberg, D.E.: Genetic Algorithms in Search, Optimization and Machine Learning. Addison-Wesley Longman Publishing, Boston, MA (1989)
3. Liu, H., Motoda, H.: Feature Selection for Knowledge Discovery Data Mining. 1 edn. Kluwer Academic Publishers, Boston, USA (1998)
4. Li, L., et al: Gene assessment and sample classification for gene expression data using a genetic algorithm/k-nearest neighbor. Method. Combinat. Chem. and High Throughput Screening **4** (2001) 727–739
5. Liu, J., Iba, H., Ishizuka, M.: Selecting informative genes with parallel genetic algorithms in tissue classification. Genome Inform **12** (2001) 14–23
6. Golub, T.R., et al: Molecular classification of cancer: Class discovery and class prediction by gene expression monitoring. Science **286** (1999) 531–537
7. de Souza, B.F., de Carvalho, A., Cancino, W.: Gene subset selection using genetic algorithm and svms. In: Proceedings of SBRN 2004, IEEE (2004) To be published.
8. Ooi, C.H., Tan, P.: Genetic algorithms applied to multi-class prediction for the analysis of gene expression data. Bioinformatics **19** (2003) 37–34
9. Kohavi, R., Sommerfield, D.: Feature subset selection using the wrapper method: Overfitting and dynamic search space topology. In: Proc. 1st Intl. Conf. on Knowledge Discovery and Data Mining, Menlo PArk, CA, AAAI Press (1995) 166–185

10. Jain, A., Dubes, R.: Algorithms for Clustering Data. Prentice Hall, Englewood Cliffs, N.J. (1998)
11. Alon, U., et al: Broad patterns of gene expression revealed by clustering analysis of tumor and normal colon tissues probed by oligonucleotide arrays. In: Proc Natl Acad Sci USA. Volume 96., National Academy of Sciences (1999) 6745–6750
12. Breiman, L., Friedman, J., Olshen, R., Stone, C.: Classification and Regression Trees. Wadsworth International, California (1984)
13. Congdon, C.B.: A comparison of genetic algorithm and other machine learning systems on a complex classification task from common disease research. Phd thesis, University of Michigan (1995)
14. Duda, R.O., Hart, P.E., Stork, D.G.: Pattern Recognition. 2nd edition edn. Wiley-Interscience (2000)
15. Vapnik, V.N.: The nature of statistical learning theory. Springer-Verlag New York, Inc. (1995)
16. Antonov, A.V., et al: Optimization models for cancer classification: extracting gene interaction information from microarray expression data. Bioinformatics **20** (2004) 644–52
17. Fu, L.M., Youn, E.S.: Improving reliability of gene selection from microarray functional genomics data. IEEE Trans Inf Technol Biomed **7** (2003) 191–6
18. Furey, T.S., et al: Support vector machine classification and validation of cancer tissue samples using microarray expression data. Bioinformatics **16** (2000) 906–14
19. ALIZADEH, A.A., et al: Distinct types of diffuse large b-cell lymphoma identified by gene expression profiling. Nature **403** (2000) 503–511
20. Li, L., et al: Gene selection for sample classification based on gene expression data: study of sensitivity to choice of parameters of the ga/knn method. Bioinformatics **17** (2001) 1131–42
21. Potamias, G., , et al: Gene selection via discretized gene-expression profiles and greedy feature-elimination. In: Proceedings of SETN 2004. Volume 3025 of LNCS., Greece, Springer Verlag (2004) 256–266
22. Kadota, K., Nishimura, S.I., Bono, H.: Detection of genes with tissue-specific expression patterns using akaike's informationcriterion procedure. Physiol. Genomics **12** (2003) 251–259
23. Li, J., Wong, L.: Identifying good diagnostic gene groups from gene expression profiles using the concept of emerging patterns. Bioinformatics **18** (2002) 1406–7
24. Khan, J., et al: Classification and diagnostic prediction of cancers using gene expression profiling and artificial neural networks. Nat Med **7** (2001) 673–9
25. Tibshirani, R., Hastie, T., Narasimhan, B., Chu, G.: Diagnosis of multiple cancer types by shrunken centroids of gene expression. Proc Natl Acad Sci U S A **99** (2002) 6567–72

Knowledgeable Clustering of Microarray Data

George Potamias[1,2]

[1] Institute of Computer Science, Foundation for Research and Technology – Hellas (FORTH), Vassilika Vouton, P.O. Box 1385, 711 10 Heraklion, Crete, Greece
[2] Dept. of Computer Science, University of Crete, 71409 Heraklion, Crete, Greece
potamias@ics.forth.gr
http://www.ics.forth.gr/~potamias/Potamias.htm

Abstract. A novel graph-theoretic clustering (GTC) is presented. The method relies on a weighted graph arrangement of the genes, and the iterative partitioning of the respective minimum spanning tree of the graph. The final result is the hierarchical clustering of the genes. GTC utilizes information about the functional classification of genes to knowledgeably guide the clustering process and achieve more informative clustering results. The method was applied and tested on an indicative real-world domain producing satisfactory and biologically valid results. Future R&D directions are also posted.

1 Introduction

The completion of DNA sequences for various organisms re-orient the related R&D agenda from static structural genomics activities to dynamic functional genomics ones. In this context, *microarray* technology offers a promising alternative towards the understanding of the underlying genome mechanisms [9], [10].

Microarray or, *gene-expression* data analysis is heavily depended on Gene Expression Data Mining (GEDM) technology, and in the very-last years a lot of research efforts are in progress. GEDM is used to identify intrinsic patterns and relationships in gene expression data, and related approaches falls into two categories: (a) *hypothesis testing*- to investigate the induction or perturbation of a biological process that leads to predicted results, and (b) *knowledge discovery*- to detect *internal structure* in biological data.

In this paper we present an integrated methodology that combines both. It is based on a *hybrid clustering* approach able to compute and utilize different distances between the objects to be clustered. In this respect the whole exploratory data analysis process becomes more *knowledgeable* in the sense that pre-established *domain-knowledge* is used to guide the clustering operations.

2 Graph-Theoretic Clustering

The microarray or, *gene expression* data are represented in a *matrix* with *rows* representing genes, *columns* representing samples (e.g., developmental stages, various tissues, treatments etc). Each cell contains a number characterizing the expression level of the particular gene in the particular sample [2], [13]. When comparing rows or columns, we can look either for *similarities* or for *differences* and accordingly form *clusters*.

J.M. Barreiro et al. (Eds.): ISBMDA 2004, LNCS 3337, pp. 491–497, 2004.

Here we present a graph-theoretic clustering – GTC methodology suited for *sequential* (e.g., developmental) gene expression data. In this case we view the expression profile of a gene as *time-series* object. Reliable time-series matching and clustering operations should take in consideration the following functions [1]: (a) ignore small or not-significant parts of the series;(b) translate the offset of the series in order to align them vertically;and (c) scale the am plitude of the series so that each of the respective segments lies within an envelope of fixed width.

2.1 Discretization of Time-Series

The above tasks could be tackled by discretizing the series. Each value of a time-series is transformed into a representative nominal one. In the present work we follow and adjust the qualitative dynamic discretization- QDD method presented in [4].

The basic idea underlying QDD is the use of statistical information about the preceding values observed from the series in order to select the discrete value that corresponds to a new continuous value from the series. A static discrete transformation measure will assign a new discrete value to each continuous one if this value exhibits a statistical-significance deviation from its preceding ones. The overall time-series discretization process is illustrated in Figure 1, below.

<u>Input</u>

(a) Set of n time-series, $TS_i(X)$, with m continuous positive-integer values each: $TS_i(X) = \{X_1, X_2 \ldots X_m\}$, $1 \le i \le n$, X_k continuous, $X_k \ge 0$, and $1 \le k \le m$;
(b) Statistical-significance level t_a ; and (**c**) number of intervals for discretization s.

<u>Discretization</u>

Check for constant time-series patterns

Compute: $TS_{i,[0-1]}(X) = \{X_{k,[0-1]} = \{X_k \;/\; \max\{TS_i(X)\}/X_k \in TS_i(X)\}$,
<u>for</u> $i = 1 \,..\, n$
Compute and set the constant time-series threshold:
$Th = \max(\min(TS_{[0-1],i})) - sd(\min(TS_{[0-1],i}))$
<u>if</u> $\min(TS_{i,[0-1]}(X)) > Th$
<u>then</u> $v_i \leftarrow s$, $1 \le i \le n$
<u>else</u> $QDD(TS_{i,[0-1]}(X))$ ... time-series discretisation with QDD; refer to [4].

<u>Output</u>

Discrete time-series transform, $TS\{V\} = \{v_1, v_2 \ldots v_n\}$

Fig. 1. Details of the time-series discretization process;notice the identification and formation of constant time-series patterns (internal dotted rectangle)

Constant Patterns: Coping with ‘Insignificant’ Changes. With the QDD method it is very-difficult to model ‘constant’ time-series, i.e., series with values fluctuating in ‘small’ or, insignificant ranges. We re fined and enhanced the QDD method by computing a threshold value in order to decide if the series should be considered as constant or not. For each time-series a test is applied that identifies a time-series as ‘constant' (internal rectangle in Figure 1). If not, the QDD discretization process is triggered (else condition in Figure 1) where, the continuous values of the series are assigned to respective nominal values.

2.2 Distances Between Time-Series

The distance between two time-series, $TS_a(X)$ and $TS_b(X)$, of m time-points both, is computed by the distance between their corresponding discretized transforms, $TS_a(V)$ and $TS_b(V)$.

$$\text{distance}(TS_a(X), TS_b(X)) = \text{distance}(TS_a(V), TS_b(V)) = \frac{\sum_{j=1}^{m} \mathbf{dist}(v_{a;j}, v_{b;j})}{m} \quad (1)$$

The (natural) definition of a distance defined over the nominal values of the series is: $\text{NOM\_dist}(v_{a;j}, v_{b;j})$ equals 1 if $v_{a;j} \neq v_{b;j}$; otherwise equals to 0. Besides this type of distance computation, in the current implementation of GTC we have implemented a variety of other distance metrics such as, the *Euclidean*;the *Pearson* linear correlation and *Rank* correlation etc. Moreover, the Value Difference Metric is also implemented.

Value Difference Metric (VDM): A Knowledgeable Distance Measure. VDM combines information about the input objects that originates from different modalities. For example, the a-priori assignment of genes to specific functional classes could be utilized. The VDM metric, given by the formula below, takes into account this information [12].

$$\mathbf{VDM}_a(V_a = x, V_a = y) = \sum_{c=1}^{C} \left| \frac{N_{a;x;c}}{N_{a;x}} - \frac{N_{a;y;c}}{N_{a;y}} \right|^2 \quad (2)$$

where, $V_a = x$: x is the value of feature a; $N_{a;x}$: the number of objects with value x for feature a; $N_{a;x;c}$: the number of class c objects with value x for feature a;and C the total number of classes.

Using VDM we may conclude into a distance arrangement of the objects that differs from the one that results when the used distance-metric does not utilize objects' class information. So, the final hierarchical clustering outcome will confront not only to the distance between the feature-based (i.e., gene expression values) description of the objects but to their class resemblance as well. As the assignment of classes to objects reflect to some form of established domain knowledge the whole clustering operation becomes more knowledgeable'.

2.3 Iterative Graph Partitioning

The GTC algorithm is realized by the following procedure:

a. *Minimum Spanning Tree* (MST) construction. Given a set E of n objects, the minimum spanning tree- MST of the fully-connected weighted graph of the objects is constructed. In the current GTC implementation we use Prims' MST construction method [8]. A basic characteristic of the MST is that it reserves the shortest distances between the objects. This guarantees that objects lying in 'close areas' of the tree exhibit low distances. So, finding the 'right' cuts of the tree could result in a reliable grouping of the objects;

b. *Iterative MST partition.* It is implemented within the following steps:
   - Step-1: *Binary Splitting.* At each node (i.e., sub-cluster) in the so-far formed hierarchical tree, each of the edges in the corresponding node's sub-MST is cut. With each cut a binary split of the objects is formed. If the current node includes `n` objects then `n-1` such splits are formed. The two sub-clusters, formed by the binary split, plus the clusters formed so far (excluding the current node) compose a potential partition;
   - Step-2: *Best split.* The *Category Utility- CU* of all formed `n-1` potential partitions are computed. The one that exhibits the highest CU is selected as the best partition of the objects in the current node – CU is an information entropic formula based on the distribution of objects' feature-values in a set of object groups (refer to [3]);
   - Step-3: *Iteration & Termination criterion.* Following a depth-first tree-growing process, steps 1 and 2 are iteratively performed. The category utility of the 'current' best partition, $CU_{current}$, is tested against the 'so-far' formed clusters, CU_{so_far}. If $CU_{current} > CU_{so\_far}$ then, the node is split (step 1), otherwise we stop further expansion of the current clustering-tree node.

The final outcome is a hierarchical clustering tree where, (by default) the termination nodes are the final clusters. Special parameters control the generalization level of the hierarchical clustering tree (e.g., minimum number of objects in each sub-cluster).

Accessing the Utility of Domain Theories and Background Knowledge. With GTC/VDM is possible to access the degree to which the experimental data parallels, i.e., confirms or, rejects specific domain theories. To do this we introduce the *Diversity Index* metric, given by formula: $\sum_{c\in C} DI_{C,c} / |C|$, where, $DI_{C,c}$ is the conditional diversity index of a specific class value [5]. Diversity index measures the descriptive power of a cluster with respect to the classes assigned to the input objects. Lower diversity indices show better descriptive power of clusters with respect to the assigned classes.

Time Complexity of GTC. In general, and for the worst case, GTC exhibits a quadratic to the total number of input objects, n, and linear to the number of features, F, and the mean number of feature values, V, time-complexity, that is, $\sim O(n^2 \times F \times V)$ (refer to [6] and [7]).

3 Experimental Evaluation

We utilized GTC on an indicative gene expression profiling domain namely, large scale gene expression profiling of central nervous system development, referred as the *Wen* case-study [11]. The respective case-study present the mRNA expression levels of 112 genes during rat central nervous system development (cervical spinal cord);

assignment of the 112 genes to four main functional classes, spitted further to fourteen class-values, is also provided.

Utilizing the VDM metric in the course of GTC five clusters were induced that exhibit, not only similar expression profiles but similar, more-or-less, functions as well. The natural interpretation of the induced clusters and their correspondence to the respective Wen 'w'aves are: EARLY / w1;MID-LATE / w2;MID / w3;LATE / w4; and CONSTANT / w5. Figure 2, below, shows the representative profiles for each of the induced clusters (the plotted patterns present the developmental-stage means over all genes in the respective cluster).

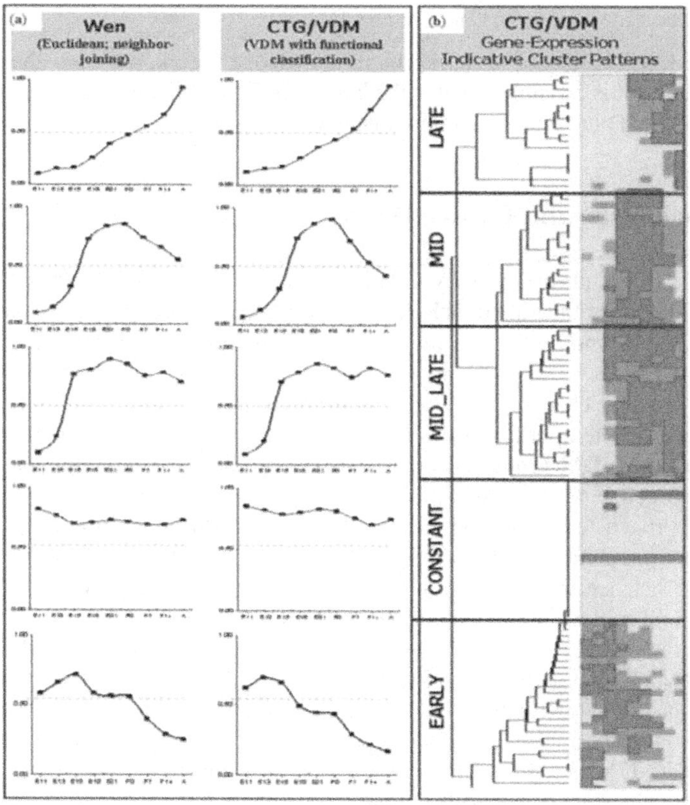

Fig. 2. Plots of the clusters' mean expression level (representative patterns) for Wen and CTG/VDM clustering

The result shows that the presented clustering approach is well-formed and reliable producing similar results with the standard joining-neighboring clustering approaches (followed by Wen).

- Moreover, for all functional classes GTC/VDM exhibits lower diversity indices figures;compared with Wen's clusteri ng a significance difference was observed on the P99%level. So, the GTC/VDM clustering approach induces more 'compact', with respect to the genes' functions, clusters.

- Furthermore, in hierarchical clustering approaches it is difficult to identify the 'borderline' patterns, i.e., genes with expression profiles that lie between two or, more clusters. This is the situation with the w2/c2112 and w3/c2111 clusters. In Wen clustering there are some genes that are assigned to cluster w2, even if their expression patterns fits more-or-less to the w3/c2111 pattern. The GTC/VDM clustering approach remedies this, and groups the genes within cluster w3/c2111. A special case of 'bordeline' cases are the 'unclassified' ones – some genes assigned to the `'neuro_glial_markers'` function remain unclassified in the Wen case study (the 'other' pattern in Wen's terminology). With CTC/VDM most of these genes are assigned to cluster w3/c2111 in which, most of the genes comes from the `'neuro_glial_markers'` function.

So, with the utilization of background-knowledge (i.e., knowledge about the function of genes) it is possible to solve the 'borderline' problem, and make the interpretation of the final clustering result more natural.

4 Conclusions and Future Work

GTC, a novel graph-theoretic hybrid clustering approach was presented that utilizes information about the functional classification of genes in order to achieve a more knowledgeable, and by though, more naturally interpretable clustering arrangements of the genes.

The presented clustering approach is based on the discrete transformation of the gene expression temporal profiles (a method appropriate for sequential / time-series data), and the VDM (value difference metric) formula for the computation of distances between gene expression profiles.

The approach was tested on an indicative real-world microarray domain, and the results are comparable with the originally published case-study. Moreover, utilizing the VDM distance metric, we were able to tackle the 'borderline' cluster assignment problem, and achieve more naturally interpretable results.

Our future research and development plans are moving towards two directions: (a) extensive and large scale experimentation with various gene-expression profiling domains in order to test the effectiveness and the scalibility of the approach - the method is already applied on a neurophysiology domain with good and biologically valid results [7], and (b) incorporation of GTC in the framework of an *integrated clinico-genomics environment* [6], aiming to achieve the operational communication as well as to provide functional links between the clinical and the genomic worlds.

Acknowledgement

The work presented is this paper was partially supported by the EU IST program under the Network of Excellence (NoE) FP6-IST-507585 project, and the PrognoChip project (funded by the Greek Secretariat for Research and Technology).

References

1. Agrawal, R., Lin, K., Sawhney, H.S., Shim, K.: Fast Similarity Search in the Presence of Noise, Scaling, and Translation in Time-Series Databases. In: Proceddings of the 21st VLDB Conf., Zurich, Switzerland (1995) 490–501
2. Bassett, D.E., Eisen, M.B., Boguski, M.S.: Gene expression informatics: it's all in your mine. Nat. Genet. 21 (1999) 51–55
3. Fisher, D.: Knowledge Acquisition via Incremental Conceptual Clustering. Machine Learning 2 (1987) 139-172
4. Lopez, L.M., Ruiz I.F., Bueno, R.M., Ruiz, F.T.: Dynamic Discretization of Continuous Values from Time Series. In: Ramon Lopez de Mantaras and Enric Plaza (eds.): Proceedings of the 11th European Conference on Machine Learning (ECML 2000), Catalonia, Spain (2000) 80–291
5. Pielou, E.C.: The Measurement of Diversity in Different Types of Biological Collections. Journ. Theoret. Biology 13 (1966) 131–144
6. Potamias, G.: Utilizing Genes Functional Classification in Microarray Data Analysis: a Hybrid Clustering Approach. In: K. Margaritis and I. Pitas (eds): Proceedings of the 9th Panhellenic Conference in Informatics, Thessaliniki, Greece, (2003) 415–430
7. Potamias, G., Dermon, C.R.: Protein Synthesis Profiling in the Developing Brain: A Graph Theoretic Clustering Approach. Computer Methods and Programs in Biomedicine, in press (2004)
8. Prim, P.: Shortest connection networks and some generalizations. Bell System Technical Journal 36 (1957) 1389–1401
9. Scena, Mark, Schena, March.: Microarray Biochip Technology. 1st edn. Eaton Pub Co; (2000)
10. Schena, M., Heller, R.A., Theriault, T.P., Konrad, K., Lachenmeier, E., Davis, R.W.: Microassays: biotechnology's discovery platform for functional genomics. Trends Biotechnol. 16:7 (1998) 301–306
11. Wen, X., Fuhrman, S., Michaels, G.S., Carr, D.B., Smith, S., Barker, J.L., Somogyi, R.: Large-scale temporal gene expression mapping of central nervous system development. Procs Natl. Acad. Sci. (PNAS) 95 (1999) 334–339
12. Wilson, D., Martinez, T.: Improved heterogeneous distance functions. Journal of Artificial Intelligence Research 6 (1997) 1–34
13. Zweiger, G.: Knowledge discovery in gene-expression-microarray data: mining the information output of the genome. Trends Biotechnol. 17:11 (1999) 429–436

Correlation of Expression Between Different IMAGE Clones from the Same UniGene Cluster

Giacomo Gamberoni[1], Evelina Lamma[1], Sergio Storari[1], Diego Arcelli[2], Francesca Francioso[2], and Stefano Volinia[2]

[1] ENDIF-Dipartimento di Ingegneria, Università di Ferrara, Ferrara, Italy
{ggamberoni;elamma;sstorari}@ing.unife.it
[2] Dipartimento di Biologia, Università di Ferrara, Ferrara, Italy
{diego.arcelli,francesca.francioso,s.volinia}@unife.it

Abstract. Through the use of DNA microarray it is now possible to obtain quantitative measurements of the expression of thousands of genes present in a biological sample. DNA arrays yield a global view of gene expression and they can be used in a number of interesting ways.
In this paper we are investigating an approach for studying the correlations between different clones from the same UniGene cluster. We will explore all possible couples of clones valuing the linear relations between the expression of these sequences. In this way, we can obtain several results: for example we can estimate measurement errors, or we can highlight genetic mutations.
The experiments were done using a real dataset, build from 161 microarray experiments about Hepatocellular Carcinoma.

1 Introduction

From DNA microarray experiments, we can obtain a huge amount of data about gene expression of different cell populations. An intelligent analysis of these results can be very useful and important for cancer research. In this paper we present a method to evaluate the relations between the expressions of sequences belonging to the same gene. This method was applied to a real dataset: a gene expression matrix about hepatocellular carcinoma.

The paper is structured as follows. In Sect. 2 we briefly describe the data source: microarray experiment results about hepatocellular carcinoma. In Sect. 3 we discuss perspectives and possible utilizations of the results of this study. In Sect. 4 we present our method for studying relations between expressions of sequences from the same gene. Results of the experiments are presented in Sect. 5, with some considerations. Finally, in Sect. 6 we discuss main results and some hypotheses of future works and developments.

2 Microarray

All living cells contain chromosomes, large pieces of DNA containing hundreds or thousands of genes, each of which specifies the composition and the structure of

J.M. Barreiro et al. (Eds.): ISBMDA 2004, LNCS 3337, pp. 498–506, 2004.

a single protein. Proteins are responsible for cellular structure and functionality and are very important during the whole cellular cycle. Even the differentiation between cells of different tissues, are due to changes in protein state, abundance and distribution. The changes in protein abundance are determined by the changes in the levels of messenger RNAs (mRNAs), which shuttle information from chromosome to the cellular components involved in protein synthesis. Those levels of mRNAs are known as gene expression

Recent technical and analytical advances make it practical to quantitate the expression of thousands of genes in parallel using complementary DNA microarrays. This mode of analysis has been used to observe gene expression variation in a variety of human tumors.

A microarray experiment consists of measurements of the relative representation of a large number of mRNA species in a set of biological samples [2, 6, 5]. Each experimental sample is compared to a common reference sample and the results for each probe is the ratio of the relative abundance of the gene in the experimental sample compared to the reference. The results of such experiments are represented in a table, where each row represents a sequence, each column a sample, and each cell the log_2 of the expression ratio of the Expression Sequence Tag (EST) [7] in the appropriate sample.

The whole microarray process is the following. The DNA samples (up to several thousands) are fixed to a glass slide, each one in a known position in the array. A target sample and a reference sample are labeled with red and green dyes, respectively, and each one is hybridized on the slide. Using a fluorescent scanner and image analysis the $log_2(green/red)$ intensities of mRNA hybridizing in each site is measured. The result is a few thousand numbers, measuring the expression level of each sequence in the experimental sample relative to the reference sample.

The data from M experiments considering N genes, may be represented as a $N \times M$ expression matrix, in which each of the N rows consists of a M-element expression vector for a single sequence.

Sequences are identified by their IMAGE [7] cloneID, that is a number coding for the sequence fixed on the slide (usually cloned from a genomic repository). Usually a gene is longer than these sequences, so we can find on the slide different sequences that are part of the same gene. In order to regroup the sequences from the same gene, we used the UniGene cluster definitions [10]. UniGene is an experimental system for automatically partitioning GenBank sequences into a non-redundant set of gene-oriented clusters. Each UniGene cluster contains sequences that represent a unique gene, as well as related information such as the tissue types in which the gene has been expressed and map location.

2.1 Hepatocarcinoma

Hepatocellular carcinoma (HCC) is the most common liver malignancy and among the five leading causes of cancer death in the world. Virtually all HCCs are associated with chronic hepatitis B virus (HBV) or hepatitis C virus infections, but the molecular nature of this association is poorly understood. HCC treatment options remain limited. Surgical resection is considered the only "curative treatment", but more than 80% of patients have widespread HCC at the time of diagnosis and are not candidates for surgical treatment. Among patients with localized HCC who undergo surgery, 50% suffer a recurrence. Standard clinical pathological classification of HCC has limited value in predicting the outcome of treatment. Clearly, molecular markers for early and accurate diagnosis and classification of HCC would address an important medical need.

The analyzed dataset regroups the results of 161 microarray experiments, divided as follows:

95 HCC
66 Liver

On the second channel (red) of each experiment, we had a common reference RNA collection. So we calculated the $log_2(green/red)$ and obtained a normalized gene expression matrix of 7449 genes for 161 experiments.

2.2 Normalization

Primary data collection and analysis were carried out using GenePix Pro 3.0 (Axon Instruments) [4]. Areas of the array with obvious blemishes were manually flagged and excluded from subsequent analysis. All nonflagged array elements for which the fluorescent intensity in each channel was more than 1.5 times the local background were considered well measured.

A normalization factor was estimated from ratios of median by GenePix Pro. We calculated the $log_2(green/red)$ and normalized, for each different array, by adding the log_2 of the respective normalization factor to the log_2 of the ratio of medians for each spot within the array, so that the average log-transformed ratio equaled zero.

The threshold for significant RNA expression changes (3.0-fold; i.e., 1.5 on the log_2 scale) was established as three times the SD of an assay, where the same RNA sample was independently retrotranscribed and labeled with both cyanines. DNA spots present in at least 75% of the arrays and with expression ratios higher than the above-defined threshold, in at least one array, were selected for the following analysis.

On the second channel (red) of each experiment, we had a common reference RNA collection. So we calculated the $log_2(green/red)$ and obtained a normalized gene expression matrix.

3 Purpose

Starting from the gene expression matrix, we will consider only groups of clones that belong to the same UniGene Cluster, in order to study the correlations between them. Examining these relation can be useful in several ways, some of which are discussed below.

3.1 Quality Control

In an ideal experiment, different clones from the same gene should be equally expressed. They should have very strong relations, that can get worse due to the experimental errors and noise.

For example, if we had a gene that is usually weakly expressed, all the spots on the slide related to his clones will have low intensity levels. In these cases the background noise is very relevant and the measurement will not be precise.

When we valuate relations between these clones, if they are badly correlated, then we can assert the information provided by the UniGene cluster and these spots are not reliable. So, measuring correlation, we can determine an useful parameter for assessing quality control of the microarray experiment.

We can evaluate the quality of the measurements for a single gene, on the base of the errors of all the relations. If all the relations have an high error, probably this is due to a systematic error on measurements.

3.2 Chromosomal Aberrations

Another interesting perspective is to use these analysis in order to find the anomalies of specific clones. In particular, we can discover if a clone loses his relations with the other ones. Deletions or insertions of sequences is very frequent in cancer genetic profiles.

For this study it is necessary to separate normal samples from cancer, and to compare the correlation between the same couple of clones in the two cases. So, we can highlight if there were some evidences of genetic mutations.

If we can observe errors regarding a single clone, or anomalies for some examples, this is probably due to a genetic mutation causing gene copy number alterations.

4 Methodology

In order to valuate all the relations between clones from the same unigene cluster, we will study all possible couples of clones in it. If we consider n clones from the same UniGene Cluster, we have $\frac{n\cdot(n-1)}{2}$ couples to study. For example, if we have 4 different clones from a given cluster, we will analyze 6 relations.

We will study all these possible relations, valuing the regression error for three models: the one computed on the entire dataset and two calculated on cancer and normal tissues separately. So, we can see relations differences between clones in these two type of cells.

4.1 Correlation

In order to find relation between variables we used a linear regression. After choosing two genes, we represent each example as a point in a plane, where on x and y axis there are the expressions of the two genes. Then, we calculate the coefficients a and b of the relation $y = ax + b$ that minimize the sum of squares of error($err = y - (ax + b)$). This is called least squares method [3].

When trying to compare errors in models for different couples of genes, the sum of squares presents two problems:

- It increases with the number of points we are considering, so we can't compare two models from two different sets of examples, or from two parts of the same set. To avoid this difficulty, it is necessary to divide it by the number of examples N, so we consider the mean of square error, instead of its sum.
- Genes have variable expression ranges, for example one can vary in $[-1; +1]$ and another in $[-5; +5]$. So, if we have on the y axis a gene with a restricted range, it will give a smaller error, because of its nature, even if that approximation is not better than the one found for a gene with a more extended range. In order to resolve this we divide the result obtained before by the variance (σ_y^2) of the gene on y axis.

So, the error value used to compare different regressions will be:

$$Err = \frac{\sum_{i=1}^{N} (y_i - P(x_i))^2}{N\sigma_y^2}. \quad (1)$$

5 Results and Discussion

The experiments were conducted using two main software tools. First, we created a MySQL database for managing queries and for merging informations coming from different sources. For example we had the gene expression matrix in a comma separated values file, while informations about the Unigene cluster were downloade from SOURCE database [8] in a tab-separated text file. The second software used is the Matlab environment: this were used for all mathematical processing, in order to fast implement flexible algorithms.

First of all, we must select from the entire gene expression matrix the groups of rows containing the EST clones from the same UniGene cluster. Focusing our

Table 1. UniGene clusters with at least 4 EST clones in the dataset.

	Clones	Possible	Total	LIV	HCC
Hs.315379	6	15	12	3	13
Hs.306864	5	10	7	4	8
Hs.381184	4	6	6	2	6
Hs.8207	4	6	2	0	2
Hs.386834	4	6	3	1	3
Hs.386784	4	6	0	0	0
Hs.355608	4	6	0	1	0
Hs.236456	4	6	1	0	2
Hs.168913	4	6	2	0	2

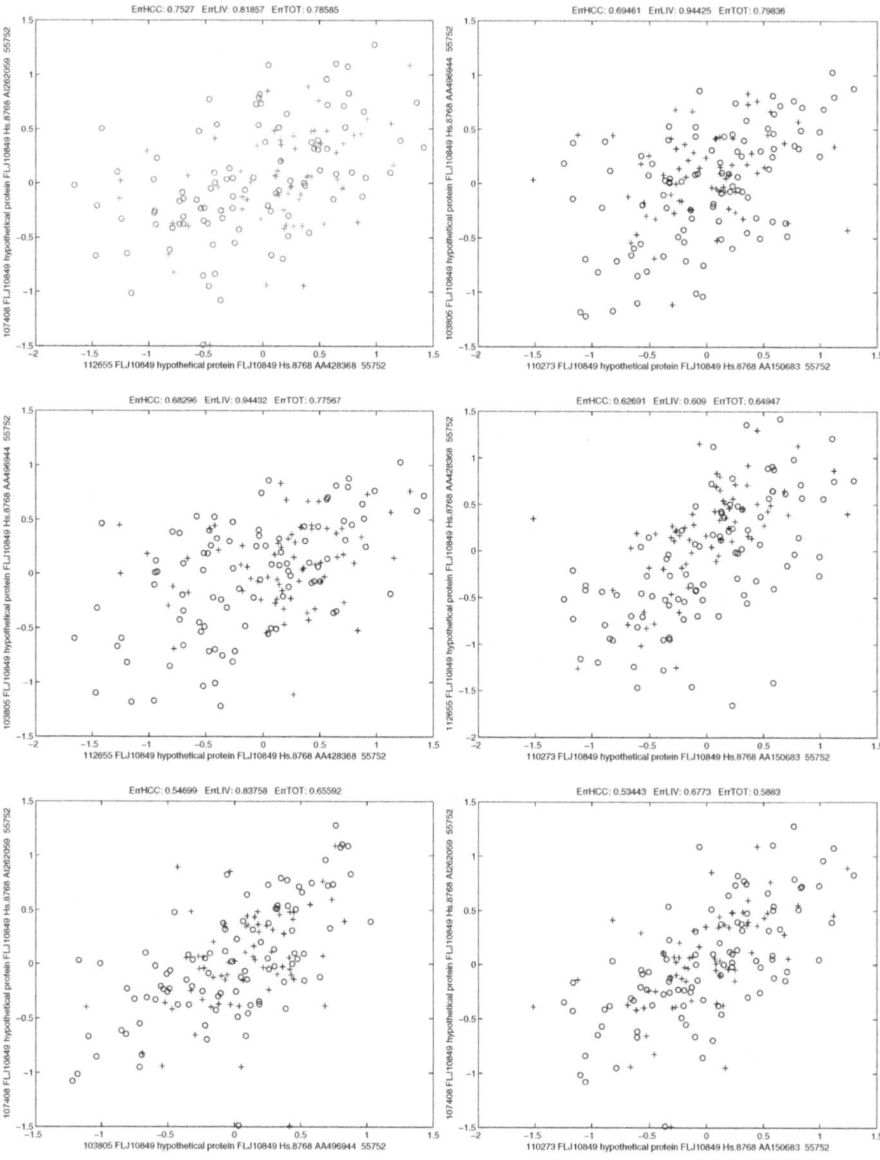

Fig. 1. Relations in Hs.386784.

attention on UniGene clusters with several ESTs clones, so we selected only clusters with 4 or more ESTs. In our dataset we found a UniGene cluster containing 6 ESTs, another one containing 5 ESTs, and 7 containing 4 ESTs.

In order to evaluate how many relations are meaningful or not in the liver or in the cancer, we can put a threshold on the error. For each UniGene cluster Tab. 1 shows the number of clones involved and the number of possible relations, then

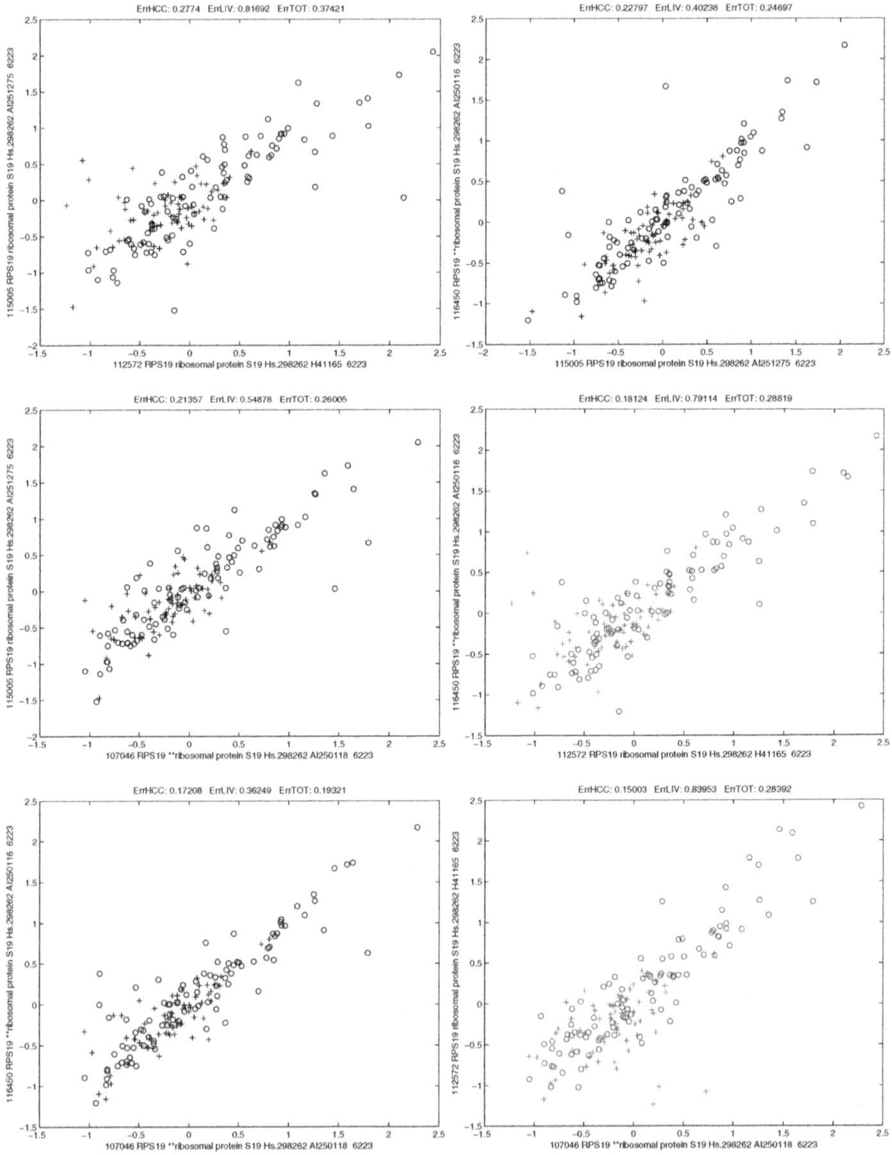

Fig. 2. Relations in Hs.381184.

the number of these relations that have error less or equal to 0.5, respectively considering the entire dataset (Total), the healthy samples (LIV) and the cancer (HCC).

We can see that many relation are better in the HCC samples than in the LIV ones. This finding is somewhat unexpected, since it indicates better intragene correlations for cancer tissues than normal liver. This trend is maintained true for all the UniGene clusters analyzed. A possible explanation is the tissue etherogeneity in the normal liver tissue, where the biopsy could be representing a number of different cell types. On the other hand, hepatocarcinoma biopsies are probably constituted by cancer cells and infiltrated endothelial cells. If this hypothesis will hold true for future analysis, it will reveal an high level of differential exon usage in different cell types, as it has been recently proposed. This would be in line with lower than expected number of human genes. Moreover, it seems that ESTs correlation will be useful as QC parameter particularly in experiments with purified tissues.

We can better analyze these results looking at the graphical representations of relations.

In the following pages we report a graphical representation of the relations regarding two genes: Hs.386784 and Hs.381184. In every diagram we have the expression level of a couple of sequences on the axes. Then we represent every sample as a point in the plane: circles are cancer samples, while crosses represent healthy liver samples.

The example in Fig. 1 shows a gene that has only bad relations between its clones: observing this figure, we can see only badly correlated couples, with no evidence of interactions between ESTs involved.

The one in Fig. 2 has a very low error level: all relations are quite good. Looking at these diagrams, we can notice that the relations involving the sequence with CloneID 112572 have an high error (≈ 0.8) in healthy livers. From the graphs we can notice that the crosses in these relation are quite grouped but they do not show any relation. In particular, we can see three liver samples that are clearly out of the overall relation. This is probably due to differential expression of these ESTs between normal and cancer tissues.

6 Conclusions and Future Works

In this paper we describe a novel method to analyze gene expression data. We applied this method to a large cDNA microarray dataset obtained from normal human liver and his cancer counterpart. We show here how, using this method, we evaluate intra-gene probe interactions.

We identified significant differences between cancer and normal tissues. We hypothesize that such differences can be due to alternative exon usage [9]. This method can be easily applied to other data sources. To better define the role of intra-gene ESTs interactions, we will perform further experiments with homogeneous source such as human leukemias. Furthermore, we are planning to expand such method in order to analyze Affymetrix [1] microarray results.

An important improvement of this method, could be to include the absolute intensity measurement in the intra-gene ESTs interaction analysis.

References

1. Affymetrix corp., see the website: http://www.affymetrix.com
2. Alizadeh, A.A., Eisen, M.B., Davis, R.E., Ma, C., Lossos, I.S., Rosenwald, A., Boldrick, J.C., Sabet, H., Tran, T., Yu, X., Powell, J.I., Yang, L., Marti, G.E., Moore, T., Hudson, J. Jr., Lu, L., Lewis, D.B., Tibshirani, R., Sherlock, G., Chan, W.C., Greiner, T.C., Weisenburger, D.D., Armitage, J.O., Warnke, R., Levy, R., Wilson, W., Grever, M.R., Byrd, J.C., Botstein, D., Brown, P.O., Staudt, L.M.: Distinct types of diffuse large B-cell lymphoma identified by gene expression profiling. Nature 403 (2000) 503–511
3. Anderson, D.R., Sweeney, D.J. and Williams, T.A. : Introduction to statistics concepts and applications, Third Edition. West Publishing Company (1994)
4. Axon instruments, see the website: http://www.axon.com
5. Eisen, M.B., Spellman, P.T., Brown, P.O., and Botstein, D. : Cluster analysis and display of genome-wide expression patterns. Proc. Natl. Acad. Sci. USA 95 (1998) 14863–14688
6. Golub, T.R., Slonim, D.K., Tamayo, P., Huard, C., Gaasenbeek, M., Mesirov, J.P., Coller, H., Loh, M.L., Downing, J.R., Caligiuri, M.A., Bloomfield, C.D., Lander, E.S.: Molecular classification of cancer: class discovery and class prediction by gene expression monitoring. Science 286 (1999) 531–537
7. IMAGE consortium, see the website: http://image.llnl.gov
8. SOURCE search engine, see the website: http://source.stanford.edu
9. Alternative splicing, see the website: http://www.exonhit.com/alternativesplicing/
10. NCBI UniGene, see the website: http://www.ncbi.nlm.nih.gov/UniGene

Author Index

Acuña, César J. 49
Alonso, Fernando 344
Alonso, Francisco Javier 281
Arcelli, Diego 498
Arregui, Miguel 368
Aslanidis, Ioannis 269

Bång, Angela 141
Barreiro, José María 418
Blanco, Rosa 212
Bolotin, Arkady 243, 251
Brause, Rüdiger W. 439
Burguillo, Juan C. 129

Cardoso, M. Luis 450
Chalmeta, Ricardo 368
Cohen, Gilles 200
Collada Ali, Laura 299
Coltell, Oscar 368
Corella, Dolores 368
Crespo, Jose 224

Dan Serbanati, Luca 299
de Carvalho, André C.P.L.F. 479
de Castro, Valeria 49
de Ledesma, Luis 67
de la Cámara, A. Gómez 224
de la Prieta, Roberto 27
del Arco, Aurora 96
Del Castillo, José María 281
Dias, Gaspar 409
Diaz, Carlos 418
Driesch, Dominik 427
Dusza, Jacek J. 259

Elbers, Armin 148
Estruch, Antonio 458

Farghali, H. 292
Fazi, Paola 299
Feres de Souza, Bruno 479
Filipec, M. 292
Francioso, Francesca 498
Friger, Michael 243

Gamberoni, Giacomo 171, 498
Garcia-Gomez, Juan M. 96
García-Remesal, M. 224
Geenen, Petra 148
Geissbuhler, Antoine 200
Gellerstedt, Martin 141
Gerlach, Joerg 427
González, Carolina 129
Guthke, Reinhard 427

Heredia, José Antonio 458
Herlitz, Johan 141
Hermosilla, Isabel 409
Hernández, C. 9
Hernández, Juan A. 1, 9, 21, 49
Hilario, Mélanie 200

Inza, Iñaki 212

Jankowski, Stanisław 259

Konias, Sokratis 313
Kosar, Karel 39, 322
Koutkias, Vassilis 378
Krajca, Vladimir 39, 322, 333
Kurzynski, Marek 105, 356

Laita, L. 67
Laita, Luis M. 67
Lamma, Evelina 171, 498
Larrañaga, Pedro 212, 388
Lhotska, Lenka 39, 322, 333
Lim, Sukhyun 60
Llamas, Martin 129
Loeffen, Willie 148
Lozano, José A. 388
Lucas, Peter 188
Luzi, Daniela 299

Magdalena, Rafael 160
Maglaveras, Nicos 313, 378
Malousi, Andigoni 378
Maojo, Victor 224, 235, 418
Marcos, Esperanza 49
Marin, Juan M. 85
Marti-Bonmati, Luís 96
Martin-Sánchez, Fernando 409, 418

Martínez, Loïc 344
Matousek, Milos 333
Mello, Paola 171
Möller, Ulrich 399
Montes, César 344
Montes Diez, Raquel 21, 85
Mora, Martha L. 1
Muñoz, Jorge 160

Neuhaus, Peter 427

Oliveira, Ilídio 409
Oliveira, José Luís 409, 450
Oręziak, Artur 259
Ordovas, Jose M. 368

Parnell, Larry 368
Pavesi, Piercamillo 171
Pérez, Aurora 344
Pérez, Gabriela 21
Pfaff, Michael 427
Pinheiro, Miguel 450
Pintado, Publio 281
Pless, Gesine 427
Potamias, George 491

Radke, Dörte 399
Riaño, David 117, 269
Ricci, Fabrizio L. 299
Rieger, Josef 39, 333
Rios Insua, David 85
Roanes-Lozano, Eugenio 67
Robles, Montserrat 96
Rocha, Hugo 450
Rocha, Patrícia 409

San Martín, José 21
Sanandrés-Ledesma, J.A. 224
Sánchez-Morgado, R. 67
Santamaría, Agustín 344
Santana, Roberto 388
Santos, Manuel A.S. 450
Sanz, Ferran 418
Sas, Jerzy 105
Schaefer, Gerald 182
Schiavi, Emanuele 1, 9
Schmidt, Rainer 79
Schmidt-Heck, Wolfgang 427
Serrano, Agustin 160
Serrano, Antonio J. 160
Shin, Byeong-Seok 60
Soria, E. 160
Sousa Pereira, António 409
Spiteri, Inmaculada 409
Storari, Sergio 171, 498
Svozilkova, P. 292
Symeonidis, Alkiviadis 468

Toepfer, Susanne 427
Toharia, Pablo 1
Tollis, Ioannis G. 468
Trocino, Giuseppe 171

Valenta, Zdenek 292
Valente, Juan Pedro 344
van der Gaag, Linda C. 148, 212
van Gerven, Marcel 188
Vicente, Javier 96, 409
Vidal, César 96
Vidal, Juan C. 129
Vignetti, Marco 299
Vila, Joan 160
Vilarinho, Laura 450
Vlahavas, Ioannis 313
Volinia, Stefano 498

Waligora, Tina 79
Wierzbowski, Mariusz 259
Wolczowski, Andrzej 356

Zeilinger, Katrin 427
Zhu, Shao Ying 182
Zvarova, J. 292

Lecture Notes in Computer Science

For information about Vols. 1–3217

please contact your bookseller or Springer

Vol. 3337: J.M. Barreiro, F. Martin-Sanchez, V. Maojo, F. Sanz (Eds.), Biological and Medical Data Analysis. XI, 508 pages. 2004.

Vol. 3323: G. Antoniou, H. Boley (Eds.), Rules and Rule Markup Languages for the Semantic Web. X, 215 pages. 2004.

Vol. 3316: N.R. Pal, N. Kasabov, R.K. Mudi, S. Pal, S.K. Parui (Eds.), Neural Information Processing. XXX, 1368 pages. 2004.

Vol. 3315: C. Lemaître, C.A. Reyes, J. González (Eds.), Advances in Artificial Intelligence – IBERAMIA 2004. XX, 987 pages. 2004. (Subseries LNAI).

Vol. 3312: A.J. Hu, A.K. Martin (Eds.), Formal Methods in Computer-Aided Design. XI, 445 pages. 2004.

Vol. 3311: V. Roca, F. Rousseau (Eds.), Interactive Multimedia and Next Generation Networks. XIII, 287 pages. 2004.

Vol. 3309: C.-H. Chi, K.-Y. Lam (Eds.), Content Computing. XII, 510 pages. 2004.

Vol. 3308: J. Davies, W. Schulte, M. Barnett (Eds.), Formal Methods and Software Engineering. XIII, 500 pages. 2004.

Vol. 3307: C. Bussler, S.-k. Hong, W. Jun, R. Kaschek, Kinshuk, S. Krishnaswamy, S.W. Loke, D. Oberle, D. Richards, A. Sharma, Y. Sure, B. Thalheim (Eds.), Web Information Systems – WISE 2004 Workshops. XV, 277 pages. 2004.

Vol. 3306: X. Zhou, S. Su, M.P. Papazoglou, M.E. Orlowska, K.G. Jeffery (Eds.), Web Information Systems – WISE 2004. XVII, 745 pages. 2004.

Vol. 3305: P.M.A. Sloot, B. Chopard, A.G. Hoekstra (Eds.), Cellular Automata. XV, 883 pages. 2004.

Vol. 3303: J.A. López, E. Benfenati, W. Dubitzky (Eds.), Knowledge Exploration in Life Science Informatics. X, 249 pages. 2004. (Subseries LNAI).

Vol. 3302: W.-N. Chin (Ed.), Programming Languages and Systems. XIII, 453 pages. 2004.

Vol. 3299: F. Wang (Ed.), Automated Technology for Verification and Analysis. XII, 506 pages. 2004.

Vol. 3298: S.A. McIlraith, D. Plexousakis, F. van Harmelen (Eds.), The Semantic Web – ISWC 2004. XXI, 841 pages. 2004.

Vol. 3295: P. Markopoulos, B. Eggen, E. Aarts, J.L. Crowley (Eds.), Ambient Intelligence. XIII, 388 pages. 2004.

Vol. 3294: C.N. Dean, R.T. Boute (Eds.), Teaching Formal Methods. X, 249 pages. 2004.

Vol. 3293: C.-H. Chi, M. van Steen, C. Wills (Eds.), Web Content Caching and Distribution. IX, 283 pages. 2004.

Vol. 3292: R. Meersman, Z. Tari, A. Corsaro (Eds.), On the Move to Meaningful Internet Systems 2004: OTM 2004 Workshops. XXIII, 885 pages. 2004.

Vol. 3291: R. Meersman, Z. Tari (Eds.), On the Move to Meaningful Internet Systems 2004: CoopIS, DOA, and ODBASE, Part II. XXV, 824 pages. 2004.

Vol. 3290: R. Meersman, Z. Tari (Eds.), On the Move to Meaningful Internet Systems 2004: CoopIS, DOA, and ODBASE, Part I. XXV, 823 pages. 2004.

Vol. 3289: S. Wang, K. Tanaka, S. Zhou, T.W. Ling, J. Guan, D. Yang, F. Grandi, E. Mangina, I.-Y. Song, H.C. Mayr (Eds.), Conceptual Modeling for Advanced Application Domains. XXII, 692 pages. 2004.

Vol. 3288: P. Atzeni, W. Chu, H. Lu, S. Zhou, T.W. Ling (Eds.), Conceptual Modeling – ER 2004. XXI, 869 pages. 2004.

Vol. 3287: A. Sanfeliu, J.F. Martínez Trinidad, J.A. Carrasco Ochoa (Eds.), Progress in Pattern Recognition, Image Analysis and Applications. XVII, 703 pages. 2004.

Vol. 3286: G. Karsai, E. Visser (Eds.), Generative Programming and Component Engineering. XIII, 491 pages. 2004.

Vol. 3285: S. Manandhar, J. Austin, U. Desai, Y. Oyanagi, A. Talukder (Eds.), Applied Computing. XII, 334 pages. 2004.

Vol. 3284: A. Karmouch, L. Korba, E.R.M. Madeira (Eds.), Mobility Aware Technologies and Applications. XII, 382 pages. 2004.

Vol. 3283: F.A. Aagesen, C. Anutariya, V. Wuwongse (Eds.), Intelligence in Communication Systems. XIII, 327 pages. 2004.

Vol. 3281: T. Dingsøyr (Ed.), Software Process Improvement. X, 207 pages. 2004.

Vol. 3280: C. Aykanat, T. Dayar, İ. Körpeoğlu (Eds.), Computer and Information Sciences - ISCIS 2004. XVIII, 1009 pages. 2004.

Vol. 3278: A. Sahai, F. Wu (Eds.), Utility Computing. XI, 272 pages. 2004.

Vol. 3274: R. Guerraoui (Ed.), Distributed Computing. XIII, 465 pages. 2004.

Vol. 3273: T. Baar, A. Strohmeier, A. Moreira, S.J. Mellor (Eds.), <<UML>> 2004 - The Unified Modelling Language. XIII, 454 pages. 2004.

Vol. 3271: J. Vicente, D. Hutchison (Eds.), Management of Multimedia Networks and Services. XIII, 335 pages. 2004.

Vol. 3270: M. Jeckle, R. Kowalczyk, P. Braun (Eds.), Grid Services Engineering and Management. X, 165 pages. 2004.

Vol. 3269: J. Lopez, S. Qing, E. Okamoto (Eds.), Information and Communications Security. XI, 564 pages. 2004.

Vol. 3266: J. Solé-Pareta, M. Smirnov, P.V. Mieghem, J. Domingo-Pascual, E. Monteiro, P. Reichl, B. Stiller, R.J. Gibbens (Eds.), Quality of Service in the Emerging Networking Panorama. XVI, 390 pages. 2004.

Vol. 3265: R.E. Frederking, K.B. Taylor (Eds.), Machine Translation: From Real Users to Research. XI, 392 pages. 2004. (Subseries LNAI).

Vol. 3264: G. Paliouras, Y. Sakakibara (Eds.), Grammatical Inference: Algorithms and Applications. XI, 291 pages. 2004. (Subseries LNAI).

Vol. 3263: M. Weske, P. Liggesmeyer (Eds.), Object-Oriented and Internet-Based Technologies. XII, 239 pages. 2004.

Vol. 3262: M.M. Freire, P. Chemouil, P. Lorenz, A. Gravey (Eds.), Universal Multiservice Networks. XIII, 556 pages. 2004.

Vol. 3261: T. Yakhno (Ed.), Advances in Information Systems. XIV, 617 pages. 2004.

Vol. 3260: I.G.M.M. Niemegeers, S.H. de Groot (Eds.), Personal Wireless Communications. XIV, 478 pages. 2004.

Vol. 3258: M. Wallace (Ed.), Principles and Practice of Constraint Programming – CP 2004. XVII, 822 pages. 2004.

Vol. 3257: E. Motta, N.R. Shadbolt, A. Stutt, N. Gibbins (Eds.), Engineering Knowledge in the Age of the Semantic Web. XVII, 517 pages. 2004. (Subseries LNAI).

Vol. 3256: H. Ehrig, G. Engels, F. Parisi-Presicce, G. Rozenberg (Eds.), Graph Transformations. XII, 451 pages. 2004.

Vol. 3255: A. Benczúr, J. Demetrovics, G. Gottlob (Eds.), Advances in Databases and Information Systems. XI, 423 pages. 2004.

Vol. 3254: E. Macii, V. Paliouras, O. Koufopavlou (Eds.), Integrated Circuit and System Design. XVI, 910 pages. 2004.

Vol. 3253: Y. Lakhnech, S. Yovine (Eds.), Formal Techniques, Modelling and Analysis of Timed and Fault-Tolerant Systems. X, 397 pages. 2004.

Vol. 3252: H. Jin, Y. Pan, N. Xiao, J. Sun (Eds.), Grid and Cooperative Computing - GCC 2004 Workshops. XVIII, 785 pages. 2004.

Vol. 3251: H. Jin, Y. Pan, N. Xiao, J. Sun (Eds.), Grid and Cooperative Computing - GCC 2004. XXII, 1025 pages. 2004.

Vol. 3250: L.-J. (LJ) Zhang, M. Jeckle (Eds.), Web Services. X, 301 pages. 2004.

Vol. 3249: B. Buchberger, J.A. Campbell (Eds.), Artificial Intelligence and Symbolic Computation. X, 285 pages. 2004. (Subseries LNAI).

Vol. 3246: A. Apostolico, M. Melucci (Eds.), String Processing and Information Retrieval. XIV, 332 pages. 2004.

Vol. 3245: E. Suzuki, S. Arikawa (Eds.), Discovery Science. XIV, 430 pages. 2004. (Subseries LNAI).

Vol. 3244: S. Ben-David, J. Case, A. Maruoka (Eds.), Algorithmic Learning Theory. XIV, 505 pages. 2004. (Subseries LNAI).

Vol. 3243: S. Leonardi (Ed.), Algorithms and Models for the Web-Graph. VIII, 189 pages. 2004.

Vol. 3242: X. Yao, E. Burke, J.A. Lozano, J. Smith, J.J. Merelo-Guervós, J.A. Bullinaria, J. Rowe, P. Tiňo, A. Kabán, H.-P. Schwefel (Eds.), Parallel Problem Solving from Nature - PPSN VIII. XX, 1185 pages. 2004.

Vol. 3241: D. Kranzlmüller, P. Kacsuk, J.J. Dongarra (Eds.), Recent Advances in Parallel Virtual Machine and Message Passing Interface. XIII, 452 pages. 2004.

Vol. 3240: I. Jonassen, J. Kim (Eds.), Algorithms in Bioinformatics. IX, 476 pages. 2004. (Subseries LNBI).

Vol. 3239: G. Nicosia, V. Cutello, P.J. Bentley, J. Timmis (Eds.), Artificial Immune Systems. XII, 444 pages. 2004.

Vol. 3238: S. Biundo, T. Frühwirth, G. Palm (Eds.), KI 2004: Advances in Artificial Intelligence. XI, 467 pages. 2004. (Subseries LNAI).

Vol. 3236: M. Núñez, Z. Maamar, F.L. Pelayo, K. Pousttchi, F. Rubio (Eds.), Applying Formal Methods: Testing, Performance, and M/E-Commerce. XI, 381 pages. 2004.

Vol. 3235: D. de Frutos-Escrig, M. Nunez (Eds.), Formal Techniques for Networked and Distributed Systems – FORTE 2004. X, 377 pages. 2004.

Vol. 3234: M.J. Egenhofer, C. Freksa, H.J. Miller (Eds.), Geographic Information Science. VIII, 345 pages. 2004.

Vol. 3233: K. Futatsugi, F. Mizoguchi, N. Yonezaki (Eds.), Software Security - Theories and Systems. X, 345 pages. 2004.

Vol. 3232: R. Heery, L. Lyon (Eds.), Research and Advanced Technology for Digital Libraries. XV, 528 pages. 2004.

Vol. 3231: H.-A. Jacobsen (Ed.), Middleware 2004. XV, 514 pages. 2004.

Vol. 3230: J.L. Vicedo, P. Martínez-Barco, R. Muñoz, M. Saiz Noeda (Eds.), Advances in Natural Language Processing. XII, 488 pages. 2004. (Subseries LNAI).

Vol. 3229: J.J. Alferes, J. Leite (Eds.), Logics in Artificial Intelligence. XIV, 744 pages. 2004. (Subseries LNAI).

Vol. 3226: M. Bouzeghoub, C. Goble, V. Kashyap, S. Spaccapietra (Eds.), Semantics of a Networked World. XIII, 326 pages. 2004.

Vol. 3225: K. Zhang, Y. Zheng (Eds.), Information Security. XII, 442 pages. 2004.

Vol. 3224: E. Jonsson, A. Valdes, M. Almgren (Eds.), Recent Advances in Intrusion Detection. XII, 315 pages. 2004.

Vol. 3223: K. Slind, A. Bunker, G. Gopalakrishnan (Eds.), Theorem Proving in Higher Order Logics. VIII, 337 pages. 2004.

Vol. 3222: H. Jin, G.R. Gao, Z. Xu, H. Chen (Eds.), Network and Parallel Computing. XX, 694 pages. 2004.

Vol. 3221: S. Albers, T. Radzik (Eds.), Algorithms – ESA 2004. XVIII, 836 pages. 2004.

Vol. 3220: J.C. Lester, R.M. Vicari, F. Paraguaçu (Eds.), Intelligent Tutoring Systems. XXI, 920 pages. 2004.

Vol. 3219: M. Heisel, P. Liggesmeyer, S. Wittmann (Eds.), Computer Safety, Reliability, and Security. XI, 339 pages. 2004.

Made in the USA
Monee, IL
18 October 2026

66037392R10289